HANDBOOK OF PAIN ASSESSMENT

HANDBOOK
of
PAIN ASSESSMENT

Dennis C. Turk
Ronald Melzack

Editors

THE GUILFORD PRESS
New York   London

Library of Congress Cataloging-in-Publication Data

Handbook of pain assessment / edited by Dennis C. Turk, Ronald
   Melzack.
       p.   cm.
    Includes bibliographical references and index.
    ISBN 0-89862-883-0
    1. Pain—Measurement. I. Turk, Dennis C.   II. Melzack, Ronald.
    [DNLM:D1. Pain—diagnosis. 2. Pain Measurement. WL 704 H243]
RB127.H355   1992
616′.0472—dc20
DNLM/DLC
for Library of Congress   92-49847
                                                              CIP

To our wives,
Lorraine Turk and Lucy Melzack,
who consistently inspire and help us

Contributors

Frank Andrasik, PhD, Department of Psychology, University of West Florida, Pensacola, Florida.

Niels Birbaumer, PhD, Department of Clinical and Physiological Psychology, University of Tübingen, Tübingen, Germany; Dipartimento di Psicologia Generale, Universita Degli Studi, Padova, Italy.

Laurence A. Bradley, PhD, Department of Psychology, and Division of Gastroenterology, University of Alabama at Birmingham, Birmingham, Alabama.

Margaret C. Brigham, PhD, Paediatric Pain Program, Child Health Research Institute and Department of Paediatrics, University of Western Ontario, London, Ontario, Canada.

Michael C. Brody, MD, Department of Anesthesiology/CCM, University of Pittsburgh Medical Center, Pittsburgh, Pennsylvania.

C. Richard Chapman, PhD, Department of Anesthesiology, University of Washington, Seattle, Washington; Pain and Toxicity Research Program, and Division of Clinical Research, Fred Hutchinson Cancer Research Center, Seattle, Washington.

Charles S. Cleeland, PhD, Pain Research Group, and Department of Neurology, University of Wisconsin Medical School, Madison, Wisconsin.

Kenneth D. Craig, PhD, Department of Psychology, University of British Columbia, Vancouver, British Columbia, Canada.

Douglas E. DeGood, PhD, Department of Anesthesiology, Pain Management Center, University of Virginia Health Sciences Center, Charlottesville, Virginia.

Gary W. Donaldson, PhD, Pain and Toxicity Research Program, and Division of Clinical Research, Fred Hutchinson Cancer Research Center, Seattle, Washington.

Samuel F. Dworkin, DDS, PhD, Department of Psychiatry and Behavioral Sciences, School of Medicine, and Department of Oral Medicine, School of Dentistry, University of Washington, Seattle, Washington.

Michael Feuerstein, PhD, Center for Occupational Rehabilitation, University of Rochester Medical Center, Rochester, New York.

Herta Flor, PhD, Department of Clinical and Physiological Psychology, University of Tübingen, Tübingen; University of Marburg, Marburg, Germany.

Robert D. Gerwin, MD, The Johns Hopkins University, Baltimore, Maryland, and Neurological Medicine, Greenbelt, Maryland.

Ruth V. E. Grunau, PhD, Department of Psychology, University of British Columbia, Vancouver; The British Columbia Children's Hospital, Vancouver, Canada.

Charles S. Greene, DDS, Northwestern University Dental School, Chicago, Illinois.

Julie McDonald Haile, BS, Department of Psychology, and Division of Gastroenterology, University of Alabama at Birmingham, Birmingham, Alabama.

Stephen W. Harkins, PhD, Department of Gerontology, Medical College of Virginia, Virginia Commonwealth University, Richmond, Virginia.

Paul F. Hickey, MEd, Center for Occupational Rehabilitation, University of Rochester Medical Center, Rochester, New York.

Mary Casey Jacob, PhD, Departments of Psychiatry and Obstetrics and Gynecology, University of Connecticut Health Center, Farmington, Connecticut.

Robert C. Jacobson, PhD, Pain and Toxicity Research Program, Division of Clinical Research, Fred Hutchinson Cancer Research Center, Seattle, Washington.

Theresa M. Jaworski, PhD, Section of Psychology, Mayo Clinic, Rochester, Minnesota.

Mark P. Jensen, PhD, Department of Rehabilitation Medicine, University of Washington, Seattle, Washington.

Paul Karoly, PhD, Department of Psychology, Arizona State University, Tempe, Arizona.

Joel Katz, PhD, Department of Psychology, The Toronto Hospital, Toronto General Division, and Department of Behavioral Science, University of Toronto, Toronto, Ontario, Canada.

Francis J. Keefe, PhD, Department of Medical Psychology, Duke University Medical Center, Durham, North Carolina.

Robert D. Kerns, PhD, Departments of Psychiatry, Neurology, and Psychology, Yale University, New Haven; Psychology Service Veterans Administration Medical Center, West Haven, Connecticut.

Daniel M. Laskin, DDS, MS, Department of Oral and Maxillofacial Surgery, Medical College of Virginia, Virginia Commonwealth University, Richmond, Virginia.

Tom G. Mayer, MD, Department of Orthopedic Surgery, University of Texas Southwestern Medical Center, Dallas, Texas.

Patricia A. McGrath, PhD, Paediatric Pain Program, Child Health Research Institute and Department of Paediatrics, University of Western Ontario, London, Ontario, Canada.

Ronald Melzack, PhD, Department of Psychology, McGill University, Montreal, Quebec, Canada.

Wolfgang Miltner, PhD, Department of Medical Psychology, University of Tübingen, Tübingen, Germany.

Peter B. Polatin, MD, Department of Psychiatry, University of Texas Southwestern Medical Center, Dallas, Texas.

Kenneth M. Prkachin, PhD, University of Waterloo, Waterloo, Ontario, Canada.

Donald D. Price, PhD, Department of Anesthesiology, Medical College of Virginia, Virginia Commonwealth University, Richmond, Virginia.

Thomas E. Rudy, PhD, Department of Anesthesiology/CCM, and Pain Evaluation and Treatment Institute, University of Pittsburgh Medical Center, Pittsburgh, Pennsylvania.

Michael S. Shutty, Jr., PhD, Department of Anesthesiology, University of Virginia Medical Center, Charlottesville, Virginia; Department of Psychology, Western State Hospital, Staunton, Virginia.

Karen L. Syrjala, PhD, Pain and Toxicity Program, Fred Hutchinson Cancer Research Center, Seattle, Washington.

Dennis C. Turk, PhD, Departments of Psychiatry, Anesthesiology/CCM, Behavioral Science, and Pain Evaluation and Treatment Institute, University of Pittsburgh Medical Center, Pittsburgh, Pennsylvania.

Sridhar V. Vasudevan, MD, Elmbrook Memorial Hospital, Brookfield, Wisconsin.

Michael Von Korff, ScD, Center for Health Studies, Group Health Cooperative/ Puget Sound, Seattle, Washington.

Gordon Waddell, MD, FRCS, Orthopaedic Department, Western Infirmary, Glasgow, Scotland.

Coralyn W. Whitney, PhD, Departments of Dental Public Health Sciences and Oral Medicine, School of Dentistry, University of Washington, Seattle, Washington.

David A. Williams, PhD, Department of Psychiatry, Georgetown University Medical Center, Washington, DC.

Preface

Pain is an integral part of life and plays an important protective function. Yet pain that is uncontrolled and prolonged can greatly compromise the quality of life. Pain is the primary symptom that prompts individuals to seek medical attention; it results from disease and tissue pathology, and may even be reported in the absence of any identifiable physical pathology. Despite the prevalence of pain, there remains much that we do not understand about it.

Everyone knows what pain is, but no one can truly know another's experience of pain. Pain has many perplexing characteristics. Why do two individuals with ostensibly the same degree of physical pathology sometimes respond so differently? Why do patients treated by the same methods to control pain show different results? What causes pain in the absence of peripheral tissue damage, as in the case of central pain states or deafferentation pain syndromes?

Pain is a perception that is experienced by the individual. According to the definition of the International Association for the Study of Pain (IASP) (1979),* "Pain is an unpleasant sensory and emotional experience associated with actual or potential tissue damage or described in terms of such damage." This definition underscores the inherent subjectivity of pain. The definition acknowledges the importance of emotional as well as sensory factors.

To understand and adequately treat pain, we need to be able to measure it. This seems at first to be quite a simple task. All that is required is that the individual respond to the question "How much does it hurt?" Unfortunately, the problem is not as simple as this question might suggest. Many factors contribute to the individual's response. There does not appear to be a simple isomorphic relationship between the amount of pain and the extent of tissue damage. As noted in the IASP definition, psychological factors are involved in the pain experience. A number of cultural, economic, social, demographic, and environmental factors, along with the individual's personal history, situational factors, interpretation of the symptoms and resources, current psychological state, as well as physical pathology, all contribute to the response to the question "How much does it hurt?" Moreover, this set of factors will influence the individual's response to pain and to the treatments that are provided.

The complexity of pain has been revealed in recent decades. Investigators and

---

*International Association for the Study of Pain. (1979). Pain terms: A list with definitions and notes on usage. *Pain, 6,* 249–252.

clinicians have learned that a diverse range of factors need to be examined in the hope of understanding the response to the simple question of how much it hurts. In this volume, we have asked a group of internationally acknowledged experts to provide a description of the available instruments and procedures for assessing pain. In addition, we asked contributors to provide practical information about the merits of the various instruments and procedures to assist a clinical investigator or health-care provider make informed decisions regarding the most appropriate methods to assess the person who is experiencing pain. We have also included contributions that provide more general discussion of the issues that need to be considered in selecting from the array of instruments and procedures that are available.

The volume is organized into six sections. The first section includes chapters that address medical and physical examination procedures that are appropriate for some of the most common pain diagnoses—back pain (Polatin & Mayer, Waddell & Turk), myofascial pain (Gerwin), and orofacial pain (Laskin & Greene). This section also includes a chapter on recent advances in assessment based on ergonomics (Feuerstein & Hickey). A general discussion of the important issues of impairment and disability (Vasudevan) closes this section.

The second section focuses specifically on the methods and instruments available to quantify pain using self-report (Price & Harkins, Jensen & Karoly, Melzack & Katz) and psychophysiological methods (Flor, Miltner, & Birbaumer).

The third section is devoted to assessment of the *individual* who experiences pain. The use of traditional psychological methods (Bradley, Haile, & Jaworski) and the most appropriate instruments designed to assess the cognitive factors believed to be important in the response to pain (DeGood & Shutty), as well as the impact of pain on the individual sufferer's life (Kerns & Jacob) are discussed in depth.

The fourth section of the volume examines the behavioral manifestations of pain—"pain behaviors." Specifically, voluntary behaviors that communicate pain, distress, and suffering (Keefe & Williams) and facial expressions associated with pain (Craig, Prkachin, & Grunau) are reviewed. Detailed methods for assessing these two broad sets of behaviors are presented.

The fifth section addresses special topics in pain assessment based on unique and potentially important individual characteristics of pain sufferers such as children (McGrath & Brigham) and the elderly (Harkins & Price). Specific assessment issues associated with diagnosis having features in need of special attention, for example, acute pain (Chapman, Donaldson, & Jacobson), cancer pain (Cleeland & Syrjala), and headache (Andrasik) patients are also included in this section.

The sixth section addresses important methodological topics that transcend the previous chapters. The chapters in this section include discussions of basic psychometrics required for all assessment instruments and procedures (Dworkin & Whitney) and advanced methods to deal both with psychometric issues and also the difficult problem of combining a diverse array of assessment information (Rudy, Turk, & Brody). Other topics covered in this section concern epidemiology and survey methods (Von Korff) and issues associated with classification of patients within groups based on comprehensive assessment findings (Turk & Rudy).

In our introductory and summary chapters, we have provided an overview of concepts of pain assessment and attempted to identify current trends as well as future directions. We hope that this volume will (1) provide a practical guide to currently available instruments and procedures, (2) suggest areas in which currently available procedures are inadequate, and (3) serve as an impetus for research to improve upon existing instruments and procedures. The achievement of these goals should enhance our understanding of pain and lead to more successful treatment. The ultimate aim of this volume is to contribute to decreased suffering and improvement in the quality of life of those who experience pain.

DENNIS C. TURK
RONALD MELZACK

Contents

PART V. SPECIAL TOPICS

PART VI. METHODOLOGICAL ISSUES

SUMMARY

INTRODUCTION

Chapter 1

The Measurement of Pain and the Assessment of People Experiencing Pain

DENNIS C. TURK, PhD
RONALD MELZACK, PhD

> Just as "my pain" belongs in a unique way only to me, so I am utterly alone with it. I cannot share it. I have no doubt about the reality of the pain experience, but I cannot tell anybody what I experience. I surmise that others have "their" pain, even though I cannot perceive what they mean when they tell me about them. I am certain about the existence of their pain only in the sense that I am certain of my compassion for them. And yet, the deeper my compassion, the deeper is my certitude about the other person's utter loneliness in relation to his experience.
>
> IVAN ILLICH (1976, pp. 147–148)

> . . . the investigator who would study pain is at the mercy of the patient, upon whose ability and willingness to communicate he is dependent.
>
> LASAGNA (1960, p. 28)

Pain is the primary symptom that instigates people to seek medical treatment and accounts for over 35 million new office visits to physicians (Knapp & Kock, 1984) and over 70 million (80%) of all office visits to physicians each year in the United States (National Center for Health Statistics, 1986). Annually, in the United States there are over 50 million trauma injuries, many associated with high levels of pain (Chapman & Turner, 1986). Furthermore, every year more than 15 million people are diagnosed with cancer in the United States, with 40–45% in the early stages of the disease and 60–85% in advanced stages of the disease reporting moderate to severe pain (Bonica, 1979).

In addition to pain associated with disease or injury, medical and surgical procedures often produce pain. For example, in 1980 over 23 million Americans underwent surgery, and more than 70% of these individuals report moderate to very severe pain (Bonica & Benedetti, 1980).

The statistics cited above are derived from physician and hospital records; however, they probably reflect only the tip of the iceberg when it comes to the prevalence of pain experienced. Many people try to self-manage their pain without seeking medical attention. Von Korff, Dworkin, LeResche, and Kruger (1988) conducted an epidemiological study of common pain conditions among adults enrolled in a health maintenance organization in Seattle, Washington (see also Von Korff, Chapter 22). They reported that the prevalence of recurrent episodes of pain was 37%, with 8% reporting severe, persistent pain. They also reported that 2.7% of the sample indicated that they experienced seven or more days of pain in the six months preceding the survey during which they were unable to carry out their usual activities.

Obviously, pain is a ubiquitous feature of life and only in the case of the extremely rare condition of congenital insensitivity do any humans escape from the aversive experience. Although pain is essential for survival, in many circumstances pain exceeds the signaling function. Given the statistics cited above, it might be expected that pain would be well understood. Unfortunately, this is not the case. Frequently, the cause of the individual's pain is poorly understood, and even when it is, the severity may not be adequately managed. The measurement of pain is essential for the study of pain mechanisms and for the evaluation of methods to control pain.

A central impediment to increased understanding and control of pain is a result of the inherent subjectivity of pain. It is difficult to describe pain and different descriptions may be used by two individuals attempting to describe what is seemingly the same phenomenon. Similarly, the language used by a patient to describe his or her subjective experience to a health-care provider may be difficult to communicate because the patient and provider have different languages, different experiences, and different frames of reference. The individual is the "experiencer" whereas the physician or investigator can only be an observer (note the quote by Illich above). In short, pain is a subjective experience, a complex perceptual phenomenon. Thus, by its very nature, pain can be assessed only indirectly.

A BROADER PERSPECTIVE ON THE PAIN SUFFERER

The complexity of pain was emphasized by Melzack and Wall (1965) and was an important impetus for their formulation of the gate control theory of pain. The landmark papers by Melzack and his colleagues (Melzack & Casey, 1968; Melzack & Wall, 1965) formulating the gate control theory expanded the conceptualization of pain from a purely sensory phenomenon to a multidimensional model that integrates motivational–affective and cognitive–evaluative components with sensory–physiological ones.

The gate control model served as an important impetus to physiological research and research on identifying and demonstrating the important modulation of psychological variables in pain perception. In the 1970s Melzack and colleagues (Melzack, 1975; Melzack & Torgerson, 1971) developed the first assessment instrument, the McGill Pain Questionnaire (MPQ), designed to measure the three components of pain postulated by the gate control theory (see Melzack & Katz, Chapter 10). The first book to focus exclusively on pain measurement was edited by Melzack (1983), and presented the state of knowledge at that time. It served as an important impetus to the expanded research in this area.

In the years after this pioneering work on pain assessment, a number of investigators have emphasized that pain that extends over time (i.e., chronic pain, acute recurrent pain, pain associated with progressive diseases) has an important impact on all domains of the sufferer's life. Since persistent pain is so prepotent, psychological factors may come to play an even greater role in influencing the subjective experience, report, and responses. The present volume builds on the original Melzack (1983) text and provides a status report of current knowledge of pain assessment and, equally important, assessment of the individual pain sufferer's multidimensional experience.

CATEGORIZING PAIN

In order to communicate, there needs to be a common language and categorization system that can be used in a consistent fashion. One common way to categorize pain is to consider it along a continuum of duration. Thus, pain associated with tissue damage, inflammation, or a disease process that is of relatively brief duration (i.e., hours, days, or even weeks), regardless of intensity, is frequently referred to as acute pain (e.g., post–surgical pain). In contrast, pain that persists for extended periods of time (i.e., months or years), that accompanies a disease process (e.g., rheumatoid arthritis), or that is associated with an injury that has not resolved within an expected period of time (e.g., low back pain, phantom limb pain) is referred to as chronic.

This duration continuum is inadequate because it does not include acute recurrent pain (e.g., migraine headaches, sickle cell anemia), tends to ignore pain associated with progressive diseases such as chronic obstructive pulmonary disease and metastatic cancer, and pain induced in a laboratory context. In the case of acute recurrent pain, individuals may suffer from episodes of acute pain interspersed with pain-free periods. In the case of pain associated with progressive diseases, certain unique features of the pain that are influenced by the nature of the disease need to be considered. Finally, in the laboratory there are a number of contextual factors that require consideration before extrapolating to the clinical context. Using these five discrete categories of pain (i.e., acute, acute recurrent, chronic, chronic progressive, and laboratory-induced) comprises a categorical approach rather than a simple continuum based on duration.

Another way to categorize pain is based on the diagnosis. For example, pain associated with headaches (see Andrasik, Chapter 20) and orofacial pain (see Laskin & Greene, Chapter 4) have been contrasted with pain associated with the low back (see Polatin & Mayer, Chapter 3, Waddell & Turk, Chapter 2). Physicians and clinical investigators have long recognized that disease categories provide minimal information about the impact of illness upon patient experiences. A diagnosis is important because it may identify a cause of symptoms and recommend treatment. Yet within a specific diagnosis, patients differ considerably in how they are affected. Consequently, these patients required assessment of not only the direct components of pain but also the patients' mood, attitudes, beliefs, coping efforts, resources, and the impact of pain on their lives (see Bradley, Haile, & Jaworski, Chapter 12, DeGood & Shutty, Chapter 13, Kerns & Jacob, Chapter 14).

Yet another continuum used to discuss pain is the age of the sufferer. For example, there has been much debate on whether children experience pain the same way as adults do (see McGrath & Brigham, Chapter 17). At the other end of the life span, there has been considerable discussion on alterations in sensory sensitivity in the later stages of life and the impact of age-related physical changes have on pain perception (see Harkins & Price, Chapter 18).

The categorizations described above are only a few examples and are definitely not exhaustive (see Turk & Rudy, Chapter 23). There is, however, no one system for categorizing pain or pain patients that has been universally accepted by clinicians or researchers.

Regardless of the way one categorizes pain, and people with pain, a number of commonalities transcend age of the sufferer, duration of pain, diagnosis, and other variables. However, before we can hope to understand pain, we need to consider how to measure this elusive phenomenon (Turk, 1989).

VERBAL MEASUREMENT OF PAIN

There is no simple thermometer that can objectively record how much pain an individual experiences. Anything that can be determined about the intensity of an individual's pain is based on what the patient verbally or nonverbally communicates about his or her subjective experience.

Often patients are asked to quantify their pain by providing a single general rating of pain: "Rate your usual level of pain on a scale from 0 to 10 where 0 equals no pain and 10 is the worst pain you can imagine." Here the patient is being asked to quantitate and average his or her experience of pain over time and situations. These ratings are retrospective, and a number of studies have reported that patients significantly overestimate their pain when asked to recall previous levels of pain (e.g., Linton & Gotestam, 1983). Moreover, pain intensity is likely to vary over time and to depend upon what the patient is doing. It has also been demonstrated that present levels of pain tend to influence memory; consequently, present pain levels may serve as anchors that influence the averaging of pain (Eich, Reeves, Jaeger, & Graff-Radford, 1985).

It is possible that patients may be unable to discriminate reliably between the points on the scale, and for some the points may not even be on the same dimensions. The anchor words of the scale may also influence the distribution of responses. Many of these points are discussed by Jensen and Karoly (Chapter 9).

Despite the concerns noted, intensity of pain, is, without a doubt, the most salient dimension of pain, and a variety of procedures have been developed to measure it. There has been tremendous interest and effort to develop reliable and valid measures to quantify pain intensity (see Jensen & Karoly, Chapter 9, and Price & Harkins, Chapter 8) and to objectively identify the causes of pain (see Polatin & Mayer, Chapter 3, Waddell & Turk, Chapter 2, Gerwin, Chapter 5, Dworkin & Whitney, Chapter 24, and Laskin & Greene, Chapter 4). However, pain is a complex, multidimensional, subjective experience. The report of pain is related to numerous variables such as cultural background, past experience, the meaning of the situation, personality variables, attention, arousal level, emotions, and reinforcement contingencies (Melzack & Wall, 1983; Turk, Meichenbaum, & Genest, 1983). Using a single dimension, such as intensity, will inevitably fail to capture the many qualities of pain and the pain experience (Melzack, 1975). In short, pain intensity, although frequently used in clinical practice to quantify the disorder, is inadequate. Moreover, pain intensity itself does not provide a good reflection of either psychological or physical disruption caused by specific disorder (Naliboff, Cohen, Swanson, Bonebakker, & McArthur, 1985; see Waddell & Turk, Chapter 2).

ASSESSMENT OF THE PHYSICAL COMPONENT OF PAIN

Physicians are often wary of patients' self-reports of pain and may prefer more "objective" measures that they believe are more valid than questionnaires. Biomedical research and advanced technology have been used in an attempt to identify the physical basis of the report of pain. The implicit assumption of this research seems to be that there would be an isomorphic relationship between the report of pain and tissue pathology. It is believed that once the nature and extent of tissue pathology are identified by using objective physical assessment, sophisticated imaging, and laboratory diagnostic procedures, the information would provide direct knowledge of the subjective state. To date, this research has been disappointing. There is little information on how to

effectively integrate the information derived from these physical procedures (see Rudy, Turk, & Brody, Chapter 25). Moreover, the relationship between pathology, physical measurements of muscle strength and range of motion, behavior, and reports of pain have not been firmly established and appear to be only weakly correlated (Deyo, 1986; Nachemson, 1976). A number of studies have demonstrated significant pathology in asymptomatic subjects, which places into question the clinical significance of these findings (e.g., Boden, Davis, Dina, Patronas, & Wiesel, 1990; Hitselberger & Witten, 1968; Wiesel, Tsourmas, Feffer et al., 1984). Conversely, little identifiable pathology may occur in patients who report severe pain (e.g., White & Gordon, 1982).

In short, the association between physical abnormalities and patients' reports of pain is often ambiguous and poorly correlated. Moreover, physical pathology has been reported not to be predictive of disability (Cats-Baril & Frymoyer, 1991; Hagglund, Haley, Reveille, & Alarcon, 1989; Waddell, 1987), return-to-work after an injury (Bigos et al., 1991), or treatment outcome (e.g., Cairns, Mooney, & Crane, 1982). One possible contributing factor to the apparent lack of correlation between pathology, symptoms, and outcome is the observation that the reliability of many physical examination procedures is questionable (e.g., Matyas & Bach, 1985; Rowe, 1969; Waddell et al., 1982; see also Dworkin & Whitney, Chapter 24, Rudy, Turk, & Brody, Chapter 25, and Waddell & Turk, Chapter 2). In addition, although physical examination measurements such as flexibility and strength may be objective, they are influenced in many cases by patients' motivation, effort, and psychological state.

A number of physicians have tried to develop systematic approaches to physical assessment and have suggested that sophisticated laboratory and imaging techniques should form the basis of pain assessment (see Rudy, Turk, & Brody, Chapter 25, and Waddell & Turk, Chapter 2). However, considerable research has demonstrated that there is no isomorphic association between physical pathology and pain. Many factors seem to mediate this association in acute (Bonica, 1990), chronic (Waddell, Bircher, Finlayson, & Main, 1984) pain, and pain associated with terminal illness (Turk & Fernandez, 1990).

In an effort to avoid the problems inherent

in self-reports of pain severity, some investigators and many clinicians suggest that the report of pain should be ignored because it is a symptom rather than an objective sign that is believed to be more reliable and valid. For example, the Social Security Administration in the United States bases disability determination solely on physical examination and imaging and laboratory diagnostic tests. It is only when these objective findings are identified that subjective report of pain is considered.

Identification of pain-specific physiological response has also met with mixed success (cf. Sternbach, 1968; Turk, 1989). The reliability of many psychophysiological parameters has been questioned (e.g., Arena, Blanchard, Andrasik, Cotch, & Meyers, 1983; see Flor, Miltner, & Birbaumer, Chapter 11). As Sternbach (1968) noted, "Because of the variability of response elicited by different pain stimuli, and because of the additional variance contributed by individual differences in response-stereotype, it is difficult to specify a pattern of physiological responses characteristic of pain" (p. 259).

ASSESSMENT OF PHYSICAL FUNCTIONING

In many patients, objective physical findings to support their complaints of pain are absent. Thus, reliable and valid measures of pain and function must be developed. A number of studies demonstrate that self-report questionnaires can be highly valid measures of functional status (e.g., Deyo & Diehl, 1983). Physical and laboratory measures are useful primarily to the degree that they correlate with symptoms and functional ability. However, self-report functional status instruments seek to quantify symptoms, function, and behavior directly, rather than inferring them (Deyo, 1988).

A great deal of research has been targeted toward the development of self-report measures designed to assess individuals' reports of their abilities to engage in a range of functional activities (e.g., Bergner, Bobbitt, Carter, & Gilson, 1981; Millard, 1989) and the pain experienced upon performance of those activities (e.g., Jette, 1987). Although, as noted above, many are skeptical of the validity of self-report measures and prefer more objective measures, studies have revealed high concor-

dances among self-report, disease characteristics, physicians' or physical therapists' ratings of functional abilities, and objective functional performance (e.g., Deyo & Diehl, 1983; Jette, 1987). Despite obvious limitations of bias, self-report instruments have several advantages. They are economical, enable the assessment of a wide range of behaviors that are relevant to the patient, and permit emotional, social, and mental functions to be assessed. More recently, investigators have developed procedures for standardized evaluation of functional capacity that directly assess the individual's physical capabilities (see Polatin & Mayer, Chapter 3, and Feuerstein & Hickey, Chapter 6).

ASSESSMENT OF THE BEHAVIORAL MANIFESTATIONS OF PAIN

Psychologists have also been concerned with the development of assessment procedures to evaluate pain in patients without depending on self-reports. Fordyce (1976) provided an important contribution by emphasizing the important role of environmental contingencies on communications of pain, distress, and suffering. Patients experiencing pain display a broad range of observable manifestations that communicate to others the fact that they are having pain, that they are distressed and suffering. These behaviors, termed pain behaviors, include verbal report, paralinguistic vocalizations, motor activity, facial expressions, gesticulations, and postural adjustments (Fordyce, 1976). Because pain behaviors, unlike pain per se, are observable, they are susceptible to influences by conditioning and learning. Patients have many opportunities to learn that the display of pain behaviors may lead to reinforcing consequences, such as attention, and the opportunity to avoid unwanted responsibilities. In some cases, these pain behaviors may be maintained by these reinforcing consequences long after the normal healing time for injury.

According to operant theory, behavior is controlled to a great extent by its consequences. With an initial injury or pathological state, these behaviors may be reflexive responses (in the language of behavioral theory, respondents); however, over time, these initially reflexive responses may be maintained by reinforcement contingencies. That is, attention or financial gain may be positively reinforcing and thereby contribute to maintenance of the behaviors long after the initial cause of pain has been resolved. These insights have led to an emphasis on the assessment of these pain behaviors (see Keefe & Williams, Chapter 16) as well as treatments designed to extinguish maladaptive pain behaviors and increase the level of activity (i.e., "well-behaviors"). Typically, methods used to assess pain behaviors had relied on patients' self-reports of their activities. For example, patients have been asked to indicate in general how much time they spend engaging in specific activities such as sitting, standing, walking ("up-time") or to complete daily monitoring forms recording the frequency of such activities. Some studies, however, have reported that patients are not accurate in their self-reports of activities and thus challenge the validity of them (e.g., Kremer, Block, & Gaylor, 1981). Keefe and his colleagues (for a review, see Keefe & Williams, Chapter 16) have developed specific behavioral observation methods to assess pain behaviors that are not dependent on patients' self-reports.

Unfortunately, none of the pain behaviors appears to be uniquely or invariably associated with the experience of pain. Craig and his colleagues (see Craig, Prkachin, & Grunau, Chapter 15) have made a strong case for the priority of nonverbal facial expression of pain for making judgments about the pain experienced by others. These investigators have conducted fine-grained observations of the facial musculature that is associated with pain.

Interestingly, Fordyce and his colleagues (1984) found a positive correlation between what patients reported and the actual physical limitations but little relationship between pain reports and pain behaviors. Thus, although physical impairment is related to disability it bares a much smaller association with reported pain. Council, Ahern, Follick, and Kline (1988) found that actual physical performance of back pain patients was best predicted by their *beliefs of their capabilities* and not pain per se. Flor and Turk (1988) examined the relationship between general and specific pain-related thoughts, convictions of personal control, pain severity, and disability levels in chronic back pain and rheumatoid arthritis patients. The general and situation-specific convictions of uncontrollability and helplessness were more highly related to pain and

disability than disease-status variables for both samples. These data suggest that it not only important to assess how much patients report they hurt but how much they are able to do.

One conclusion that seems incontrovertible is that there are no isomorphic relationships among reports of pain, disability, and tissue pathology (e.g., World Health Organization, 1980). Many individuals report significant degrees of pain but have minimal or no objective physical findings, or the reported pain appears to be disproportionate to the extent of physical pathology that is identified. Moreover, few objective physical findings have been shown to be associated with injured workers with back pain who return to work (Gallagher et al., 1989; Murphy, Sperr, & Sperr, 1986). This is a very perplexing and frustrating state of affairs for physicians who prescribe treatments for patients and for third-party payers who are asked to pay for these treatments.

ASSESSMENT OF PSYCHOLOGICAL CONTRIBUTIONS TO PAIN EXPERIENCE

Although biomedical factors appear to instigate the initial report of pain, psychosocial and behavioral factors may exacerbate and maintain high levels of pain and subsequent disability. It is important to acknowledge that disability is not solely a function of the extent of physical pathology (impairment) or reported pain severity (e.g., Fordyce et al., 1984; Gallaher et al., 1989, Naliboff et al., 1985; Waddell et al., 1984). Disability is a complex phenomenon that incorporates tissue pathology, the individual response to the physical insult, and environmental factors that can serve to maintain the disability and associated pain even after the initial physical cause has resolved. Pain that persists over time should be viewed not as caused by either solely physical or solely psychological determinants; rather, a set of biomedical, psychosocial, and behavioral factors contribute to the total experience of pain.

Health-care providers have long considered pain as synonymous with nociception and as a symptom of pathology. It is important, however, to make a distinction between nociception, pain, pain behavior, and suffering. Nociception is the processing of stimuli that are defined as related to the stimulation of nociceptors and capable of being experienced as pain. Pain, because it involves conscious awareness, selective abstraction, appraisal, ascribing meaning, and learning, is best viewed as a perceptual process comprised of the integration and modulation of a number of afferent and efferent processes (Melzack & Casey, 1968). Thus, the experience of pain should not be equated with peripheral stimulation. Suffering, which includes interpersonal disruption, economic distress, occupational problems, and myriad other factors associated with pain's impact on life, is largely associated with the interpretive processes and subsequent response to the perception of pain. Reesor and Craig (1988) demonstrated that maladaptive cognitive processes appeared to amplify or distort patients' experience of pain and suffering. In sharp contrast to the nociceptive model, operant pain behaviors can occur in the absence of and thus may be independent of nociception.

There are some similarities in the distinction between objective impairment and subjective disability and between nociception and pain. Gallagher et al. (1989) reported that few objective physical or biomechanical measures predicted return-to-work at 6 months, whereas a number of psychosocial variables (e.g., perceived control) were significant predictors of work status. The data suggest that exclusive reliance on the physical examination to determine level of disability, without consideration of psychosocial conditions, is not empirically justifiable. Furthermore, Waddell (1987) indicated that the correlation between objective physical impairment and pain was modest, but the correlation between impairments and self-reported restrictions in activity (disability) and between pain and restrictions were substantially greater.

The failure to find a relationship between reported pain and pathology has led some writers to suggest that personality factors may be the cause of pain and may influence reports of pain that are disproportionate to the identified pathology. The search for a "pain-prone personality" (e.g., Blumer & Heilbronn, 1982) and psychogenic pain has been futile. The many variables that have been perceived to be part of a personality constellation related to psychogenic pain may actually be reactions to illness independent of psychiatric diagnosis.

It is important to distinguish between the role of psychological factors as causal agents in pain and the role of psychological factors in the maintenance and exacerbation of pain. Regardless of the initial cause of nociception, as described by the gate control model of pain, a range of cognitive and affective factors can modulate the experience. In the case of chronic pain, these modulating psychological factors may come to play an even greater role than in acute pain. Thus, evaluation of the sufferer requires that attention be given to assessing the range of psychological factors—behavioral, cognitive, and affective—that contribute to the experience.

As might be expected, the first attempts to examine psychological factors associated with pain relied on the traditional psychological instruments such as the Minnesota Multiphasic Personality Inventory (MMPI) (see Bradley, Haile, & Jaworski, Chapter 12) that were never standardized on populations of pain sufferers, so that the generalizability of these instruments must be viewed as somewhat suspect. Furthermore, many of the commonly used psychological instruments have not demonstrated clear utility in either diagnostic or treatment outcome predictions (Turk, 1990). Additional research has begun to appear that will help in the development of normative information specific to the population of pain patients that can be serve as a basis for understanding the role of psychological factors. One of the major advances since the publication of Melzack's (1983) volume has been the rapid development of assessment instruments designed specifically to assess psychological factors associated with reports of pain (see Keefe & Williams, Chapter 16, Kerns & Jacob, Chapter 14, and DeGood & Shutty, Chapter 13).

SOME PROSPECTIVE CAVEATS

In this volume, detailed discussions and descriptions are provided of a broad range of assessment techniques and measures. These chapters represent a status report of current knowledge of assessment methods and methodology. At this point it seems appropriate to provide some cautions that may serve to inoculate the reader as he or she studies each of the chapters. One of us (DCT) is reminded of the examination question he gave to the graduate students in his course on Tests and Measurements: "Imagine that you read a journal article describing a new assessment battery and you believe it is the answer to your prayers for the research study that you are proposing in a grant application. Describe how you would go about convincing your collaborators and the grant reviewers that this battery should be used."

We must balance the tendency to focus on variables for which there are existing reliable and valid measures against the need to examine what is truly important. Clinicians and researchers should also guard against picking instruments blindly "off the shelf" simply because they are well known, popular, or have received extensive validation. It is essential that the instrument or procedure under consideration has been standardized on the population of interest. It should not be assumed that because an instrument or procedure has been demonstrated to have good psychometric properties on one population, it can be applied to another population without first demonstrating the psychometric properties of the instrument on the new population.

Currently, there are many competing instruments and procedures for evaluating pain. Each investigator or clinician develops his or her assessment package by selecting from the many available techniques or develops an assessment instrument, often without giving sufficient attention to the psychometric properties of the instruments. This practice makes it difficult to compare results across studies. There needs to be some agreement on the set of instruments and procedures that will be used as the standards for each relevant domain of assessment. But this is something of a double-edged sword, and we must be careful to prevent the need for consensus to interfere with the discovery of important new techniques and information.

Most of what is known about chronic pain patients has been learned by studying patients referred to specialized pain clinics or laboratory volunteers. The samples of patients represent a very small percentage of those who experience chronic pain—that is, they have gone through a selective filtering process (Turk & Rudy, 1990). The degree to which this segment of patients is representative of the larger population of people with chronic pain is highly questionable. Epidemiological surveys suggest that the pain-clinic sample differs in many ways from community samples. For example, the association between psychological abnormality and pain frequently noted in pain clinics is less frequently observed in epidemiological studies (Crook, Weir, & Tunks, 1989).

The issue of generalization from laboratory

volunteers is not new and has been debated for a long time (Chapman, 1983). There are a number of contextual factors (e.g., meaning of the situation, level of affective distress, motivation) that argue against generalizing from the laboratory to the clinic. There are, however, some important advantages to the laboratory context, most notably the precision of control of the nociceptive stimuli. Thus, when we consider current knowledge, we must acknowledge the limitations imposed by the existing databases.

Because of the subjectivity and the lack of reliable and valid techniques for measurement, pain is difficult to prove, disprove, or quantify in a satisfactory manner. Moreover, pain is impossible to study in isolation. A conscious individual will perceive pain in an idiosyncratic fashion depending upon a range of psychological as well as physical factors. The primary purpose of this volume is to provide a comprehensive review of the advances in the measurement of pain and the assessment of people who experience pain. The hope is that the reader will, upon examination of each contribution, be better able to develop a psychometrically acceptable and sufficiently comprehensive set of procedures to evaluate the pain population of interest.

REFERENCES

Arena, J.G., Blanchard, E.B., Andrasik, F., Cotch, P.A., & Meyers, P.E. (1983). Reliability of psychophysiological assessment. *Behaviour Research and Therapy, 21*, 447–460.

Bergner, M., Bobbitt, R.A., Carter, W.B., & Gilson, B.S. (1981). The Sickness Impact Profile: Development and final revision of a health status measure. *Medical Care, 19*, 787–805.

Bigos, S.J., Battie, M.C., Spengler, D.M., Fisher, L.D., Fordyce, W.E., Hansson, T.H., Nachemson, A.C., & Wortley, M.D. (1991). A prospective study of work perceptions and psychosocial factors affecting the report of back injury. *Spine, 16*, 1–6.

Blumer, D., & Heilbronn, D. (1982). Chronic pain as a variant of depressive disease: The pain-prone disorder. *Journal of Nervous and Mental Disease, 170*, 381–406.

Boden, S.D., Davis, D.O., Dina, T.S., Patronas, N.J., & Wiesel, S.W. (1990). Abnormal magnetic-resonance scans of the lumbar spine in asymptomatic subjects. *Journal of Bone and Joint Surgery, 72-A*, 403–408.

Bonica, J.J. (1979). Cancer pain: Importance of the problem. In J.J. Bonica and V. Ventafridda (Eds.), *Advances in pain research and therapy* (Vol. 2, pp. 1–12). New York: Raven Press.

Bonica, J.J. (1990). Postoperative pain. In J.D. Loeser (Ed.), *The management of pain* (Vol. 1, pp. 461–480). Philadelphia: Lea & Febiger.

Bonica, J.J., & Benedetti, C. (1980). Post-operative pain. In R.E. Condon & J.J. DeCosse (Eds.), *Surgical care: A physiological approach to clinical management*. Philadelphia: Febiger.

Cairns, D., Mooney, V., & Crane, P. (1982). Spinal pain rehabilitation: Inpatient and outpatient treatment results and development of predictors for outcome. *Spine, 9*, 91–95.

Cats-Baril, W.L., & Frymoyer, J.W. (1991). Identifying patients at risk of becoming disabled because of low back pain. The Vermont Engineering Center Predictive Model. *Spine, 16*, 605–607.

Chapman, C.R. (1983). On the relationship of human laboratory and clinical pain research. In R. Melzack (Ed.), *Pain measurement and assessment* (pp. 243–249). New York: Raven Press.

Chapman, C.R., & Turner, J.A. (1986). Psychological control of acute pain in medical settings. *Journal of Pain and Symptom Management, 1*, 9–20.

Council, J.R., Ahern, D.K., Follick, M.J., & Kline, C.L. (1988). Expectancies and functional impairment in chronic low back pain. *Pain, 33*, 323–331.

Crook, J., Weir, R., & Tunks, E. (1989). An epidemiological follow-up survey of persistent pain sufferers in a group family practice and specialty pain clinic. *Pain, 36*, 49–61.

Deyo, R.A. (1986). The early diagnostic evaluation of patients with low back pain. *Journal of General Internal Medicine, 1*, 328–338.

Deyo, R.A. (1988). Measuring the functional status of patients with low back pain. *Archives of Physical Medicine and Rehabilitation, 69*, 1044–1053.

Deyo, R.A., & Diehl, A.K. (1983). Measuring physical and psychosocial function in patients with low-back pain. *Spine, 8*, 635–642.

Eich, E., Reeves, J. Jaeger, B., & Graff-Radford, S.B. (1985). Memory for pain: Relation between past and present pain intensity. *Pain, 23*, 375–379.

Flor, H., & Turk, D.C. (1988). Chronic back pain and rheumatoid arthritis: Predicting pain and disability from cognitive variables. *Journal of Behavioral Medicine, 11*, 251–265.

Fordyce, W.E. (1976). *Behavioral methods for chronic pain and illness*. St. Louis, MO: Mosby.

Fordyce, W.E., Lansky, D., Calsyn, D.A., Shelton, J.L., Stolov, W.C., & Rock, D.L. (1984). Pain measurement and pain behavior. *Pain, 18*, 53–69.

Gallagher, R.M., Rauh, V., Haugh, L.D., Milhous, R., Callas, P.W., Langelier, R., McClallen, J.M., & Frymoyer, J. (1989). Determinants of return-to-work among low back pain patients. *Pain, 39*, 53–67.

Hagglund, K.J., Haley, W.E., Reveille, J.D., & Alarcon, G.S. (1989). Predicting individual impairment among patients with rheumatoid arthritis. *Arthritis and Rheumatism, 32*, 851–858.

Hitselberger, W.E., & Witten, R.M. (1968). Abnormal myelograms in asymptomatic patients. *Journal of Neurosurgery, 28*, 204–206.

Illich, I. (1976). *Medical nemesis: The exploration of health*. Harmondsworth, UK: Penguin Books.

Jette, A.M. (1987). The Functional Status Index: Reliability and validity of a self-report functional disability measure. *Journal of Rheumatology, 14*(Suppl. 14), 15–19.

Knapp, D.A., & Koch, H. (1984). *The management of new pain in office-based ambulatory care. National Ambulatory Medical Care Survey*. National Center for Health Statistics, 1980 and 1981. *Advance Data from Vital and Health Statistics*, No. 97 (DHHS Publication No. PHS 84-1250). Hyattsville, MD: Public Health Service.

Kremer, E.F., Block, A., & Gaylor, M.S. (1981). Behavioral approaches to treatment of chronic pain: The inaccuracy of patient self-report measures. *Archives of Physical Medicine and Rehabilitation, 62*, 188–191.

Lasagna, L. (1960). Clinical measurement of pain. *Annals of the New York Academy of Science, 86*, 28–37.

Linton, S.J., & Gotestam, K.G. (1983). A clinical comparison of two pain scales: Correlation, remembering chronic pain and a measure of compliance. *Pain, 17*, 57–66.

Matyas, T.A., & Bach, T.M. (1985). The reliability of selected techniques in clinical arthrometrics. *Australian Journal of Physiotherapy, 31*, 173–197.

Melzack, R. (1975). The McGill Pain Questionnaire: Major properties and scoring methods. *Pain, 1*, 277–299.

Melzack, R. (Ed.) (1983). *Pain measurement and assessment*. New York: Raven Press.

Melzack, R., & Casey, K.L. (1968). Sensory, motivational, and central control determinants of pain: A new conceptual model. In D. Kenshalo (Ed.), *The skin senses* (pp. 423–443). Springfield, IL: Chas C. Thomas.

Melzack, R., & Torgerson, W.S. (1971). On the language of pain. *Anesthesiology, 34*, 50–59.

Melzack, R., & Wall, P.D. (1965). Pain mechanisms: A new theory. *Science, 150*, 971–979.

Melzack, R., & Wall, P.D. (1983). *The challenge of pain*. New York: Basic Books.

Millard, R.W. (1989). The Functional Assessment Screening Questionnaire: Application for evaluating pain-related disability. *Archives of Physical Medicine and Rehabilitation, 70*, 303–307.

Murphy, J.K., Sperr, E.V., & Sperr, S.J. (1986). Chronic pain: An investigation of assessment instruments. *Journal of Psychosomatic Research, 30*, 289–296.

Nachemson, A.L. (1976). The lumbar spine: An orthopedic challenge. *Spine, 1*, 59–71.

Naliboff, B.D., Cohen, M.J., Swanson, G.A., Bonebakker, A.D., & McArthur, D.L. (1985). Comprehensive assessment of chronic low back pain patients and controls: Physical abilities, level of activity, psychological adjustment and pain perception. *Pain, 23*, 121–134.

National Center for Health Statistics, Koch, H. (1986). *The management of chronic pain in office-based ambulatory care: National Ambulatory Medical Care Survey. Advance Data from Vital and Health Statistics*, No. 123 (DHHS Publication No. PHS 86-1250). Hyattsville, MD: Public Health Service.

Reesor, K.A., & Craig, K.D. (1988). Medically incongruent chronic back pain: Physical limitations, suffering, and ineffective coping. *Pain, 32*, 35–45.

Rowe, M. (1969). Low back pain in industry—a position paper. *Journal of Occupational Medicine, 15*, 476–478.

Sternbach, R. (1968). *Pain: A psychophysiological analysis*. New York: Academic Press.

Turk, D.C. (1989). Assessment of pain: The elusiveness of latent constructs. In C.R. Chapman and J.D. Loeser (Eds.), *Advances in pain research and therapy: Vol. 12. Issues in pain measurment* (pp. 267–279). New York: Raven Press.

Turk, D.C. (1990). Customizing treatments for chronic pain patients: Who, what and why. *Clinical Journal of Pain, 6*, 255–270.

Turk, D.C., & Fernandez, E. (1990). On the putative uniqueness of cancer pain: Do psychological principles apply? *Behaviour Research and Therapy*, *28*, 1–13.

Turk, D.C., Meichenbaum, D., & Genest, M. (1983). *Pain and behavioral medicine: A cognitive-behavioral perspective*. New York: Guilford Press.

Turk, D.C., & Rudy, T.E. (1990). Neglected factors in chronic pain treatment outcome studies—referral patterns, failure to enter treatment, and attrition. *Pain*, *43*, 7–26.

Von Korff, M., Dworkin, S.G., LeResche, L., & Kruger, A. (1988). An epidemiologic comparison of pain complaints. *Pain*, *32*, 33–40.

Waddell, G. (1987). A new clinical method for the treatment of low back pain. *Spine*, *12*, 632–644.

Waddell, G., Bircher, M., Finlayson, D., & Main, C.J. (1984). Symptoms and signs: Physical disease or illness behavior? *British Medical Journal*, *289*, 739–741.

Waddell, G., Main, C.J., Morris, E.W., Venner, R.M., Rae, P.S., Sharmy, S.H., & Galloway, H. (1982). Normality and reliability in the clinical assessment of backache. *British Medical Journal*, *284*, 1519–1523.

White, A.A., & Gordon, S.L. (1982). Synopsis: Workshop on idiopathic low-back pain. *Spine*, *7*, 141–149.

Wiesel, S.W., Tsourmas, N., & Feffer, H. (1984). A study of computer-assisted tomography. 1. The incidence of positive CAT scans in an asymptomatic group of patients. *Spine*, *9*, 549–551.

World Health Organization. (1980). *International classification of impairments, disabilities and handicaps: A manual of classification relating to the consequences of disease*. Geneva: WHO.

I

MEDICAL AND PHYSICAL EVALUATION OF PAIN PATIENTS

Chapter 2

Clinical Assessment of Low Back Pain

GORDON WADDELL, MD, FRCS
DENNIS C. TURK, PhD

Back pain is one of the commonest presenting symptoms to the physician. A number of epidemiological surveys have reported 50–70% of people have an episode of low back pain at some time in their adult lives (Anderson, Pope, & Frymoyer, 1984; Frymoyer, Pope, Rosen, & Goggin, 1980; Nagi, Riley, & Newby, 1973). Based on the U.S. National Health and Nutrition Survey (NHANES), Deyo and Tsui-Wu (1987) found that almost 14% of the large sample indicated that they had experienced back pain lasting more than two weeks. Fortunately, for the large majority the pain is relatively mild and transient. When asked to rate the intensity of pain, only 18–22% of those reporting back pain indicated that it was severe to excruciating (Frymoyer et al., 1980; Nagi et al., 1973).

Perhaps more important than the prevalence of symptoms is the impact of pain on activities. It has been estimated that 11.7 million Americans are significantly impaired (Holbrook, Grazier, Kelsey, & Staufer, 1984), with 2.6 million temporarily disabled by their pain and 2.6 million permanently disabled (National Center for Health Statistics, 1981). A particularly disturbing trend is the observation that between 1957 and 1976, the rate of disability due to back pain increased at a rate 14 times faster than the U.S. population (Fordyce, 1985). The cost of compensation and medical payments for occupationally related back disorders, in the United States, has been estimated at $7.2 billion (Frymoyer & Cats-Baril, 1987).

A serious problem exists when the statistics cited above are considered in the light of current methods available to assess back pain. It has been suggested that for as many as 85% of back pain episodes, the cause of pain is unclear (White & Gordon, 1982). Contributing to the failure to identify the etiology of back pain may be the dubious reliability, sensitivity, specificity, and utility of many common examination and laboratory tests used in the diagnosis of back pain (Bernard & Kirkaldy-Willis, 1987). As a consequence, there are a large number of patients reporting back pain for whom we are unable to demonstrate objective findings.

Conversely, sophisticated imaging procedures may reveal objective abnormalities in asymptomatic individuals. Moreover, similar abnormalities in symptomatic patients may be identified but these may not necessarily be the source of the patient's pain. Thus, we must be cautious not to over-interpret either the presence or absence of objective findings.

ASSESSING THE PHYSICAL CONTRIBUTION TO THE REPORT OF PAIN

Difficulties in assessing the physical contributions to chronic pain are well recognized and there are no universal criteria for scoring the presence, absence, or importance of a particular sign (e.g., positive radiographs, distorted gait, limitation of spinal mobility), quantifying the degree of disability, or establishing the association of these findings to treatment outcome (see Rudy, Turk, & Brody, Chapter 25, as well as Vasudevan, Chapter 7). Interpretation of biomedical findings relies on clinical judgments and medical consensus based on the physician's experience and, in some instances, quasi-standardized criteria (e.g., Brena & Koch, 1975).

There remains a good deal of subjectivity both in the manner in which physical examinations are performed and diagnostic findings are interpreted, and in the extent of functioning that is established (Rudy, Turk, & Brena, 1988; Rudy, Turk, & Brody, Chapter 25; however, see Polatin & Mayer, Chapter 3). This should hardly be surprising when we consider, for example, that functional assessment of a back pain patient may include such physical examination procedures as "active forward flexion" and "straight leg raising" without any specific instructions regarding how these procedures should be conducted, how motivation should be maximized, or how the patient's performance should be scored.

The inherent subjectivity of physical examination is most evident when it is noted that agreement between physicians may be better for items of patient history than for some items of the physical examination (Wood, Diehr, Wolcott, Slay, & Tompkins, 1979). The reproducibility of clinical findings even among experienced physicians is low (e.g., Nelson, Allen, Clamp, & deDombal, 1979), and medical judgment as to organic versus nonorganic pain has only a moderate level of reliability across raters (Agre, Magness, Hull, Wright, & Baxter, 1987; Fordyce, Brena, & Holcomb, 1978; Nelson et al., 1979; Waddell et al., 1982; Wood et al., 1979). Furthermore, the interob-

server agreement in rating spine motion and muscle strength, even when using dynamometers, may be surprisingly poor (Agre et al., 1987). Moreover, the discriminative power of common objective signs of pathology has been questioned. For example, Rowe (1969) reported that the prevalences of leg-length differences, increased lumbosacral angles, spondylolisthesis, transitional lumbosacral vertebra, and spina bifida occulta in back pain patients were not significantly different from those of an asymptomatic control group.

Some of the variability in results of physical examination are associated with the patient's behavior during the assessment. Measures of flexibility, strength, or timed activities (e.g., obstacle courses) often reflect nonphysical, highly subjective states as much as actual physical capabilities. Thus, although physical measurements are more objective than patient reports, they are probably influenced in many cases by a patient's motivation, effort, and psychological state (Pope, Rosen, Wilder, & Frymoyer, 1980; see Polatin & Mayer, Chapter 3).

Most physicians make no attempt to carry out any formal assessment of how the patient is reacting to and coping with the pain but rely on their general "clinical impression" to detect any gross psychological disturbance. Such a typical medical interview and examination provide an inadequate basis for either diagnosis or management. There is clearly room for improvement in the clinical assessment of the patient with low back pain (see also Polatin & Mayer, Chapter 3).

Frustration with the inherent subjectivity in clinical examination has often led to overreliance on radiological investigations and laboratory tests, but this is unjustified. Substantial interobserver variability has also been documented for the more "objective" imaging and laboratory tests, including simple lumbar spine radiographs (Deyo, McNiesh, & Cone, 1985; Koran, 1975). However, the sensitivity, specificity, and predictive value of myelography (Hiltselberger & Witten, 1968; Hudgens, 1970), x-rays (Rockey, Tompkins, Wood, & Wolcott, 1978; Torgerson & Dotter, 1976), and magnetic resonance imaging (MRI) (Boden, Davis, Dina, Patronas, & Wiesel, 1990; Powell, Wilson, Szypryt, Symonds, & Worthington, 1986) in the evaluation of back pain patients, all common strategies for assessing pathology, have been questioned. A significant problem noted for imaging procedures is the high rate of false-positives, particularly in older patients.

In short, routine clinical assessment of the patient with low back pain is frequently subjective and unreliable (McCombe, Fairbank, Cockersole, & Pynsent, 1989). It is usually not possible to make any precise pathological diagnosis or even to identify the anatomical origin of the pain. Despite these limitations, the patient's history and physical examination remain the basis of medical diagnosis and may be the best defense against over-interpreting results from sophisticated imaging procedures (Laros, 1991).

In this chapter we consider three aspects of clinical assessment, with an emphasis on specific strategies for improving physical examination of low back pain patients. First, we outline a simple algorithm for making a differential diagnosis of simple low back pain, nerve root pain, and serious spinal pathology. The remainder of the chapter concentrates on the clinical assessment of the patient with low back pain. In the second section we consider assessment of severity in terms of pain, disability, and physical impairment. Finally, we consider a broader biopsychosocial assessment of cognitive factors, affective disturbance, and illness behavior. Throughout this chapter, the emphasis is on methods suitable for routine clinical assessment rather than on research techniques.

DIFFERENTIAL DIAGNOSIS

Most medical textbooks provide a long list of differential diagnoses for low back pain but many of these conditions are rare. Moreover, attempting to match the presentation of a particular patient to a vaguely recalled series of such "thumbnail" clinical sketches is an illogical and inefficient clinical strategy.

Analysis of a series of 900 patients referred to an orthopedic outpatient clinic (Waddell, 1982) suggests that an alternative approach, using clinical history and examination, can be used to separate patients into three broad diagnostic groups: (1) simple mechanical low back pain, (2) nerve root pain, and (3) serious spinal pathology. The term "mechanical" is used simply to indicate that the pain is related to physical activity. Serious pathology includes tumor, infection, or inflammatory conditions. Major structural deformities such as scoliosis or kyphosis and widespread neurological disorders involving more than one nerve root should be obvious in even the most cursory examination. Such major structural deformities introduce completely different issues of differential diagnosis and will not be considered further here. The differential diagnosis between low back pain, nerve root pain, and serious pathology, however, is fundamental to the management and prognosis of low back disorders.

Most patients with low back disorders present to the physician with symptoms of pain located generally in the region of the lower back, with or without radiation of pain to the legs. These patients less commonly present with neurological symptoms or significant spinal deformities. Neurological aspects of low back disorders are commonly confined to a single dermatome or myotome. Similarly, the common deformity associated with low back pain is a simple sciatic list due to muscle spasm. Differentiation of these presenting symptoms depends on two fundamental decisions that are based largely on careful assessment of the symptoms supplemented by the clinical examination. The first question to consider is whether any leg pain reported is an indication of nerve root involvement or is simply referred pain. The second question concerns suspicion of serious spinal pathology. We will address these two questions below.

The Interpretation of Leg Pain and Identification of Nerve Root Involvement

It is wrong to assume that all leg pain is "sciatica" and that it is due to pressure on a nerve root or that it must be due to a disc prolapse. Percutaneous needle stimulation of most of the structures of the back either electrically or by injection of hypertonic saline solution can initiate referred pain spreading to the buttocks and thighs, usually posterior and only occasionally spreading much below the knees (Kellgren, 1938, 1939). This dull, aching, ill-localized referred pain arising from the ligaments, muscles, facet joints, peridural structures, or disc itself (but not due to pressure on the nerve root) may be regarded simply as a spread of low back pain.

Clinically, this radiating pain is quite different from the root pain produced when a needle hits a nerve. In that case the pain is described as sharper and shooting. Moreover, it at least approximates a dermatomal pattern, often contains an element of paresthesia, and at the common L5 and S1 levels, usually radiates to the ankle or foot. The first clinical decision is to decide if leg pain is root pain or simply referred pain. Referred pain can be classified, investigated, and treated together with low back pain.

Examination findings of root irritation and root compression signs provide additional evidence of nerve root involvement. The earliest signs are those of nerve root irritation that can be demonstrated by maneuvers that stretch or press upon an irritable nerve to reproduce radiating root pain and paresthesia.

Despite widespread use, the straight leg raising (SLR) test is still commonly misinterpreted. Limitation of SLR due to low back pain is simply an index of severity of low back pain and is not in itself a sign of nerve involvement. The specific sign of nerve irritation on SLR is limitation due to reproduction of radiating leg pain. Root irritation may also be demonstrated by reproduction of symptomatic leg pain by direct pressure on the irritable nerve in the bowstring test or by cross-over pain from SLR of the asymptomatic leg.

Actual compression of the nerve interferes with electrical function to give muscle wasting, motor weakness, sensory disturbance, or depressed tendon reflexes that approximate the myotome and dermatome supplied by a single nerve root. Nerve function is usually only depressed rather than absent and classical anesthesia or total paralysis is rare, so that examination for minor neurological changes should be based on comparison with the normal leg.

Final confirmation of nerve root involvement depends on integration of clinical and radiological criteria:

1. Pattern of root pain
2. Root irritation signs
3. Root compression signs
4. Matching radiology by computed tomography (CT) or magnetic resonance imaging (MRI)

In a prospective surgical series of 175 patients, we have demonstrated that the four criteria listed above provide accurate prediction of surgical findings and distinguished nerve root involvement due to disc prolapse from bony entrapment (Morris, DiPaola, Vallance, & Waddell, 1986). Diagnosis based on logical interpretation of a limited number of salient criteria was shown to be more accurate than either a "total clinical picture" or overreliance on radiology alone.

Screening for Possible Spinal Pathology

The second essential feature of differential diagnosis is to have a simple, rapid, yet efficient method of identifying patients who require further investigation for possible spinal pathology or, alternatively, one that permits confident reassurance that there is no sign of any serious disease. Analysis of 900 patients (Waddell, 1982) identified the following suspicious features:

• Age—less than 20 or more than 55 years.
• Thoracic pain—rather than cervical or lumbosacral pain
• Nonmechanical pain—unrelated to physical activity or time
• Previous medical history—particularly a primary neoplasm
• Systemic symptoms—particularly weight loss
• Limited lumbar flexion
• Major spinal deformity or widespread neurological disorder
• Raised sedimentation rate
• Abnormalities on plain x-rays

Summary of Clinical Approach

The basic clinical observations and decisions described above allow differential diagnosis of the three main categories of simple mechanical low back pain, nerve root problems, and possible spinal pathology, each with quite different significance for investigation, management, and prognosis. Several studies have confirmed the normality, reliability, validity, and clinical utility of both the methods of clinical history and examination and the diagnostic classification (Waddell et al., 1982).

We suggest that the approach to differential diagnosis of low back pain described above and outlined in Table 2.1 provides a logical basis for clinical assessment that is simple, reliable, and dependable. From the most basic medical student level to a specialized back pain clinic, it forms a fundamental framework for clinical decision making and helps to remove some of the confusion and doubt that too often obscures our approach to low back pain.

TABLE 2.1. Differential Diagnosis of Low Back Pain

Presenting symptoms	Diagnostic decision	Major clinical problem

Back pain ⟶

Leg pain
— Referred pain
— Radicular pain

Neurological
— Single root
— Widespread

Deformity
— Muscle spasm list
— Structural deformity

Mechanical ⟶ Simple low back pain

Nonmechanical ⟶ ? Serious pathology

⟶ Nerve root levels

Note. Adapted from Waddell (1982), page 191. Copyright 1982 *British Journal of Hospital Medicine.* Adapted by permission.

ASSESSMENT OF SEVERITY

Assessment of the severity of low back pain is fundamental to decisions about treatment, monitoring progress, and the provision of support. Severity can be assessed in terms of pain, disability, and physical impairment. Physicians are frequently asked to provide a medical evaluation of disability although the ultimate determination of disability is rarely a purely medical decision. The disability determination process is predicated on a fundamental assumption: that disability bears a one-to-one relationship to specific impairments. Unfortunately, the impairment–disability link has not been unequivocally demonstrated (see Vasudevan, Chapter 7). It is therefore important to make a very clear conceptual and clinical distinction between pain and disability and between disability and physical impairment.

Definitions

Pain is "an unpleasant sensory and emotional experience associated with actual or potential tissue damage, or described in terms of such damage" (Merskey, 1979, p. 249). Impairment, and disability are fundamentally different concepts. *Physical impairment* is "an anatomical, pathological, or physiological abnormality of structure or function leading to loss of normal bodily ability," and *disability* is the resulting "diminished capacity for everyday activities and gainful employment" or the "limitation of a patient's performance compared to a fit person's of the same age and gender" (Waddell, Allan, & Newton, 1991; Waddell & Main, 1984). Thus, impairment is a tissue damage-based concept in contrast to disability which is a task-based concept.

Ideally, there should be a close correspondence between physical impairment and disability. If this were the case then the task of awarding disability compensation would be relatively easy. Unfortunately, this is often not the case. Moreover, current physical status is a poor predictor of future disability. In a prospective study of the subsequent status of a sample of back patients, Gallagher et al. (1989) reported that few objective physical or biomechanical measures were associated with return-to-work 6 months after a work-related injury. Interestingly, a number of psychosocial variables (e.g., perceived control, psychological distress) were more significant predictors of return-to-work.

Thus, although disability is predicated on objective determination of what the patient can or cannot do, this depends to a great extent on what the patient reports that he or she cannot do, and these reports are determined as much by the patient's attitudes, beliefs, and motivation as by objective physical pathology. We will return to a consideration of psychosocial variables in assessment of back pain patients later in this chapter.

Assessment of impairment is based on objective structural limitation and is solely a medical responsibility whereas clinical assessment of pain and disability is based largely on the patient's subjective report. Disability rating and compensation awards, however, are ultimately an administrative or legal, not a medical, responsibility, and are based both on the patient's report of disability and the physician's assessment of impairment. There are presently no completely objective means for measuring pain or impairment or for determining disability (Andersson, 1991), nor is there consensus regarding how to determine unequivocally the extent of disability. Commenting on the current state of affairs, Minnesota's Workers/Compensation Division to Study Schedules of Disability (1983) noted at a meeting of medical disability evaluation specialists that "it was the conclusion of all present that no system currently exists that accurately and adequately assesses permanent loss of flexibility, strength, and endurance in a permanently injured individual."

ASSESSMENT TECHNIQUES

Pain

We have found it useful to consider the following in routine clinical assessment of the pain of low back pain patients. As noted in the report of the Quebec Task Force on Spinal Disorders (1987), the simplest and most reliable strategy for assessing pain is based on anatomical distribution. This derives from the patient's report of low back pain alone, low back pain with referred pain into the thigh but not below the knee, and nerve root pain with or without neurological deficit.

The pattern of pain over time is also a useful distinction. Specifically, does the patient describe his or her pain as acute, recurrent, or chronic? Acute and chronic pain are fundamentally different in kind (Sternbach, 1977). Acute pain bears a more straightforward relationship to peripheral stimulus and tissue damage. There may be some anxiety about the meaning and consequences of the pain, however; acute pain, acute disability, and acute illness behavior are usually proportionate to the physical findings. Appropriate treatment directed at the underlying physical problem usually relieves acute pain. Chronic pain, chronic disability, and chronic illness behavior, by way of contrast, become increasingly dissociated from the physical problem. There may be very little evidence of any remaining tissue damage. Instead, chronic pain and disability become increasingly associated with psychological distress, depression, disease conviction, and illness

behavior. The patient seems to adapt to chronic disability.

Chronic pain may become a self-sustaining condition that does not respond to traditional medical management (Fordyce, 1976). Physical treatment directed to hypothetical but unidentified tissue damage may not only be unsuccessful but may cause further damage. Failed treatment may then reinforce and aggravate pain, psychological distress, illness behavior, and disability.

Perhaps the simplest and most useful clinical method for measuring the severity of pain is some form of visual analogue pain scale. We have found a pain thermometer to be particularly useful (see Figure 2.1). It is simple to administer and to score. The major difficulty lies in interpreting exactly what the pain scale measures.

Verbal rating scales are frequently used to describe the severity of pain. It is, however, difficult to define the exact severity of each adjective used and the "steps" on the scale may not be equal. The fundamental limitation of both a visual analogue scale (VAS) and the rating of pain severity is that no unidimensional scale can adequately effect the complexity of the pain experience.

The quality of pain can be assessed to some extent by the use of descriptive adjectives. The most widely used method is the McGill Pain Questionnaire (MPQ) (Melzack, 1975; see Melzack & Katz, Chapter 10). This was originally administered as an interview but is now generally used as a self-report questionnaire. The adjectives used to describe the pain

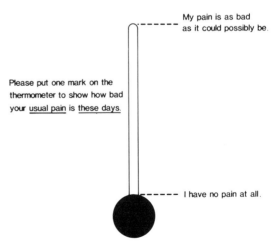

FIGURE 2.1. Pain thermometer.

can be separated into sensory, affective, and evaluative dimensions that provide some assessment of different qualities of the pain. The affective and cognitive dimensions bear similarities to other clinical measures of psychological distress. The evaluative dimension on the MPQ is often supplemented by other cognitive measures (see DeGood & Shutty, Chapter 13). For routine use in medical practice the short-form MPQ (Melzack, 1987) is much simpler and more practical.

Ratings on any self-report pain rating scales are in no sense an absolute or objective measure of pain and the patient's reports of pain intensity on these scales may bear very little relationship to any physiological or pathological change. The patient's self-report of pain may include physical sensation, distress, pain behavior, and communication. With these qualifications, it is obviously important not to overinterpret patients' pain severity ratings but to accept them as a measure of how patients choose to communicate their experience. How patients communicate is important because it serves as a cue for responses from significant others including health-care providers. We will return to the importance of patient communications when we discuss pain and illness behavior below.

Disability

Disability is a complex phenomenon that incorporates physical pathology, the individual's response to that physical insult, and environmental factors that can serve to maintain the disability and associated pain even after the initial physical cause has been resolved. It is important to keep in mind Cailliet's (1969) assertion that "Evaluation is not of disability; it is evaluation of a patient who is disabled" (p. 1380). Clinical assessment of disability must concentrate on loss of function rather than pain. The question is not, "Is that activity painful?" but rather "Are you actually restricted in that activity?" "Does your back limit how much you do or do you now require help with that activity?"

Although disability is predicated on objective determination of what patients can or cannot do, this usually depends on what patients report, and their reports are determined as much by patients' attitudes, beliefs, and motivations as by objectively determined physical pathology. Consequently, disability deter-

mination will always be highly subjective, based on both physicians' attitudes and beliefs concerning the associations between physical pathology and ability to engage in specific physical functions, and the credibility they give to patients' subjective reports (Turk, 1991).

To illustrate the subjectivity of physicians' making disability determinations, the results of a recent study can be examined. Carey et al. (1988) asked physicians to rate disability of simulated case vignettes of U.S. Social Security Administration disability claimants. The vignettes were constructed so that the simulated claimant did *not even approximate* the statutory prerequisites for a disability award under Social Security guidelines. The mean certainty of disability for the individual vignettes ranged from .08 to .43. In addition, the mean certainty estimates across physicians ranged from 0 to .61, indicating substantial variability in how physicians determined disability. This is likely related to physicians' data interpretation and their conceptualizations of impairment and consequent disability. For example, Carey et al. reported that approximately one-half of the physicians surveyed indicated that disabled applicants tended to exaggerate their symptoms and that they could work if they "tried hard enough."

The common or usual effect of an impairment should be assessed, discounting occasional limitations or special efforts. Our studies (Waddell & Main, 1984) have shown that disability in activities of daily living can be assessed reliably during clinical interview and the following limits to be most applicable in low back disorders. The patient can be asked:

Bending and lifting: Do you require help or avoid heavy lifting, for example, 30 to 40 lb, a heavy suitcase, or a 3- to 4-year-old child?

Sitting: Can you sit in an ordinary chair for more than 30 minutes at a time before you need to get up and move around?

Standing: Can you stand in one place generally for 30 minutes or more at a time before you need to move around?

Walking: Is walking generally limited to less than 30 minutes or 1–2 miles at a time before needing to rest?

Traveling: Can you travel in a car or bus for 30 minutes or more at a time before you need to stop and have a break?

Social life: Do you regularly miss or curtail social activities and normal social mobility (excluding sports)?

Sleep: Is your sleep regularly disturbed by your low back pain (i.e., two or three times per week)?

Sex life: Have you reduced the frequency of your usual sexual activity because of pain?

Dressing: Do you regularly require help with footwear—tights, socks, or shoelaces?

Alternatively, disability in activities of daily living can be assessed by self-report questionnaires. A number of self-report measures of functional capacity are available. One of the best developed and established is the Roland and Morris Disability Questionnaire derived from the Sickness Impact Profile (SIP; Roland & Morris, 1983; see Appendix 2.A). In an unpublished study we have found this to have better factor structure, score distribution, and clinical utility than the Oswestry Disability Scale (Fairbank, Couper, Davies, & O'Brien, 1980).

Physical Impairment

The aim of assessing physical impairment is to provide objective medical evidence of impairment that is reliable, is distinguishable from nonorganic and behavioral features, distinguishes patients with low back pain from normal asymptomatic subject, and is related to functional disability. Waddell and Main (1984) identified the following structural factors that were associated with permanent impairment: structural deformity of the spine, structural damage such as fracture or spondylolisthesis, surgical damage and scarring, and longstanding neurological deficit. None of these is applicable to the patient with simple low back pain with no nerve root involvement and no previous surgery.

More recently we have developed a comprehensive clinical evaluation of current physical impairment applicable to the patient with simple low back pain (Waddell, Sommerville, Henderson, & Newton, in press-b). It should be stressed that this is a measure of current rather than permanent impairment (Cox, Keeley, Barnes, Gatchel, & Mayer, 1988). Moreover, although it is based on objective clinical findings it assesses restriction of function due to pain rather than any anatomical or structural impairment.

In terms of the World Health Organization (1980) definition, our clinical evaluation may be best regarded as a measure of physiological impairment. Because, as noted above, many physical examination procedures have proven unreliable, it is important that any attempt to develop strategies with improved reliability include specific details of the examination. Examiners should be calibrated in the use of each of the examination components prior to assessing the reliability of the test to prevent unreliability due to procedural variation (see Dworkin & Whitney, Chapter 24). In the next section we describe the methods we suggest for each examination technique.

Examination Technique

The first step is to identify the anatomical landmarks (Ohlen, 1989; Spangfort, 1989; Troup, 1989). They can be palpated most easily with the patient lying prone with relaxed muscles.

- Horizontal marks are made on the skin in the midline at S2 and T12/L1. For S2 palpate the inferior border of the posterior superior iliac spines that lie at the bottom of the posterior part of the iliac crest just below and lateral to the dimples of Venus.
- Then count up to the spinous processes of T12/L1 checking that the iliac crests approximate to the L4/5 level. Make additional vertical marks in the midline over the spinous processes of T12 and T9.
- Have the patient perform warm-up exercises (Keeley et al., 1986): flexion/extension twice, left/right rotation twice, left/right lateral flexion twice, and one more full flexion/extension.
- It is then necessary to standardize the examination positions (Ohlen, 1989; Spangfort, 1989; Troup, 1989). We found particular difficulty in achieving a consistent erect position but this is essential because reliable measurement of movement depends on a standard starting point. After personal discussion with Spangfort (1989) and Troup (1989), we finally found the most satisfactory position to be bare feet, heels together, knees straight with the weight borne evenly on the two legs, looking straight ahead, arms hanging at the sides, relaxed. If there is severe muscle spasm then ask the patient to get as close to that position as they can hold comfortably for several minutes. The supine position is lying relaxed flat on the back, head lying on the couch without a pillow, arms at the sides with hips and knees ex-

tended as fully as possible without tension. The prone position is lying with no pillow, head and shoulders relaxed on the table, arms by the side.

The only equipment required is a ballpoint pen, a small spring-loaded centimeter tape from any clothing store, and an inclinometer. Although not essential, we have found an electronic inclinometer more convenient (manufactured by Cybex Division of Lumex Inc., 100 Spence Street, New York, NY 11706; see Polatin & Mayer, Chapter 3).

The following tests can be carried out in whatever order the examiner prefers; however, we generally arrange them in sequence in the erect, prone, and supine positions:

1. *Flexion* is measured with the inclinometer (Mayer, Tencer, Kristoferson, & Mooney, 1984). With the patient in the erect position recordings are made at S2 and then at T12/L1. Next instruct the patient to bend forward and reach down with the fingertips of both hands as far as possible toward the toes. Make sure the patient keeps the knees straight. Keep the patient fully flexed and obtain the third recording at T12/L1 and the fourth recording at S2. These four readings permit simple calculation of true lumbar flexion, pelvic flexion, and total combined flexion.

2. *Lumbar extension* is measured at T12/L1 (Mayer et al., 1984; see Polatin & Mayer, Chapter 3). Obtain the first reading with the patient in the erect position. Then instruct the patient to arch backward as far as possible while looking up to the ceiling. Support the patient with your free hand on one shoulder to maintain his or her balance and to give some feeling of security. Tell the patient to hold this position and obtain the second reading. Simple subtraction gives the measure of total extension.

3. *Lateral lumbar flexion* is also measured at T12/L1. A longer bar is needed on the inclinometer. Obtain the first inclinometer reading with the inclinometer bar lined up tangentially with the spine processes at T9 and T12. Then instruct the patient to lean straight over to one side as far as possible with their fingertips reaching straight down the side of the thigh. Avoid flexing forward or twisting around. Support the patient's shoulder with a hand and make sure that both feet stay flat on the ground. Repeat to the other side.

4. *Straight leg raising* (SLR) is carried out with the patient supine, making sure that the head remains relaxed and that the patient does not look up to watch what is happening (modified from Brieg & Troup, 1979; Mayer et al., 1984). Hold the foot with one hand and make sure that the hip is in neutral rotation. Position the inclinometer on the tibial crest just below the tibial tubercle with the other hand and set to zero. Passively raise the leg and at the same time hold the inclinometer in position with the other hand that also holds the knee fully extended. Raise the leg slowly to the maximum tolerated SLR (not the onset of pain) and record the maximum reading obtained. If SLR is less than 75 degrees then note if it is limited by back pain, hamstring discomfort, or radiating leg pain (Edgar & Park 1974). Limited SLR on formal examination should always be checked with distraction at a later stage of the examination (Waddell, McCulloch, Kummel, & Venner, 1980).

5. Reliable examination of *tenderness* can only be achieved by particularly careful standardization. This is carried out with the patient prone and it is important to make sure the muscles are relaxed. Palpation should be done slowly without sudden pressure and without hurting the patient unduly. Start by making sure that there is no superficial tenderness to light skin pinch: this is behavioral in nature and invalidates palpation for deep tenderness (Waddell et al., 1980). Local tenderness to firm pressure is then sought with the ball of the thumb over the spinous process or interspinous ligaments within 1 cm of the midline from T12 to S2. It is important to use specific wording: "Is that painful?" Any response apart from a specific "No" is taken as positive. Any qualified response such as "only a little bit" is counted positive. If the patient is doubtful or does not answer then repeat the question "Is that painful when I do that?" Widespread nonanatomical tenderness is again discounted as behavioral (Waddell et al., 1980).

6. *Bilateral active SLR* is tested in the supine position (modified from Biering-Sorensen, 1983). Ask the patient to lift both legs together 6 inches off the examination table and hold that position for 5 sec. Only count as positive if both calves and heels are clear of the examination table. Do not count aloud or use verbal encouragement. Do not allow the patient to use his or her hands to lift the legs. Record if he or she fails to lift the legs clear of the couch at

all, can lift clear but for less than 5 sec or can manage to hold the position for a full 5 sec.

7. *Active sit-up* is again tested in the supine position (modified from Biering-Sorensen, 1983; Lloyd & Troup, 1983; National Institute for Occupational Safety and Health, 1988). Flex the knees to 90 degrees and place the soles of the feet flat on the couch. The examiner should hold down both feet with one hand. Instruct the patient to reach up with the fingertips of both hands to touch (not hold) both knees and hold that position for 5 sec. Only count as successful if the fingertips of both hands reach the patellae. Again record if he or she fails to reach his or her knees, is able to reach his or her knees but for less than 5 sec, or is able to hold the position for the full 5 sec.

Scoring

These seven items are simply scored 0/1 on a scale from 0 to 7 (see Table 2.2).

Summary of Assessment of Severity

When pain, physical impairment, and disability are all proportionate, then together they provide an good measure of clinical severity. However, when there is significant disproportion between the patient's report of pain, disability and work loss, the physician's assessment of the underlying pathology, and objective physical impairment, then a more comprehensive assessment is required of the cognitive, affective, and behavioral dimensions of the illness.

TABLE 2.2. Objective Clinical Evaluation of Physical Impairment[a]

Total flexion	<87°
Total Extension	<18°
Average lateral flexion (left and right)	<24°
Average straight leg raising	
Female	<71°
Male	<66°
Spinal tenderness	positive
Bilateral active straight leg raising	<5 seconds
Sit-up	<5 seconds

[a]Each scored 0/1 to give a total score out of 7.
Note. Adapted from Waddell, Allan, and Newton (1991). Copyright 1991 Raven Press Books, Ltd. Adapted by permission.

BIOPSYCHOSOCIAL ASSESSMENT

It is important to acknowledge that by its very nature, chronic pain extends over time. Biomedical factors, in the majority of cases, appear to instigate the initial report of pain. With the prolonged course, psychosocial and behavioral factors may serve to exacerbate and maintain levels of pain and disability. Moreover, secondary physical factors may come to play an important role with physical deconditioning contributing to weakened muscles, loss of muscle flexibility, and reduced physical endurance. The longer the pain persists, the greater the disability. Thus, pain that persists over time should not be viewed as solely physical or as solely psychologically caused; rather, a set of biomedical, psychosocial, and behavioral factors contribute to the experience of pain.

Clinical assessment of the patient with low back pain should provide not only a physical assessment and diagnosis but also a comprehensive evaluation of the patient's pain, his or her attitudes and beliefs about the pain, the affective dimension of the pain, the pattern of illness behavior that has developed, and the disability that results. The most systematic approach is to consider each component of a biopsychosocial model of illness: sensory, cognitive, affective, and behavioral (see Figure 2.2).

In clinical practice, however, these are generally assessed in the reverse order: behavioral symptoms and signs are present at clinical interview and examination and often provide

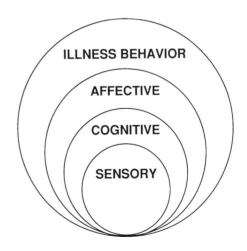

FIGURE 2.2. A biopsychosocial model of chronic pain and disability.

the first clinical clue that further psychological assessment is required; affective disturbance may be detected on closer clinical assessment and measured by standard psychological assessment; the underlying cognitive factors are buried most deeply and have been hardest to elucidate.

ILLNESS BEHAVIOR

All good clinicians use the clinical interview and examination not only to diagnose physical disease but also to learn about the patient and his or her response to illness. First, we must recognize that the patient is ill, not only by what he or she tells us but also by changes in the whole pattern of behavior that we recognize as "sick" or "illness behavior." Unfortunately, medical training concentrates on disease and assessment of the patient is learned by experience and is largely based on subconscious impressions that are unreliable, difficult to validate, and impossible to teach. What we need to do now is to distinguish the symptoms and signs of illness behavior from those of physical disease.

The Pain Drawing

Clinical observation of illness behavior is most simply illustrated by the pain drawing (Figure 2.3). Patients willingly record their pain on an outline of the body, but the *way* they draw the pain is strongly influenced by emotional distress (Ransford, Cairns, & Mooney, 1976).

Poorly localized, widespread and nonanatomical drawings, expansion or magnification of pain to other areas of the body and additional emphasis or comment on the severity of the pain all reflect the patient's distress rather than the physical characteristics of the pain. So the patient's description of pain communicates both physical information about the pain and psychological information about his or her response to the pain (contrast drawings A and B in Figure 2.3).

It is not a question of deciding whether the pain is physical or psychogenic and has nothing to do with the origin of the pain, but rather of recognizing that parts of the clinical description of pain are physical and that others are part emotional in nature and then interpreting them appropriately.

Mark the areas on your body where you feel these sensations. Use the symbols. Mark all the affected areas.

Numbness	= = =		Pins	O O O O
	= = =		&	O O O O
	= = =		Needles	O O O O

Ache	xxxxx	Pain	/ / / / /
	xxxxx		/ / / / /
	xxxxx		/ / / / /

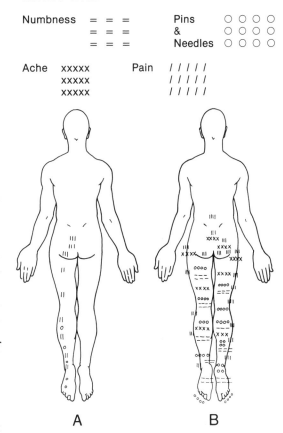

A   B

FIGURE 2.3. Pain drawing.

BEHAVIORAL SYMPTOMS

Interpretation of a medical history is based on the occurrence of common and hence recognizable patterns of symptoms. The way most patients describe their symptoms approximates anatomical and pathological patterns of disease. Occasionally, however, patients offer descriptions that clearly do not fit clinical experience. These "behavioral" symptoms and signs are vague and ill localized and fit what Walters (1961) has described as regional or body-image patterns rather than neuroanatomical patterns. They lack the normal relationship to time and physical activity and are difficult to fit to any reasonable anatomical or pathological mechanism.

Of course our knowledge is limited and the fact that we cannot understand a physical problem does not mean that it is psychological.

It is only reasonable to consider psychological factors as present when symptoms reported actually contradict normal anatomy and pathology.

We have been able to identify a group of such symptoms that are physically inappropriate and more closely related to psychological distress (Waddell, Main, Morris, DePaola, & Gray, 1984):

1. *Pain at the tip of the tailbone*: Coccydynia can be caused by local direct injury. Coccydynia in a patient with low back pain, however, is often associated with other behavioral symptoms.

2. *Whole leg pain*: The whole leg is reported to become painful in a stocking distribution usually from the groin down or below the knee. Such regional patterns of pain do not fit any nerve anatomy.

3. *Whole leg numbness*: The whole leg goes numb or dead in a stocking distribution. It usually comes and goes. The distribution again contradicts normal nerve anatomy.

4. *Whole leg giving way*: The whole leg gives way or collapses although very few patients actually fall to the ground. Again, the essential feature is the regional nature of the symptoms that is clearly different from a localized muscle weakness.

5. *Complete absence of any periods without pain*: Pain that has persisted for many years and become progressively worse without the normal variation and remissions with time.

6. *Intolerance and reactions to treatments*: Our treatment for low back pain is not very effective so we should not blame the patient if the pain does not improve. Side effects of treatment are also quite common but are usually minor. Beware, however, of the patient in whom every treatment has to be stopped because it aggravates the pain or causes severe side effects or subjective complications.

7. *Emergency admissions to hospital*: Simple low back pain is so severe that the patient has to be rushed to the hospital. This may be inappropriate behavior on the part of the doctor who refers him to hospital or the one who admits him rather than by the patient himself. Nevertheless, it is a measure of the patient's distress and emotional reaction to the pain.

These behavioral symptoms are clearly separate from the common symptoms of physical disease and have been shown to be closely related to psychological distress (Waddell et al.,

1984). They are simple and reliable to assess as part of the routine clinical history. Indeed, most of them are elicited by the standard medical interview and it is simply a matter of recognizing that these are behavioral rather than physical symptoms. They form a closely interrelated homogeneous group of symptoms that must be considered as a whole. Assessment should be based on the whole clinical picture, and isolated symptoms should be ignored. No physician would diagnose a disk prolapse solely on an absent ankle reflex, and it is equally important not to make a psychological diagnosis on isolated clinical observations. In rare cases these behavioral symptoms can occur in relation to serious spinal pathology such as tumor, infection, or paraparesis. This particular group of symptoms is therefore only inappropriate in the case of simple low back pain or sciatica and may not be inappropriate in other situations. They should not be regarded as behavioral until serious spinal pathology has been excluded.

NONORGANIC SIGNS OR BEHAVIORAL RESPONSES TO EXAMINATION

In the same way, we have identified and standardized a group of nonorganic signs or, more precisely, behavioral responses to examination (Waddell et al., 1980). Physical findings on medical examination are frequently regarded as objective. But when one human being examines another human being who is in pain and in the process deliberately elicits pain, for example, when looking for tenderness or testing straight leg raising, then the examination should not only detect objective physical abnormality but also provide information about the patient's response to pain. Behavioral responses to examination include:

1. *Tenderness*: Tenderness related to physical disease is usually localized to a particular skeletal or neuromuscular structure. Nonorganic tenderness may be superficial or nonanatomical (Figure 2.4).

1a. *Superficial tenderness*: The skin is tender to light pinch over a wide area of lumbar skin. A localized band in a posterior primary ramus distribution may be caused by nerve irritation and should be accepted as physical.

1b. *Nonanatomical tenderness*: Deep tenderness over a wide area is not localized to any musculoskeletal anatomy but extends to the thoracic spine, sacrum, or pelvis.

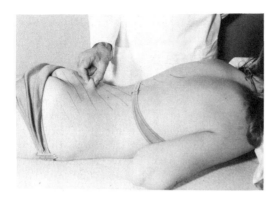

FIGURE 2.4. Nonorganic tenderness showing technique of testing superficial skin tenderness and the area (shaded) frequently involved in widespread nonorganic tenderness. From Waddell et al. (1980), page 118. Copyright 1980 Harper & Row. Reprinted by permission of J.B. Lippincott.

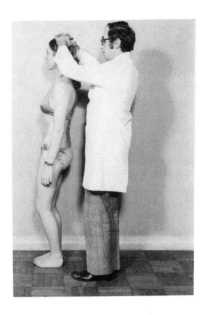

FIGURE 2.5. Axial loading: Back pain on vertical loading on the standing patient's head. From Waddell et al. (1980), page 118. Copyright 1980 Harper & Row. Reprinted by permission of J.B. Lippincott.

2. *Simulation tests*: These give the impression that a particular maneuver is being carried out when in fact it is not. Usually this is based on movement producing pain. On formal examination a particular movement causes the patient to report pain. That movement is then simulated without actually being performed. If pain is reported it is physically inappropriate. It is essential to minimize suggestion.

2a. *Axial loading*: Low back pain may be reported on vertical loading over the patient's skull by the examiner's hands (Figure 2.5). Neck pain is common and should be accepted as physical, but organic lumbar pain is surprisingly rare even in the presence of serious spinal pathology such as tumor or infection.

2b. *Simulated rotation*: Back pain is reported when the shoulders and pelvis are passively rotated together in the same plane as the patient stands relaxed with the feet together (Figure 2.6). In the presence of nerve irritation, leg pain may be produced and should be accepted as physical.

3. *Distraction tests*: A positive physical finding is demonstrated in the routine manner, and this finding is then checked while the patient's attention is distracted. Distraction must be nonpainful, nonemotional, and nonsurprising. In its simplest and most effective form, this consists of indirect observation—simply observing the patient throughout the period that he or she is in the examiner's presence, when he or she is unaware of being examined. During examination, parts of the body other than the particular part being for-

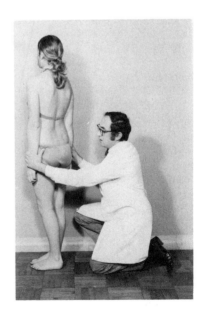

FIGURE 2.6. Simulated rotation: Back pain when shoulders and pelvis are passively rotated in the same plane. From Waddell et al. (1980), page 119. Copyright 1980 Harper & Row. Reprinted by permission of J.B. Lippincott.

mally tested should also be observed. Any finding that is consistently present is likely to be physically based. Findings that are present

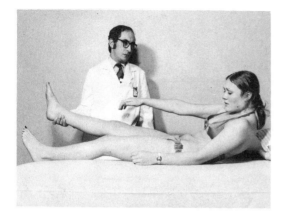

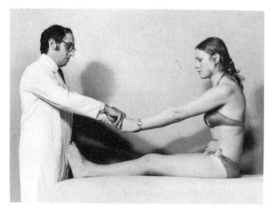

FIGURE 2.7. *Top:* Overreaction to examination: Disproportionate verbalization, facial expression, muscle tension and tremor, collapsing or sweating. *Bottom:* Straight leg raising improving with distraction. From Waddell et al. (1980), page 119. Copyright 1980 Harper & Row. Reprinted by permission of J.B. Lippincott.

muscle groups that cannot be explained on a localized neurological basis.

4b. *Sensory:* Sensory disturbances include altered sensation to light touch, pinprick, and sometimes other modalities fitting a "stocking" rather than dermatomal pattern (Figure 2.8).

Giving way and sensory changes commonly affect the same area and there may be associated nonanatomical regional tenderness. Care must be taken, particularly in patients with spinal stenosis or who have had repeated spinal surgery, not to mistake multiple nerve root involvement for a regional disturbance.

These nonorganic or behavioral signs are again clearly separable from the standard signs of physical disease and are closely related to emotional distress. Although they can occur in a medicolegal context, they are also commonly seen in the pain clinic and tertiary back clinic in patients with no legal proceedings or compensation claims. These nonorganic signs form part of complex emotional and behavioral patterns. They must not be over-interpreted simplistically as faking or malingering and it is essential to assess the whole clinical picture before drawing conclusions. Rather, they should be regarded as the clinical presentation of psychological distress, as a form of patient–doctor communication of the patient's cry for help.

only on formal examination and disappear at other times are more likely to be behavioral.

3a. *Straight Leg Raising:* SLR is the most useful distraction test. A patient with distress or limited pain tolerance may show marked improvement in SLR on distraction compared with formal testing (Figure 2.7). There are several variations based on sitting. This is commonly known in North America as the "flip test."

4. *Regional disturbances:* Regional disturbances involve a widespread region of neighboring parts such as the leg below the knee. The essential feature is divergence from accepted neuroanatomy.

4a. *Weakness:* Weakness is demonstrated on formal testing by a jerky "giving way" of many

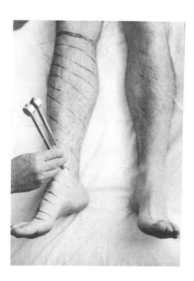

FIGURE 2.8. Nonorganic sensory alteration in a "stocking" distribution affecting light touch, pinprick, and sometimes other modalities. From Waddell et al. (1980), page 119. Copyright 1980 Harper & Row. Reprinted by permission of J.B. Lippincott.

OVERT PAIN BEHAVIOR

The operant model of chronic pain proposes that when an individual is exposed to a nociceptive stimulus that creates tissue damage, the immediate response is withdrawal and attempts to escape from pain. This may be accomplished by avoidance of activity believed to cause or exacerbate pain (e.g., work, movement) or help seeking (e.g., complaining) to reduce the symptoms. The operant model does not concern itself with the subjective experience of pain but with "pain behaviors." Pain behaviors are observable communications of pain, distress, and suffering (e.g., moaning, grimacing, limping). Overtime, avoidance of activity, or distorted ambulation and posture may lead to greater disability. Moreover, attention to these behavioral reactions by environmental reinforcers (e.g., attention, compensation) may lead to maintenance of the pain behaviors even when the initial cause of the pain is no longer present.

We (Waddell et al., 1980) originally included a clinical judgment of overreaction to examination as one of the nonorganic signs but found that this was open to considerable observer bias. The most systematic approach to the quantification of pain behaviors is reflected in the work of Keefe and his colleagues. Keefe and Block (1982; see also Keefe & Williams, Chapter 16) have developed a coding system for the observation of five overt pain behaviors commonly displayed by patients with low back pain in static and dynamic conditions. We have confirmed that after careful training these can be assessed by physicians during routine clinical examination (Waddell & Richardson, 1992). Briefly, these include observation of:

Guarding: Abnormally stiff, interrupted or rigid movement when moving from one position to another.

Bracing: A stationary position in which a fully extended limb supports and maintains an abnormal distribution of weight.

Rubbing: Any contact between hand and back (i.e., touching, rubbing or holding the affected area of pain).

Grimacing: Obvious facial expression of pain that may include furrowed brow, narrowed eyes, tightened lips, corners of mouth pulled back, or clenched teeth.

Sighing: Obvious exaggerated exhalation of air usually accompanied by shoulders first rising and then falling. The patient's cheeks may be expanded.

These are all methods of assessing illness behavior or, more specifically, illness presentation in the context of a medical interview and examination. Illness behavior in low back pain can now be assessed in a variety of ways that can be combined in factor analysis (Waddell & Richardson, 1992):

- Pain drawing (Ransford et al., 1976)
- Behavioral symptoms (Waddell et al., 1984)
- Nonorganic or behavioral signs (Waddell et al., 1980)
- Overt pain behavior (Keefe & Block 1982; see also Keefe & Williams, Chapter 16)
- Use of walking aids
- Downtime—the average number of hours spent lying down between 7 A.M. and 11 P.M.

DISTRESS

Fordyce (1988) has emphasized the distinction between pain and suffering. The best definition and measure of suffering may be psychological distress.

From an extensive review of previous work (Engel, 1959; Merskey & Spear, 1967; Szasz, 1968) and his own detailed clinical studies (Sternbach 1974; Sternbach, 1977; Sternbach & Timmermans, 1975; Sternbach, Wolf, Murphy, & Akerson, 1973a, 1973b), Sternbach concluded that the most important psychological disturbances associated with pain were anxiety in acute pain and depression in chronic pain.

In our own analysis of chronic low back pain and disability (Main & Waddell, 1982; Waddell et al., 1984), we found that the most important psychological features were increased bodily awareness (Modified Somatic Perception Questionnaire, MSPQ; Main, 1983, see Appendix 2.B), which appears to be related to anxiety and depressive symptoms.

Increased bodily awareness completely overshadowed other psychological measures of personality traits or fears and beliefs about illness. In particular, increased awareness and reporting of bodily functioning appeared to be a much more powerful clinical concept than theories of hypochondriasis, whereas depressive symptoms appeared to be part of a normal affective dimension of pain rather than a primary psychiatric illness (Sternbach & Timmermans, 1975; Waddell, Morris, DiPaola, Bircher, & Finlayson, 1986). Anxiety, increased bodily awareness, and depression are best regarded clinically as forms of distress, a simple emotional reaction to pain and disability (see Bradley, Haile, & Jaworski, Chapter 12).

Psychological distress cannot be assessed reliably by the general physician's or surgeon's "clinical impressions." The senior author of this chapter (GW) is a spinal surgeon who has had 15 years' research experience in this field. Recently he studied a series of 120 patients and attempted to rate depression from his general clinical interview. This rating was then compared with the patient's score on a psychological questionnaire measuring depressive symptoms. His experienced clinical judgment was *hopelessly inaccurate*. Psychological distress can however be measured easily and reliably by simple questionnaires such as the MSPQ Perception (Main, 1983) described above to assess anxiety, and either the Beck Depression Inventory (BDI) (Beck, Ward, Mendelson, Mock, & Erbaugh, 1961) or Zung Depression Inventory (Zung, 1965) can be used to assess level of dysphoric mood.

COGNITION

Persistent pain, like any chronic condition, extends over time and affects all domains of the patient's life: familial, marital, social, psychological, as well as physical. Thus, pain behavior and disability ultimately depend on the patient's attitudes and beliefs about pain, his or her coping resources, his or her plight, the health-care system, and the medical-legal system (Turk & Rudy, 1992).

One of the earliest attempts to explore cognitive factors in low back pain was the Illness Behavior Questionnaire (IBQ) (Pilowsky & Spence, 1983), but this dealt with clinical features of hypochondriasis and illness behavior rather than primary cognitions. Over the past decade a number of questionnaires have been developed to measure cognitive factors and coping strategies (e.g., Flor & Turk 1988; Main, Wood, Spanswick, Roberts & Robson, 1991; Rosensteil & Keefe, 1983; Wallston, Wallston, & Devellis, 1978; see Jensen, Turner, Romano, & Karoly, 1991, and DeGood & Shutty, Chapter 13, for reviews).

Interestingly, Reesor and Craig (1988) demonstrated that the primary difference between chronic low back patients who were referred because of the presence of many nonorganic signs and those who did not display these signs was maladaptive thoughts. There were no difference between these groups on the number of surgeries, compensation, litigation status, or employment status. Their maladaptive cognitive processes may amplify or distort patients' experiences of pain and suffering and influence disability.

Clinically, the most important cognitive factor identified from these questionnaires appears to be "catastrophizing" (Rosensteil & Keefe, 1983; Turk & Rudy, 1992), which is closely linked to depressive symptoms (Rudy, Kerns, & Turk, 1988) and low back disability (Main & Waddell, 1991).

Waddell, Sommerville, Henderson, Newton, & Main (in press-a) have argued that the available cognitive measures are too general and thus have recently developed a Fear-Avoidance Beliefs Questionnaire (FABQ) (see Appendix 2.C). The FABQ was based on fear theory and avoidance behavior (Lenthem, Slade, Troup, & Bentley, 1983) and focused specifically on the patient's beliefs about how physical activity and work would or might affect his or her low back pain. Fear-avoidance beliefs about work appeared in this study to be the most specific and powerful cognitive factor yet identified to explain work loss due to low back pain. Additional research with this instrument is required to demonstrate the generality of our results. However, it does appear that fear-avoidance beliefs may be detected by a few simple questions in routine clinical interview or measured more accurately by a simple one-page questionnaire. And these beliefs do appear to predict specific behaviors of back pain patients, most notably, return-to-work.

CONCLUSION

Assessment of back pain requires care and systematic physical examination to arrive at a diagnosis and treatment plan. It is essential that reliable and valid procedures be employed. In order to accomplish this, a great deal of attention has to be given to the manner in which the physical examination is performed. This chapter has described a detailed strategy for physical examination.

It is important to acknowledge that for *chronic* back pain, physical examination by itself is not sufficient. A number of psychological and behavioral factors also need to be considered as there is no simple one-to-one association among physical pathology, pain, and disability. A number of psychological assessment instruments are available and many of these are discussed throughout this volume. Clinicians should be careful to select instruments that have demonstrated good reliability, validity, and utility.

Acknowledgments. Preparation of this paper was supported in part by the Chief Scientist Office, Scottish Home and Health Department and the MacTaggart Trust awarded to the first author and Grant 2R01AR38698 from the National Institute of Arthritis and Musculoskeletal and Skin Diseases and Grant 2R01DE07514 from the National Institute of Dental Research awarded to the second author.

APPENDIX 2.A
Roland and Morris Disability Questionnaire*

When your back hurts, you may find it dificult to do some of the things you normally do.

These are some sentences that people have used to describe themselves when they have back pain. When you read them, you may find that some stand out because they describe you *today*. As you read the list, think of yourself *today*. When you read a sentence that describes you today circle YES. If that sentence does not describe you today circle NO. Remember, only answer YES if you are sure that the sentence describes you today.

1 I stay at home most of the time because of my back. YES / NO

2 I change position frequently to try and get my back comfortable. YES / NO

3 I walk more slowly than usual because of my back. YES / NO

4 Because of my back I am not doing any of the jobs that I usually do around the house. YES / NO

5 Because of my back, I use a handrail to get upstairs. YES / NO

6 Because of my back, I lie down to rest more often. YES / NO

7 Because of my back, I have to hold on to something to get out of an easy chair. YES / NO

8 Because of my back, I try to get other people to do things for me. YES / NO

9 I get dressed more slowly than usual because of my back. YES / NO

10 I only stand up for short periods of time because of my back. YES / NO

11 Because of my back, I try not to bend or kneel down. YES / NO

12 I find it difficult to get out of a chair because of my back. YES / NO

13 My back is painful almost all the time. YES / NO

14 I find it difficult to turn over in bed because of my back. YES / NO

15 My appetite is not very good because of my back pain. YES / NO

16 I have trouble putting on my socks (or stockings) because of the pain in my back. YES / NO

17 I only walk short distances because of my back pain. YES / NO

18 I sleep less well because of my back. YES / NO

19 Because of my back pain, I get dressed with help from someone else. YES / NO

20 I sit down for most of the day because of my back. YES / NO

21 I avoid heavy jobs around the house because of my back. YES / NO

22 Because of my back pain, I am more irritable and bad tempered with people than usual. YES / NO

23 Because of my back, I go upstairs more slowly than usual. YES / NO

24 I stay in bed most of the time because of my back. YES / NO

Score: Total of all items answered YES.

*From Roland and Morris (1983), page 144. Copyright 1983 Harper & Row. Reprinted by permission of J.B. Lippincott.

APPENDIX 2.B
Modified Somatic Perception Questionnaire*

Please describe how you have felt during the PAST WEEK by making a check mark ($\checkmark$) in the appropriate box. Please answer all questions. Do not think too long before answering.

	Not at all	A little/ Slightly	A great deal Quite a bit	Extremely/ Could not have been worse
Heart rate increase				
Feeling hot all over**	0	1	2	3
Sweating all over**	0	1	2	3
Sweating in a particular part of body				
Pulse in neck				
Pounding in head				
Dizziness**	0	1	2	3
Blurring of vision**	0	1	2	3
Feeling faint**	0	1	2	3
Everything appearing unreal				
Nausea**	0	1	2	3
Butterflies in stomach				
Pain or ache in stomach**	0	1	2	3
Stomach churning**	0	1	2	3
Desire to pass water				
Mouth becoming dry**	0	1	2	3
Difficulty swallowing				
Muscles in neck aching**	0	1	2	3
Legs feeling weak**	0	1	2	3
Muscles twitching or jumping**	0	1	2	3
Tense feeling across forehead**	0	1	2	3
Tense feeling in jaw muscles				

*From Main (1983), page 114. Copyright 1983 Pergamon Press. Reprinted by permission.
**Only these 13 items are scored.

APPENDIX 2.C
Fear-Avoidance Beliefs Questionnaire

Here are some of the things which other patients have told us about their pain. For each statement please circle any number from 0 to 6 to say how much physical activities, such as, bending, lifting, walking or driving affect or would affect *your* back pain.

	COMPLETELY DISAGREE			UNSURE		COMPLETELY AGREE	
1 My pain was caused by physical activity.........	0	1	2	3	4	5	6
2 Physical activity makes my pain worse...........	0	1	2	3	4	5	6
3 Physical activity might harm my back	0	1	2	3	4	5	6
4 I should not do physical activities which (might) make my pain worse	0	1	2	3	4	5	6
5 I cannot do physical activities which (might) make my pain worse.................................	0	1	2	3	4	5	6

The following statements are about how your normal work affects or would affect your back pain.

	COMPLETELY DISAGREE			UNSURE		COMPLETELY AGREE	
6 My pain was caused by my work or by an accident at work	0	1	2	3	4	5	6
7 My work aggravated my pain	0	1	2	3	4	5	6
8 I have a claim for compensation for my pain	0	1	2	3	4	5	6
9 My work is too heavy for me......................	0	1	2	3	4	5	6
10 My work makes or would make my pain worse	0	1	2	3	4	5	6
11 My work might harm my back....................	0	1	2	3	4	5	6
12 I should not do my normal work with my present pain	0	1	2	3	4	5	6
13 I cannot do my normal work with my present pain	0	1	2	3	4	5	6
14 I cannot do my normal work till my pain is treated	0	1	2	3	4	5	6
15 I do not think that I will be back to my normal work within 3 months	0	1	2	3	4	5	6
16 I do not think that I will ever be able to go back to that work	0	1	2	3	4	5	6

Scoring:

Scale 1: fear-avoidance beliefs about work—items 6, 7, 9, 10, 11, 12, 15.
Scale 2: fear-avoidance beliefs about physical activity—items 2, 3, 4, 5.

REFERENCES

Andersson, G.B.J. (1991). Impairment evaluation issues and the disability system. In T.G. Mayer, V. Mooney, & R.J. Gatchel (Eds.). *Contemporary conservative care for painful spinal disorders* (pp. 531–535). Philadelphia: Lea & Febiger.

Agre, J.C., Magness, J.L., Hull, Wright, K.C., & Baxter, T.L. (1987). Strength testing with portable dynamometer: Reliability for upper and lower extremities. *Archives of Physical Medicine and Rehabilitation, 68,* 454–458.

Anderson, G.B.J., Pope, M.H., Frymoyer, J.W. (1984). Epidemiology. In M.H. Pope & J.W. Frymoyer (Eds.), *Occupational low back pain* (pp. 115–124). New York: Praeger.

Beck, A.T., Ward, C.H., Mendelson, M.M., Mock, J., & Erbaugh, J. (1961). An inventory for measuring depression. *Archives of General Psychiatry, 4,* 561–571.

Bernard, T.N., Jr., & Kirkaldy-Willis, W.H. (1987). Recognizing specific characteristics of nonspecific low back pain. *Clinical Orthopaedics, 217,* 266–280.

Biering-Sorensen, F. (1984). Physical measurements at risk indicators for low back trouble over a one year period. *Spine, 9,* 106–119.

Boden, S.D., Davis, D.O., Dina, T.S., Patronas, N.J., & Wiesel, S.W. (1990). Abnormal magnetic-resonance scans of the lumbar spine in asymptomatic subjects. *Journal of Bone and Joint Surgery, 72-A,* 403–408.

Breig, A., & Troup, J.D.G. (1979). Biomechanical considerations in the straight-leg-raising test. *Spine, 3,* 242–250.

Brena, S.F., & Koch, D.L. (1975). A "pain estimate" model for quantification and classification of chronic pain states. *Anesthesia Review, 2,* 8–13.

Caillet, R. (1969). Disability evaluation. *Southern Medical Journal, 62,* 1380–1382.

Carey, T.S., Hadler, N.M., Gillings, D., Stinnett, S., & Wallsten, T. (1988). Medical disability assessment of the back pain patient for the Social Security Administration: The weighting of presenting clinical features. *Journal of Epidemiology, 41,* 691–697.

Cox, R., Keeley, J., Barnes, D., Gatchel, R., & Mayer, T. (1988). Effects of functional restoration treatment upon Waddell impairment/disability ratings in chronic low back pain patients. Paper presented to the International Society for the Study of the Lumbar Spine, Miami, Florida.

Deyo, R.A., McNiesh, L.M., & Cone, R.O., III (1985). Observer variability in interpretation of lumbar spine radiographs. *Arthritis and Rheumatism, 28,* 1066–1070.

Deyo, R.A., & Tsui-Wu, Y.J. (1987). Descriptive epidemiology of low back pain and its related medical care in the United States. *Spine, 12,* 264–271.

Edgar, M.A., & Park, W.M. (1974). Induced pain patterns on passive straight-leg raining in lower lumbar disc protrusion. *Journal of Bone and Joint Surgery* [BR], *56,* 658–667.

Engel, G.L. (1959). "Psychogenic" pain and the pain-prone patient. *American Journal of Medicine, 26,* 899–918.

Fairbank, J.C.T., Couper, J., Davies, J.B., & O'Brien, J.P. (1980). The Oswestry Low Back Pain Disability Questionnaire. *Physiotherapy, 66,* 271–273.

Flor, & Turk, D.C. (1988). Chronic back pain and rheumatoid arthritis: Predicting pain and disability from cognitive variables. *Journal of Behavioral Medicine, 11,* 251–265.

Fordyce, W.E. (1976). *Behavioral methods for chronic pain and illness.* St. Louis, MO: Mosby.

Fordyce, W.E. (1988). Pain and suffering: A reappraisal. *American Psychologist, 43,* 276–282.

Fordyce, W. E., Brena, S. F., & Holcomb, R. (1978). Relationship of semantic pain descriptions to physicians' diagnostic judgments, activity levels measures, and MMPI. *Pain, 5,* 292–303.

Frymoyer, J.W., & Cats-Baril, W. (1987). Predictors of low back pain disability. *Clinical Orthopaedics and Related Research, 221,* 89–98.

Frymoyer, J.W., Pope, M.H., Rosen, J., & Goggin, J. (1980). Epidemiologic studies of low back pain. *Spine, 5,* 419–428.

Gallagher, R.M., Rauh, V., Haugh, L.D., Milhous, R., Callas, P.W., Langelier, R., McCallen, J.M., & Frymoyer, J. (1989). Determinants of return-to-work among back pain patients. *Pain, 39,* 55–67.

Hitzelberger, W.E., & Witten, R.M. (1968). Abnormal myelograms in asymptomatic patients. *Journal of Neurosurgery, 28,* 204–208.

Holbrook, T.L., Grazier, K., Kelsey, J.L., & Stauffer, R.N. (1984). *The frequency of occurrence, impact and cost of selected musculoskeletal conditions in the United States.* Park Ridge, IL: American Academy of Orthopaedic Surgeons.

Hudgens, R.W. (1970). The predictive value of myelography in the diagnosis of ruptured lumbar disc. *Journal of Neurosurgery, 32,* 151–162.

Jensen, M.P., Turner, J.A., Romano, J.M., & Karoly, P. (1991). Coping with chronic pain: A critical review of the literature. *Pain, 47,* 249–284.

Keefe, F.J., & Block, A.R. (1982). Development of an observation method for assessing pain behavior in chronic low back pain patients. *Behavior Therapy, 13,* 363–375.

Keeley, J., Mayer, T.G., Cox, R., Gatchel, R.J., Smith, J., & Mooney, V. (1986). Quantification of lumbar function. Part 5: Reliability of range of motion measures in the sagittal plane and in vivo torso rotation measurement technique. *Spine, 11,* 31–35.

Kellgren, J.H. (1938). Observations on referred pain arising from muscle. *Clinical Science, 3,* 173–190.

Kellgren, J.H. (1939). On the distribution of pain arising from deep somatic structures with charts of segmental pain areas. *Clinical Science, 4,* 35–46.

Koran, L.M. (1975). Reliability of clinical methods, data, and judgements. *New England Journal of Medicine, 293,* 642–646, 695–701.

Laros, G.S. (1991). Differential diagnosis of low back pain. In T.G. Mayer, V. Mooney, & R.J. Gatchel (Eds.), *Contemporary conservative care for painful spinal disorders* (pp. 122–130). Philadelphia: Lea & Febiger.

Lenthem, J., Slade, P.D., Troup, J.D.G., & Bentley, G. (1983). Outline of a fear-avoidance model of exaggerated pain perception. *Behavior Research and Therapy, 21,* 401–408.

Lloyd, D.C., & Troup, J.D. (1983). Recurrent back pain and its prediction. *Journal of Social and Occupational Medicine, 33,* 66–74.

Main, C.J. (1983). The Modified Somatic Perception Questionnaire. *Journal of Psychosomatic Research, 27,* 503–514.

Main, C.J., & Waddell, G. (1982). Chronic pain, distress

and illness behavior. In C.J. Main (Ed.), *Clinical psychology and medicine* (pp. 1–52). New York: Plenum.

Main, C.J., & Waddell, G. (1989). The assessment of pain. *Clinical Rehabilitation*, *3*, 267–274.

Main, C.J., & Waddell, G. (1991). A comparison of cognitive measures in low back pain: Statistical structure and clinical validity at initial assessment. *Pain*, *46*, 287–298.

Main, C., Wood, P.L.R., Spanswick, C.C., Roberts, A.P., & Robson, J. (1991). *The Pain Locus of Control Questionnaire*. Manuscript submitted for publication.

Mayer, T.G., Tencer, A.F., Kristoferson, S., & Mooney, V. (1984). Use of noninvasive techniques for quantification of spinal range-of-motion in normal subjects and chronic low-back dysfunction patients. *Spine*, *9*, 588–595.

McCombe, P.F., Fairbank, J.C.T., Cockersole, B.C., & Pynsent, P.B. (1989). Reproducibility of physical signs of low-back pain. *Spine*, *14*, 908–918.

Melzack, R. (1975). The McGill Pain Questionnaire: Major properties and scoring methods. *Pain*, *1*, 277–299.

Melzack, R. (1987). The short-form McGill Pain Questionnaire. *Pain*, *30*, 191–197.

Merskey, H. (1979). Pain terms: A list with definitions and notes on usage. *Pain*, *6*, 249–252.

Merskey, H., & Spear, F.G. (1967). *Pain: Psychological and psychiatric aspects*. London: Bailliere, Tundall, & Cassell.

Minnesota Workers/Compensation Division Committee to Study Schedules of Disability. (1983). *Report to the legislature*. St. Paul, MN: State of Minnesota Printing Office.

Morris, E.W., DiPaola, M., Vallance, R., & Waddell, G. (1986). Diagnosis and decision making in lumbar disc prolapse and bony entrapment. *Spine*, *11*, 436–439.

Nagi, S.Z., Riley, L.E., & Newby, L.G. (1973). A social epidemiology of back pain in a general population. *Journal of Chronic Disease*, *26*, 769–773.

National Center for Health Statistics (1981). *Prevalence of selected impairments, United States—1977*. (DHHS Series 10, No. 134; DHHS Publication No. PHS 81-1562). Hyattsville, MD: U.S. Government Printing Office.

Nelson, M.A., Allen, P., Clamp, S.E., deDombal, F.T. (1979). Reliability and reproducibility of clinical findings in low-back pain. *Spine*, *4*, 97–101.

National Institute for Occupational Safety and Health. (1988). *National Institute for Occupational Safety and Health low back atlas*. Morgantown, WV: United States Department of Health and Human Services.

Ohlen, G. (1989). *Spinal sagittal configuration and mobility. A kyphometer study*. [MD thesis] Stockholm, Sweden: Karolinska Institute.

Pilowsky, I., & Spence, N.D. (1983). *Manual for the Illness Behaviour Questionnaire (IBQ)* (2nd Ed) Adelaide: University of Adelaide.

Pope, M.H., Rosen, J.C., Wilder, D.G., & Frymoyer, J.W. (1980). Relation between biomechanical and psychological factors in patients with low back pain. *Spine*, *5*, 173–178.

Powell, M.C., Wilson, M., Szypryt, P., Symonds, E.M., & Worthington, B.S. (1986). Prevalence of lumbar disc degeneration observed by magnetic resonance in symptomless women. *Lancet*, *2*, 1366–1367.

Quebec Task Force on Spinal Disorders. (1987). Scientific approach to the assessment and management of activity-related spinal disorders. *Spine*, *12*(Suppl. 1), S1–S59.

Ransford, A.O., Cairns, D., & Mooney, V. (1976). The pain drawing as an aid to the psychological evaluation of patients with low back pain. *Spine*, *1*, 127–134.

Reesor, K.A., & Craig, K. (1988). Medically incongruent chronic back pain: Physical limitations, suffering and ineffective coping. *Pain*, *32*, 35–45.

Rockey, J.S., Tompkins, R.K., Wood, R.W., & Wolcott, B.W. (1978). The usefulness of X-ray examinations in the evaluation of patients with back pain. *Journal of Family Practice*, *7*, 455–465.

Roland, M., & Morris, R. (1983). A study of the natural history of back pain. Part I: Development of a reliable and sensitive measure of disability in low back pain. *Spine*, *8*, 141–144.

Rosensteil, A.K., & Keefe, F.J. (1983). The use of coping strategies in chronic low back pain: Relationships to patient characteristics and current adjustment. *Pain*, *17*, 33–44.

Rowe, M.L. (1969). Low back pain industry: A position paper. *Journal of Occupational Medicine*, *11*, 161–169.

Rudy, T.E., Kerns, R.D., & Turk, D.C. (1988). Chronic pain and depression: Toward a cognitive-behavioral mediational model. *Pain*, *35*, 129–140.

Rudy, T.E., Turk, D.C., & Brena, S.F. (1988). Differential utility of medical procedures in the assessment of chronic pain patients. *Pain*, *34*, 53–60.

Spangfort, E.V. (1989). Personal communication.

Sternbach, R.A. (1974). *Pain patients: Traits and treatment*. New York: Academic Press.

Sternbach, R.A. (1977). Psychological aspects of chronic pain. *Clinical Orthopaedics*, *129*, 150–155.

Sternbach, R.A., & Timmermans, G. (1975). Personality changes associated with reduction of pain. *Pain*, *1*, 177–182.

Sternbach, R.A., Wolf, S.R., Murphy, R.W., & Akeson, W.H. (1973a). Aspects of chronic low back pain. *Psychosomatics*, *14*, 52–56.

Sternbach, R.A., Wolf, S.R., Murphy, R.W., & Akeson, W.H. (1973b). Traits of pain patients: The low-back "loser." *Psychosomatics*, *14*, 226–229.

Szasz, T.S. (1968). The psychology of persistent pain: A portrait of l'homme douloureux. In A. Souairac, J. Cahm, & J. Charpentier (Eds.), *Pain* (pp. 93–113). New York: Academic Press.

Torgerson, W.R., & Dotter, W.E. (1976). Comparative roentgenographic study of the asymptomatic and symptomatic lumbar spine. *Journal of Bone and Joint Surgery*, *58A*, 850.

Troup, J.D.G. (1989). Personal communication.

Turk, D.C. (1991). Evaluation of pain and dysfunction. *Journal of Disability*, *2*, 1–20.

Turk, D.C., & Rudy, T.E. (1992). Cognitive factors and persistent pain: A glimpse into Pandora's box. *Cognitive Therapy and Research*, *16*, 99–122.

Waddell, G., McCulloch, J.A., Kummel, E., & Venner, R.M. (1980). Nonorganic physical signs in low back pain. *Spine*, *5*, 117–125.

Waddell, G. (1982). An approach to backache. *British Journal of Hospital Medicine*, *28*, 187–219.

Waddell, G., Allan, D.B., & Newton, M. (1991). Clinical evaluation of disability in low back pain. In J.W. Frymoyer, (Ed.), *The adult spine* (pp. 155–166). New York: Raven Press.

Waddell, G., & Main, C.J. (1984). Assessment of severity in low back pain disorders. *Spine*, *9*, 204–208.

Waddell, G., Main, C.J., Morris, E.W., Venner, R.M., Rae, P.S., Sharmy, S.H., & Galloway, H. (1982).

Normality and reliability in the clinical assessment of backache. *British Medical Journal, 284,* 1519–1523.

Waddell, G., Main, C.J., Morris, E.W., DiPaola, M., & Gray, I.C. (1984). Chronic low-back pain, psychologic distress, and illness behavior. *Spine, 9,* 209–213.

Waddell, G., Morris, E.W., DiPaola, M.P., Bircher, M., & Finlayson, D. (1986). A concept of illness tested as an improved basis for surgical decisions in low back disorders. *Spine, 11,* 712–719.

Waddell, G., Sommerville, D., Henderson, I., Newton, M., & Main, C.J. (in press-a). Pain disability and fear-avoidance. *Pain.*

Waddell, G., Sommerville, D., Henderson, I., & Newton, M. (in press-b). Objective clinical evaluation of physical impairment in chronic low back pain. *Spine.*

Waddell, G., & Richardson, J. (1992). Observation of overt pain behavior by physicians during routine clinical examination of patients with low back pain.

Journal of Psychosomatic Research, 36, 77–87.

Walters, A. (1961). Psychogenic regional pain alias hysterical pain. *Brain, 84,* 1–18.

Wallston, K.A., Wallston, B.S., & DeVellis, R. (1978). Development of the multidimensional health locus of control (MHLC) scales. *Health Education Monographs, 6,* 160–170.

White, A.A., & Gordon, S.L. (1982). Synopsis: Workshop on idiopathic low-back pain. *Spine, 7,* 141–149.

Wood, R.W., Diehr, P., Wolcott, B.W., Slay, L., & Tompkins, R.K. (1979). Reproducibility of clinical data and decisions in management of upper respiratory illnesses: Comparison of physicians and nonphysician providers. *Medical Care, 17,* 767–779.

World Health Organization (1980). *International classification of impairments, disability and handicaps.* Geneva: Author.

Zung, W.W.K. (1965). A self-rating depression scale. *Archives of General Psychiatry, 12,* 63–70.

Chapter 3

Quantification of Function in Chronic Low Back Pain

PETER B. POLATIN, MD
TOM G. MAYER, MD

Chronic low back pain is the "most expensive benign condition in America" (Mayer et al., 1987). Approximately 80% of Americans will suffer a serious episode of low back pain during their lives, and 4% of the population undergo such an episode each year (Andersson, 1981). In certain occupations, the risk of back injury is as high as 15% per annum (Andersson, 1981). Although more than 50% of such episodes resolve within 2 weeks, and 90% resolve within 3 months, those patients who remain symptomatic after that period of time have the poorest prognosis and cost the most in health dollars (Mayer & Gatchel, 1988). Surgery may be of benefit for only 1% or 2% of patients with a low back episode (Mayer et al., 1987). It therefore falls within the province of conservative care to manage the majority of these patients.

In the interest of establishing objective guidelines for assessment, treatment, and therapeutic goal setting, the utilization of measures to quantify lumbar function has been found to be useful (Mayer, 1987; Mayer et al., 1987; Mayer, Barnes, & Kishino, 1988; Mayer, Barnes, Nichols et al., 1988; Mayer & Gatchel, 1988, 1989; Mayer, Gatchel et al., 1986; Mayer, Gatchel, Barnes, Mayer, & Mooney, 1990; Mayer,

Kishino, Keeley, Mayer, & Mooney, 1985; Mayer, Smith et al., 1985; Mayer & Polatin, in press; Mayer, Tencer, Kristoferson, & Mooney, 1985). Functional deficits have also been found to be predictive of and associated with disability (Biering-Sorensen, 1984; Cady, Bischoff, O'Connell, Thomas, & Allen, 1979; Chaffin, 1978; Nachemson, 1983).

WHY QUANTIFY FUNCTION?

Pain perception has been one of the primary indices used in the documentation of human suffering. However, it is a subjective phenomenon influenced by multiple factors (Beals, 1984; Fordyce, Roberts, & Sternbach, 1985; Turk, Meichenbaum, & Genest, 1983; White & Gordon, 1982). Furthermore, similar lesions may produce very different pain reports in different individuals (Gatchel, Mayer, Capra, Diamond, & Barnett, 1986; Mooney, Cairns, & Robertson, 1976). Therefore, although standardized measures of pain are clinically useful, their primary benefit is for intraindividual comparison.

Disability, a direct outcome of chronic pain,

is more easily defined objectively in a behavioral context. Within the socioeconomic sphere, it is measured by *decreased productivity*, and represents a major loss for society (Gatchel et al., 1986; see also Vasudevan, this volume). Physically, it presents as *impaired performance of functional tasks*, and is frequently accompanied by psychological symptoms such as depression, anxiety, somatization, and alcohol and drug abuse (Kinney, Polatin, & Gatchel, 1990; Lillo, Gatchel, Polatin, & Mayer, 1991), which are all well established concomitants of chronic pain, but which themselves are also significant causes of disability. Legally, it is associated with claims for *financial compensation* based on alleged inability to work, suffering as a result of injury, and the defining of fault with others.

Defining disability within the context of *physical function* has advantages. It is far less subjective than self-report, as long as certain criteria are met. Initial measures provide a baseline that may define the disabled state as an existing physical entity, *the deconditioning syndrome* (Kondraske, 1986; Mayer & Gatchel, 1989; Mayer & Polatin, in press), which the patient can more easily accept than traditional concepts of functional pain. This makes him or her more accessible to not only corrective functional restoration, but to educational and psychotherapeutic interventions as well. Agencies involved in the definition and treatment of disability may be more responsive to human performance measures that directly address the disabled state within the context of the workplace. And finally, outcome may be more objectively defined by posttreatment functional capacity measures, whereas modification of self-report of pain *alone* does not necessarily lead to elimination of low back disability (Sturgis, Schaefer, & Sikora, 1984).

The term "deconditioning syndrome" refers to the cumulative physical changes found in chronically disabled patients suffering from spinal dysfunction that have occurred *as a result of disuse* (Mayer & Gatchel, 1989). Repetitive microtrauma, spinal soft tissue disruption, and perhaps surgery have precipitated scarring, and this has been accompanied by immobilization and inactivity. Muscle atrophy is not as easily discernible in the low back as it is in a dysfunctional extremity, which is readily compared to the unimpaired side. Nevertheless, atrophy of the abdominal flexor and trunk extensor muscle groups has been identified even at a relatively early stage of immobilization (Deyo,

Diehl, & Rosenthal, 1986; Hadler, 1986; Mayer, & Gatchel, 1988). The lumbar facet joints typically involved in back extension become immobilized with inactivity, causing progressive loss of joint function and range of motion. With disuse, cardiovascular fitness and neuromuscular coordination deteriorate. These physical changes result in a patient who is actually exercise-intolerant, with true muscular weakness, lumbar stiffness, poor endurance, and impaired fine motor coordination (Polatin, 1990). These changes themselves have therefore exacerbated and perpetuated a state of physical disability *that may be individually defined* through functional quantification measures. Subsequent efforts at correction through functional restoration represent a valid alternative treatment approach for this patient group.

CRITERIA FOR QUANTIFICATION TESTING

Physical measures of human performance must adhere to certain basic requirements to be useful (Mayer & Gatchel, 1988, 1989; Polatin, 1990). A test must be *physiologically relevant* (i.e., measure a specific and defined capacity and not reflect extraneous information). For example, strength of a specific muscle group such as trunk extensors is not accurately measured by a whole body task such as lifting (Gracovetsky & Farfan, 1986). The test must be *valid*: the measurement device must be accurate in its measurement. There must be *reproducibility* such that repeatable and precise measurements of a clinical variable are possible, by the same tester (*intertest reliability*) and by different testers (*interrater reliability*). A valid test may not be reproducible and vice versa. Although an invalid test is useless, problems of reproducibility may be corrected by altering the test protocol (see Dworkin & Whitney, Chapter 24, and Rudy, Turk, & Brody, Chapter 25).

A relevant, valid, reproducible, and reliable functional test of human performance will have no clinical value unless it can identify *suboptimal effort*. Otherwise, invalid low readings may be interpreted as true functional deficits when actually they may be more reflective of poor motivation, pain sensitivity, emotional distress, or malingering. Therefore, each individual test of function must have a built-in mechanism to assess effort.

A relevant, large *normative database* is required for a test of human performance in order for any meaningful clinical interpretive statement to be made. The larger the database, the more specific the interpretation may be. With very large databases one is able to extract meaningful information with regard to such variables as age, gender, occupation, structural lesion, or postsurgical status (Mayer, Gatchel, Keeley, & Mayer, 1991; Mayer, Gatchel, Keeley, Mayer, & Richland, 1991). Because of the proliferation of different test protocols and testing devices in recent years, the size of the normative database must be carefully assessed. Many of the newer devices have almost no database as of yet, although they may in a few years, so, for the clinician attempting to provide relevant treatment, this may present a short-term problem.

TESTS OF FUNCTIONAL CAPACITY IN THE LUMBAR SPINE

There is no single test that can adequately assess lumbar function, but evaluation of separate physical capabilities may be combined to give a statement of functional capacity. *Range of motion*, particularly in the sagittal plane, provides important information about the functioning of the intervertebral disc and facet joints. *Trunk strength* is controlled by a number of specific muscle groups moving the lumbar spine in flexion and extension, as well as in rotation and abduction/adduction. These include the intrinsics (erector spinae, multifidus, quadratus lumborum, psoas, and deep interspinalis and intertransversalis) as well as the extrinsics (abdominals, glutealis, latissimus dorsi, and posterior thigh muscles). When the lumbopelvic unit is isolated by some sort of restraint, the strength of the intrinsic extensors and extrinsic flexors is being measured without the contribution of other extrinsic groups, to give information about isolated trunk strength. Tests of task performance involving the lumbar spine are typically *lifting tests*, in which the trunk is not isolated. Some give information about maximum weight lifted under defined conditions, while others address frequent, repetitive capability to lift over time. The former may address occasional lifting capacity, while the latter delineate lifting endurance. *Other tests of work capacity* may address other functional tasks less directly related to the low back, such as

sitting tolerance, crawling, stooping, bending, or shifting. Assessment of *cardiovascular endurance* provides important information about overall physical conditioning, as delineated by the work capacity of the body's most important muscle, the heart.

To measure strength and lifting capacity, different technologies may be utilized (Mayer & Gatchel, 1988). *Isometric* testing measures the maximum force a muscle or group of muscles can generate in contraction. It is the most well established technique, particularly for lifting capacity, but lacks dynamic measurement capability. There is also greater risk for muscle strain with truly maximal exertions. *Isokinetic* testing has the advantage of providing a measurement of dynamic performance with methodology that "locks in" the speed and acceleration variables so that they become known quantities. Then, torque or force becomes the only independent variable, making calculation of both inter- and intraindividual differences relatively easy. Other dependent variables, such as work and power, can be derived from computer-generated curves. *Isodynamic* testing measures torques and position changes occurring about multiple centers. No motion is permitted until a preselected minimum torque is produced, after which the acceleration and velocity increase in proportion to the degree to which a torque exceeds the preset minimum. Therefore, as torque varies, acceleration and velocity also vary without control. Finally, *isotonic* or *isoinertial* testing holds the mass constant or progresses it while the subject does a whole body motion (lifting) sequentially, and velocity is not controlled. We have found the isokinetic and isotonic testing most helpful in assessing the strength and lifting capacity aspects of lumbar function.

Range of Motion

Many of the techniques currently used to measure range of motion in the lumbar spine fail to fulfill necessary criteria of validity, relevance, reproducibility, and effort assessment. Gross lumbar flexion and extension actually consist of motion at the hips as well as at the five lumbar motion segments. Conventional "fingertip to floor" and goniometric techniques fail to separate out this compound motion and are therefore invalid. Additionally, there is intertest and interrater variability and no effort assessment.

The *two inclinometer technique* has proven to be the most useful in measuring spinal mobility (see Figure 3.1), and has been accepted as the preferred test in the recently revised *American Medical Association Guides to the Evaluation of Permanent Impairment* (Engelberg, 1988). An inclinometer is a circular fluid-filled disc with a weighted gravity pendulum that remains oriented in the vertical direction, readily obtainable in hardware stores, but also now marketed specifically for mobility testing. There is also a more expensive computerized version (the EDI-320) (Figure 3.4).

With the patient standing erect, the T12-L1 interspace is identified, as is a point over the convex surface of the sacrum. The first inclinometer is applied over the sacrum, parallel to the spine. The second inclinometer is aligned in the sagittal plane, bridging the T12-L1 spinous processes. The trunk must be in the neutral position while the inclinometers are "zeroed out." The patient is then asked to flex forward maximally while maintaining the knees

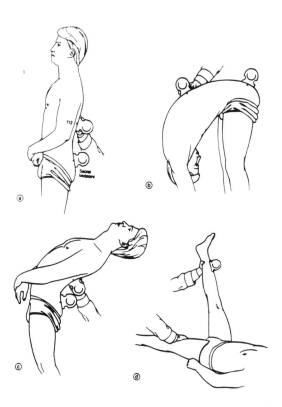

FIGURE 3.1. Use of inclinometer to measure spinal mobility. From Engelberg (1988), page 92. Copyright 1990 American Medical Association. Reprinted by permission.

in extension, and at full flexion the two inclinometers are read. The upper (T12-L1) inclinometer gives the "gross flexion" reading, while the lower (sacral) inclinometer gives hip flexion. True lumbar flexion is obtained by subtracting hip flexion from gross flexion and represents motion at the five lumbar segments.

After returning the patient to the neutral position, he or she is asked to extend maximally, and similar readings are taken, thereby deriving gross lumbar extension, hip extension, and true lumbar extension.

This technique has demonstrated relevance and validity. Sagittal measurements correlate accurately with true lumbar flexion/extension readings obtained on lumbar flexion and extension x-rays (Mayer, Kishino, et al., 1985). Intra- and intertester reliability have been established as well as a normative database (Keeley et al., 1986). The assessment of effort is provided by measuring maximal supine straight leg raising (SLR) bilaterally. The inclinometer is placed on each tibial spine with both knees extended. In a supine straight leg raise, hamstrings are initially stretched to maximal extensibility, and then the pelvis starts to flex until it is restrained by maximum hyperextension of the contralateral hip. Therefore, SLR should be very close to hip motion, and if the tightest SLR exceeds total sacral (hip) motion by more than 10 degrees, effort has been suboptimal.

In the two-inclinometer technique, a compound motion is being measured, and values are being derived for each component of that motion (i.e., hip and true lumbar flexion and extension). A linear relationship between true lumbar flexion and hip flexion has been demonstrated through the gross lumbar flexion arc for normal subjects (Figure 3.2) (Mayer et al., 1984) Therefore, even with identified suboptimal effort and limited gross lumbar flexion, it is still possible to identify structural abnormality by comparing the ratio of true lumbar flexion to hip flexion.

For example, one patient gives the following readings on measurement of lumbar mobility by the two-inclinometer method: gross lumbar flexion: 50 degrees, gross lumbar extension: 15 degrees; sacral (hip) flexion: 20 degrees; sacral (hip) extension: 5 degrees; true lumbar flexion: 30 degrees; true lumbar extension: 10 degrees; and bilateral SLR: 70 degrees. In this case, the SLR exceeds hip mobility by 45 degrees, thereby indicating suboptimal effort. However, the ratio of true lumbar to hip flexion is

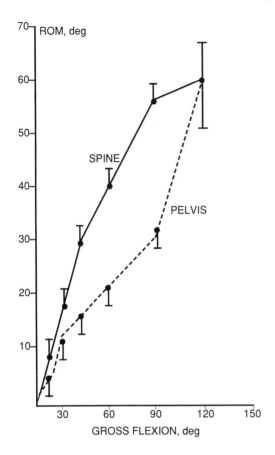

FIGURE 3.2. Linear relationship between true lumbar flexion and hip flexion demonstrated through gross lumbar flexion arc for normal subjects. From Mayer, Tencer, et al. (1984), page 592. Copyright 1984 J. B. Lippincott. Reprinted by permission.

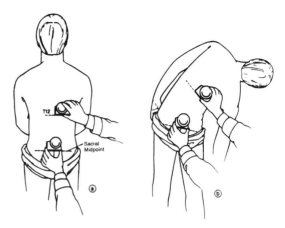

FIGURE 3.3. Two-inclinometer technique for measurement of lateral bend in the lumbar spine. From Engelberg (1988), page 93. Copyright 1990 American Medical Association. Reprinted by permission.

Trunk Strength Testing

The various devices for measuring trunk strength are tools with proven research and clinical usefulness. However, they are expensive and require training to be used properly to generate meaningful data. The lumbopelvic unit must be isolated in either the standing, sitting, side-lying, prone, or supine position, thus offering a variety of physiologically induced motion restriction and gravity effects (Mayer & Gatchel, 1989). The isokinetic devices, although not "true to life," do allow accurate measurement of torque, with proven validity and repeatability (Langrana & Lee, 1984; Smith, Mayer, Gatchel, & Becker, 1985).

Trunk flexion, extension, and right and left torso rotation-peak torque can be generated, as well as specific curve shape, from which average-points curve, maximum-points curve, best work-repetition curve, and power numbers may be derived (see Figure 3.5). By analyzing the discrepancy between the same points on three separate test curves produced under identical testing conditions, the computer may also generate the "average-points variance" (APV), which has proven to be an assessment of effort on the test (Figure 3.6). An APV greater than 20 degrees is indicative of suboptimal effort on the testing equipment we use, which are the Cybex Isokinetic TEF (torso extension/flexion) and TR (torso rotation) devices (see Figure 3.7). Different testing devices have been on the market for different periods of time, with varying normative databases.

within normal limits, even if the gross flexion was "held back," thereby indicating that there is no disruption of the normal spine/hip ratio during this flexion movement.

This technique also allows accurate measurement of lateral bend in the lumbar spine (see Figure 3.3). Maintaining the same positions for inclinometers one and two, the patient then is asked to bend the trunk maximally to the right after "zeroing out" the inclinometers, then resume neutral position and bend maximally to the left.

The measurement of compound lumbar motion may be adopted for the use of a single inclinometer by conducting each measurement separately, or similarly for the use of the computerized EDI-320 (Figure 3.4).

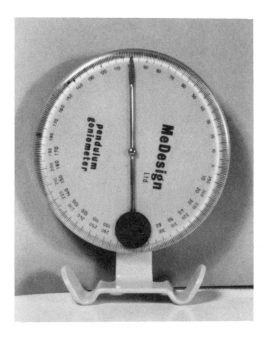

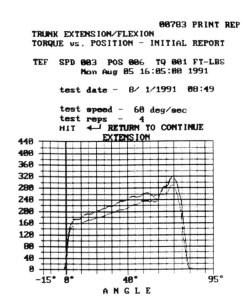

FIGURE 3.5. Cybex® TEF extension curves at 60 deg/sec. Reprinted courtesy of PRIDE.

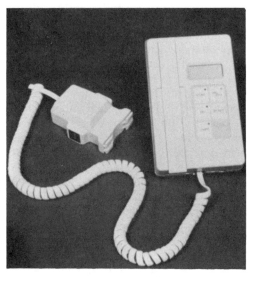

FIGURE 3.4. *Top:* Inclinometer. *Bottom:* EDI-320. Courtesy of PRIDE.

SPEED (deg/sec)	R 60
REPETITIONS	4
BODY WEIGHT (lbs)	
PEAK TORQ (ftlbs)	285
PEAK TORQ % BW	175%
ANGLE OF PEAK TORQ	63
TORQ @ DEGREES	
TORQ @ DEGREES	
ACCEL. TIME (secs)	.03
TOTAL WORK (BWR,ftlbs)	302
TOTAL WORK (BWR) %BW	186%
AVG.POWER (BWR,WATTS)	302
AVG.POWER (BWR) %BW	186%
AVG.POINTS VARIANCE	3%
TAE (ftlbs)	67.7

FIGURE 3.6. Data printout of Cybex® TEF. Reprinted courtesy of PRIDE.

Tests of Lifting Capacity

Unlike the isolated trunk strength tests, lift testing devices do not stabilize the body above and below the lumbopelvic musculoskeletal unit. Isometric and isokinetic lift tests are not "natural" or "whole-body" tests in that they impose some restrictions on lifting that remove certain variables present in actual lifting tasks, such as speed/acceleration or position, to allow more precise and reproducible measurements. For instance, the isometric devices used in industry by the National Institute for Occupational Safety and Health (NIOSH) standardize a lift by having the patient pull at a bar at a predetermined height above the ground in a straight-back, bent-knee position ("leg lift"), or a straight-knee, bend-back position ("torso lift"). Isokinetic devices allow lifting in a more dynamic way, substituting a lifting handle on a

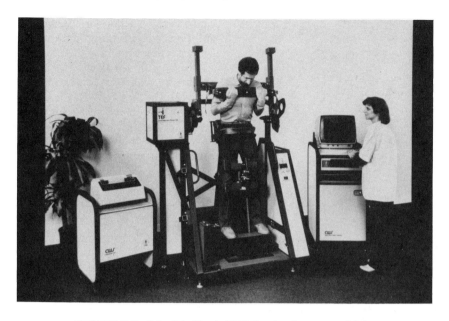

FIGURE 3.7. Cybex® isokinetic TEF. Reprinted courtesy of Cybex.

cable attached to a dynamometer and thereby permitting a wider selection of body positions and lifting styles during a test protocol. As in the isokinetic trunk strength testing, with acceleration and speed controlled, the force exerted along the cable and in line with the dynamometer is what is recorded and allows the derivation of peak force, curve shape, work performed, power consumed, and APV as an effort assessment (Figures 3.8 and 3.9).

Again, normative databases are essential in using these devices, with previously defined standardized protocols. Our clinical experience has been with the Cybex Liftask (Figure 3.10), utilizing a 3-speed (18 in./sec, 30 in./sec, and 36 in./sec) testing protocol (Kishino et al., 1985). The normative database has been expanded to include workers in different job categories, as well as comparative norms (Mayer et al., 1991).

However, dynamic psychophysical tests, in which no restriction of activity occurs, are also useful, and more directly address such aspects of performance as task endurance and neuromuscular coordination. The Progressive Isoinertial Lifting Evaluation (PILE) is one such test (Mayer, Barnes, Kishino, et al., 1988; Mayer et al., 1990) (see Figure 3.11). The protocol involves the lifting of weights in a plastic box from floor to waist (0–30 in.) and waist to shoulder height (30–54 in.). Women begin with a 5-lb load, while men begin with a 10-lb load, and weight is increased by an

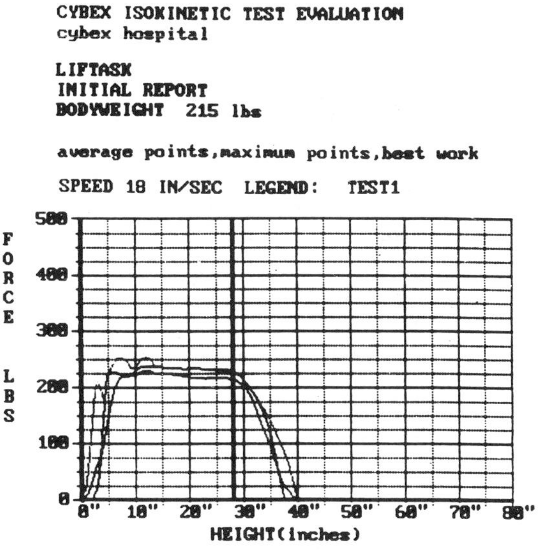

CYBEX ISOKINETIC TEST EVALUATION
cybex hospital

LIFTASK
INITIAL REPORT
BODYWEIGHT   215 lbs

average points,maximum points,best work

SPEED 18 IN/SEC   LEGEND: TEST1

FIGURE 3.8. Liftask data curves. Reprinted courtesy of PRIDE.

amount equal to the initial weight every 20 sec, with a rate of *8 lifting movements* (4 lifting cycles) in each 20 sec period. A lifting cycle consists of 2 lifting movements to return to the starting point (i.e., from floor to waist to floor).

The patient is "blind" to the actual amount of weight in the box. The test is terminated when the first of the following end points is achieved: (1) fatigue or pain (psychophysical

```
        INITIAL REPORT
REPORT DATE:Fri Jul 26 15:26:16 1991
cybex hospital

LIFTASK - FLX KNEES/FLX BACK
CYBEX TEST DATE(S)      7/ 3/1991

SPEED (in/sec)         R 18
REPETITIONS               3
START HEIGHT (in.)       00
END HEIGHT (in.)         28
BODY WEIGHT (lbs)

PEAK FORCE (lbs)        252
PEAK FORCE % BW        117%
HEIGHT OF PEAK FORCE    12
FORCE @     INCHES
FORCE @     INCHES


TOTAL WORK (BWR,ftlbs)  467
TOTAL WORK (BWR) %BW   217%
AVG.POWER (BWR,WATTS)   448
AVG.POWER (BWR) %BW    206%
AVG.FORCE (BWR,lbs)     198
AVG.FORCE (BWR) %BW     92%
AVG.POINTS VARIANCE      4%

TOTAL WORK SET 1(ftlbs)
  1st SAMPLE 1 (TW)
  2nd SAMPLE 1 (TW)
  ENDURANCE RATIO 1
TOTAL WORK SET 2(ftlbs)
  1st SAMPLE 2 (TW)
  2nd SAMPLE 2 (TW)
RECOVERY RATIO
AVG.LIFT DISTANCE (in.)  35
MAX.LIFT DISTANCE (in.)
```

FIGURE 3.9. Liftask data printout. Reprinted courtesy of PRIDE.

end point), (2) achievement of 85% of age-determined "maximum heart rate," unless cardiac precautions are in force (aerobic end point), or (3) predetermined safe limits of 45–55% of body weight (safety end point).

Results are expressed as (1) maximum weight lifted at the lumbar and cervical levels (floor to waist and waist to overhead), (2) the endurance time to discontinuation for each test, and (3) the final heart rate. Because distance and repetitions are also known, calculations of work and power consumption are possible and may be normalized to body weight. A normative database exists for this test. An assessment of effort is provided by comparing the final heart rate with the target. With the endurance factor incorporated in the test, it gives a repeatable and objective measure of *frequent lifting capacity*, which can be translated to job requirements or utilized in training protocols.

TESTS OF AEROBIC CAPACITY (CARDIOVASCULAR ENDURANCE)

The most commonly used measure to define aerobic fitness is maximum aerobic capacity (V_{O_2} max), usually estimated indirectly by means of a step test, bicycle ergometer, or treadmill protocol. Because heart rate increases with increasing oxygen uptake or workload (Astrand & Rodahl, 1979), heart rate may be paired with workloads to predict V_{O_2} max. Because maximum tests have more intrinsic risks and require more careful monitoring, submaximal tests are more applicable. Both bicycle ergometer and treadmill protocols have demonstrated reliability and validity. Although the treadmill is preferable for maximum tests, the advantage of one over the other for submaximal tests is minimal (Battie, 1991). Patients with back pain have been found to better tolerate the bicycle ergometer, however, and so we use this type of protocol (Mayer & Gatchel,

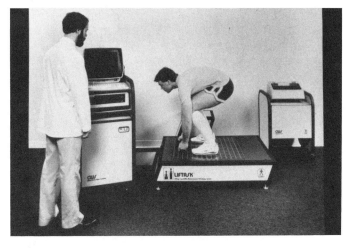

FIGURE 3.10. Cybex® Liftask. Reprinted courtesy of PRIDE.

Task-Specific Testing

Although human performance evaluation can be very sophisticated, its clinical applicability to functional assessment is still somewhat limited. Ease of administration and cost of the testing are the major problems for the most valid, reliable, and accurate protocols. However, functional task performance is an essential element of occupational therapy and is generally used in *work hardening*, a rehabilitation treatment that focuses on repetitive task training for specific job activities to develop stamina, neuromuscular coordination, and appropriate vocational behaviors.

In the assessment of spinal function, no specific task performance devices stand out as universally applicable at the present time. The multiple-task obstacle course is currently being used in several spine centers (Mayer & Gatchel, 1988). Task performance is measured on a structured progression of physical activities that simulate job demands at the workplace delineated on form CA-17 of the Department of Labor Duty Status Report. There are other devices, in various stages of development, that serve a similar function.

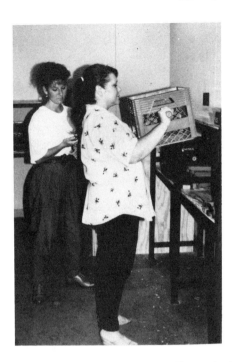

FIGURE 3.11. Progressive Isoinertial Lifting Evaluation. Reprinted courtesy of PRIDE.

1988). Testing begins at a predetermined work rate and progresses at regular intervals until the target heart rate (85% of age-related maximum) is reached. The result is expressed as final work rate, the time for the test, and ratio of final heart rate to target (as a measurement of effort).

An identical test has been devised, with similarly established normative database, utilizing repetitive cycling motion of the arms instead of the legs. This is the Upper Body Ergometer (UBE) but is less a test of cardiovascular capacity than of upper extremity strength and endurance because the blood vessels supplying the upper extremities are of significantly smaller diameter than those supplying the lower extremities such that the cardiovascular demand is less. Nevertheless, in an individual with impaired lower extremity function, it may provide the only useful endurance test obtainable, with similarly built-in validity, reliability, and some effort assessment. As an upper extremity endurance test, it also has intrinsic value, particularly in the context of rehabilitation (Mayer & Gatchel, 1988).

USES OF QUANTIFICATION

For tests of lumbar function to be useful, the results must be expressed in relation to deviation from normal, with a medical interpretive summary that integrates the results of the various tests previously described. Such a report is shown in Figure 3.12, which in our center is termed a Quantified Functional Evaluation (QFE).

As an initial evaluation, functional quantification defines the *current physical capabilities of the patient's lumbar spine, assuming good effort on testing*. By reviewing the effort factor for each individual test, the overall level of effort can be accurately delineated. But even with suboptimal or poor effort, an initial QFE is a clinical statement of *how functional this patient will allow himself or herself to be*. Consistently poor effort has meaning in itself, as does inconsistent effort. Therefore, an initial QFE allows an identification of functional level and raises the issue of psychosocial barriers to functional recovery that may subsequently be identified by further information gathering.

As a *statement of disability*, only the range of

```
Patient Name:
SS#       :
DOI       : 03/06/1990
PT/OT Test : 06/27/1991  06/27/1991 PRE
```

THORACOLUMBAR QUANTITATIVE FUNCTIONAL EVALUATION

This individual underwent a Quantitative Functional Evaluation which is a battery of tests of spinal physical capacity. This information may be used to determine medical impairment of function. % Normal ratings are based on a limited clinical sample; a large standardized normative database is being assembled and constantly updated.

SELF-REPORT SCORES

		PHYSICAL CAPACITY	
Beck Depression	0	Physical Status	R / L
Pain Drawing		Neurological Deficit	- / -
Intensity Score	1/10	FABER	- / -
Trunk	2/72	DEFORMITY/POSTURE	
Extremities	0/136	Surgical Scar:	Yes
Disability Analog	24/150		

LUMBAR RANGE OF MOTION

	SAGITTAL DEGREES		CORONAL DEGREES	
	FLEX(% norm)/ EXT(% norm)		RIGHT(% norm)/LEFT(% norm)	
Gross Motion	92 (76%) / 26 (57%)		40 (114%) / 34 (97%)	
True Lumbar	57 (87%) / 22 (73%)		22 (88%) / 22 (88%)	
Hip Motion	35 (63%) / 4 (26%)		20 (200%) / 12 (120%)	
Str.Leg Raise R/L	57 (76%) / 59 (78%)			

True Spine/Hip Flex Ratio: 162%: Normal ratio probably normal spine flexibility

Effort Factor   Fair

TRUNK STRENGTH (CYBEX)

Isokinetic Sagittal	PEAK TORQUE (ft-lb)		WORK (lb-ft)	
	FLEX(% norm)/ EXT(% norm)		FLEX(% norm) / EXT(% norm)	
60/second	199 (75%) / 180 (52%)		223 (77%) / 185 (48%)	
120/second	120 (45%) / 149 (46%)		108 (40%) / 149 (44%)	
150/second	180 (69%) / 161 (54%)		163 (64%) / 146 (50%)	
HSD (Work)	(150/60)		73% (abn) / 79% (nor)	
F/E Ratios (Work)	(60/120/150) 120%(abn) /		72% (NL) / 111% (abn)	
Avg. Pts. Variance	(F/E) at 60/sec.	24	/ 25	

CARDIOVASCULAR ENDURANCE

	BICYCLE ERGOMETRY	UPPER BODY ERGOMETRY
Work Rate(Watts)/End. Time	125 / 9:00	131 / 5:15
Heart Rate/Target	124 / 161	96 / 161
mVO2(ml/kg/min)/Mets [Calories]	61 / 17	[50]
Fitness Level/Effort Factor	High	Poor

OCCUPATIONAL CAPACITY

Working ?	No
Job Demand Category (Previous / Anticipated)	4 / N.A.

Patient Name: Test Date: 06/27/1991

Job Lifting Requirements	FLOOR-WAIST	WAIST-OVERHEAD
Frequent (lbs)	50	50
Occasional (lbs)	100-120	100-120

Frequent Lifting Capacity	FLOOR-WAIST	WAIST-OVERHEAD
Final Force (lbs) (% norm)	33 (35%)	33 (43%)
Total Work (lb-ft) (% norm)	1380 (16%)	1104 (20%)
End.Time (sec) / Power (watts)	60 / 31.3	60 / 25.0
Final HR / Effort	88 / Poor	84 / Poor

Isometric Lifting Capacity	MAX-FORCE
Leg Lift Capacity (lbs) (% norm)	275(91%)
Torso Lift Capacity (lbs) (% norm)	217(72%)
Arm Lift Capacity (lbs) (% norm)	N.A.

Dynamic Isokinetic Lift	PEAK FORCE / POWER		
	Lbs.(%n)/WATTS(%n)	Lbs.(%n)/WATTS(%n)	Lbs.(%n)/WATTS(%n)
	18 in/sec.	30 in/sec.	36 in/sec.
Lumbar	240(71%)/ 370(70%)	199(61%)/ 516(65%)	185(58%)/ 566(63%)
Avg. Pts. Variance	(Lumbar/Cervical) at 18 in/sec.	28	/

GLOBAL SCORES

CUMULATIVE SCORE:	THIS TEST	
Average Test (%)	66	
TEST VALIDITY/EFFORT	Physical Therapy	Occupational Therapy
	GOOD	GOOD

SUMMARY

Mild pain/disability self-report in a patient with mild true lumbar mobility deficits associated with severe extensor trunk strength deficits with a reversed extensor/flexor ratio and high aerobic capacity. The patient's lifting capacity is at moderately deficient range with drop-off particularly where endurance is required, but with good effort indicating a patient who should be a good candidate for functional restoration.

Test Interpretation By:
Tom G. Mayer, M.D.

TGM:ptb

FIGURE 3.12. Quantified Functional Evaluation.

motion test of the QFE has recognized validity as defined by the revised *AMA Guides to the Evaluation of Permanent Impairment* (Engelberg, 1988). However, in this context, validity has to be strictly controlled. The measurements must be repeated three times and must be consistent within 10% or 5 degrees, whichever is greater. The difference between the tightest straight leg raise and hip/flexion plus extension must be less than 10 degrees on each of these repetitions. If valid, this measurement may be used in correlating a whole-body *medical impairment rating*.

An initial QFE has additional usefulness in *defining treatment goals* for functional restoration to correct the deconditioning syndrome delineated and to educate the patient about the existence of these initial functional deficits. Having completed testing, he or she is far more easily able to understand the results and may even be surprised at how poorly he or she has done.

Serial quantification, however, provides additional uses. For the patient and the treatment team, retests after a period of rehabilitation provide objective *feedback of progress*. For the team, serial QFEs help to *identify compliance problems and psychosocial barriers* in patients who may be giving only lip service to functional recovery. Lack of progress can primarily be a result of lack of optimal effort. Mobility, strength, endurance, and neuromuscular coordination *always* improve if the appropriate physical training is taking place. These objective data, then, allow the treatment team to confront a resistent patient in spite of his or her denial, and then to help him or her overcome whatever barrier may be interfering with the training effort.

A patient who has progressed in functional restoration always shows an improved effort on testing at the end of rehabilitation. This posttreatment QFE, then, is a valid statement of functional capacity and will allow the treatment team to *delineate functional capability to return to a particular job* or to "fine tune" a patient's functional profile for a particular job.

Finally, tracking during a 2-year period after functional restoration, with QFE's repeated at 3 months, 6 months, 12 months, and 24 months after treatment, allows the physician and treatment team to follow these patients in a meaningful way and *to identify functional deficits if they reoccur* as a result of "slacking off" on prescribed home exercise programs. A normal functional profile is the back patient's best defense against recurrent injury, and serial testing allows preventive screening to be enforced (Mayer & Gatchel, 1987).

SUMMARY

Quantification of function in chronic low back pain introduces objectivity into the clinical assessment and treatment of a problematic patient group. In so doing, it may enhance the effectiveness of more traditional pain modulation techniques. It serves to define the initial deconditioning state, to document functional improvements in rehabilitation, and to delineate an end point from which the patient can resume a normal life. Thereafter, quantification may delineate recurrent risk factors for reinjury, so that preventive measures may be taken. Therefore, quantification of function is a tool to define disability in physical and ergonomic terms, to guide rehabilitation to correct functional deficits, and to establish a therapeutic end point from which this disability may end. In utilizing these techniques of measurement, traditional pain management therapies and physical rehabilitation techniques may be integrated into an interdisciplinary program with enhanced effectiveness.

REFERENCES

Andersson, G. (1981). Epidemiologic aspects of low back pain in industry. *Spine, 6*, 50–53.

Astrand, P.O., & Rodahl, K. (1979). Textbook of work physiology. In *Physiological basis for exercise* (2nd ed, pp. 333–365). New York: McGraw-Hill.

Battie, M. (1991). Aerobic fitness and its measurement. *Spine, 16*, 677–678.

Beals, R. (1984). Compensation and recovery from injury. *Western Journal of Medicine, 104*, 233–237.

Biering-Sorensen, F. (1984). Physical measurements as risk indicators for low back trouble over a one year period. *Spine, 9*, 106–119.

Cady, L., Bischoff, D., O'Connell, E., Thomas, P., & Allen, J. (1979). Strength and fitness and subsequent back injuries in fire fighters. *Journal of Occupational Medicine, 21*, 269–272.

Chaffin, D. (1978). Pre-employment strength testing, updated position. *Journal Occupational Medicine, 10*, 105–110.

Deyo, R., Diehl, A., & Rosenthal, M. (1986). How many days of bed rest for acute low back pain. *New England Journal of Medicine, 315*, 1064–1070.

Engelberg, A. (Ed.). (1988). *American Medical Association guides to the evaluation of permanent impairment* (3rd Ed., rev.). Chicago: American Medical Association.

Fordyce, W., Roberts, A., & Sternbach, R. (1985). The behavioral management of chronic pain: A response to critics. *Pain, 22*, 113–125.

Gatchel, R., Mayer, T., Capra, P., Diamond, P., & Barnett, J. (1986). Quantification of lumbar function, Part VI: Use of psychological measures in guiding physical functional restoration, *Spine, 10*, 36–42.

Gracovetsky, S., & Farfan, H. (1986). The optimum spine. *Spine, 11*, 543–573.

Hadler, N. (1986). Regional back pain. *New England Journal of Medicine, 315*, 1090–1092.

Keeley, J., Mayer, T., Cox, R., Gatchel, R., Smith, J., & Mooney, V. (1986). Quantification of lumbar function: Part V. Reliability of range of motion measures in the sagittal plane and in vivo torso rotation measurement technique. *Spine, 11*, 31–35.

Kinney, R., Polatin, P., & Gatchel, R. (1990). The high incidence of psychiatric disorder in chronic low back pain patients. Proceedings of the International Society for the Study of the Lumbar Spine, Annual Meeting, Boston.

Kishino, N., Mayer, T., Gatchel, R., Parrish, M., Andersson, C., Gustin, L., & Mooney, V. (1985). Quantification of lumbar function Part 4: Isometric and isokinetic lifting simulation in normal subjects and low back dysfunction patients. *Spine, 10*, 921–927.

Kondraske, G. (1986). Towards a standard clinical measure of postural stability. In G. Kondraske & C. Robinson (Eds.), *Proceedings of the 8th Annual Conference of the IEEE Engineering in Medicine and Biology Society, 3*, 1579–1582.

Langrana, N., & Lee, C. (1984). Isokinetic evaluation of trunk muscles. *Spine, 9*, 171–175.

Lillo, E., Gatchel, R., Polatin, P., & Mayer, T. (1991). The prevalence of major psychiatric disorders in chronic low back pain patients: A replication study. Proceedings of the North American Spine Society, Annual Meeting, Keystone, CO.

Mayer, T., Barnes, D., Kishino, N., Nichols, G., Gatchel, R., Mayer, H., & Mooney, V. (1988). Progressive isoinertial lifting evaluation I: A standardized protocol and normative database. *Spine, 13*, 993–997.

Mayer. T., Barnes, D., Nichols, G., Kishino, N., Coval, K., Piel, B., Hoshino, D., & Gatchel, R. (1988). Progressive isoinertial lifting evaluation II: A comparison with isokinetic lifting in a disabled chronic low back pain industrial population. *Spine, 13*, 998–1002.

Mayer, T., & Gatchel, R. (1988). *Functional restoration for spinal disorders: The sports medicine approach to low back pain*. Philadelphia: Lea & Febiger.

Mayer, T., & Gatchel, R. (1989). Functional restoration for chronic low back pain, Part I: Quantifying physical function. *Pain Management*, March/April, 67–73.

Mayer, T., Gatchel, R., Barnes, D., Mayer, H., & Mooney, V. (1990). Progressive isoinertial lifting evaluation, erratum notice. *Spine, 15*, 5.

Mayer, T., Gatchel, R., Kishino, N., Keeley, J., Mayer, H., Capra, P., & Mooney, V. (1986). A prospective short term study of chronic low back pain patients utilizing novel objective functional measurement. *Pain, 25*, 53–68.

Mayer, T., Gatchel, R., Keeley, J., Mayer, H., & Richland, D. (1991, June). Building industrial databases: Physical capacity measurements specific to major job categories in U.S. railroads. Proceedings of international society for the study of the lumbar spine, Annual Meeting, Heidelberg, Germany.

Mayer, T., Gatchel, R., Mayer, H., Kishino, N., Keeley, J., & Mooney, V. (1987). A prospective two year study of functional restoration in industrial low back injury, an objective assessment procedure. *Journal of the American Medical Association, 258*, 1763–1767.

Mayer, T., Kishino, N., Keeley, J., Mayer, H., & Mooney, V. (1985). Using physical measures to assess low back pain. *Journal of Musculoskeletal Medicine, 6*, 44–59.

Mayer, T., & Polatin, P. (in press). *Spinal rehabilitation*. In S. Halderman (Ed.), *Modern developments in the principles and practice of chiropractic* (2nd ed.). Norwalk, CT: Appleton & Lang.

Mayer, T., Smith, S., Kondraske, G., Gatchel, R., Carmichael, T., & Mooney, V. (1985), Quantification of lumbar function: Part 3. Preliminary data on isokinetic torso rotation testing with myoelectric spectral analysis in normal and low back pain subjects *Spine, 10*, 912–920.

Mayer, T., Tencer, A., Kristoferson, S., & Mooney, V. (1984). Use of noninvasive techniques of quantification of spinal range-of-motion in normal subjects and chronic low-back dysfunction patients. *Spine, 9*, 588–595.

Mooney, V., Cairns, D., & Robertson, J. (1976). A system for evaluating and treating chronic back disability. *Western Journal of Medicine, 124*, 370–376.

Nachemson, A. (1983). Work for all. *Clinical Orthopedics and Related Research, 179*, 77–82.

Polatin, P. (1990). The functional restoration approach to chronic low back pain. *Journal of Musculoskeletal Medicine, 7*, 17–30.

Smith, S., Mayer, T., Gatchel, R., & Becker, T. (1985). Quantification of lumbar function: Part I. Isometric and multi-speed isokinetic trunk strength measure in sagittal and axial planes in normal subjects. *Spine, 10*, 757–764.

Sturgess, E., Schaefer, C., & Sikora, T. (1984). Pain center follow-up study of treated and untreated patients. *Archives of Physical Medicine and Rehabilitation, 65*, 301–303.

Turk, D., Meichenbaum, D., & Genest, M. (1983). *Pain and behavioral medicine: A cognitive–behavioral perspective*. New York: Guilford Press.

White, A., & Gordon, S. (1982). Synopsis: Workshop on idiopathic low back pain. *Spine, 7*, 141–149.

Chapter 4

Assessment of Orofacial Pain

DANIEL M. LASKIN, DDS, MS
CHARLES S. GREENE, DDS

The physical proximity of numerous complex structures capable of giving rise to pain, plus the similarities in signs and symptoms produced by many of the conditions that can affect these structures, makes the assessment of orofacial pain a difficult task. The situation is complicated even further by the unique patterns of referred pain in the orofacial region, as well as by the diffuse nature of many of the pains that occur. Finally, compared to other sites in the body, there is a paucity of reliable diagnostic technology and testing methods available. Thus, the clinician ultimately must rely mainly on a detailed history and careful clinical examination to establish the correct diagnosis. Inherent in this approach is a thorough understanding on the part of the clinician of the various conditions that can give rise to orofacial pain and of the subtle differences in the history and signs and symptoms that help distinguish these conditions (Table 4.1).

DENTOALVEOLAR PAIN

Orofacial pain arising from pathologic conditions of the teeth and periodontal tissues constitutes a major source of human suffering. Fortunately, many of the conditions causing such pain can be detected by direct observa-

tion, but others cannot be properly diagnosed without using some type of clinical test. These tests may range in complexity from the simple acts of tapping on teeth, placing ice chips on them, or probing the gums, to sophisticated radiographic imaging techniques.

ODONTOGENIC PAIN

Teeth are innervated by simple pain fibers that are part of the dental pulp tissues. These fibers cannot discriminate among the various stimuli that are capable of producing a painful response; they simply transmit a message of pain to the CNS that is passed on to higher centers for interpretation and response. In the absence of local anesthesia, all dental nerves will experience a painful response to an adequate stimulus; for example, drilling on the tooth or extreme temperatures. A nerve that is hypersensitive (usually because of a hyperemic pulp) will respond excessively to minimal stimulation, whereas a more severely inflamed nerve may ache spontaneously. The three major sources of such nerve inflammation are: (1) dental caries with its bacterial toxins; (2) dental drilling and filling, which stimulate the nerve through heat, air drying, and temperature conductivity of metal filling materials; and (3)

TABLE 4.1. Differential Diagnosis of Orofacial Pain.

Disorder	Limitation	Muscle tenderness	Diagnostic features
Pulpitis	No	No	Mild to severe ache or throbbing; intermittent or constant; aggravated by thermal changes; eliminated by dental anesthesia; positive X-ray findings
Pericoronitis	Yes	Possible	Persistent mild to severe ache; difficulty swallowing; possible fever; local inflammation; relieved with dental anesthesia;
Otitis media	No	No	Moderate to severe earache; pain constant; fever; usually history of upper respiratory infection; no relief with dental anesthesia
Parotitis	Yes	No	Constant aching pain, worse when eating; pressure feeling; absent salivary flow; ear lobe elevated; ductal suppuration
Sinusitis	No	No	Constant aching or throbbing; worse when change head position; nasal discharge; often molar pain not relieved by dental anesthesia
Trigeminal neuralgia	No	No	Sharp stabbing pain of short duration; trigger zone; pain follows nerve pathway; older age group; often relieved by dental anesthesia
Atypical (vascular) neuralgia	No	No	Diffuse throbbing or burning pain of long duration; often associated autonomic symptoms; no relief with dental anesthesia
Temporal Arteritis	No	No	Constant throbbing preauricular pain: artery prominent and tender; low grade fever; may have visual problems; elevation sedimentation rate
Trotter's syndrome (nasopharyngeal carcinoma)	Yes	No	Aching pain in ear, side of face, lower jaw; deafness; nasal obstruction; cervical lymphadenopathy
Eagle's syndrome (elongated styloid process)	No	No	Mild to sharp stabbing pain in ear, throat, retromandible; provoked by swallowing, turning head, carotid compression; usually posttonsillectomy; styloid process longer than 2.5 cm

Note: Modified from Laskin and Block (1986), page 77. Copyright 1986 Mosby-Year Book, Inc. Reprinted by permission.

trauma. Following necrosis of the dental pulp, the dental nerve loses all capacity to respond to stimuli; however, toxins from this necrotic tissue can become the source of a painful condition in the bone surrounding the apex of the tooth.

Symptoms

The most common pain pattern in toothache is a mild to severe aching or throbbing. It can be constant with fluctuations, or it can be intermittent. The pain is often poorly localized, particularly when it is intense, and sometimes the patient feels it in one jaw when the problem is actually in the other (referred pain). When periapical inflammation occurs, however, localization of the pain becomes more accurate.

If the dental pulp and nerve are still vital, responses to temperature change can occur; in some cases, heat or cold will precipitate or aggravate the pain, while in other cases they will ameliorate it. If the pulp is necrotic, these responses will not occur. Injection of a local anesthetic will block the pain completely, but this is not a unique characteristic of odontogenic pain.

Distinguishing Clinical Findings

The teeth are unique among most body structures in their response to moderate temperature changes. If a patient reports a painful response to hot or cold foods and liquids, it is almost certain that the pain is coming from a dental nerve. Less clear are the painful symptoms reported when biting on hard objects or elicited by tapping on teeth with metal instruments, because a positive response may be due not only to a degenerating or necrotic pulp, but also to a cracked tooth, a defective filling, or a periodontal infection.

Diagnosis

After obtaining a detailed history of the pain patterns and responses noticed by the patient, the clinician can perform a variety of simple tests on the suspected teeth in an attempt to duplicate the pain. These may include the application of ice chips and hot instruments, tapping on the teeth, and having the patient bite on a tongue blade. Infiltration of a local anesthetic, or a nerve block in the area of the suspected tooth, can also be used in an attempt to eliminate the pain and confirm the diagnosis. A radiograph that includes the periapical tissues is almost always indicated in these situations to examine for pathologic changes in the surrounding bone. If doubt remains about the vitality of one or more dental pulps, they can be tested by using an electrical stimulator. Unfortunately, neither positive nor negative results from this test are absolutely reliable, because an inflamed or degenerating nerve may not give a vital response, whereas a vital pulp in one root of a multirooted tooth with an otherwise necrotic pulp can still give a positive response. Nevertheless, differences in the response of the various teeth may be quite informative. When a high probability of pulpal disease or necrosis exists, the ultimate test is to drill into the pulp chamber for direct observation and treatment (root canal therapy).

In addition to the true toothache of dental origin, several kinds of nondental pathology can also produce unilateral pain that appears to be coming from one or more of the teeth. The misdiagnosis of these problems frequently leads to the use of irreversible dental treatments, including endodontic therapy, apical surgery, and tooth extraction, all of which prove to be unsuccessful. Among the conditions to be considered when the dental findings are essentially negative are sinusitis, vascular headaches, cardiac infarcts, intracranial tumors or infarcts, myofascial pain, psychogenic pain, and trigeminal and pretrigeminal neuralgia (Graff-Radford, 1991). Consideration should also be given to the possibility of atypical odontalgia

when there is no obvious organic cause of the toothache (see page 53).

Periodontal Pain

Periodontal problems are generally painless conditions. Although inflammation of the gum margin may cause it to bleed during eating or toothbrushing, this condition (gingivitis) is usually not painful. Likewise, pockets that develop as the periodontal attachment is destroyed by disease (periodontitis) rarely produce symptoms that would alert the patient to their existence. This unfortunate characteristic of periodontal problems is largely responsible for their high prevalence without detection, especially in people who visit dentists infrequently. Nevertheless, there are some painful periodontal conditions that need to be considered.

The most likely reasons for periodontal pain are direct mechanical trauma to the gums or an acute flare-up of a chronic periodontal condition. Obviously, even a person with healthy gums can have pain if a piece of food impacts between two teeth, or if a sharp cracker or a hot pizza injures the tissues directly. For people with chronic periodontal disease, however, there is a greater chance of food impacting into a pocket, or of bacterial toxins becoming trapped (periodontal abscess) and exacerbating the condition enough to produce pain.

Symptoms

The pain from subacute periodontal problems is generally felt as an aching soreness, qualitatively different from a toothache. In the acute stage, however, the pain can have a more throbbing character. Pain of periodontal origin ordinarily tends to be better localized than toothache, although occasionally the patient may report difficulty in isolating it to a specific spot. Usually the pain will be increased by biting on one or more teeth in the affected area and the teeth will be painful to percussion. Unlike with toothache, periodontal pain is not significantly affected by thermal changes.

Distinguishing Clinical Findings

The most useful clinical findings are likely to result from periodontal probing, which should reveal an exquisitely tender pocket that is the main source of the problem. A major visual clue may be the presence of a swollen and red gingival margin or papilla, or a gingival abscess. Routine dental radiographs may show loss of alveolar bone adjacent to the tooth, which correlates clearly with the problem, and also can help in discriminating between periapical and periodontal bony pathology.

Diagnosis

There are no specific tests that can be used to definitively establish a diagnosis of periodontal pain. Several technological tests such as DNA probes, crevicular fluid analysis, and bacterial assays are being developed to differentiate active periodontal defects from passive ones, but these are not likely to be helpful in the diagnosis of periodontal pain. In the final analysis, the diagnostic challenge in these dental pain situations is to utilize all the findings from the history and clinical examination in order to differentiate between odontogenic and periodontal pain.

Pain from Pathology in the Jawbones

Nearly all of the pathologic processes that affect other bones in the body can affect the jawbones. In addition, there are a few special types of pathology that arise from embryologic remnants of the dental structures. Although it is beyond the scope of this chapter to discuss all of these possibilities, it should be recognized that many of these conditions may produce pain at some point in their development. Regardless of whether the conditions are benign or malignant, they generally need to be treated, and pain is often the first sign of their existence. Techniques for the assessment of pathologic conditions in the jawbones include a variety of imaging procedures such as panoramic radiography, skull films, CT scans, and scintigraphy, as well as biopsy and needle aspiration of fluids to establish a final diagnosis.

Trigeminal Neuralgias

Trigeminal neuralgia, as the name implies, is a painful disorder involving one or more branches of the fifth cranial nerve, which may be of central or peripheral origin. Although most frequently the term "trigeminal neuralgia" is used synonymously with the terms "tic douloureux" and "idiopathic" or "primary trigeminal neuralgia," there are other condi-

tions that can cause a neuralgic pain in the fifth nerve that must be considered in the differential diagnosis. These include multiple sclerosis, postherpetic neuralgia, tumors, posttraumatic neuralgia, dental pathology, lesions or inflammation of the nasal and paranasal sinuses, and temporomandibular (TMJ) joint disorders. The neuralgic pain from these conditions is referred to as secondary rather than primary trigeminal neuralgia because there is a known etiology.

Idiopathic Trigeminal Neuralgia (Tic Douloureux, Primary Trigeminal Neuralgia)

Symptoms

This condition is characterized by a sharp, paroxysmal, lancinating pain of unknown origin, lasting for seconds to minutes, that can frequently be provoked by stimulation of the facial skin or oral mucosa (trigger zone), but that usually arises spontaneously. Between attacks, the patient may be pain free, or there may be a background burning or aching pain. The most common trigger zones are located in the nasolabial fold, on the upper lip, on the lateral aspect of the lower lip, and on the alveolar gingiva.

Distinguishing Clinical Findings

Idiopathic trigeminal neuralgia generally occurs in middle-aged or older patients and has a unilateral distribution, although some bilateral cases have been reported. The maxillary division is affected most frequently, the mandibular division next most frequently, and the ophthalmic division least frequently. More than one division at a time can be involved. The pain occurs more commonly on the right side and in females. It characteristically follows the nerve pathway(s), in contrast to an atypical facial neuralgia, which has a more diffuse, less well localized distribution. There are no associated sensory nerve deficits, and the presence of such changes or any peripheral pathology should lead one to suspect another diagnosis.

Diagnosis

There are no diagnostic tests for idiopathic trigeminal neuralgia, and the diagnosis is usually made on the basis of the character of the pain, the presence of a trigger zone, and the lack of regional pathology. In contrast to atypical neuralgia, the pain from idiopathic trigeminal neuralgia can be stopped temporarily with a peripheral anesthetic nerve block of the involved branch(es). It will also generally respond favorably to a trial of carbamazepine (Tegretol) or phenytoin (Dilantin).

Secondary Trigeminal Neuralgias

Multiple Sclerosis

The pain of multiple sclerosis duplicates the pain of idiopathic trigeminal neuralgia. There are also trigger zones present. Women are affected more than men, but the age of onset is earlier than with tic douloureux (20–40 years vs. 50 or older). It also differs from the latter in being associated with paresthesia of the face, the trunk, and the extremities, as well as with a variety of motor and autonomic nerve dysfunctions. Nystagmus, intention tremor, and scanning speech are common in advanced stages of the disease.

Postherpetic Neuralgia

This condition follows a herpes zoster infection of the trigeminal nerve, and the history and character of the pain establish the diagnosis. The pain generally has a burning quality and may be associated with hyperalgesia. Paresthesia and masticatory muscle weakness have also been reported. The maxillary division is most commonly involved. The pain may persist for more than a year following the acute attack, although it usually subsides after a few weeks or months.

Neuralgia Due to Tumors

Neoplasms involving the gasserian ganglion as well as the cerebellopontine angle can cause pain having the characteristics of trigeminal neuralgia. Carcinomas originating in the nose, sinuses, and pharyngeal space may also cause such pain. The chronic nature of the pain, the presence of progressive numbness in the face, and the occasional motor involvement should lead one to suspect such lesions.

Posttraumatic Neuralgia

Fractures of the jaws and facial bones, surgery of the jaws, and traumatic facial injuries can cause neuralgias that may begin weeks after the injury and last for years. Usually there is a continuous ache, with acute exacerbations of lancinating or burning pain. However, in some patients the pain may resemble idiopathic trigeminal neuralgia and be associated with a trigger zone. Common sites of pain are the infraorbital region, the chin, and the lower lip. A history of trauma to the region is usually the basis for establishing the diagnosis.

Glossopharyngeal Neuralgia

Glossopharyngeal neuralgia has all of the characteristics of idiopathic trigeminal neuralgia except for its location and the fact that men are affected more often than women.

Symptoms

The pain has a paroxysmal, stabbing character and arises either spontaneously or is precipitated by such movements as chewing, swallowing, or talking. It usually starts at the base of the tongue, or in the pharynx or soft palate, and radiates to the ear or down the anterolateral aspect of the neck. Trigger zones are located in the tonsil, pharyngeal wall, base of the tongue, and the ear.

Diagnosis

The diagnosis is based on the location of the pain, its characteristics, precipitation of an attack by having the patient swallow or by touching the trigger zone with a cotton applicator, and temporarily eliminating the pain by application of a topical anesthetic to the lateral pharyngeal wall.

ATYPICAL FACIAL PAIN

Atypical Odontalgia

As the name implies, this condition resembles a toothache but is not of pulpal origin. Therefore, the clinician must constantly be on guard against assuming every toothache is a dental problem and engaging in inappropriate therapy. Typically, the patients are female in the fourth or fifth decade. Most often the pain is located in the maxillary premolar or molar region and has an aching, burning, or throbbing character. Although the pain is not relieved with local anesthesia, it often responds to a sympathetic nerve block and serotonergic and antidepressant medications (Reik, 1984).

The currently recognized inclusionary criteria are (1) no obvious local cause, (2) no abnormality on x-ray, (3) continuous (or nearly continuous) pain in a tooth and surrounding alveolar bone, (4) pain present for more than 4 months, (5) associated hyperesthesia, and (6) equivocal response to a somatic nerve block (Graff-Radford & Solberg, 1986). The most frequently mentioned theories of etiology are psychogenic, vascular, and deafferentation, but little objective evidence exists for any of them.

The diagnostic assessment of atypical odontalgia depends heavily on clinical interpretation of the findings. Although there may frequently be a positive response to sympathetic nerve blocks and serotonergic and antidepressant drugs, and a negative reaction to local anesthetics, these tests are not always reliable. Thermography has shown some positive correlation between localized heat sites and atypical odontalgia (Gratt, Sickles, Graff-Radford, & Solberg, 1989), indicating a possible vascular component, but the clinical utility of this test has not been established.

Atypical Facial Neuralgia

This condition, often described as lower-half headache, is characterized by a diffuse, burning, throbbing, or nagging ache in the face, sometimes referring to the forehead, the temporal region, around the ear, and to the neck and shoulder girdle. The pain is poorly localized and does not conform to the anatomic boundaries of the sensory nerve supply (e.g., as in trigeminal neuralgia). Usually the ache is constant, unaffected by external factors, with acute exacerbations lasting for hours or days. The focal point of this midface pain is in the deeper structures of the cheek, the upper jaw, the teeth, and the zygomatic arch. In terms of differential diagnosis, it must be discriminated from atypical odontalgia, other common types of headache, odontogenic pain, and true neuralgias (Bell, 1985).

From an etiologic viewpoint, it has been proposed that this type of "neuralgia" is actually caused by an irritation of the sympathetic

pathways. This hypothesis is supported by the frequent finding of associated symptoms such as facial flushing, rhinorrhea, and lacrimation, and by the failure to obtain relief of pain with sensory nerve blocks (Moskowitz, 1984). An alternative viewpoint is that either obvious or concealed depression is a major factor in the etiology of this condition, but it is not clear whether this is a cause of the symptoms or a consequence of them. Nevertheless, psychopharmacologic treatment of the depressive symptoms often produces significant relief of the pain.

Neuralgia-Inducing Cavitational Osteonecrosis (Painful Jawbone Cavities)

A controversial explanation for many cases of atypical facial pain (as well as many cases of trigeminal neuralgia) has been offered by a number of investigators, beginning with Ratner in 1979. According to this concept, a dental procedure (usually extraction or endodontics) may be responsible for creating conditions within the jawbones that ultimately produce chronic pain. Initially, it was proposed that a deafferentation phenomenon ("amputation neuroma") could occur unpredictably following tooth extraction or pulpectomy, resulting in a continuously painful site ("phantom tooth pain," atypical odontalgia). This concept was later expanded to include the development of a necrotic cavitational process inside the jawbone following certain dental procedures. These cavitations, or "holes in bone," are thought to be sites of chronic infection surrounded by a sclerotic bony wall that impedes the blood flow required for healing. Currently, the term neuralgia-inducing cavitational osteonecrosis (NICO) is used to describe this phenomenon (Ratner, Langer, & Evins, 1986). The treatment proposed is to eradicate the area by aggressive curettage, usually followed by an intensive course of antibiotic therapy.

From a diagnostic point of view, this has proved to be a difficult subject. The cavities are usually not detectable on the radiographs, and use of diagnostic nerve blocks, as recommended by Ratner (Ratner et al., 1986; Ratner, Person, Kleinman, Shklar, & Socransky, 1979), depends heavily on interpretation of the response. At present, it is not possible to draw any clear conclusions about the validity of this entire concept. Its advocates claim to obtain high levels of clinical success, but many critics have been unable to replicate their results. A review of the clinical papers on this topic reveal a lack of controlled studies, with strong suggestions of positive bias on the part of those involved in the projects.

TEMPOROMANDIBULAR JOINT PAIN

The TMJ is prone to development of the same pathologic conditions that can involve any joint in the body. These include congenital and developmental anomalies, traumatic injuries, neoplastic disease, ankylosis, internal derangements, and various forms of arthritis. Of the numerous conditions, however, the only ones associated with chronic pain are the internal derangements and the arthritides. Trauma can result in chronic pain, but it does so only indirectly by producing secondary arthritic changes or internal derangement.

TEMPOROMANDIBULAR JOINT ARTHRITIS

Although the TMJ can be affected by any of the numerous types of arthritis involving other joints, the most common are degenerative arthritis (osteoarthritis) and rheumatoid arthritis.

Degenerative Arthritis

Degenerative arthritis of the TMJ can be divided into primary and secondary forms. Primary degenerative joint disease tends to involve persons 50 years of age or older and is related to the normal wear and tear of aging. Secondary arthritis usually occurs in persons 20–40 years of age, although it can occur in younger persons, and represents an acceleration of the degenerative process. It is generally seen in patients with chronic masticatory muscle pain and dysfunction (primary masticatory myalgia, MPD syndrome), especially whose with chronic clenching and tooth-grinding habits. Trauma is also a frequent etiologic factor.

Symptoms

The pain of degenerative arthritis tends to be of a dull, aching character, located in the preauricular region. Although initially it is usually intermittent, being exacerbated by function, it later becomes more constant. With chewing there is often sharp, shooting pain as well as the aching background pain. Patients who have an internal derangement associated with their arthritis may exhibit clicking or popping sounds in the joint. In the later stages of degenerative arthritis, crepitant sounds may be heard.

Patients with degenerative arthritis will often have tenderness of the joint on both lateral and intrameatal palpation. There may also be masticatory muscle tenderness. This will be more severe in patients with MPD, although all patients with degenerative joint disease will have some masticatory muscle tenderness due to the physiologic splinting of the mandible as a self-protective mechanism. Associated with the joint pain and muscle dysfunction, there is usually varying degrees of limitation of mouth opening.

Distinguishing Clinical Findings

Degenerative arthritis can be distinguished from rheumatoid arthritis by the fact that it is generally unilateral rather than bilateral, and usually involves only the TMJ. A history of trauma or myofascial pain and tenderness associated with chronic clenching or tooth grinding is often elicited. Crepitus in the joint is another pathognomonic sign of degenerative arthritis.

Degenerative arthritis can be distinguished from chronic masticatory myalgia (MPD syndrome) by the more localized quality of the pain, by the frequent presence of joint tenderness, and when present, by the existence of crepitant sounds. However, when the two conditions are present simultaneously, the chronology of the symptoms helps to determine which is the primary condition or whether the two are unrelated.

Diagnosis

In addition to the clinical findings, other diagnostic aids include the use of radiographs, which may show subcondylar sclerosis, condylar flattening and lipping, and osteophyte formation or erosions on the articular surface, and radionuclide scans, which may show increased cellular activity even before it is visible radiographically.

Rheumatoid Arthritis

Patients with rheumatoid arthritis will frequently have involvement of the TMJ. The disease affects both children and adults. In children, destruction of the condylar growth site can result in facial deformity. Ankylosis is another common sequela of rheumatoid arthritis, particularly in the child or young adult.

Symptoms

Pain of an aching character, joint tenderness and stiffness, and redness and swelling are the common findings in patients with rheumatoid arthritis. Multiple joints are usually affected, including hands, wrists, elbows, feet, and ankles, but any joint can be involved.

Distinguishing Clinical Findings

Rheumatoid arthritis is distinguished from degenerative arthritis by the presence of symmetrical joint symptoms, involvement of multiple joints, the frequent presence of low-grade fever and anemia, and the more severe destructive changes that occur in the condyle. It is also characterized by periods of remission and recrudescence rather than by a steady, slow progression of the symptoms. Onset in the adult form usually occurs between ages 25 and 50.

Diagnosis

In contrast to degenerative arthritis, laboratory tests can be used to establish the diagnosis of rheumatoid arthritis. The erythrocyte sedimentation rate is increased in 90% of the patients, and the presence of the so-called rheumatoid factor can be detected by the latex fixation test in 70% of cases. The test for antinuclear antibodies may also be positive. A normochromic or slightly hypochromic, normocytic anemia is found in 80% of patients.

Internal Derangement

An internal derangement is characterized by an abnormal relationship between the intraarticular disc and the mandibular condyle when the teeth are in occlusion. Usually this involves an anterior or anteromedial displacement, with the disc returning to its normal position during the opening movement, accompanied by a clicking or popping sound (anterior displacement with reduction, open lock), or with the disc remaining permanently in a forward position due to extreme laxity of the capsule and TMJ ligament, and/or the presence of adhe-

sions, and causing inability to open the mouth normally (anterior displacement without reduction, closed lock).

When the disc assumes a forward position, the highly innervated retrodiscal tissues are pulled into the articulating zone and compressed by the condyle. This, plus the synovitis that occurs in response to the liberation of tissue breakdown products, results in pain that is exacerbated with function. Compression of the retrodiscal tissues can also eventually lead to a tear or perforation in these tissues, resulting in bone-to-bone contact.

In some patients with limited ability to open the mouth, however, the disc is not anteriorly displaced but instead becomes adherent to the glenoid fossa, due either to a change in the consistency and flow properties of the synovial fluid or to the formation of actual adhesions. In these situations, translation of the condyle is prevented and mouth opening is restricted just as it is when there is an anteriorly displaced, nonreducing disc. However, when pain is present, it is not due to compression of the retrodiscal tissue, but rather it results from a stretching of the capsule (capsulitis) and a synovitis.

Symptoms

Internal derangement produces a dull, aching, well-localized, preauricular pain that is exacerbated by function. Tenderness is usually present when the joint is palpated either laterally or intrameatally. When the disc reduces on mouth opening, there is an accompanying clicking or popping sound. When reduction does not occur, or when disc mobility is restricted, the pain is accompanied by limitation of mouth opening. If a perforation or tear exists in the retrodiscal tissue, grating sounds may be heard.

Diagnosis

Clicking or popping sounds in the temporomandibular joint are generally pathognomonic of an anteriorly displaced, reducing intraarticular disc. The one exception is clicking or popping caused by disc irregularity or deformity. In the latter instance, both opening and closing sounds usually occur at the same point in the cycle. In the former situation, a closing sound often is not heard, but when present, it occurs at a different point from the opening sound.

Magnetic resonance imaging (MRI) is the preferred method for distinguishing between disc displacement and possible disc irregularity or deformity. It is also used to help distinguish anterior disc displacement or adhesions from other causes of limited mouth opening. A perforation is difficult to visualize with MRI, but arthrography can be used for this purpose.

Sophisticated sound recording machines have been used to study TMJ noises that occur during mandibular movement, and attempts have been made to correlate the various sounds with different types of intraarticular pathology. Because of the difficulty in demonstrating distinct differences between the various sound patterns and the inability to reliably relate specific sounds to specific diseases or disorders, sonography has not proved to be a reliable diagnostic aid (Mohl, Lund, Widmer, & McCall, 1990; Widmer, 1989).

MASTICATORY MYALGIA

Primary Masticatory Myalgia (Myofascial Pain Dysfunction Syndrome)

The most common condition affecting the masticatory muscles (which move the mandible) is MPD (Laskin et al., 1983). As the name implies, this condition includes both the pain of muscle fatigue, spasm, or hyperemia and a dysfunction of mandibular movement. In the past, this has been referred to as a type of "TMJ" problem, but in recent classification systems for temporomandibular disorders it has been distinguished from true intracapsular joint problems.

Within the dental profession, concepts about the etiology and treatment of MPD have undergone continuous revision. Originally, it was thought that overclosure of the jaws due to missing teeth was responsible for MPD symptoms, whereas subsequent theories emphasized the minute details of dental occlusion (bite). Malposition and malalignment of the mandibular condyle were frequently described and treated, and it was not uncommon to see major procedures such as full-mouth restorations, orthodontics, and orthognathic surgery done for the sake of eliminating MPD.

Today, these mechanistic theories have been largely replaced by a medical orthopedic model of muscle dysfunction that includes a significant component of psychophysiologic stress as an etiologic agent. As a result, treatments have become more conservative and reversible, with behavioral factors being considered throughout the diagnostic and treatment process (Greene & Laskin, 1983; McNeill, 1990).

Symptoms

The major symptom of MPD is a dull, aching pain in one or more of the masticatory muscles, especially the masseter and temporalis. This pain generally is diffuse, and may be accompanied by tenderness to palpation of the affected muscle(s) and limitation of mouth opening. Attempts to open the mouth widely, chew, speak, and yawn will usually precipitate or exacerbate the pain. If the patient is engaging in nightly tooth grinding and/or clenching activity (bruxism), jaw stiffness and pain on awakening will frequently be reported; on the other hand, if the patient is engaging in daytime clenching or grinding, has poor postural work habits, or is involved in stressful situations, the pain may start in the morning and increase throughout the day. In some patients, both situations may exist, and they complain of constant pain.

Distinguishing Clinical Findings

The diagnosis of MPD requires two important negative findings in addition to the preceding symptoms: (1) absence of major local or systemic intracapsular TMJ pathology and (2) absence of significant degenerative changes on TMJ radiographs (Laskin, 1969). There are no absolutely clear pathognomonic findings for MPD, but one would expect to elicit pain on masticatory muscle palpation, and also to see limited opening and lateral movements, with inability to open the mouth further without pain. There is often a history of bruxism, exposure to stressful life events, and aggravation of the symptoms when eating hard foods, gum chewing, and so forth.

Diagnosis

The "gold standard" procedure for diagnosing MPD is a thorough history and physical examination, which cover all of the considerations previously discussed (Goulet & Clark, 1990; Laskin & Greene, 1990). However, there are some who advocate a technological approach to either discover or confirm this diagnosis. Because the condition involves muscle dysfunction, it is claimed that an electromyogram (EMG) can detect abnormal patterns of muscle behavior and validate the diagnosis. In addition, it is claimed that the abnormal muscle behavior will produce characteristic aberrations of jaw movement and that these can be recorded by jaw-tracking machines (Cooper & Rabuzzi, 1984). Although it is true that these machines can record such phenomena (and they have been widely used to do so in various research projects), it has not been demonstrated that they are useful in the clinical setting (Mohl, Lund et al., 1990; Mohl, McCall, Lund, & Plesh, 1990). This is due mainly to their inability to discriminate between normal and clinically abnormal variations of jaw movement and muscle behavior. Even in clearly identified MPD patients, a wide variety of findings have been reported by researchers using these instruments (Widmer, Lund, & Feine, 1990). For these reasons, their use is not recommended at this time (Greene, 1990).

Those clinicians who subscribe to the concept of occlusal problems as a cause of MPD often use intraoral acrylic appliances (biteplate, splint, night guard, mandibular orthopedic repositioning appliance) as diagnostic tools on the basis that they eliminate direct contact of the teeth. Thus, if the pain and dysfunction are relieved, it is assumed that a correct diagnosis has been made and that the occlusal problems are causative. Although such appliances have been shown to be very effective, there are other reasons, including control of parafunction, restoration of muscle length, and placebo response, that explain the therapeutic effect.

Thermography has also been recommended as a diagnostic test for MPD. Currently, however, it has not been shown to be useful for this purpose. At best, it merely shows an altered temperature in a painful muscle (Gratt & Sickles, 1991). Unfortunately, muscle tenderness on palpation, a much more sensitive test, often fails to show a positive correlation with thermography.

Secondary Masticatory Myalgia

Muscle Splinting Pain

Muscle splinting is a normal protective neurophysiologic process that develops in response to regional tissue pain. In the orofacial region, it frequently accompanies painful conditions involving the TMJ such as arthritis or disc displacement. The chronically increased contractile activity in the muscle causes an accumulation of metabolic by-products, resulting in myalgia. Thus, a primary joint disorder leads to secondary muscle pain. Such pain is often confused with that of primary masticatory myalgia (MPD), but generally can be distinguished by the presence of associated joint pathology. When MPD is associated with degenerative joint disease, the history helps to determine which was the primary condition.

Referred and Spreading Pain

It is generally recognized that muscle pain can be associated with characteristic patterns of referred pain. This phenomenon was originally demonstrated in the head and neck region by Travell and Rinzler (1952) nearly 40 years ago when they injected hypertonic saline into all the head and neck muscles. They found reproducible distributions of pain to other sites, and this information has been quite valuable to diagnosticians.

It is common to see muscles becoming involved in a "spreading" of pain. For example, lower back pain of muscular origin often affects other nearby back muscles and muscles of the buttocks and thighs. This same phenomenon occurs in the head and neck region, with the most common manifestations being sore neck, and shoulder muscles accompanying MPD. Clark, Seligman, Solberg, and Pulinger (1990) have shown that it is frequently necessary to treat both the neck and masticatory muscles to help these patients.

Trigger Point Pain

A more controversial theory of referred muscular pain is the concept of muscle trigger points. As described by Fricton (1991), "a trigger point is a localized, deep tenderness in a taut band of skeletal muscle that is responsible for the pain in the zone of reference and, if treated, will resolve the resulting pain" (p. 1). Because it is nearly impossible to directly demonstrate these trigger points in living muscle, a series of indirect arguments have been made to support this concept (Simons & Travell, 1991; see also Gerwin, Chapter 5). Although it is beyond the scope of this chapter to discuss this matter at length, one should be aware of the possibility of trigger points contributing to the overall head and neck pain problem.

Injection of a suspected trigger point with a local anesthetic without a vasoconstrictor can be used as a diagnostic procedure to help localize the source of the pain. If the diagnosis is correct, the pain will be relieved for at least as long as the anesthesia lasts, but often the relief will last for months. Although some clinicians suggest adding a corticosteroid to the local anesthetic, this has been shown to produce long-lasting muscle damage (Guttu, Page, & Laskin, 1990).

Fibromyalgia

Fibromyalgia is a descriptive term for a generalized muscular pain condition; several other labels such as fibrositis, nonarticular rheumatism, and systemic myofascial pain also have been used to describe this condition (see Gerwin, Chapter 5). Recently, Wolfe et al. (1990) established diagnostic criteria for fibromyalgia that include (1) generalized ache or stiffness involving 3 or more anatomic sites for at least three months; (2) exclusion of other conditions that may cause similar symptoms; and (3) the presence of reproducible tenderness in 11 out of 18 specific sites.

Most clinicians who see a large number of head and neck pain patients have seen some of these fibromyalgia patients in their practice because they may also have facial pain. It is crucial to distinguish these people from the patients who merely have regional myofascial pain, not only because some of the treatment approaches are different, but also because of the potentially poorer prognosis.

SUMMARY

Despite the complexity of the orofacial region and the various painful conditions that affect it, an accurate diagnosis can generally be established on the basis of a thorough history and clinical examination. Where indicated, this method can be supplemented by the use of established diagnostic techniques such as local anesthetic blocks, appropriate drug trials, and various forms of hard and soft tissue imaging. When problems in the assessment of orofacial pain occur, it is generally not because of the inadequacy of the existing diagnostic ap-proaches, but rather it is from the inappropriate use of unproven diagnostic technology leading to a wrong conclusion.

REFERENCES

Bell, W.H. (1985). *Orofacial pains—Classification, diagnosis, and management* (3rd ed.). Chicago: Yearbook Publishers.

Clark, G.T., Seligman, D.A., Solberg, W.K., & Pullinger, A.G. (1990). Guidelines for the treatment of temporomandibular disorders. *Journal of Craniomandibular Disorders, 4*, 80–87.

Cooper, B.C., & Rabuzzi, D.S. (1984). Myofascial pain dysfunction syndrome: A clinical study of asymptomatic subjects. *Laryngoscope, 94*, 68–75.

Fricton, J.R. (1991). Clinical care for myofascial pain. *Dental Clinics of North America, 35*, 1–28.

Goulet, J-P., & Clark, G.T. (1990). Clinical TMJ examination methods. *California Dental Association Journal, 18*, 25–33.

Graff-Radford, S.B. (1991). Headache problems that can present as toothache. *Dental Clinics of North America, 35*, 155–170.

Graff-Radford, S.B., & Solberg, W.K. (1986). Atypical odontalgia. *California Dental Association Journal, 14*, 27–32.

Gratt, B.M., & Sickles, E.A. (1991). Future applications of electronic thermography. *Journal of the American Dental Association, 122*, 29–36.

Gratt, B.M., Sickles, E.A., Graff-Radford, S.B., & Solberg, W.K. (1989). Electronic thermography in the diagnosis of atypical odontalgia: A pilot study. *Oral Surgery, Oral Medicine, Oral Pathology, 68*, 472–481.

Greene, C.S. (1990). Can technology enhance TM disorder diagnosis? *California Dental Association Journal, 18*, 21–24.

Greene, C.S., & Laskin, D.M. (1983). Long-term evaluation of treatment for myofascial pain-dysfunction syndrome: A comparative analysis. *Journal of the American Dental Association, 107*, 235–238.

Guttu, R.L., Page, D.G., & Laskin, D.M. (1990). Delayed healing of muscle after injection of bupivacaine and steroid. *Annals of Dentistry, 49*, 5–8.

Laskin, D.M. (1969). Etiology of the pain-dysfunction syndrome. *Journal of the American Dental Association, 79*, 147–153.

Laskin, D.M., & Greene, C.S. (1990). Diagnostic methods for temporomandibular disorders: What we have learned in two decades. *Anesthesia Progress, 37*, 66–71.

Laskin, D.M., Greenfield, W., Gale, E.N., Rugh, J.D., Neff, P., Alling, C., & Ayers, W.A. (Eds.). (1983). *The president's conference on the examination, diagnosis, and management of temporomandibular disorders*. Chicago: American Dental Association.

McNeill, C. (Ed.). (1990). *Craniomandibular disorders: Guidelines for evaluation, diagnosis, and management*. Chicago: Quintessence Publishing Company.

Mohl, N.D., Lund, J.P., Widmer, C.G., & McCall, W.D. Jr. (1990). Devices for the diagnosis and treatment of temporomandibular disorders. Part II: Electromyography and sonography. *Journal of Prosthetic Dentistry, 63*, 332–335.

Mohl, N.D., McCall, W.D., Jr., Lund, J.P., & Plesh, O. (1990). Devices for the diagnosis and treatment of temporomandibular disorders. Part I: Introduction, scientific evidence and jaw tracking. *Journal of Prosthetic Dentistry, 63*, 198–201.

Moskowitz, M.A. (1984). The neurobiology of vascular head pain. *Annals of Neurology, 16*, 157–168.

Ratner, E. J., Langer, B., & Evins, M. (1986). Alveolar cavitational osteopathosis: Manifestations of an infectious process and its implications in the causation of chronic pain. *Journal of Periodontology, 57*, 593–603.

Ratner, E.J., Person, P., Kleinman D.J., Shklar, G., & Socransky, S.S. (1979). Jawbone cavities and trigeminal and atypical facial neuralgias. *Oral Surgery, Oral Medicine, Oral Pathology, 48*, 3–20.

Reik, L. (1984). Atypical odontalgia: A localized form of atypical facial pain. *Headache, 24*, 222–224.

Simons, D.G., & Travell, J. (1981). Myofascial trigger points, a possible explanation. *Pain, 10*, 106–109.

Travell, J., & Rinzler, S.H. (1952). Scientific exhibit: The myofascial genesis of pain. *Postgraduate Medicine, 11*, 425–433.

Widmer, C.G. (1989). Temporomandibular joint sounds: A critique of techniques for recording and analysis. *Journal of Craniomandibibular Disorders Facial and Oral Pain, 3*, 213–217.

Widmer, C.G., Lund, J.P., & Feine, J.S. (1990). Evaluation of diagnostic tests for TMD. *California Dental Association Journal, 18*, 53–60.

Wolfe, F., Smythe, H.A., Yunus, M.B., Bennett, R.M., Bombardier, C., Goldenberg, D.L., Tugivell, P., Campbell, S.M., Abeles, M., & Clark, P. (1990). The American College of Rheumatology 1990 criteria for the classification of fibromyalgia. *Arthritis and Rheumatism, 33*, 160–172.

Chapter 5

The Clinical Assessment of Myofascial Pain

ROBERT D. GERWIN, MD

The individual with pain has a story to tell. It is our task to listen, to extract the signs of dysfunction and disease, and to create a reasonable hypothesis explaining the problem from the observations presented to us by the patient. That is the essence of medical history taking. The theories that we then construct on the basis of the story are put to the test in the physical examination and are further confirmed or rejected by appropriate laboratory tests. This traditional approach to diagnosis applies particularly well to the area of myofascial pain.

Myofascial pain syndrome (MPS) is among the most common causes of pain that we see in our clinics (Fricton, 1990; Rosomoff, Fishbain, Goldberg, Santana, & Rosomoff, 1989). Myofascial trigger points (MTrPs) are a frequent cause of low back pain, a condition that afflicts about 60% of the population over a lifetime (Bierring-Sorenson, 1982). Headache, neck, and shoulder pain are common consequences of active MTrPs. The unrelenting daily headache, and the failed low back pain syndrome each may have its origin in the MTrP. Several studies have identified a high incidence of myofascial pain among groups of individuals complaining of pain in a general medical clinic, or in persons evaluated for undiagnosed pain at a major pain center (Rosomoff, Fishbain, Gold-

berg, & Rosomoff, 1990; Skootsky, Jaeger, & Oye, 1989).

The diagnosis of MPS proceeds in steps:

1. Determine that there is a MPS present and note the muscles that are involved with MTrPs.
2. Identify the factors that perpetuate the MPS.
3. Define the factors that need to be corrected in order to avoid recurrences.
4. When evaluating chronic pain, uncover the mechanical or structural stresses and the medical illnesses that impede recovery.

In this way, the diagnosis of MPS proceeds from a particular region in what may be an acute or chronic pain problem, to a chronic more generalized problem that requires uncovering perpetuating factors.

Myofascial pain is pain of muscle origin. The term "myofascial" was coined by Dr. Janet G. Travell after she observed a muscle fiber twitch in response to light stroking of the muscle fascia at open biopsy. The MTrP is the essential feature of the MPS (Travell, & Simons, 1983, 1992; Sola & Bonica, 1990). MTrPs are locally tender regions in taut bands of muscle that usually refer pain, tenderness, and dysesthesias (unpleasant sensations) to distant areas. Once established, they may persist long after the initiating event has subsided. MPS is a regional disorder. It can become secondarily widespread when associated with other illnesses such as fibromyalgia, rheumatoid arthritis, or hypothyroidism, or in the presence of postural and structural imbalances. In chronic MPS, multiple areas of the body may develop signs and symptoms of active MTrPs.

FUNCTIONAL MOTOR UNIT

Knowledge of the concept of the functional motor unit is essential in order to understand the regional nature of myofascial pain. A functional motor unit is a group of muscles that are linked by reciprocal reflexes, that act together synergistically as agonists, or that act in opposition as antagonists. They extend the direction of force of the primary muscle, or act to stabilize body parts. An example of a functional unit is that of the adductor and internal rotator of the arm, the subscapularis muscle, in which the teres major, latissimus dorsi, and pectoralis major muscles are synergists that also adduct and internally rotate the arm, and the infraspinatus and teres minor muscles are the antagonists that oppose internal rotation of the arm. MTrPs commonly spread from the muscle primarily involved to other muscles of the functional unit through the development of secondary MTrPs.

MYOFASCIAL TRIGGER POINT

(Simons, 1988, 1989). The MTrP produces pain that is experienced at a distant site, a phenomenon known as referred pain. Stimulation of the tender region of the taut band *triggers* pain in a distant site, hence the name trigger point (TrP). MTrPs also develop in the zone of referred pain, producing *satellite* TrPs. Once established, secondary and satellite TrPs may persist and refer pain to their own pain reference zones, thereby extending the areas of the body involved in the MPS, until multiple regions are affected.

The features of the MTrP that help to identify and diagnose the condition are:

1. Localized tenderness in a taut band of muscle. Stimulation of the tender area reproduces the patient's pain.

2. Local twitch response (LTR) when the taut band is stimulated. The LTR has both a spinal reflex and a local muscle component (Dexter & Simons, 1981; Fricton, Auvinen, Dykstra, & Schiffman, 1985; Hong & Simons, 1988). It is easily seen in superficial muscles as a pronounced contraction but may be more difficult to appreciate in deeper muscles.

3. Restriction of motion—the result of increased tension in the taut bands of muscle—limits muscle stretch and thereby limits movement of a body part. For example, rotation of the head is limited by active TrPs in the levator scapulae muscle, and extension at the waist is limited by MTrPs in the quadratus lumborum muscle.

4. Weakness occurs perhaps as a result of chronic muscle overload, perhaps as a result of pain, as a result of muscle dysfunction caused by irregular sarcomere length in affected muscle fibers, or by the mechanical disadvantage inherent in contracting shortened muscle fibers. There is no atrophy and no alteration of tendon reflexes in muscles with MTrPs.

5. Referred pain is a major feature of the MTrP. The patterns of referred pain zones are reproducible from patient to patient and for a single patient from visit to visit. Referred pain patterns can be confusing because they do not follow the usual pathways of peripheral nerves or of dermatomes, blood vessels, or sclerotomes. Referred pain from muscle has been well known since Kellgren (1938) reported his studies about 50 years ago. Sessle (1990; Sessle, Hu, Amano, & Zhong, 1986) and Mense (1990; Mense & Meyer, 1988) have demonstrated that visceral and somatic afferents carrying impulses from peripheral nociceptive stimuli in muscle can modulate the excitability of nociceptive receptor neurons so that they shift the mechanical threshold of these cells into the innocuous range. Normally nonpainful mechanical stimulation thereby elicits painful nociceptive responses.

The receptive fields of dorsal horn neurons can also be modulated and altered by peripheral stimulation. Convergence of afferent inputs from cutaneous, visceral, and motor nociceptive receptors occurs in spinal and trigeminal somatosensory neurons. Responsiveness of central sensory neurons to converging afferent input from different peripheral sites of origin can be enhanced by peripheral nociceptive input. A noxious or painful lesion in muscle widens the receptive field of the nociceptive neuron in the dorsal horn, and sensitizes it to respond to normally innocuous mechanical stimulation. Thus, non-noxious stimuli may be interpreted by the brain as painful and as coming from other areas of the body that share a common pathway to the spinal cord and brain when they travel via afferents that arise in the wide-dynamic-range neuron. Other explanations for the phenomenon of referred pain have been put forth (Selzer & Spencer, 1969), but as yet none has been as well supported by experimental evidence as the convergence-projection theory described above.

DIAGNOSTIC STEPS

History

The initial step in the evaluation of the patient is the determination of the nature and distribution of the pain. The history or story of the problem always includes a general medical history identifying factors that potentially contribute to the persistence of chronic MTrPs. The description of the initiating event is, of course, essential. In addition, a review of daily recreational and work activities should highlight physical and postural stresses that bear on activation of MTrPs. Medications, including birth control pills, dietary habits, and smoking and drinking habits are also important in the identification of causes of persistent pain.

Patients are often unaware of the relationship of posture to activity. Therefore, care must be taken to obtain a detailed description of actual physical activity related to daily tasks in order to understand the stresses that contribute to muscle overload and muscle fatigue. Information gathered from the patient sometimes may be obtained only with persistence on the part of the examiner. A secretary once told me that she worked with a word processor, a typewriter, telephones, and adding machines. I found that her cluttered desk forced her to turn her head sharply to the left for long periods of time in order to read material that was placed behind and to the left of her chair. Her work postures created an overload and fatigue of the levator scapulae and sternocleidomastoid mus-

cles. It is not enough just to ask what someone's occupation is or what he or she does for a living. The examiner needs a description of actual body positions and movements. Photographs of the workplace can be quite enlightening in this regard.

The history must explore social upheavals caused by the pain syndrome, and it must provide insight into the nature of the family support or the disruption of family relationships in order for the practitioner to have a concept of the effect of the pain syndrome on the economic and social life of the patient, and to understand the psychological strengths and weaknesses that influence recovery (see Kerns & Jacob, Chapter 14).

A body diagram upon which the patient draws a picture of his pain, noting the more severe, persistent painful areas and the milder, lesser affected areas, and areas of dysesthesias and paresthesias, is extremely helpful to the clinician. Colored pencils may be used to highlight important points in the drawing. The drawing can be prepared prior to the physician entering the examining room, or it may be completed jointly by the physician and the patient (Figure 5.1).

Physical Examination

The physical examination of a patient being evaluated for pain must include an assessment of the muscles for active MTrPs. However, the approach should never be one of assuming that MPS is or is not the cause of the pain. The history and physical examination approach the problem as an unknown and are meant to discover the causes of discomfort or dysfunction. The examination, therefore, is comprehensive beginning with an evaluation of the mental state of the patient (for depression, anger, resignation, motivation, etc.) (see Bradley, Haile, & Jaworski, Chapter 12).

Bodily asymmetries and postural imbalances—factors that may produce stress on axial or limb muscles—are noted even while the history is being obtained. Gait is evaluated for evidence of hip and shoulder imbalance (tilt) caused by a leg-length discrepancy or scoliosis, and for excessive pronation, supination, and internal or external rotation of the foot. Scoliosis is noted if present, and a determination is made as to whether it is pseudoscoliosis due to spasm of the quadratus lumborum muscle that

A.

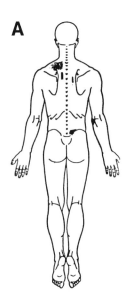

FIGURE 5.1. A. Copy of a drawing made by a 47-year-old man with a 30-month history of left shoulder pain, localized to the trapezius muscle. In addition, he noted areas of low back pain. He reported having polio affecting his neck and upper back at age eight.

B. Copy of the drawing made by the examiner at the time of physical examination. The left leg is smaller and shorter than the right, the left iliac crest is lower than the right, and an S-shaped scoliosis is present. The left shoulder is lower than the right shoulder. Myofascial trigger points (X's) are noted in both infraspinatus muscles, in the left upper and lower trapezius and in the left teres minor muscles, in both quadratus lumborum and gluteus maximus muscles, and in the left serratus anterior muscle. A lift under the left buttock when sitting and under the left heel when standing reduced the scoliosis and shoulder tilt. The diagnosis in this patient is regional myofascial pain syndrome involving the left trapezius, infraspinatus, teres minor and serratus anterior muscles, perpetuated by a structural imbalance caused by a leg length discrepancy and secondary scoliosis. When the structural asymmetry was corrected, the MTrPs were easily inactivated.

C. A body diagram prepared by a young woman showing bilateral neck, shoulder and arm pain with distal limb numbness. She had bilateral MTrPs in the neck and shoulders with referred pain and paresthesias in the wrists and hands. Eventual complete resolution of her problem was accomplished by dental treatment of MTrPs of the neck and jaw, and correcting stresses in neck and shoulder muscles created by unusually awkward working postures.

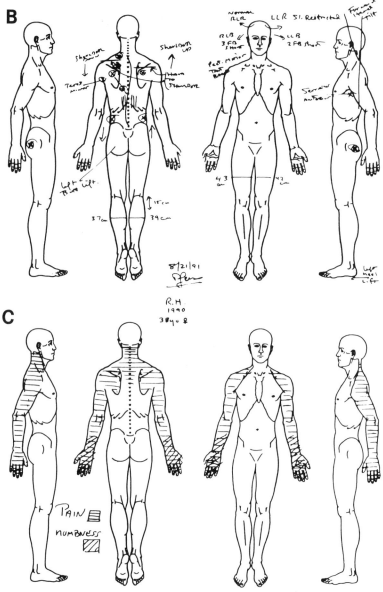

attaches superiorly to the lower rib cage and inferiorly to the iliac crest, or to the shortening of the piriformis muscle, an external rotator of the leg. These muscles are stretched using intermittent cold, or vapocoolant spray, and stretch (Nielson, 1978; Travell, 1952). Sitting posture is likewise evaluated for shoulder tilt and spinal curvature, possibly indicating a small half-pelvis.

In the *short leg syndrome* (Travell & Simons, 1983, 1992) there is a leg-length discrepancy that produces a pelvic tilt, the pelvis on the side of the short leg being lower, which in turn produces a tilt of the lumbar spine to the side of the short leg (see Figure 5.2). A compensatory curve to the opposite side rights the torso, the spine thus forming a C-shape, convex to the short leg side, thereby elevating the shoulder ipsilateral to the short leg. *Hence, the side of the high shoulder is often the side of the short leg.* An S-shaped spinal curvature frequently develops if the leg-length discrepancy is greater than 1/2 in. Use of a heel lift under the appropriate foot or a butt lift under the appropriate ischial prominence of the pelvis can eliminate a postural asymmetry that causes musculoskeletal stress. Diagnostically, many

persons experience relief within minutes following the use of a heel lift or a butt lift, confirming the clinical suspicion that the imbalance is clinically relevant to the painful state.

In persons with low back or lower extremity MPS, the foot should be examined for a long second metatarsal bone and a relatively short first metatarsal bone, the foot configuration described by Morton (1935). This configuration shifts the body weight when walking from the head of the first metatarsal to the head of the second metatarsal bone. The foot is pronated, the leg internally rotated at the knee and hip. MTrPs are activated in the peroneus longus muscle, which refers pain to the ankle; the vastus medialis, which refers pain to the knee; and the gluteus medius, which refers pain to the low back. Calluses under the head of the second metatarsal bone and along the medial aspect of the great toe and foot indicate that weight-bearing is abnormal.

Neurologic examination is performed to identify cervical or lumbar radiculopathy, peripheral nerve entrapment, or peripheral neuropathy, and yields clues concerning nutritional deficiency states and other underlying pathologic conditions. Sensory loss in a dermatomal distribution, with loss of deep tendon reflexes and weakness of appropriate muscles, indicates a radiculopathy or peripheral neuropathy. Pain and paresthesias elicited by percussion over a peripheral nerve (Tinel's sign) indicate a focal compressive neuropathy. A symmetrical distal sensory loss, often with loss of Achilles tendon reflexes, is seen in many neuropathies, including nutritional deficiencies. However, selective loss of vibration and position sense in the legs, but with hyperactive reflexes and often with the Babinski toe sign, signifies vitamin B12 deficiency. A small, weak limb with absent reflexes but with normal sensation suggests past polio.

Examination of the muscles is a hands-on procedure that initiates the therapeutic relationship between the practitioner and the patient. The direct contact of palpation can have a confidence-building effect as well as a bonding effect when the examiner is gentle and nonthreatening. For this reason, palpation and manipulation are often best begun in a nonpainful or less painful area of the body to put the patient at ease and to avoid guarding. The patient should be comfortable and warm, with the arms and legs well supported.

Range of motion is evaluated prior to palpa-

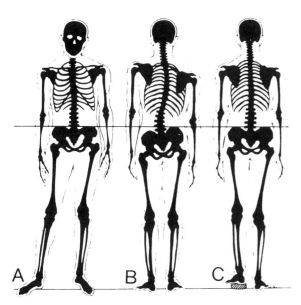

FIGURE 5.2. Structural imbalance caused by a short leg. In this illustration, a short left leg causes the pelvis to tilt producing a secondary scoliosis which is corrected by a heel lift. Note that the shoulders are tilted as well as the pelvis. From Travell and Simons (1983), page 650. Copyright 1983, the Williams & Wilkins Co., Baltimore. Reprinted by permission.

tion of muscle. Results of this aspect of the exam as well as of subsequent examination for TrPs, are recorded on a body chart during the examination. This provides a visual record of inestimable value in reviewing examinations at a later date. The diagrams can also be reviewed with patients to demonstrate progress or changes in their physical status. Range of motion is examined for the head and neck, the shoulder, the waist, the hips, and the smaller joints.

Restriction of motion is noted, and is used to identify muscle groups or functional units that are likely to harbor active MTrPs. Restriction of head rotation occurs with MTrPs in the levator scapulae and sternocleidomastoid muscles. Limitation of external (lateral) rotation of the arm at the shoulder, attempting to bring the arm around behind the head, and the hand to the opposite side of the mouth (the mouth wraparound test) occurs when the subscapularis muscle or the biceps brachii muscle contains active TrPs. Inability to internally (medially) rotate the arm fully to bring the hand behind the back to the opposite scapula (hand to scapula test) is seen with infraspinatus and teres minor MTrPs. Limited bending at the waist results from MTrPs in the quadratus lumborum, a muscle that is a common, but often overlooked, cause of low back pain. Limited internal rotation of the leg at the hip indicates active piriformis muscle TrPs, the piriformis muscle being a major external rotator of the leg.

The MTrP is an objective physical sign that is identified by palpation of muscle. Patients have reported that previous examiners had not performed a manual examination and therefore did not find MTrPs. The muscle to be examined should be placed under slight tension to facilitate palpation of the taut band and the production of the LTR. The taut band and LTR cannot easily be elicited on a fully shortened or fully lengthened muscle. Examination of an individual muscle may be done using either a pincer grasp or by using flat palpation. The pincer grasp in which the muscle is gently rolled and palpated between the fingertips (Figure 5.3) is used for such muscles as the sternocleidomastoid and the latissimus dorsi (Figure 5.4).

Muscles that overlie bone and that cannot be palpated using a pincer grasp are examined with flat palpation, gently rolling the muscle over the underlying bone to identify the taut band

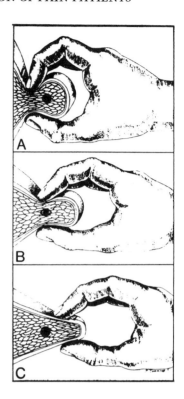

FIGURE 5.3. Pincer palpation showing the trigger point being rolled between the palpating fingers. From Travell and Simons (1983), page 61. Copyright 1983, the Williams & Wilkins Co., Baltimore. Reprinted by permission.

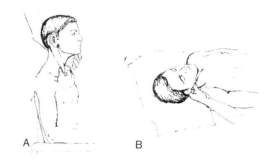

FIGURE 5.4. Examination of the sternocleidomastoid muscle for MTrPs using pincer palpation. From Travell and Simons (1983), page 211. Copyright 1983, the Williams & Wilkins Co., Baltimore. Reprinted by permission.

and to elicit LTRs. Infraspinatus, longissimus lumborum, and gluteal muscles are examples of muscles well examined by flat palpation. The muscle is examined for the presence of taut bands, and both observed and palpated for LTRs. The patient is asked if the muscle is tender and, if so, if pain is felt elsewhere and if it is like the spontaneous pain that is usually experienced. Radiation of pain to pain reference zones is noted and recorded.

Muscles in the functional motor unit are examined for *secondary* MTrPs. Muscles in the zone of referred pain are examined for *satellite* MTrPs. In each case, the MTrPs may persist after the initiating muscle is treated, and therefore need to be identified in order to inactivate them in the treatment phase of management.

The diagnosis of the MPS depends upon the skill of the examiner and the care taken to assess each muscle. With practice, taut bands can be identified with confidence, and LTRs elicited without difficulty. Stretch the muscle following the examination using intermittent cold and stretch and then warm the muscle with moist heat in order to diminish the pain and discomfort produced by manipulation and palpation of sore muscle.

MTrPs can be found in many asymptomatic individuals. They may be spontaneously active causing pain at rest (phase I). A less irritable TrP causes pain only on movement (phase II TrP). Latent MTrPs restrict motion and cause stiffness and referred pain or tenderness but are painful when injected (phase III TrP). The normal muscle without pain or tenderness has no TrPs (phase IV) (Travell, 1990). Many people have phase III MTrPs with no real complaint of pain. The taut band and LTR can be found in a phase III TrP.

A single-muscle MPS is very likely to be acute, as there is a tendency for the MPS to spread, with time, through activation of MTrPs in functional motor units and in zones of referred pain. Single-muscle syndromes are less complicated than widespread MPS, but nonetheless they require examination of the entire functional motor unit and of the common areas of referred pain. As MPS becomes chronic, extension of MTrPs along a chain of muscles will cause multiple regions of myofascial pain to develop. For example, the subscapularis-latissimus dorsi-quadratus lumborum chain of muscles acts as a muscular link connecting the shoulder girdle muscles with those of the hip and low back.

Systematic identification of the muscles involved in widespread MPS is done by applying the principles of examination described for a single muscle to the entire functional motor unit and to the muscles in the zone of referred pain. The patient may complain of diffuse pain, or of pain in an entire side, but the examiner may find widespread latent or inactive TrPs that are painful only when examined and that may not have been appreciated by the patient prior to the examination.

The diagnostic process is not confined to identification of MTrPs. As pointed out in the discussion of the medical history, the diagnostic process includes uncovering the physical stresses that initiate the process and that cause it to persist. This requires attending to the details of daily routine. The schoolteacher who was found to have bilateral trapezius TrPs habitually carried shopping bags of craft supplies to and from school daily. The church organist who had bilateral trapezius, levator scapulae, and supra- and infraspinatus muscle TrPs, held her arms unsupported while playing the organ for long periods of time. A dentist chronically elevated his right shoulder when working from the side of his patient, and a trombonist raised his left shoulder tucking his ear against his shoulder while playing his instrument. Each of these individuals had prominent levator scapulae MTrPs. Persons who cradle the telephone receiver between their ear and shoulder also risk activating levator scapulae and scalene TrPs.

Obvious sources of MTrPs and development of the MPS are seen in postsurgical patients, including patients treated for lumbar radiculopathy who no longer have neurologic signs of sensory loss or reflex change, but who have gluteal or quadratus lumborum MTrPs instead, causing persistent pain. MTrPs can also occur in the abdominal wall after abdominal or pelvic surgery. Treatment should then proceed to inactivate them, thereby reducing postoperative pain.

Laboratory Tests

There are no general laboratory tests that are specific for MPS. Blood counts and blood chemistries, urinalyses, and stool examinations are used to identify coexistent and contributory illnesses such as gout and rheumatoid arthritis, infections, hypothyroidism (Sonkin, 1988), nutritional deficiencies, and iron deficiency (Beard & Borel, 1988; Beard, Green, Miller, & Finch, 1984). X-ray imaging, bone scans, CT scans, and MRI do not identify the MTrP, but will identify herniated disc, intrathecal tumors, ligamentous tears, Paget's disease, osteoporotic changes of bone, and degenerative changes of joints, which either produce pain themselves or which aggravate or perpetuate myofascial pain. Electromyography and nerve conduction tests show no specific abnormality in MPS, but can identify other neuromuscular disorders.

Two laboratory tests are of value in the evaluation of MPS. They are thermography and pressure threshold algometry (Fischer, 1988; Jaeger & Reeves, 1986). The thermogram shows a "hot spot" in the vicinity of the MTrP. The pressure threshold for pain is reduced in the same vicinity as the hot spot. Clinical examination of these areas shows that the combination of the hot spot and the reduced pressure threshold required to cause pain correlates well with the presence of the MTrP. In addition, the thermogram may show changes in heat emission indicative of reflex sympathetic disfunction, which can coexist with MPS, be induced by the MTrP, or perpetuate the MTrP.

Perpetuating Factors

Many patients have a long history of pain, rather than an acute problem. In such instances, the practitioner must find out why there has not been improvement as expected following the usual effective treatments. I have already touched upon some of the postural factors that tend to prevent normal recovery, such as the short leg and the small hemipelvis syndrome. Short upper arms, where the elbow does not extend to the iliac crest, can also cause problems through lack of support of the shoulder girdle when sitting. The arms will not reach the armrests of most chairs and will therefore be unsupported, stressing the trapezius muscles in particular. Chronic muscle compression also perpetuates MTrPs. A woman with pendulous breasts frequently has the trapezius muscles compressed by the shoulder straps of her brassiere, with a readily identifiable indentation in the muscles of the shoulder. Even the tight elastic tops of socks can compress the calf muscles enough to perpetuate MTrPs.

Systemic or general medical factors that lead to muscular stress because of nutritional, metabolic, or hormonal abnormalities act as perpetuating factors. Noting coexistent conditions that may aggravate or promote MTrP development and that need treatment is most important.

Hypothyroidism (Wilke, Sheeler, & Makarowski, 1981) produces a state of chronic fatigue and muscle weakness. Highly sensitive TSH determinations are a sensitive way of evaluating thyroid function and should be used in suspect cases. Iron is essential for cytochrome oxidase function (required for oxidative phosphorylation) and for nonshivering-related thermal regulation (Beard & Borrel, 1988; Beard et al., 1984). When individuals complain of chronic, widespread muscle pain, of feeling cold when others feel comfortable, and of cramping following exercise, then hypothyroidism and iron insufficiency (as determined by the serum ferritin test) should be considered. Symptoms of folic acid insufficiency include restless legs, headache, muscular irritability, myalgias, diarrhea, and cold intolerance (Herbert & Coleman, 1988). The weakness, abnormal gait, and body asymmetry of old polio commonly produce MTrPs. Gouty arthritis and rheumatoid arthritis are other systemic disorders associated with MPS. MPS is a treatable cause of nonmalignant pain in persons with cancer. Identifying the underlying causes of chronic MPS allows correction of those factors which perpetuate the syndrome and which impede recovery and inactivation of the MTrPs.

Fibromyalgia

A chronic, painful muscular disorder often discussed in association with MPS, fibromyalgia (FM) must be distinguished from MPS conceptually and clinically. FM is diffusely painful, affecting the body as a whole. The generalized nature of FM is well illustrated by the observation that identification of 11 of 18 specific points as tender (defined as complaint of pain alone, pain with grimace or flinch, adversive withdrawal, or pain so severe as to render palpation intolerable) was the most sensitive, specific, and accurate diagnostic test found by the Multicenter Study for the Classification for Fibromyalgia (Wolfe et al., 1990). The finding of 11 tender points out of 18 sites assures the examiner that muscle tenderness is widespread and is present in both the right and left sides of the body and in the upper and lower regions of the body. In addition to widespread pain, a nonrestorative sleep pattern with morning fatigue, pain and stiffness is found in most patients with FM. The non-REM sleep disorder is an intrusion of alpha activity into Stage IV or delta sleep, thereby reducing total Stage IV sleep time. The alpha-delta sleep disturbance is not confined to FM, but is seen in other conditions, including sleep-related myoclonus, rheumatoid arthritis, and ankylosing spondylitis. Frequently seen in FM, but less commonly than the sleep disorder, are irritable bowel syndromes, SICCA syndrome, Raynaud's phenomenon, paresthesias, headaches and anxiety. These symptoms, however, are not essential to the diagnosis of FM (Bennett, 1990; Russell, 1989; Wolfe, 1989; Wolfe et al., 1990).

FM is a generalized and widespread disorder; MPS is regional, not systemic, even when more than one region is involved. If FM is chronic, MPS may be acute or chronic. FM can be primary or secondary (although it is more often primary); MPS is usually secondary, to trauma, for example. MTrPs are not necessary for the diagnosis of FM, although they can be found in patients who have FM. Nonrestorative sleep is common in FM, but sleep is generally normal and less disturbed by pain in MPS. FM requires long-term management and tends to be persistent, while MPS is potentially curable.

In practice, one must question the patient about sleep disturbance, easy fatiguability, distribution of pain, and associated medical disorders such as irritable bowel syndrome, dry eyes, and dry mouth. The examination of the patient must involve evaluation of the characteristic sites for tender spots, and a generalized survey of muscles including palpation for TrPs and examination for restricted movement with active or passive movement of parts of the body in order to determine whether the disorder is generalized or regional.

In conclusion, diagnosis of MPS requires knowing in what circumstances MPS is likely to occur, identifying those circumstances through the history, evaluating the restricted motion at the affected joint and in the affected muscle, palpating the muscle in order to identify MTrPs, and identifying MTrPs in the functional motor unit and in the referred pain zone (secondary and satellite TrPs respectively). Finally, the clinician must consider why certain persons do not recover as expected and must then search for the mechanical and general medical abnormalities that delay recovery and that perpetuate the MPS.

Acknowledgments. The author thanks Teresa Menendez for her assistance in preparation of the manuscript, and Cathy Cumbo of the Washington Adventist Hospital Medical Library, Takoma Park, Maryland.

REFERENCES

Beard, J., & Borel, M. (1988). Iron-deficiency and thermoregulation. *Nutrition Today, 23,* 41–45.

Beard, J., Green, W., Miller, L., & Finch, C. (1984). Effect of iron-deficiency anemia on hormone levels and thermoregulation during cold exposure. *American Journal of Physiology, 247,* 114–119.

Bennett, R.M. (1990). Myofascial pain syndromes and the fibromyalgia syndrome: A comparative analysis. In J.R. Fricton & E.A. Awad (Eds.), *Myofascial pain and fibromyalgia. Advances in pain research and therapy* (Vol. 17, pp. 43–66). New York: Raven Press.

Bierring-Sorenson, F. (1982). Low back trouble in a general population of 30-40-50 & 60-year-old men and women. *Danish Medical Bulletin, 29,* 289–299.

Dexter, J.R., & Simons, D.G. (1981). Local twitch response in human muscle evoked by palpation and needle penetration of a trigger point. *Archives of Physical Medicine & Rehabilitation, 62,* 521 (Abstract).

Fischer, A.A. (1988). Documentation of myofascial trigger points. *Archives of Physical Medicine & Rehabilitation, 69,* 286–291.

Fricton, J., Auvinen, N., Dykstra, D., & Schiffman, E. (1985). Myofascial pain syndrome: Electromyographic changes associated with local twitch response. *Archives of Physical Medicine & Rehabilitation, 66,* 314–317.

Fricton, J. R. (1990). Myofascial pain syndrome: Characteristics and epidemiology. In J.R. Fricton & E.A. Awad (Eds.). *Myofascial pain and fibromyalgia. Advances in pain research and therapy* (Vol. 17, pp. 107–128). New York: Raven Press.

Herbert, V.D., & Coleman, N. (1988). Folic acid & vit. B12. In M.E. Shills & B.R. Young (Eds.), *Modern nutrition in health and disease.* (7th ed., pp. 388–416). Philadelphia: Lea & Febiger.

Hong, C-Z., & Simons, D.G. (1988). Persistence of local twitch response with loss of conduction to and from spinal cord. *Archives of Physical Medicine and Rehabilitation, 69,* 789 (Abstract).

Jaeger, B., & Reeves, J.L. (1986). Quantification of changes in myofascial trigger point sensitivity with the pressure algometer following passive stretch. *Pain, 27,* 203–210.

Kellgren, J.H. (1938). A preliminary account of referred pains arising from muscle. *British Medical Journal, 1,* 325–327.

Mense, S. (1990). Physiology of nociception in muscles. In J.R. Fricton and E. A. Awad (Eds.), *Myofascial pain and fibromyalgia. Advances in pain research and therapy* (Vol. 17, pp. 67–86). New York: Raven Press.

Mense, S., & Meyer, H. (1988). Bradykinin induced modulation of the response behavior of different types of feline group iii and iv muscle receptors. *Journal of Physiology, 398,* 49–63.

Morton, D.J. (1935). *The human foot.* New York: Columbia University Press.

Nielson, A.J. (1978). Spray and stretch for myofascial pain. *Physical Therapy, 58,* 567–569.

Rosomoff, H.L., Fishbain, D.A., Goldberg, M., & Rosomoff, R.S. (1990). Myofascial findings with patients with "chronic intractable benign pain" of the back and neck. *Pain Management*, *3*, 114–118.

Rosomoff, H.L., Fishbain, D.A., Goldberg, M., Santana, R., & Rosomoff, R.S. (1989). Physical findings in patients with chronic intractable benign pain of the neck and/or back. *Pain*, *37*, 279–287.

Russell, I.J. (1989). Neurohormonal aspects of fibromyalgia syndrome. *Rheumatic Disease Clinics of North America*, *15*, 149–168.

Selzer, M., & Spencer, W.A. (1969). Convergence of visceral and cutaneous afferent pathways in the lumbar spinal cord. *Brain Research*, *14*, 331–348.

Sessle, B.J. (1990). Central nervous system mechanisms of muscular pain. In J.R. Fricton and E.A. Awad (Eds.), *Myofascial pain and fibromyalgia. Advances in pain research and therapy* (Vol. 17, pp. 86–106). New York: Raven Press.

Sessle, B.J., Hu, J.W., Amano, N., & Zhong, G. (1986). Convergence of cutaneous tooth pulp visceral neck and muscle afferents onto nociceptive and non-nociceptive neurons in trigeminal subnucleus caudalis (medullary dorsal horn) and its implications for referred pain. *Pain*, *27*, 219–235.

Simons, D.G. (1988). A myofascial pain syndrome due to trigger points. In J. Goodgold (Ed.), *Rehabilitation medicine* (pp. 686–723). St. Louis: Mosby.

Simons, D.G. (1989). Single muscle myofascial pain syndromes. In C.D. Tollison (Ed.), *Handbook of chronic pain management* (pp. 490–508). Baltimore: Williams & Wilkins.

Skootsky, S. A., Jaeger, B., & Oye, R.K. (1989). Prevalence of myofascial pain in general internal medicine practice. *Western Journal of Medicine*, *151*, 157–160.

Sola, A.E., & Bonica, J.J. (1990). Myofascial pain syndromes. In J.J. Bonica (Ed.), *The management of pain* (2nd ed., pp. 352–367). Philadelphia: Lee & Febiger.

Sonkin, L.S. (1988). Myofascial pain in metabolic disorders. In H. Kraus (Ed.), *Diagnosis and treatment of muscle pain* (pp. 91–96). Chicago: Quintessence Books.

Travell, J. (1952). Ethyl chloride spray for painful muscle spasm. *Archives of Physical Medicine*, *33*, 291–298.

Travell, J.G. (1990). Chronic Myofascial Pain Syndromes: Mysteries of the history. In J.R. Fricton and E.A. Awad (Eds.), *Myofascial pain and fibromyalgia. Advances in pain research and therapy* (Vol. 17, pp. 129–137). New York: Raven Press.

Travell, J.G., & Simons, D.G. (1983). *Myofascial pain and dysfunction: The trigger point manual* (Vol. 1). Baltimore, Williams & Wilkins.

Travell, J.G., & Simons, D.G. (1992). *Myofascial pain and dysfunction: The trigger point manual* (Vol. 2). Baltimore, Williams & Wilkins.

Wilke, W.S., Sheeler, L.R., & Makarowski, W.S. (1981). Hypothyroidism with presenting symptoms of fibrositis. *Journal of Rheumatology*, *8*, 626–630.

Wolfe, F. (1989). Fibromyalgia: The clinical syndrome. *Rheumatic Disease Clinics of North America*, *15*, 1–17.

Wolfe, F., Smythe, H.A., Yunus, M.B., Bennett, R.M., Bombardier, C., Goldenberg, D.L., Tudwell, P., Campbell, S.M., Ables, M., Clark, P., Fam, A.G., Farber, S.J., Fiechtner, J.J., Franklin, C.M., Gatter, R.A., Hamaty, D., Lessard, J., Lichtbroun, A.S., Masi, A.T., McCain, G.A., Reynolds, W.J., Romano, T.J., Russell, I.J., & Sheon, R.P. (1990). The American College of Rheumatology 1990 criteria for the classification for fibromyalgia. Report of the Multi-Center Criteria Committee. *Arthritis and Rheumatism*, *33*, 160–172.

Chapter 6

Ergonomic Approaches in the Clinical Assessment of Occupational Musculoskeletal Disorders

MICHAEL FEUERSTEIN, PhD
PAUL F. HICKEY, MEd

Pain related to the musculoskeletal system is the most frequent cause of clinic visits in primary care settings (Deyo & Tsui-Wu, 1987; Knapp & Koch, 1984; National Center for Health Statistics, 1984, 1986). Although the specific etiologies of these various musculoskeletal pain problems remain an enigma, evidence suggests that workplace factors can play a role in the initiation, exacerbation, and maintenance of pain associated with these various musculoskeletal disorders (Kelsey & Golden, 1987; Putz-Anderson, 1988). Data from the United States suggest that disorders of the musculoskeletal system that involve damage to the tendons, tendon sheaths and related bones, muscles, and nerves of the hands, wrists, elbows, arms, back, or legs represent a relatively high percentage of all occupational illnesses/injuries (Bureau of Labor Statistics, 1991). These problems have significantly increased in incidence over the past decade (Bureau of Labor Statistics, 1991). It is commonly assumed that these disorders are associated with occupations that involve forceful exertions, awkward postures, and repetitive motions (Chaffin & Anderson, 1990; Putz-Anderson, 1988). These disorders typically include activity-related spinal disorders of the upper, middle, and lower spine (Spitzer, LeBlanc, & Dupuis, 1987) and the upper extremity cumulative trauma disorders (UECTDs) including a range of nerve entrapment and tendinitis-related disorders (Putz-Anderson, 1988). Although for the majority of cases and disorders symptoms are self-limiting, if acute medical management efforts are not successful and pain persists these problems can result in chronic pain and disability (Feuerstein, 1991).

For those cases where an occupational musculoskeletal disorder of either an acute or chronic nature is associated with work disability, an increased emphasis has been placed on recovery of function with particular focus on return-to-work. This approach is in contrast to the earlier focus on pain or symptom relief or management. Over the past decade, clinicians and researchers have indicated the utility of such an active approach to rehabilitation and rapid, safe return-to-work, providing the patient has obtained maximal medical recovery despite the absence of complete pain relief for low back pain cases (Mayer et al., 1987; Mitchell & Carmen, 1990) and upper extremity disorders (Flinn-Wagner, Mladonicky, & Goodman, 1990; Mitchell & Carmen, 1990). This emphasis on return-to-work suggested the need for a comprehensive conceptual model that identifies the multiple factors that can contribute to work disability and form the basis for an integrated evaluation and rehabilitation approach to occupational musculoskeletal disorders, applicable to subacute (1–3 months) and chronic (3–22 months) cases where pain persists. Feuerstein (1991) recently proposed such a conceptual model based upon available epidemiological and clinical research. This model is illustrated in Figure 6.1 below.

The model proposes four broad factors that can influence the work reentry process. These include the medical status of the individual, particularly in the musculoskeletal, neurologic, and cardiovascular systems. The physical capabilities of the individual represents the second component. This area includes the physical status or degree of strength, flexibility, and endurance in specific muscle groups as well as the aerobic capacity of the individual. Physical capabilities also include the work tolerances characteristic of the individual which may include lifting, walking, standing, sitting, climb-

ing, and reach capabilities among others. The third component includes the work demands of the job the individual is returning to, both physiologic demands including both biomechanical and aerobic demands as well as the psychological demands of the work. The last component of the model includes psychological and behavioral factors including worker traits, psychological readiness to return to work (e.g., expectation to return to work, work environment, and family support), and the ability to manage pain and symptoms. These psychological factors can influence the work reentry process independently or through their impact on the interaction between physical capabilities and work demands. (Refer to Figure 6.1.)

It is assumed that, if these multiple factors contribute to work disability, a comprehensive assessment should consider each of these areas. Such an evaluation includes (1) assessment of the patient's medical status as it impacts the capacity for work, (2) physical capabilities of the individual in relation to work demands, and (3) evaluation of the potential psychological and behavioral factors that can influence the return-to-work process. This chapter emphasizes the assessment of work demands with a focus on the clinical application of ergonomics. It is important to emphasize, however, that this area should be considered in the broader context of the multiple factors that can present barriers to work reentry in patients with occupational musculoskeletal disorders.

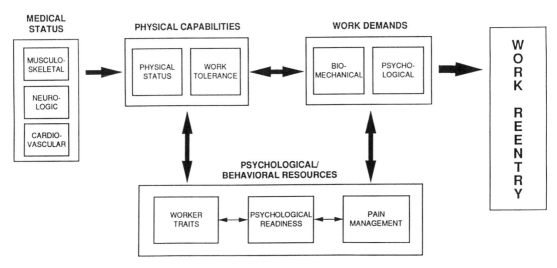

FIGURE 6.1. Factors potentially affecting work disability associated with the occupational musculoskeletal disorders. From Feuerstein (1991), page 10. Copyright 1991 Plenum Press. Reprinted by permission.

Ergonomics represents an area that is inadequately addressed in the assessment of pain, particularly in cases with persistent pain. As briefly discussed above, given the magnitude of musculoskeletal-related pain problems, and the role that work factors may play in these disorders, assessment of the workplace from an ergonomic perspective in a given patient represents an important component of a comprehensive pain assessment.

Ergonomics has been defined as "that branch of science and technology that includes what is known and theorized about human behavioral and biological characteristics that can be validly applied to the specification, design, evaluation, operation, and maintenance of products and systems to enhance safe, effective, satisfying use by individuals, groups and organizations" (Christensen, Topmiller, & Gill, 1988, pp. 7–8). Ergonomics is a diverse field with multiple methodological approaches. In the context of health and safety, the goals of ergonomics are typically reduced risk of trauma in the workplace and improved performance. This focuses on the use of ergonomic principles and methodologies in the comprehensive assessment of the patient with a musculoskeletal pain disorder in which occupational factors are assumed to play a role. Ergonomic assessment and subsequent ergonomic consultation in this clinical context are directed at returning the individual to some form of safe, productive work.

This chapter first provides a review of ergonomic factors that may contribute to discomfort, pain, and disability in those with occupational musculoskeletal disorders, particularly back disorders and the UECTDs. Following this, a brief discussion of the difference between the classic ergonomics approach and the use of ergonomics in the clinic is presented. The next section orients the clinician to some of the assessment approaches used in ergonomics and provide examples of selected methods. Representative ergonomic job analysis protocols are then reviewed, and case examples of the application of ergonomic principles to the assessment of patients with persistent low back pain and medial epicondylitis are illustrated. The purpose of this chapter is to provide an introduction to certain principles and techniques in ergonomics that can be applied in the clinical context to develop a rehabilitation program that more accurately considers the work environment in its broadest definition, with the assumption that such consideration facilitates a more timely and safe work reentry.

ERGONOMIC FACTORS ASSOCIATED WITH INCREASED RISK OF MUSCULOSKELETAL PAIN

There is an extensive literature on workplace factors that have been associated with increased risk of activity-related spinal disorders (Pope, Andersson, Frymoyer, & Chaffin, 1991; Spitzer et al., 1987) and UECTDs (Putz-Anderson, 1988). A detailed review of the workplace epidemiology of the occupational musculoskeletal disorders is beyond the scope of this chapter. The authors will, therefore, focus on six generic categories of ergonomic risk factors (Keyserling, Armstrong, & Punnett, 1991) as the basic factors the clinician involved in ergonomic assessment of the injured worker should attend to when considering the potential role of the workplace in the initiation, exacerbation, and/or maintenance of pain. These factors include: (1) forceful exertions, (2) awkward work postures, (3) localized contact stresses, (4) whole-body or segmental vibration, (5) temperature extremes, and (6) repetitive motions or prolonged activities. The authors add psychosocial job stress to the list, given findings indicating the importance of such factors as perceived work environment on pain (Feuerstein, Sult, & Houle, 1985), work disability (Gallagher et al., 1989) and the influence of quality of work-life on reports of work-absence related to back pain (Bigos et al., 1991). This section briefly reviews each of these factors. It is important to realize that these factors have been observed in a variety of jobs both in the manufacturing and service industries (Bureau of Labor Statistics, 1991). As well, these risk factors can occur in what, on the surface, appears to be a relatively low risk job. Extreme metabolic demands were also included as potential ergonomic risk factors.

Forceful Exertions

Lifting, pushing, and pulling are among the activities that are considered to be forceful whole-body exertions. A certain amount of muscle force is required, particularly in the lumbar or low back area, to move (lift, push, or pull) an outside object or load. The muscle force required to overcome the load can result in compressive forces on the structures of the lower back such as the intervertebral discs and vertebrae. The size and shape of the load, the weight of the load, as well as the position of the load relative to the spine, can affect compressive forces on the spine (Figure 6.2). In other words, high muscle forces can create an increase in disc compression forces that can lead to disc-related injury risk.

The National Institute for Occupational Safety and Health (NIOSH) (U.S. Department of Health and Human Services, 1981) has developed a method to predict the compressive forces on the lumbar spine during occasional lifting. This early work reported that compres-

sion forces on the disc above 650 kg are associated with an eight times greater relative risk of back disorders. Chaffin and Park (1973) have indicated a high incidence of low back pain associated with heavy (repetitive) lifting (Figure 6.3). Additionally, Magora (1972) refers to sudden, unexpected maximal efforts as being harmful to the low back. Several researchers have associated heavy physical work, such as heavy lifting, pushing, and pulling, with an increase in low back pain.

The upper extremities are at risk of injury due to forceful exertion while using the hands. Jobs that require the use of hand tools and other objects such as knives and scissors increase the risk of certain UECTDs (Putz-

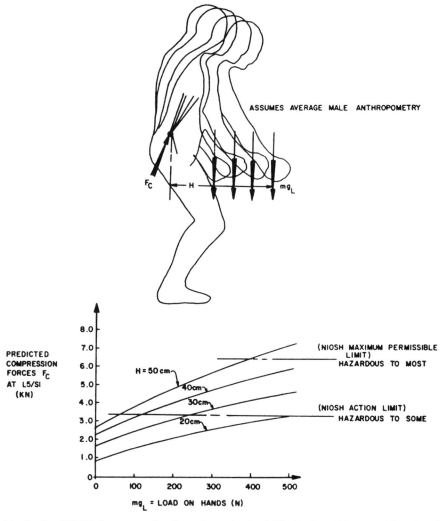

FIGURE 6.2. Predicted L5/S1 disc compression forces for varying loads lifted in four different positions from body. H = horizontal distance from L5/S1 disc; N = newtons; KN = kilonewtons. From Chaffin and Andersson (1991), page 228. Copyright 1991 John Wiley & Sons. Reprinted by permission.

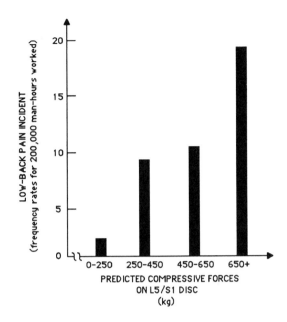

FIGURE 6.3. Relation between low back pain and peak compression forces. From Chaffin and Park (1973), page 521. Copyright 1973 American Industrial Hygiene Association. Reprinted by permission.

Anderson, 1988). Hand tools that require pinch grip, are heavy to hold, or are slippery or slick as well as tools that vibrate, and knives or scissors that have become dull can increase the amount of force required to use the particular instrument. Additionally, if the job requires the use of gloves due to such environmental factors as cold, there is an increased risk of developing certain UECTDs. The use of gloves increases the need for forceful grip of the tool or object (Eastman Kodak Company Ergonomics Group, 1986).

Awkward Postures

Keyserling et al. (1991) suggest that awkward posture at any articulation can result in transient fatigue and discomfort. They further state that remaining in an awkward posture for prolonged periods can lead to a variety of potentially disabling injuries and disorders of musculoskeletal tissue and/or peripheral nerves. Figure 6.4 presents graphically certain trunk and shoulder postures associated with reports of fatigue, pain, or discomfort, (Keyserling, 1986; Keyserling, Punnett, & Fine, 1988) as well as awkward postures of the wrist, hand, and forearm (Putz-Anderson, 1988).

Magora (1972) has found that prolonged sitting or standing postures among workers increase the risk of low back pain through increased intervertebral disc pressure. Figure 6.5 illustrates the relationship between various seated postures and disc pressure as compared to standing erect (Chaffin, Herrin, Keyserling & Garg, 1977). Additional awkward postures that increase the risk of low back pain have been reported (Snook, 1978). Snook observed that particularly when combined with lifting, awkward trunk postures such as forward bending, side bending, and twisting increased the likelihood of back pain.

With regard to the upper extremities, Byelle, Hagberg, and Michaelsson (1979) reported that workers who worked with their hands above acromion (shoulder) height had a higher risk of injury than those who worked below shoulder height. Armstrong (1986a) has suggested that awkward or extreme postures of the hand, wrist, elbow, and shoulder can increase the risk of UECTDs. Extreme or awkward positions include wrist flexion and extension, ulnar and radial deviation, forearm supination and pronation (Figure 6.4b), as well as pinch grips that are too wide or too narrow (Armstrong, 1986a; Putz-Anderson, 1988). Extended reaches in front or away from the body whether standing or seated may also increase the risk of related symptoms (Armstrong, 1986b).

Several workplace factors including workstation layout, equipment design, and the shape and orientation of handles of some hand tools can affect the postures necessary to complete a set of job tasks. These workplace factors can set the stage for the development and exacerbation of a variety of upper extremity–related symptoms (Keyserling et al., 1991).

Localized Contact Stresses

Keyserling et al. (1991) define localized contact or mechanical stresses as those caused by physical contact between body tissue and an object or a tool in the workplace. Examples of these contact stresses include resting the arms on the edge of a desk or table that may be sharp and unpadded using the hand or fist as a "hammer" and using tools that may be poorly designed for a given individual (right hand-dominant scissors used by a left-hand dominant person). Armstrong (1986a) suggests that these contact stresses may increase the risk of

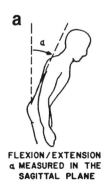
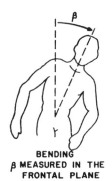
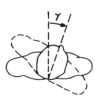

a

FLEXION/EXTENSION
α MEASURED IN THE
SAGITTAL PLANE

BENDING
β MEASURED IN THE
FRONTAL PLANE

TWISTING
γ IS ROTATION ABOUT THE
LONG AXIS OF THE TRUNK

NEUTRAL OCCURS WHEN THE TRUNK IS WITHIN 20 DEGREES OF
THE VERTICAL WITH LESS THAN 20 DEGREES OF TWISTING

STANDARD TRUNK POSTURES	
1. STAND-EXTENSION (α < 20°)	6. LIE-ON BACK OR SIDE
2. STAND-NEUTRAL	7. SIT-NEUTRAL
3. STAND-MILD FLEXION (20° ≤ α ≤ 45°)	8. SIT-MILD FLEXION
4. STAND-SEVERE FLEXION (α > 45°)	9. SIT-TWISTED/BENT
5. STAND-TWISTED/BENT (β OR γ > 20°)	

b

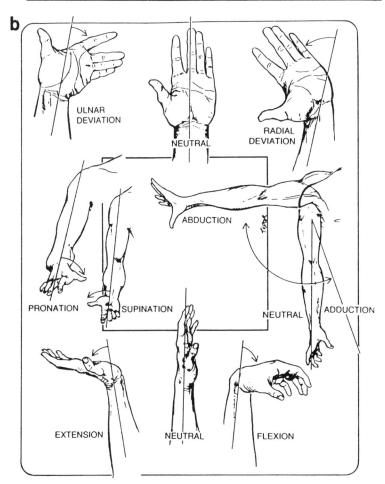

FIGURE 6.4. a. Trunk postures associated with back pain. From Keyserling (1986), page 642. Copyright 1986 American Industrial Hygiene Association. Reprinted by permission. **b.** Upper extremity postures (deviations from neutral position) that can initiate and/or exacerbate pain and discomfort. From Putz-Anderson (1988), page 116. Copyright 1988 Taylor & Francis Ltd. Reprinted by permission.

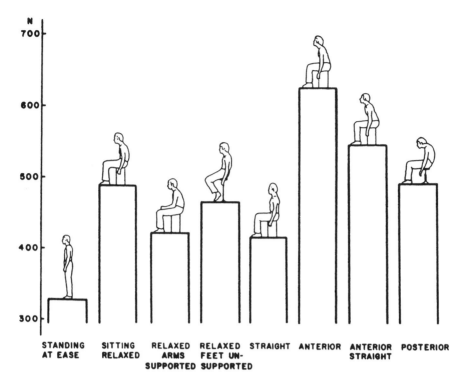

FIGURE 6.5. Disc pressure measurements in standing and unsupported sitting postures. From Andersson et al. (1974), page 108. Copyright 1974 *Scandinavian Journal of Rehabilitation Medicine*. Reprinted by permission.

UECTD such as carpal tunnel syndrome and other problems of the nerves as well as circulatory and/or tendon problems. Localized contact stresses are not limited to upper extremity problems as in the case of a poorly fit chair, which may affect the blood flow to the legs.

Vibration

Vibration or mechanical oscillations, produced by either regular or irregular periodic movements of a body about its resting posture (Grandjean, 1988), represent another potential workplace risk. For the purposes of ergonomics, vibration is divided into two areas: whole-body vibration, which typically acts on workers who are sitting or standing through a supporting surface (such as a truck), and segmental or localized vibration, which is transmitted to a body segment such as the hands and arms. The effects of vibration are dependent on the direction of the vibration input, the location of the various body segments, the level of fatigue of the worker, and the presence of external body supports (Chaffin & Andersson, 1991). Pope, Andersson, and Chaffin (1991) indicate that

selected frequencies (4–6; 9–12Hz) of whole-body vibration may increase the risk of low back pain. Kelsey and Hardy (1975) have reported that truck driving increased the risk of back pain four times that of normal, whereas tractor driving and commuting in a car (20 miles or more per day) doubled the risk. Vibration may also interfere with the nutrition of the disc, which may lead to premature degenerative changes (Sandover, 1983). Vibration exposure has been associated with a variety of symptoms as indicated in Table 6.1.

The use of hand-held power tools and the vibration associated with certain hand-held power tools has been reported to increase the risk of UECTDs (Armstrong, 1983). Cannon, Bernacki, and Walter (1981) reported the use of vibratory tools as a possible factor in carpal tunnel syndrome. Vibration exposure of the upper extremities occurs when the hand grasps a tool or any object that vibrates. Armstrong, Fine, Goldstein, Lifshitz, and Silverstein (1987) suggest that an increased amount of force is needed to control a vibrating tool. Because forceful exertion is a risk factor in itself, at this point it is difficult to isolate the contri-

TABLE 6.1. Symptoms Due to Whole Body Vibration and the Frequency Range at Which They Occur

Symptoms	Frequency (Hz)
Influence on breathing movements	4–8
General feeling of discomfort	4–9
Muscle contractions	4–9
Abdominal pain	4–10
Chest pains	5–7
Lower jaw symptoms	6–8
Urge to urinate	10–18
"Lump in throat"	12–16
Head symptoms	13–20
Increased muscle tone	13–20
Influence on speech	13–20

Note: Adapted from Chaffin and Andersson (1991). Adapted by permission.

bution of vibration independent of forceful exertion; however, for the purposes of this chapter, it should be recognized that both factors can contribute to the report of symptoms.

Temperature Extremes

There are several principle components associated with indoor climates: (1) air temperature, (2) the temperature of surrounding surfaces, (3) air humidity, (4) air movements, and (5) air quality (Grandjean, 1988). It is generally assumed that a comfort zone exists for work and that deviations from this zone can adversely affect work. Discomfort due to temperature changes can shift to pain, particularly in the extremities, due to significant vasoconstriction. Warmer environments can lead to weariness and fatigue, whereas cold can bring on restlessness; both may affect alertness and concentration (Grandjean, 1988). In addition, working in cooler temperatures may require the use of gloves. As discussed earlier, glove use requires increased force when gripping, pinching, and using hand tools that in turn can increase the risk of arm and hand discomfort. Working in colder temperatures can also lead to temporary loss of finger flexibility that may affect productivity (Eastman Kodak Company, Ergonomics Group, 1983).

Repetitive Motions and Sustained Effort

Certain workplace risk factors such as awkward postures and forceful exertions may not become a problem for the worker unless they are repeated or sustained throughout the day to the point where tendons, ligaments, and muscles become exposed to significant degrees of mechanical stress. It is assumed that repeated cumulative exposure to these factors increases the risk of injury. Repetitive motions of the extremities have been cited as a risk factor associated with UECTD in various hand-intensive jobs (Keyserling et al., 1991). Both Silverstein, Fine, and Armstrong (1987) and Armstrong et al. (1987) observed that simple tasks requiring less than 30 seconds to complete, performed over half of the working day increase the risk of developing tendinitis and carpal tunnel syndrome.

In a study of 189 cases of tenosynovitis of the upper extremity, Kurppa, Warris, and Kokkanen (1979) found that high repetitive work rates of 7,600 to 12,000 cycles per shift were a significant risk factor. Armstrong et al. (1987) reported that a combination of high repetition and high force had a 12 times greater risk of UECTD-related symptoms. However, the association between workplace risk and UECTD symptoms is controversial (Hadler, 1989). Typically, one would think of an assembly line as a repetitive job by nature in which a certain quota is produced per shift. It is important to emphasize that several jobs involve repetitive and/or sustained efforts (e.g., keyboarding, data entry, grocery checking).

Repetitiveness is a potential risk factor for areas other than upper extremity problems. Repetitive bending of the trunk has been associated with low back pain (Andersson, 1979). It is typically a combination of risk factors such as awkward posture (bending forward or twisting), high force (lifting a high load), and repeated exposure (i.e., several times per hour throughout the work shift) that increases the risk for symptoms.

Sustained effort or exertion also represents a potential work-related risk. Sustained posture can lead to localized muscle fatigue. The amount of effort relative to the maximal strength required to maintain a muscular contraction is related to the length of time the effort can be sustained. A maximal voluntary contraction (MVC) of a muscle group can be maintained for only about 6 seconds (Rohmert, 1978). As seen in Figure 6.6, an individual working at 50% of MVC can maintain a sustained effort for approximately 1 minute, while a muscle contraction requiring less than

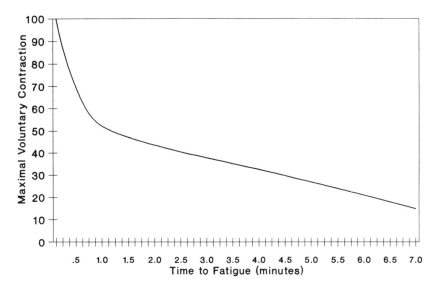

FIGURE 6.6. Relation between percentage of maximum voluntary contraction and time to fatigue. Data from Rohmert (1973).

15% of maximum could be sustained for several hours before fatigue. Fatigue during sustained muscular contraction can produce discomfort and in some occasions pain (Astrand & Rodahl, 1986). With proper breaks, intermittent maximal contractions can be performed indefinitely. However, Stull and Clark (1971) report that as the MVC reaches 60%, the time required to recover from a particular contraction becomes greater than the time to actually perform the contraction. For example, a voluntary contraction of 40–70% of maximum effort sustained for only 15 seconds would require a rest period of 33 seconds in order for the muscle to recover fully. It follows that this effort can only be repeated without fatigue approximately 1.2 times per minute. Consideration of the relationship among effort intensity, continuous-effort time, and recovery time can be a useful guide for establishing adaptive work pace and effort (Rodgers, 1988). Table 6.2 provides a guide for determining work-recovery cycles. Percentage of MVC can be divided into three basic efforts: light, approximately 0–30% MVC; moderate, approximately 40–60% MVC; and heavy, approximately 70–100% MVC.

If a job is not highly repetitive or does not require significant sustained exertions, it does not mean the job is completely risk free. Magora (1972) indicated that jobs that require constant or sustained sitting or standing can increase the risk of low back pain. Andersson

TABLE 6.2. Intensity, Duration, and Frequency Relationships for Static Muscle Effort

Effort intensity	Continuous effort time (sec)	Recovery time required (sec)	Highest efforts per minute without fatigue
Light	3	0	20.0
	6	0	10.0
	15	2	3.5
	20	5	2.4
	30	15	1.3
	60	60	0.5
Moderate	3	1	15.0
	6	5	5.4
	15	33	1.2
	20	58	0.8
	30	190	0.3
	60	400	0.1
Heavy	3	4	8.6
	6	19	2.4
	15	135	0.4
	20	220	0.25
	30	570	0.1

Note: From Rodgers (1988), page 229. Copyright 1988 Hanley and Belfus, Inc. Reprinted by permission.

(1987) has studied muscle activity in the low back area in seated individuals. Findings suggest that the position of the individual plays an important role in the resultant muscle activity and possible fatigue. The use of lumbar support, arm supports, and an increase in back-rest inclination appear to decrease the amount of muscle activity of the back. Workers whose jobs require remaining in one position may experience localized muscle fatigue in supporting muscle groups. As muscle fatigue increases, pain may increase as well.

Extreme Metabolic Demands

Different types of work can be classified by the metabolic demands required to perform that job. *The Dictionary of Occupational Titles* (U.S. Department of Labor, 1977) lists generic job demands ranging from sedentary to extremely heavy. Each classification deals with the generic amount of weight typically lifted or carried throughout the working day. Additionally, each classification carries with it a metabolic demand that is a multiple of a resting state (1 MET = the approximate rate of oxygen consumption of a seated individual at rest) that is also referred to as required aerobic or cardiovascular capacity. Table 6.3 lists the various levels of metabolic demand for each level of job demand.

Astrand and Rodahl (1986) have indicated that no more than 30–40% of maximal aerobic power, on average, can be exerted during an 8-hour workday without developing symptoms of fatigue. If the demand placed upon the worker is too high in relation to the individual's capacity for sustained physical work, fatigue will develop. This holds true for both whole-body and upper-body work. Therefore, it is useful to measure the *rate* at which the work is being completed (metabolic demand) and to assess whether this demand is within the worker's capacity to complete such work (i.e., aerobic or cardiovascular capacity) in order to reduce the likelihood of fatigue. Although such

TABLE 6.3. Metabolic Demands for Different Job Classifications

	Upper body work	Whole body work
Light effort	>1.4	.8–2
Moderate	<1.4–2.1	<2–3
Heavy	<2.1–3.4	<3–4.8
Very heavy	<3.4–5.7	<4.8–8
Extremely heavy effort	<5.7	<8

Note: Values expressed as METs. Based on data from Eastman Kodak Company, Ergonomics Group (1986).

a relationship is fairly strong in a healthy worker not encumbered by a musculoskeletal pain disorder, it must be emphasized that such a relationship is affected by multiple variables in the case of the work-disabled patient. It is currently unknown whether achieving required capacity is a necessary or sufficient condition for safe return-to-work in such workers. Although research is required to substantiate this, it may be more critical for jobs with significant metabolic demands (e.g., certain types of materials-handling jobs). The concept serves as a useful guide but should not be used as the sole criterion for determining fitness for work in injured workers.

Psychological Factors

It has become increasingly evident that a range of psychological factors related to the psychosocial aspects of work, psychological style of the worker, the specific job demands the worker is exposed to, and how these factors interact can affect the level of pain and symptoms experienced in the musculoskeletal system as well as the extent of work disability. The impact of the physical work environment itself on behavioral and psychophysiological responses of the worker is an area of significant concern for those involved in identifying ergonomic risk (Gamberale, Kjellberg, Akerstedt, & Johansson, 1990). The psychosocial aspects of work (e.g., work design and organizational problems, workload control, pacing, social support, rest periods, management of change) have been reported to play an important role in affecting health status at the workplace (World Health Organization, 1989).

A factor that can exacerbate perceived levels of stress and associated job dissatisfaction and potential increase in reported symptoms is the degree to which a job is perceived as monotonous. Svensson and Andersson (1983) reported that monotony on the job was associated with increased duration of work disability in cases of low back pain. This finding may be related to the repetitive nature of the job (Cox, 1980) as well as the lack of control over aspects of the job (perceived or actual). Perceived control over stress can play a role in reducing the impact of stressors in a variety of contexts (Feuerstein, Labbé, and Kuczmierczyk, 1986). These findings suggest the importance of assessing the patient's perceived work climate and providing the worker with strategies to exert greater control over the work while considering such concerns as production rates and quality.

Another psychological factor that may contribute to exacerbation of symptoms is the work style of the patient; that is, how the individual interacts with existing work demands (e.g., self-paced, deliberate vs. nonpaced, intense). This factor may represent a behavioral response to increased work demands or a style that is transituational and not specific to the work setting or to a high work demand situation. Regardless of its origin, this style can interact with work-specific ergonomic risks factors to increase the likelihood of symptoms (Feuerstein & Fitzgerald, 1992). A consideration of this factor in the overall assessment of the patient should be made.

Summary

This general review illustrates the potential role of a set of factors present in a variety of jobs that patients with musculoskeletal pain disorders may be required to return to following a pain management or active rehabilitation intervention. These ergonomic factors, depending upon level and duration of exposure, can set the stage for heightened discomfort, pain, and fatigue, thus exacerbating an existing pain problem and reducing the likelihood of a positive outcome of return-to-work. Therefore, comprehensive rehabilitation efforts require an evaluation of the presence of these factors in a given patient's work environment with the intent of determining whether (1) exposure to such factors exceeds the physical and psychological capabilities of the patient, (2) exposure to these factors should be modified so that the worker can effectively complete required job tasks without increasing the likelihood of an exacerbation of symptoms (i.e., ergonomic modification), and/or (3) a comprehensive occupational rehabilitation program can reduce the impact of such factors through physical conditioning, work conditioning, and training in work practices that may reduce the impact of exposure on symptoms and work-related pain and stress management. It is also important to consider exposure to these factors during nonwork. Such activities as knitting, prolonged driving, and athletic activities can also expose the individual to ergonomic risks; therefore, these should be considered as well in the overall evaluation.

BRIDGING THE GAP BETWEEN CLASSIC ERGONOMICS AND THE CLINIC

Within the context of classic occupational health and safety, ergonomic principles and techniques have been applied as an approach to reducing the risk of occupational musculoskeletal disorders by reducing exposure to suspected risk factors. This approach is typically utilized on a case by case basis (e.g., McAtee, 1987; Wick, 1987) or in large work groups (McKenzie, Stormet, Van Hook, & Armstrong, 1985; Sauter, Dainoff, & Smith, 1990) with the goal of identifying ergonomic risk and implementing modifications in the job to reduce the likelihood of developing musculoskeletal disorders in unaffected workers. This approach is proactive; emphasizes the need for a team including specialists in occupational health and safety, ergonomics, the employee/ worker and the supervisor; and is typically targeted toward reducing exposure to a large group of workers. Another characteristic of this approach, particularly when a consultation is requested, is that it may be the consequence of an increased incidence of work-related symptoms or the consequence of a governmental health and safety inspection of a particular workplace (e.g., inspection and citation by the Occupational Safety and Health Administration). Although this approach represents the classic use of ergonomics in health and safety, a trend in practice has emerged where clinicians from various disciplines involved in the evaluation and rehabilitation of the injured worker with an occupational musculoskeletal disorder (e.g., occupational medicine, nursing, physical therapy, occupational therapy, behavioral medicine/health psychology, exercise physiology) have begun to apply the principles and techniques of ergonomics to the assessment and management of the individual case in an effort to facilitate a safe work reentry. This use of ergonomics is markedly different from its classic intent. These differences are briefly elaborated below.

A fundamental goal of ergonomics is the modification of the job to fit the worker. The underlying assumption is that there exists a body of knowledge that characterizes safe work: work in which symptoms of fatigue, pain, and general discomfort can and should be prevented if the workplace and the job are engineered correctly. It is assumed that if such an approach is taken there is minimal need to modify the worker to meet the demands of the job because the work demands will be designed to meet the capabilities of the worker. Within this position there is acknowledgment for the need to match work demands to worker capabilities. In practice this typically occurs through a self-selection process. The legal system prohibits job discrimination based upon physical attributes. In addition, certain companies have implemented programs directed at increasing physical capacities of workers under the rationale that such an increase might reduce the risk for overexertion, particularly in highly demanding jobs (Snook, 1987).

When considering the injured or restricted worker in the context of the classic ergonomic approach to health and safety, it is important to acknowledge a set of assumptions: (1) the injured worker is typically perceived by management as "one employee with an injury," and the job itself is not typically viewed as high risk or problematic; (2) certain employers may be unclear as to why an analysis of a job needs to be completed, and concerns regarding liability even in a worker's compensation case may be present; (3) the ergonomic job assessment is not completed at the request of the company with the goal of identifying and reducing suspected workplace risk or within the larger context of prevention; and (4) medical management and rehabilitation are typically emphasized. The optimal goal of the clinical ergonomic job assessment (i.e., injured worker) should be the identification and modification of ergonomic and worker-related barriers to a timely safe return-to-work. This may involve modification of aspects of the work or workplace as well as the worker. This is generally accomplished with the injured worker as the focal point; however, positive consequences in terms of overall risk reduction in the workplace, in general, can occur.

In sum, the purpose of the clinical ergonomic job assessment (i.e., applied to the injured worker) differs from the classic function of ergonomic analysis. The specific goals of the clinical ergonomic job assessment are as follows:

1. Determine the presence and extent of ergonomic risk factors (former job; future job if it differs from former job).
2. Determine the degree to which (a) such risk factors on the job can be eliminated or (b)

the degree to which the patient can work around such factors (e.g., pacing).
3. Use information to assess discrepancy between physical capabilities and work tolerances in relation to work demands (functional capacity evaluation).
4. Use information to develop light duty, accommodated work, or in the case of subacute or chronic cases, to establish a work simulation/conditioning protocol.

METHODOLOGIES FOR ASSESSING ERGONOMIC RISK

The application of various methodologies in ergonomics used to assess the jobs of injured/ disabled workers is in its infancy. Although the generalization of these methodologies from the healthy to injured worker possesses face validity, many questions remain regarding the psychometric properties of the various assessment approaches. Extensive data regarding reliability and validity of various measures used with healthy or injured workers are unavailable. It is important to emphasize that the use of ergonomics in the clinic setting represents a relatively new area of application. It is the authors' position that the recognized role of ergonomic risk factors in the etiology and potential exacerbation and maintenance of symptoms associated with musculoskeletal pain disorders (e.g., fatigue, pain, distress) justifies the cautious use of these methodologies in an effort to facilitate safe work reentry of the injured worker. However, it is scientific support for such approaches that will ultimately determine the extent of application in the clinic and workplace in relation to clinical management of these cases.

A variety of measurement methodologies are available to assess the degree to which a given individual is exposed to an ergonomic risk. A detailed review of these methods is beyond the scope of this chapter. Several sources present such information (Ayoub & Mital, 1989; Borg, 1990; Eastman Kodak Company, Ergonomics Group, 1983, 1986; Frazer, 1989; Kroemer, Kroemer, & Kroemer-Elbert, 1990; Salvendy, 1987; Wilson & Corlett, 1990). Wilson and Corlett (1990) provide an excellent review of the multiple methods available for the evaluation of human work. These authors have developed a classification of methods, techniques, and measures used in ergonomics that can provide the clinician with a ready guide to existing approaches. Although there are a number of options available to the clinician, the use of videotape analysis of specific job tasks, simple measurement of forces using spring scales and torque wrenches, measurement of weights, heights, reach distances and workstations, and assessment of postural angles using goniometers, protractors, and inclinometers, in conjunction with visual analogue scales (VASs) that measure perceived fatigue, exertion, discomfort, and various symptoms in relation to certain job tasks appear to be at present the most common approaches used in applied ergonomics. It is important to emphasize that any method used should be evaluated in relation to the following criteria: (1) reliability (i.e., consistently repeatable); (2) validity (i.e., the method measures the risk factor it is assumed to measure); (3) clinical validity (i.e., the factor measured has been associated with increased symptom reporting); (4) relative simplicity of use (measurement protocol is easy to learn and time required to record and analyze data is reasonable given clinical demands); and (5) clinically utility (method generates information that can be easily translated into clinical management strategies).

Although these criteria can serve as a useful guide for determining an appropriate clinical ergonomic job analysis (EJA) methodology, at present very little data in relation to these criteria are available to guide the choice of the various methods in existence. Therefore, it is helpful if the clinician considers the choice of methods used for the clinical EJA within the broader context of how the information will assist in facilitating a safe return-to-work in the individual who experiences residual pain associated with a specific musculoskeletal disorder or may be at greater risk for a recurrence of symptoms by nature of the type of disorder (e.g., tendinitis or carpal tunnel syndrome). When the EJA is placed within this framework, choice of measures and protocols become more apparent. The next section reviews a number of such protocols.

REPRESENTATIVE PROTOCOLS

The Center for Ergonomics at the University of Michigan has contributed significantly to the knowledge base in ergonomics in general and its application to prevention of occupational musculoskeletal disorders. Chaffin, Arm-

strong, Herrin, Keyserling, and others have generated many of the concepts and approaches used in applied ergonomics in relation to the musculoskeletal disorders (Chaffin & Armstrong, 1991). The Center's model of occupational ergonomics forms the basis for the approaches the Center takes to EJA; although the focus differs somewhat among faculty members and the set of problems that represent their primary area of interest (e.g., low back pain, UECTD, postural stress, application of quality control principles to occupational health).

The generic model of occupational ergonomics proposed by the Michigan group (Chaffin & Armstrong, 1991) is presented in Figure 6.7. The major focus from this group's perspective is the development and implementation of ergonomic principles to identify and solve "worker-hardware mismatch" problems. The model focuses on three broad categories—job task requirements, environmental conditions at the workplace such as exposure to noise, heat, vibration, and the worker-hardware system. This latter system includes a subsystem—the individual worker who, in the course of completing job requirements, must incorporate the functions of perception, processing, organizing responses, and performing certain behaviors. The hardware subsystem includes such components as machines, tools, materials, and workplace layout. According to this model problems occur when a mismatch between worker and hardware subsystems emerges at the level of information interaction such as problems in display design or instru-

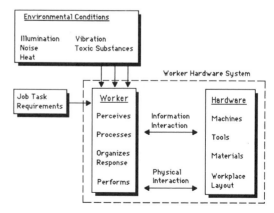

FIGURE 6.7. University of Michigan, Center for Ergonomics—Model of Occupational Ergonomics. From Chaffin and Armstrong (1991), page 1. Copyright 1991 University of Michigan. Reprinted by permission.

ment control placements or functions or between human–computer operations; essentially where information processing becomes difficult due to a mismatch. In addition to the information interaction, problems can occur at the level of physical interaction where the physical characteristics of a tool or object are such that a mismatch is evident, resulting in fatigue, symptoms, injury, and/or decrement in performance. Examples include excessive weights and sizes of objects handled, seat design, and size and grip of hand tools.

This general model proposes that if such mismatches can be eliminated or significantly reduced, the probability of various occupational musculoskeletal disorders or symptoms of fatigue, pain, and discomfort should be reduced. The group recognizes that the field of occupational ergonomics is relatively new and that enhanced knowledge requires the input of multiple disciplines. The problems are complex, involving medical, ergonomic, workplace-organizational, and psychological factors to name but a few.

The two approaches to assessing jobs reviewed in this section will be those developed by Armstrong (1991) and the NIOSH/Michigan analysis of lifting developed by Chaffin et al. (1977). These two approaches can be divided into strategies to assess jobs potentially related to initiation, exacerbation and/or maintenance of UECTDs (i.e., jobs requiring repetitive, forceful actions in awkward postures—the Armstrong Protocol) or jobs potentially associated with activity-related spinal disorders or work involving materials handling (the NIOSH Lifting Guidelines).

The Armstrong Protocol

This protocol proposes a set of occupational factors that have been associated in clinical and epidemiological research to increase the likelihood of symptoms related to tendinitis and/or nerve entrapment disorders. Armstrong (1991) presents a comprehensive review of this literature for each of the suspected factors, including repetitiveness, forceful exertions, mechanical stresses, postures, low temperatures, and vibration. It is important to emphasize that this literature is not without controversy regarding methodology (e.g., retrospective vs. prospective, clear definitions of disorders, reliable and valid measurement of disorders, and workplace risk); however, the literature is strongly sugges

tive of the potential role of these factors in the etiology of certain upper extremity disorders, and evidence continues to emerge supporting this position. The major issue in relation to the use of the EJA protocol in clinical cases, as the present authors see it, is that these workplace factors can serve to reestablish a set of symptoms and exacerbate any residual symptomology that is present following treatment, thus maintaining a certain level of symptoms that can increase distress in the worker, potentially contributing to further medical problems, development of work disability, lower productivity, compromised quality of work life, and quality of life in general.

The objective of Armstrong's job analysis is to identify and rank specific risk factors, design interventions, and evaluate such interventions in relation to reduction in ergonomic stressors and symptoms, if present. The procedure typically includes four components: (1) documentation, (2) ergonomic assessment, (3) design of control measures, and (4) evaluation of control measures. Armstrong offers a methodology that represents one of the more comprehensive approaches to the analysis of jobs involving the upper extremities available to date. The approach combines quantitative measurement of movements/exertions based upon videotape analysis, calculation of pinch forces (Armstrong, 1985), postural analysis (Armstrong, 1986b) and biomechanical analysis of posture–work station interactions considering anthropometric factors in determining optimal work area design. Armstrong also incorporates the use of psychophysical rating scales of perceived comfort, perceived effort associated with postures, and various aspects of tool use (Armstrong, Punnett, & Ketner, 1989; Ulin, Armstrong, & Radwin, 1990; Ulin, Ways, Armstrong, & Snook, 1990) as well as observer ratings of such factors as repetitiveness and postural stress. A summary of the components of the job analysis data collection form of Armstrong is provided in Table 6.4.

The final two components of the job analysis involve the design and evaluation of control measures. Design measures relate to a number of factors including tools, workplace (location/ orientation of work), fixtures used to secure the work, maintenance of tools, quality control of unit items (size of parts), materials used, product specifications such as edges or smoothness of surfaces, seating and work methods or procedures in relation to sequence of work,

TABLE 6.4. Components of the Job Analysis Data Collection Form of Armstrong

I. DOCUMENTATION
    A. Objective of job
    B. Production standard
    C. Staffing
    D. Work method
    E. Workstation and equipment
    F. Materials
    G. Tools
    H. Environment
    I. Personal protective equipment

II. ERGONOMIC ASSESSMENT
    A. Repeated and sustained exertions
       1. Exertions per unit time =
          (production units/time × elements/
          production unit) × (exertions/
          elements)
       2. Specify rate/pace (high, medium, low)
       3. Position for prolonged period
       4. Distances walked or carriers
    B. Forceful exertions
       1. Specify job tasks that require exertion to
          overcome gravity, friction or reaction
          forces
       2. Each job task evaluate
          a. intensity of force (e.g., torque)
          b. friction (low, medium, high)
          c. number and position of hands
          d. gloves (interfere or assist)
          e. shoes
    C. Localized Mechanical Stresses
       1. List all job tasks where body contacts hard/
          sharp edge
       2. For each job task identify
          a. body location
          b. force (weight of limb, impact force)
          c. contact area (sharp, flat)

D. Postural stresses
   1. List all job tasks where worker places ex-
      tremity in following positions
      a. reach overhead
      b. reach behind body
      c. fully flex elbow
      d. rotate forearm to "extremes"
      e. flex or fully extend wrist
      f. deviate wrist side to side
      g. bend trunk more than 20°
   2. Specify duration and frequency of the exer-
      tion (e.g., repeated or sustained)
E. Vibration exposure
   1. List all job tasks where worker holds or
      grasps
      a. vibrating tool
      b. vibrating part
      c. impact tool
      d. vibrating control
   2. List activities that expose worker to whole
      body vibration
   3. Indicate duration of exposure
F. Thermal extremes exposure
   1. List all elements where worker exposed to
      cold air (<75°F) from atmosphere, air tools
      or cold parts
   2. Assess temperature conductivity of material
      handled rate high (water/metal) or low
      (plastic/paper)
   3. Assess high temperatures based upon safe
      exposure criteria

III. REPORT
     1. List generic and job specific risk factors by
        category above
     2. Indicate suspected workplace causes of phys-
        ical stress
     3. Provide overall simple brief summary

Note: From Chaffin and Armstrong (1991). Copyright 1991 University of Michigan. Reprinted by permission.

and influence of work methods on posture. Lastly, Armstrong emphasizes the importance of evaluation of control measures and indicates that this can be accomplished through the use of several approaches including drawing board analysis or assessment using computer-aided design (CAD) technology (Ulin, Armstrong, & Radwin, 1990), mock-ups, and prototypes of the modified work tasks, job analysis, worker and supervisor assessments, and worker health or symptom patterns.

In terms of the clinical implications of Armstrong's approach to job analysis and redesign in restricted workers or individuals with a UECTD, it must be emphasized that at present there are no controlled systematic investigations of the application of this approach to

clinical cases. There are anecdotal reports and case histories of individual workers, but, to the authors' knowledge this comprehensive approach has not yet been subjected to the rigors of scientific clinical investigation. The approach provides a number of assessment methodologies for each of the suspected risk factors ranging from quantitative measurement of work demands to subjective rating forms. Given the relative recency in the use of such methods with clinical cases, it is best for the reader to consider this approach as providing a schema for an ergonomic evaluation of the workplace of the injured worker highlighting various measurement options. Another strength of this approach is the logical transition from assessment of suspected risk to design, implementation, and evaluation of control or risk reduction methods. Although Armstrong and colleagues have generated several low-cost strategies for reducing risk, perhaps more importantly, the evaluation approach itself facilitates the generation of potential workplace modifications by identifying risk in specific work elements in an organized sequential manner. The workplace modifications that arise from such a process can potentially greatly assist in the safe return of the injured worker.

NIOSH Evaluation of Manual Lifting

In 1981, following the work of Chaffin, Herrin, and others at the University of Michigan, NIOSH proposed a set of guidelines for the handling of manual materials that was designed to assist in managing the problem of low back pain in industry (U.S. Department of Health and Human Services, 1981). As illustrated in Figure 6.8, these lifting guidelines consider several attributes of the lift including: (1) the load's horizontal distance from the worker's spine (H), (2) the vertical distance from the floor where the load is originally grasped (V), and (3) the distance that the load travels from where it is picked up to where it is set down (D). Measures of these factors are taken in the context of an ergonomic job analysis of materials-handling tasks. These factors are then entered into a formula along with a constant of 90 pounds (40 kg) as indicated below:

$$AL \text{ (kg)} = 40(15/H)(1 - 0.004[V - 75])(0.7 + 7.5/D)$$

$$AL \text{ (lb)} = 90(6/H)(1 - 0.01[V - 30])(0.7 + 3/D)$$

$$MPL = 3(AL)$$

For repeated lifts, a frequency factor can be added to the equation. Three risk categories are then determined from the equation: (1) Lift falls within acceptable limits; (2) lift requires some administrative controls (i.e., lifting training) in an attempt to lower the risk (action limit, or AL); or (3) lift appears to be hazardous and requires some engineering controls (i.e., workplace redesign) in an attempt to lower the risk (maximal permissible limit, or MPL).

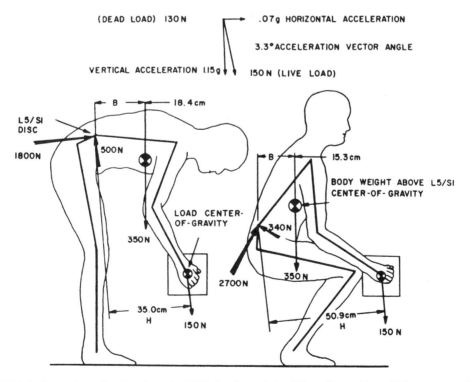

FIGURE 6.8. Comparison of predicted reactive L5/S1 disc forces during lifting of large object which cannot pass between the knees and weighs. 130 Newtons. From Chaffin and Andersson (1991), page 229. Copyright 1974 *AIIE Transactions*. Reprinted by permission.

If the load to be lifted weighs less than the AL, then the lift is considered to be acceptable. This suggests that 99% of the male population and 75% of the female population could perform this lift with minimal risk of injury. If the load to be lifted falls above the AL but below the MPL (Figure 6.9), then the job would fall into the administrative controls categories. That is, some members of the work force would be at an increased risk and some methods (e.g., training) as well as workplace modifications should be introduced. If the load is above the MPL, then the job is considered to be hazardous and it is assumed that only 25% of the male population would be able to accomplish the lift. Engineering changes would be the only acceptable method to reduce the risk of injury in this category.

There are certain limitations with this method. Assumptions related to the determination of risk (two-handed lift, lift in front of body with no twisting) are conditions that are not consistently observed in the workplace. In addition, the approach assumes the load is balanced, there are good hand-holds, and the load is less than 30 inches wide. It is also assumed that the worker has good footing, is working in an acceptable work environment (i.e., temperature, humidity, lighting), and is unrestricted with regard to body movements. Considering these limitations as well as the emphasis on static versus dynamic lifting, the NIOSH guidelines were re-evaluated and new guidelines advanced. These guidelines are believed to represent an improvement and will soon be made available by NIOSH.

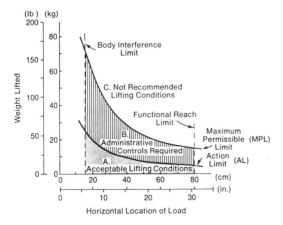

FIGURE 6.9. Nomogram for occasional lifts in the sagittal plane. From: National Institute for Occupational Safety and Health (1981)

Rodgers Protocol

Rodgers (1988) has developed an EJA protocol that focuses on the assessment of functional capacity for work in relation to the physical effort requirements of a given job. The concept of work capacity is central to Rodgers' approach. Rodgers argues that an individual's capacity for physical work is determined by such factors as the duration of continuous effort required, frequency of repeated efforts, environmental and psychological stressors, age, level of fitness, skill level for the task, and the number and size of muscle groups required for the specific work. The focus of the evaluation is on the assessment of capacity to perform work requiring specific muscle groups and aerobic capacity, although the emphasis in the Rodgers (1988) protocol is primarily on capacity of the musculoskeletal system relative to work demands. The variables considered in the protocol include (1) identification of active muscle groups, (2) effort intensity ratings or strength of the muscle groups active in specific job tasks relative to the maximum strength for specific working postures, (3) duration of continuous effort such as continuous holding time, (4) recovery time between efforts or work pace, and (5) duration of muscular effort over the workshift. Rodgers uses a combination of videotape-analysis, force-gauge measurements, heart-rate monitoring, and subjective worker ratings.

The specific protocol involves videotaping of the job and interviews with worker(s) and supervisors. An analysis of the videotape is conducted in order to generate ratings for each of three categories and each of six major muscle groups involved in the job task(s) as indicated in Figure 6.10. The three categories include effort level or intensity (heavy, 7–10 on a rating of perceived exertion (RPE) (Borg, 1982); time of *continuous* muscle effort (<6 sec; 6–20 sec; >20 sec) and efforts per minute (<1 cycle/min; 1–5 cycles/min; >5 cycles/min). By entering numbers corresponding to the usual effort levels, continuous effort times, and efforts per minute for each muscle group on the job analysis form, it is possible to determine a priority for change score indicating the necessity to modify the job in order to reduce the risk of on overexertion injury.

The priority-for-change determinations shown in Figure 6.10 list moderate, high, and very high priorities for change options. It is proposed by Rodgers that as the priority-

Ergonomic Job Analysis

Body Part	Effort Level	Continuous Effort Time	Efforts/ Minute	Priority	Effort Categories
Neck/Shoulders	——	——	——	——	1 = Light 2 = Moderate 3 = Heavy
Back	——	——	——	——	Continuous Effort Time Categories 1 = <6 secs 2 = 6 to 20 secs 3 = >20 secs
Arms/Elbows	——	——	——	——	Efforts/Minute Categories 1 = <1/min 2 = 1 to 5/min 3 = >5/min
Wrists/Hands/ Fingers	——	——	——	——	
Legs/Knees	——	——	——	——	
Ankles/Feet/ Toes	——	——	——	——	

Priority for Change		
Moderate =	1 2 3	
	1 3 2	
	2 1 3	
	2 2 2	
	2 3 1	
	2 3 2	
	3 1 2	
High =	2 2 3	
	3 1 3	
	3 2 1	
	3 2 2	
	3 2 3	
Very High =	3 3 1	
	3 3 2	

Job Title: _____

Specific Task: _____

Job Number: _____

Department: _____

Location: _____

Contact Person(s): _____

    Phone: _____

Analyst: _____

    Phone: _____

Date of Analysis: _____

FIGURE 6.10. Ergonomic job analysis. From Rodgers (1988), page 225. Copyright 1988 Hanley and Belfus Inc. Reprinted by permission.

for-change increases from moderate to very high, the muscle group activity becomes increasingly more fatiguing for the worker. If the ratings do not appear in the priority-for-change list, there is a low priority to modify the job for that specific muscle group. Each muscle group can be evaluated separately in an attempt to establish effective job modifications for that particular muscle group or as a whole.

This approach appears to hold potential for use in a clinical setting given the relative simplicity of the procedure. In addition, the approach leads to recommendations regarding change that help to identify the most problematic components of a job and by considering all major muscle groups in the analysis, which potentially reduces the likelihood that a job change recommendation would result in increased strain in other muscle groups. Despite its widespread use and anecdotal success in reducing risk and symptoms in a large number of varied work sites (Rodgers, 1988), the approach awaits systematic analysis of reliability and validity. The approach is relatively simple to learn and implement, and facilitates identification of problem areas at the workplace that require attention in order to reduce the likelihood of symptom development and/or exacerbation.

The Drury Protocol

Drury and Wick (1984) developed a protocol to evaluate jobs for repetitive-motion injury potential at first for a return-to-work program for a shoe manufacturer, subsequently for an apparel manufacturer, and ultimately applied to a number of jobs in varied workplaces (Drury, 1987). Drury proposed that based upon clinical and epidemiological studies, risk factors of a given job that should be assessed include high force, frequency or highly repetitious rates of movement, and posture or large deviations of joint angles from a neutral position. Drury argues that in the absence of specific data on the degree of exposure (dose) to these factors and the probability of injury (response), the basic assumption regarding workplace safety vis-à-vis UECTDs can be characterized as that which reduces required force, frequency of extremity movements, and postural stress. Drury also points out the importance of using the proposed methodology as a means for analyzing and comparing different jobs and to evaluate the impact of job modifications on such suspected risk factors despite the absence of absolute standards.

The criteria Drury proposes for his EJA methodology include (1) simplicity—easily taught to others and applied in a relatively short duration, (2) sufficient specificity—to reduce the likelihood of misinterpretation, and (3) facilitation of the identification of high risk jobs. The methodology to be described was designed to be implemented in a pre–post manner; initially to identify risk and propose recommendations regarding ergonomic modifications and following the implementation of such modifications (2–5 days postinitial trials with new design) to assess whether such modifications have reduced exposure to suspected risk factors.

Specifically, Drury divides the protocol into five stages: task description, task analysis, task requirements, evaluation, and implementation. For the purposes of this chapter, the authors focus on the initial four stages. Under task description, the goal is to identify the job and operator(s) to be analyzed. In the clinical setting, the ideal situation would be to assess the job that is identical to the one that the injured worker is expected to return to. In Drury's approach, one with a focus on primary prevention, the goal is to identify one to three operators with "adequate" experience. High quality videotaping of several cycles of the task from five varying approaches is then initiated. These approaches include (1) front 75% view from above operator's head height, (2) direct left side view, (3) direct right side view, (4) direct front view, and (5) direct rear view.

It is suggested that a minimum of two cycles at a wide angle setting should be used to assess gross body posture followed by a minimum of two additional work cycles of a close-up of the upper extremities. There is a need to define the subtasks of a given job to estimate cycle times of a typical repetitive task. As illustrated in Figure 6.11, the data sheet used includes the anatomical location under investigation (back, neck, shoulder, elbow, forearm, wrist, legs) in which the "extreme" angle about each axis of rotation is recorded for each subtask (up to eight subtasks on the present form). These angles can be generally measured from the video through the use of protractors, goniometers, or artist or designer mannequins. Additional details regarding measurement of rotation are provided in Drury (1987). The reverse side of the form provides an analysis of general posture and specific grip forces, general forces, vibration, shock, and lighting. Postural discomfort is measured using a Body-Part Discomfort Scale (Corlett & Bishop, 1976) and a General-Comfort Rating Scale (Schackel, Chidsey, & Shipley, 1979).

The second stage in the analysis is the transformation of the raw data on angles, forces, and discomfort to a categorization of angles at each joint in relation to extent of deviation from neutral. Drury divides the joint range of motion into three zones: no exposure—neutral ±10% of range; low exposure—±10% to ±25% of range; moderate exposure—±25% to ±50% of range; severe exposure—> ±50% of range. The joint range-of-motion averages for the U.S. population were used (National Aeronautics and Space Administration, 1978). The frequency of high risk (e.g., moderate to severe exposure) can then be calculated for a given job considering cycle time typically in seconds and a work duration in total hours per day. This can be calculated for several subtasks and problem components of a job identified.

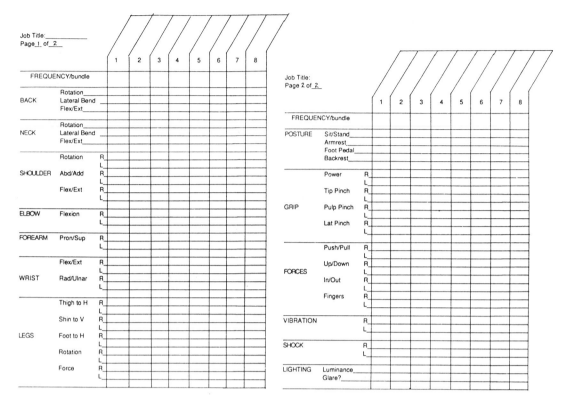

FIGURE 6.11. Task analysis form. From Drury (1987), page 43. Copyright 1987 Thieme Medical Publishers Inc. Reprinted by permission.

Data from the body-part discomfort scale are also analyzed by counting the incidence of nonzero ratings for each body area and dividing by the total number of times the scale was administered during the evaluation. Such a measure provides an index of areas in which discomfort is experienced relative to total number of queries. Drury plots the general comfort rating over the duration of time the ratings were obtained. Redesign represents the next phase and includes a team approach involving the operator, supervisor, health and safety personnel, and design engineers. Following this, a reanalysis of the job using the identical methodology along with a pre–post analysis of the impact of the redesign on symptoms or discomfort are completed.

This methodology is characteristic of the approach taken by applied ergonomists. The approach is highly individualized to a given job and worker or a group of workers. The approach involves the specification of the job tasks, quantification of posture, force, frequency or repetitiveness of a task, and some general relationship of these suspected factors to discomfort or symptoms. Although these approaches appear to have much face validity, as with the other approaches available, little is known about the reliability and validity of the measurement approach, particularly in the clinical context. The approach is used in the field by Drury and others to solve ergonomic problems at the workplace using pre–post assessments completed following consultation.

The Drury method appears to have some direct clinical applicability, particularly in those cases where extent of extremity deviation is a major concern. The approach holds promise in cases of carpal tunnel syndrome or lateral and medical epicondylitis where repeated exposure to severe wrist or forearm deviations could significantly exacerbate symptoms upon return-to-work. The methodology is well detailed (Drury, 1987), which should allow others to use the procedure and determine its use in clinical applications. Suggestions for simple workplace modifications to reduce such exposure should help to facilitate the safe reentry of the injured worker. Through such methodology it might also be possible to determine the level of workload such that symptoms do not reappear and use such information to redesign the job in an effort to reduce risk in the restricted worker. Although this is a unique application of the methodology, it does represent a potential clinical use of the approach to help facilitate return to accommodated work. Such an approach would require consistent periodic monitoring of the worker to ensure that the accommodation was effective in reducing the likelihood of symptoms.

The Rochester Protocol

The Rochester Protocol used for conducting an EJA is based in part upon the conceptual model of work disability presented in the introduction of this chapter and summarized in Feuerstein (1991). The approach our group takes to an EJA, in regard to the management of an individual with a recurrent or chronic work disability associated with an occupational musculoskeletal disorder, in contrast to the use of an EJA for primary prevention, relates to the need to identify factors that may present barriers to return-to-work or long-term work reentry (i.e., prevent relapse) following report of persistent symptoms, particularly pain.

The potential work reentry barriers tend to fall into three broad categories: (1) discrepancies between work demands (biomedical, metabolic, psychological) and capabilities of the individual in terms of strength, flexibility, endurance, aerobic capacity, work tolerance, and psychological coping resources; (2) moderate or high-risk work demands characteristic of the job in general; and (3) the manner in which the job has been accomplished to date by the injured worker (high-risk work style). Information regarding each area is used in the context of rehabilitation to facilitate a reduction in the physical-capability/work-demand discrepancies that may exist through enhancement of physical capabilities and inspection and modification of ergonomic and work-style risks in an effort to reduce the probability of symptom reoccurrence, exacerbation, or maintenance upon return to work.

The procedure includes a description of the work with a breakdown of symptom—risk-relevant task elements. This is accomplished through a combination of on-site observation, videotaping when feasible, and interview with patient, supervisor, and co-workers. Measurement of major work demands characteristic of

the job or jobs the patient is expected to return to or positions the patient may move into depending upon the outcome of rehabilitation is then initiated. The EJA is conducted using a standardized form for recording data regarding work demands. Measurement of the following work demands are possible: forward reaching (sitting), forward reaching (standing), overhead reach, crouching, repetitive squat, lifting, carrying (bilateral), carrying (one hand), dynamic pushing, dynamic pulling, static pushing, static pulling, sitting interval, standing interval, climbing stairs, climbing ladder, kneeling, walking, required manual dexterity, and required hand and pinch grip strengths. Measurements of perceived efforts and other perceived work demands are also obtained. Emphasis is placed on measurement of work demands and work tolerances that are reported to be associated with pain and discomfort (symptom-relevant tasks) or are suspected risk factors (risk-relevant tasks). The data collection form (refer to Figure 6.6 for an example of a subsection of the form) is included in the overall worksheet clinicians use to measure physical and work capabilities at the time of initial evaluation. The clinician completes the EJA ideally paying particular attention to workplace factors that might be modified to facilitate return-to-work. A summary of the steps of the clinical EJA developed at the Center for Occupational Rehabilitation is provided in Table 6.5.

Due to time and staff constraints, the EJA is not completed on *all* initial evaluations of potential work rehabilitation cases. It is used in those cases where the job demands are particularly unclear, jobs in which high risk is suspected, or in cases where the physical capabilities or extent of pathology is such that information regarding work demands is essential to generate a conclusion regarding the likelihood to return to a specific job.

The following case studies illustrate the application of the clinical EJA.

CASE EXAMPLE: DEGENERATIVE DISK DISEASE

Brief History

Forty-six-year-old female, work-disabled for 10 months. Degenerative disc disease with no current symptoms of nerve root compression, evidence of prior disc herniation. Reported severe stiffness and pain in the upper and lower back,

TABLE 6.5. Steps in Conducting a Clinical Ergonomic Job Analysis (EJA)

1. Identify Purpose of EJA
   - Estimate whether individual can return to a specific job or set of jobs.
   - Establish physical and work conditioning goals for rehabilitation program (based on physical capability/work demand discrepancies)
   - Assist in determining certain pain and stress management goals (e.g., need to modify work style)
   - Identify ergonomic risks to target in ergonomic consultation to reduce workplace risk and facilitate safe work re-entry

2. Specify scope of EJA
   - Former job
   - Potential new job (if known)
   - Determine job elements to analyze

3. Specification of risk factors
   - Develop rationale for choice of factors in a given case (e.g., pattern of symptoms)

4. Identification of measurement options and estimate time required
   - Video tape
   - Direct observation
   - Supervisor interview
   - Co-worker interview
   - Physical measurement devises (e.g., force gauges)
   - Psychological measurement devises (self report, visual analogue scales)

5. Quantification and data analyses (if necessary)

6. Provide an independent brief report or include in initial evaluation

7. Discuss findings and recommendations with worker, supervisor, clinical staff and others involved. Use problem solving approach

8. Follow up after patient returns to work
   - Workplace walkthru
   - Interview with worker/supervisor

neck, and shoulders, which appeared to be a reoccurrence of a whiplash injury from a motor vehicle accident 5 years prior to the lower back pain.

Job

Metal Press Operator—operates press that cuts, punches, or stamps metal objects of various sizes and shapes. Obtains materials to be stamped from nearby bins. Places materials in bed of stamping press. Presses switches, with both hands, to lower ram and stamp material. Removes product from press, examines for quality, and places into another nearby bin.

Current Work Demands

- Frequent bending
- Constant twisting of trunk
- Reaching forward, overhead, and below waist
- Handling and carrying objects up to 20 pounds
- Lifting floor to waist (frequently)
- Standing at workstation
- 8-hour workday, two 15-minute breaks, and 30-minute lunch

Job Demands/Work Tolerance

The data form and findings from the work tolerance evaluation and clinical ergonomic job analysis are presented in Table 6.6.

Recommendations

1. Work conditioning component of the active work rehabilitation program should include as its goals the improvement of:
   - Overhead reach tolerance
   - Lifting tolerance
   - Carrying tolerance
   - Standing tolerance

2. Particular attention should be given to certain workplace factors that can be potentially modified (low or no cost to the employer). For example, there were several presses in the same work area where the on-switches were located at waist height rather than above shoulder height. It is recommended that the worker be moved to one of these machines in an attempt to avoid constant, repetitive overhead reaching. Future consideration should be given to lowering controls on all units. Also, the bin that the material is selected from sits on a pallet. The bottom of the bin is 6 inches above the floor, requiring the worker to bend and reach below knee level to select material as the bin becomes empty. It is recommended that a second pallet be inserted to raise the lowest bin depth to 12 inches above floor level. This modification would reduce the extent of forward bending at the waist needed to select materials from the bottom of the bin.

CASE EXAMPLE: BILATERAL MEDIAL EPICONDYLITIS AND TRICEP TENDINITIS

Brief History

Twenty-three-year-old female, frequent prolonged work absences over 8-month period. History of medial epicondylitis of both arms and tricep tendinitis. Reported constant pain in elbows and wrists that increases following work and at night. Bilateral nerve conduction studies were

TABLE 6.6. Work Tolerance/Work Demands Discrepancy Worksheet: Metal Press Operator

Forward reach (standing)	Meets job demands: YES

Describe activity: Places material in bed of stamping press, then removal of material from press

Observed work tolerances	*Required work demands*
Reach distance: 12–18 in.	Reach distance: 20 in.
Duration: 180 sec	Duration: 2–5 sec
	Frequency: 8 reaches/min (throughout shift)
	Surface height: 48 in.

Overhead reach	Meets job demands: NO

Describe activity: Presses switch with both hands, to lower press

Observed work tolerances	*Required work demands*
Reach distance: 67 in.	Reach distance: 66 in.
Duration: 45 sec	Duration: 2–5 sec
	Frequency: 4 reaches/min (throughout shift)
	Surface height: 66 in.

Comments: Reports of back and shoulder pain.

Lifting floor to waist level[a]	Meets job demands: NO

Describe activity: Reaching deep into pallet (bin) container | *Item*: Metal material for stamping

Observed work tolerances	*Required work demands*
Weight: 5 lb	Weight: 1–5 lb
(Waist height: 34 in.)	Surface height: 6–36 in. (depending on materials
Frequency: 1/min	used from bin)
	Frequency: 4/min (4 times/shift)

Comments: Reports significant back pain with extreme bending. Position represents major problem at this time.

Carrying (bilateral)	Meets job demands: NO

Describe activity: Carrying jigs and dyes weighing up to 20 lb | *Item*: Jig

Observed work tolerances	*Required work demands*
Weight: 5 lb	Weight: 20 lb
Distance: 40 ft	Distance: 50 ft
	Frequency: 3/week

Comments: Reports of back pain.

Standing interval	Meets job demands: NO

Describe activity: Operating press | Type of floor surface: concrete with rubberized mat

Observed work tolerances	*Required work demands*
Observed time: 15 min	Interval: 120 min

Comments: Reports of back pain.

[a]Hand placement during lifting in front of body: 26-in. space between hand placement on weight tray; 12 in. above the base of weight tray (width of tray = 6 in.).

normal. Neurological exam was normal. No wasting of the muscles was noted.

Job

Assembler—wire harness subassembly. Lays wire around pegs on harness board and ties wires together to form harness (cable) used in electronic equipment. Selects wires of color, marking, or length specified by wire lists or diagrams, and loops them between guide pegs on board, following colored lines or numbers marked on board. Laces wires together at specified points by wrapping and tying with plastic strips. Applies sealing varnish to laces with brush to secure knots. Solders ends of cable wires to terminal strip or multiple-pin plug, using soldering iron. Inserts cable in plastic tubing to protect cable from dust and moisture. Paints identifying colors on wires. Fastens units in specified locations; cuts, strips, bends, and mounts wires using wrenches/pliers, screwdrivers wire strippers, crimping tools, and air gun/nut runners. Assembles 2.5 units per hour, or 21 units per 8-hour shift. Obtains materials from nearby bins to be used in the assembly.

Current Work Demands

- Repetitive and sustained forward reaching
- Frequent repetitive wrist movements
- Frequent gripping and pinching
- Prolonged standing at work station
- Frequent forward bending
- Occasional lifting, 25 to 40 pounds
- Constant twisting
- 8-hour workday with two 15-minute breaks and 30-minute lunch break. May be required to work overtime hours on a weekly basis

Job Demands/Work Tolerance

The data form and findings from the work tolerance evaluation and clinical EJA are presented in Table 6.7.

TABLE 6.7. Work Tolerance/Work Demands Discrepancy Worksheet: Assembler

---

Forward reach (standing)   Meets job demands: NO
_____

Describe activity: Assembly procedure for wire harness subassembly as detailed in job description

Observed work tolerances	*Required work demands*
Reach distance: 29 in.	Reach distance: 18–30 in.
Duration: 30 sec	Duration: up to 180 sec
	Frequency: 15/hr (throughout shift)
	Surface height: 36 in.

Comments: Reported increased bilateral elbow pain and left shoulder pain.

Lifting floor to waist level[a]   Meets job demands: NO
_____

Describe activity: Lifting of completed wire harness off mount/jig   *Item*: Wire harness

Observed work tolerances	*Required work demands*
Weight: 17.5 lb	Weight: 25–40 lb
(Waist height: 42 in.)	Surface height: 36–24 in.
	Frequency: 21/shift

Comments: Reported right elbow pain.

Carrying (bilateral)   Meets job demands: NO
_____

Describe activity: Carrying supplies to be used in assembly process   *Item*: Supplies, wire harness

Observed work tolerances	*Required work demands*
Weight: 20 lb	Weight: 25–40 lb
Distance: 40 ft	Distance: 20 ft
	Frequency: 3–4/shift

Comments: Reported bilateral arm pain.

Hand tool use   Meets job demands: NO
_____

Describe activity: Secures fasteners to wire harness

Observed work tolerances	*Required work demands*
Tool: Screw gun	Tool: Air gun/nut driver
Surface height: 48 in.	Principal hand used: R __X__ / L _____ / B _____
Reach distance: 20 in.	Balancer: R _____ / L _____ / B _____ / none __X__
Duration: 1.5 min	Wrist orientation: Neut _____ / Flex _____ / Ext __X__ /
	UD _____ / RD _____
Perceived grip rating[b]: R __6__ / L _____ / B	Tool weight.: 3 lb
	Surface height: 42–50 in. (height of worker = 66 in.)
	Reach distance: 15–22 in.
	Duration: 3–5 min
	Frequency: 3/hr (throughout shift)
	Perceived grip Rating[b]: R __6__ / L _____ / B _____

Right Hand/*Comments*: Reports of pain in right elbow, unable to complete task.

---

[a]Hand placement lifting in front of body: 26-in. space between hand placement on weight tray; 12 in. above the base of weight tray (width of tray = 6 in.).
[b]0–10 Scale; 0 = very comfortable; 5 = somewhat comfortable; 10 = very uncomfortable.

Recommendations

1. The work conditioning component of the active work rehabilitation program should include as its major goals the improvement of:
   - Forward reaching (standing)
   - Lifting tolerance
   - Carrying tolerance
   - Hand-tool use tolerance
2. Particular attention should be given to certain workplace factors that could be potentially modified (low or no cost to the employer). For example, include tilting the top of the mount (holding the wire harness) up and toward the worker in an attempt to reduce the forward reach distance and potential strain on the forearms and shoulders. When replacing certain tools (i.e., those that contribute toawkward deviation of the wrist and forearm) such as the pliers, wrenches, crimper, manual screwdriver, consider ergonomically designed tools. This should help reduce extreme wrist deviations and associated discomfort.

It should be noted that if certain recommended workplace modifications are implemented, the work-conditioning prescription would require a change in certain treatment goals to consider such workplace changes. The *overall* evaluation of both patients suggested that a multicomponent rehabilitation program including physical conditioning, modified work conditioning, and work-related pain and stress management should prove useful in facilitating a safe work reentry.

The reliability and validity of this approach require investigation. Although our group has operationalized the procedure and anecdotally the procedure appears to improve the quality of the evaluation and rehabilitation of the chronic work-disabled patient, specific determination of the psychometric properties of the multiple components of the approach and the validity of the decision-making algorithms await further investigation. From a clinical perspective, the approach appears to have assisted our rehabilitation efforts in this complex group of patients.

QUESTIONNAIRES AND CHECKLISTS

A number of questionnaires and checklists have been developed to assist in the analysis of ergonomic risks in the workplace and their relationship to symptoms. A comprehensive, yet simple, questionnaire has been developed by Kemmlert & Kilbom (1986). This technique was developed for large scale implementation by labor inspectors in Sweden. The questionnaire requires an identification of symptoms in select anatomical locations and then directs the observer to suspected workplace factors that may be contributing to the symptoms. The approach is simple and can be used as a point of departure for more detailed ergonomic assessment, if necessary, or as a mechanism to suggest areas requiring potential workplace modifications. Figure 6.12 provides an illustration of the form.

NIOSH has developed various questionnaires and surveys used in certain Health Hazard Appraisals (e.g., Burt, Hornung, Fine, Silverstein, & Armstrong, 1990). These questionnaires may be particularly useful in evaluating office-work risk and risk specifically associated with keyboarding in relation to upper extremity symptomatology.

CONCLUSIONS

The past decade has witnessed a greater emphasis on functional restoration rather than symptom management in patients with musculoskeletal pain disorders presumed to be associated with work. This focus on function is partly based upon the observation that given our current level of understanding of pain, the pain itself may not totally subside and that it is not necessary to wait for total pain relief before resuming normal functioning, providing the patient is medically stable or has reached maximum medical improvement. In addition, much has been reported on the importance of returning to and maintaining a certain degree of activity in that such activity may actually facilitate healing and reduce the likelihood of the negative physical and psychosocial consequences that can occur when the patient with persistent pain is isolated from daily functioning.

For those experiencing work-related musculoskeletal pain disorders and/or work disability where some aspect of the job or a work-related accident precipitated the onset and maintenance of pain and discomfort, returning to work represents a particular challenge. Work-

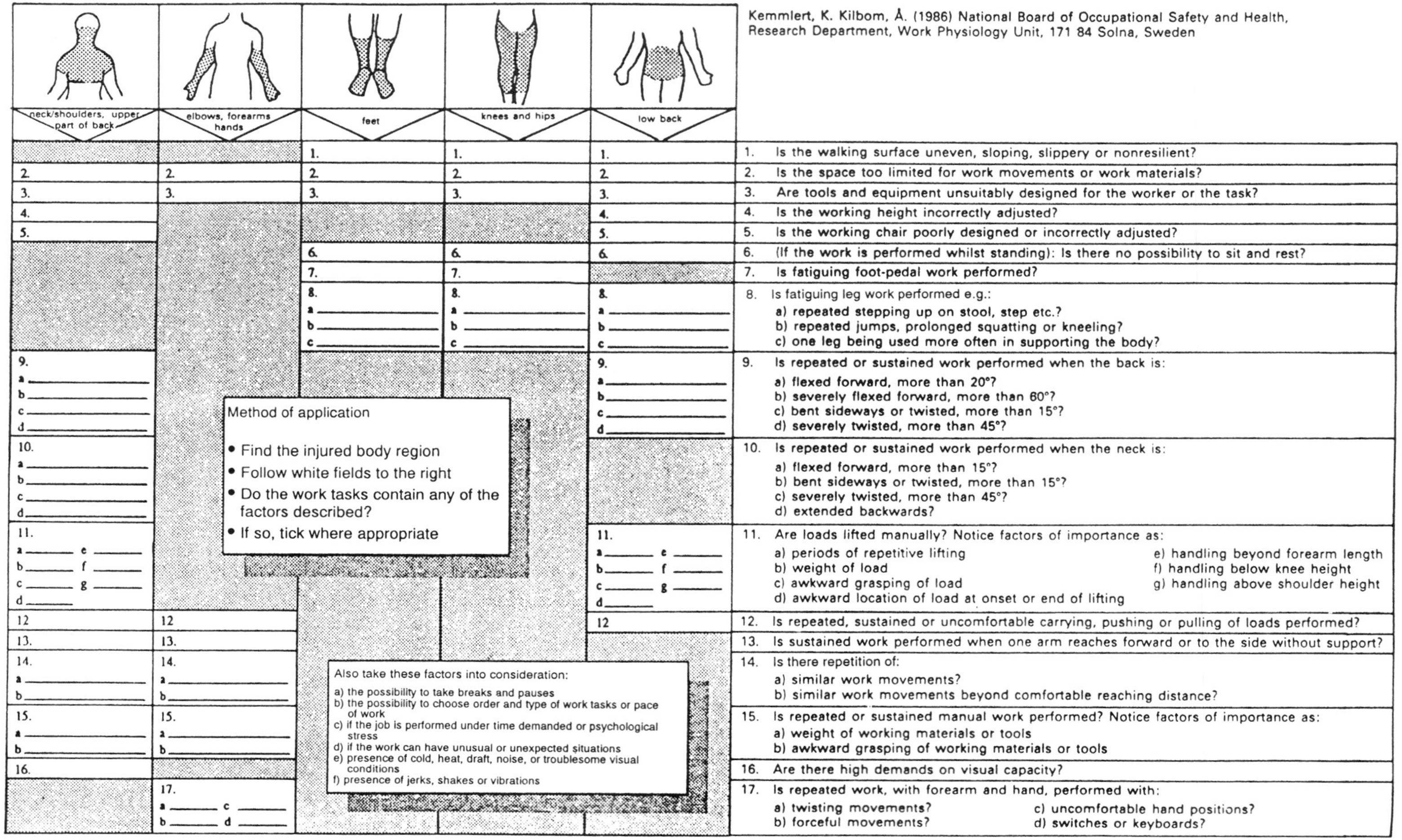

Kemmlert, K. Kilbom, A. (1986) National Board of Occupational Safety and Health, Research Department, Work Physiology Unit, 171 84 Solna, Sweden

Body regions (columns): neck/shoulders, upper part of back | elbows, forearms hands | feet | knees and hips | low back

Method of application
- Find the injured body region
- Follow white fields to the right
- Do the work tasks contain any of the factors described?
- If so, tick where appropriate

1. Is the walking surface uneven, sloping, slippery or nonresilient?
2. Is the space too limited for work movements or work materials?
3. Are tools and equipment unsuitably designed for the worker or the task?
4. Is the working height incorrectly adjusted?
5. Is the working chair poorly designed or incorrectly adjusted?
6. (If the work is performed whilst standing): Is there no possibility to sit and rest?
7. Is fatiguing foot-pedal work performed?
8. Is fatiguing leg work performed e.g.:
   a) repeated stepping up on stool, step etc.?
   b) repeated jumps, prolonged squatting or kneeling?
   c) one leg being used more often in supporting the body?
9. Is repeated or sustained work performed when the back is:
   a) flexed forward, more than 20°?
   b) severely flexed forward, more than 60°?
   c) bent sideways or twisted, more than 15°?
   d) severely twisted, more than 45°?
10. Is repeated or sustained work performed when the neck is:
    a) flexed forward, more than 15°?
    b) bent sideways or twisted, more than 15°?
    c) severely twisted, more than 45°?
    d) extended backwards?
11. Are loads lifted manually? Notice factors of importance as:
    a) periods of repetitive lifting
    b) weight of load
    c) awkward grasping of load
    d) awkward location of load at onset or end of lifting
    e) handling beyond forearm length
    f) handling below knee height
    g) handling above shoulder height
12. Is repeated, sustained or uncomfortable carrying, pushing or pulling of loads performed?
13. Is sustained or uncomfortable work performed when one arm reaches forward or to the side without support?
14. Is there repetition of:
    a) similar work movements?
    b) similar work movements beyond comfortable reaching distance?
15. Is repeated or sustained manual work performed? Notice factors of importance as:
    a) weight of working materials or tools
    b) awkward grasping of working materials or tools
16. Are there high demands on visual capacity?
17. Is repeated work, with forearm and hand, performed with:
    a) twisting movements?
    b) forceful movements?
    c) uncomfortable hand positions?
    d) switches or keyboards?

Also take these factors into consideration:
a) the possibility to take breaks and pauses
b) the possibility to choose order and type of work tasks or pace of work
c) if the job is performed under time demanded or psychological stress
d) if the work can have unusual or unexpected situations
e) presence of cold, heat, draft, noise, or troublesome visual conditions
f) presence of jerks, shakes or vibrations

FIGURE 6.12. Method for identifying symptom–workplace risk for occupational musculoskeletal disorders. From Kemmlert and Kilbom (1986).

place factors may indeed reestablish, exacerbate, and/or maintain symptoms and, therefore, consideration of such workplace risk factors represents an important component of a comprehensive clinical pain assessment in those individuals with an occupational musculoskeletal pain disorder. Such workplace analyses are completed by a number of healthcare and workplace safety professionals in an effort to facilitate the rehabilitation of the injured worker. These analyses range from a listing of "generic" job demands for particular sets of jobs based upon such databases as the *Dictionary of Occupational Titles* to a comprehensive on-site quantitative and qualitative assessment of task elements, suspected risks, suggested workplace modifications, and evaluation of the impact of such modifications.

The use of EJA in whatever form, conducted on a single workstation or work area in an *individual* worker experiencing symptoms and functional limitations, will significantly increase over the next decade in an effort to provide information to supervisors and human resources personnel to assist them with compliance to the recent Americans with Disabilities Act of 1990 (Morrisey, 1991). Efforts to curb rising workers' compensation costs associated with musculoskeletal disorders by facilitating return-to-work in injured workers and reducing reinjury once back at work should also serve to increase the use of the clinical EJA. These factors, coupled with an increased emphasis on primary prevention in which ergonomics plays an essential role, the development of guidelines for industry to reduce the risk of CTDs (e.g., U.S. Department of Labor, 1990; National Safety Council, 1990), and a general increased awareness on the part of labor and management facilitated by government regulatory agencies such as the Occupational Safety and Health Administration (OSHA), all suggest that the role of ergonomics in workplace safety and health is expanding. Thus, the use of such approaches to facilitate a safe return-to-work should find continuing and increasing support among workers, supervisors, and senior management. It is no longer an esoteric exercise.

However, despite a supportive climate for such an approach, the clinician faced with the task of returning the injured worker to the workplace meets with a number of challenges. Although there are a variety of measurement techniques available, the cost-effectiveness, reliability, and validity associated with the use of these techniques within a clinical context remain to be determined. Despite these limitations, the use of such methods and the general approach to considering the workplace in the evaluation and rehabilitation of the patient with an occupational musculoskeletal disorder represent a logical addition to the armamentarium of the clinician involved in the management of these complex cases.

Acknowledgments. This chapter was supported in part by a grant from the National Institute on Disability and Rehabilitation Research, Grant Number H133A00040. Address requests for reprints to: Michael Feuerstein, Ph.D., Center for Occupational Rehabilitation, University of Rochester Medical Center, 2337 Clinton Avenue South, Rochester, NY 14618.

REFERENCES

Andersson, G.B.J., Ortengren, R., Nachemson, A., & Elfstrom, G. (1974). Lumbar disc pressure and myoelectric back muscle activity during sitting. I. Studies on an experimental chair. *Scandinavian Journal of Rehabilitation Medicine, 6*, 104–114.

Andersson, G.B.J. (1979). Lowback pain in industry: Epidemiological aspects. *Scandinavian Journal of Rehabilitation Medicine, 11*, 163–168.

Andersson, G.B.J. (1987). Biomechanical aspects of sitting: an application to VDT terminals. *Behavior and Information Technology, 6* 257–269.

Armstrong, T.J. (1983). *An ergonomic guide to carpal tunnel syndrome.* Akron, OH: American Industrial Hygiene Association.

Armstrong, T.J. (1985). Mechanical considerations of skin in work. *American Journal of Industrial Medicine, 8*, 463–472.

Armstrong, T.J. (1986a). Ergonomics and cumulative trauma disorder. *Hand Clinics, 2*, 553–565.

Armstrong, T.J. (1986b). Upper extremity posture: Definition, measurement and control. In N. Corlett, J. Wilson, & I. Manenica (Eds.), *The ergonomics of working postures.* London: Taylor & Francis.

Armstrong, T.J. (1991). *Job analysis data collection form.* University of Michigan, Ann Arbor.

Armstrong, T.J., Fine, L.J., Goldstein, S.A., Lifshitz, Y.R., & Silverstein, B.A. (1987). Ergonomics consideration in hand and wrist tendinitis. *Journal of Hand Surgery, 12A* Pt. 2:830–837.

Armstrong, T.J. Punnett, L., & Ketner, P. (1989). Subjective worker assessments of hand tools used in automobile assembly. *American Industrial Hygiene Association Journal, 50*, 639–645.

Astrand, P.O., & Rodahl, K. (1986). *Textbook of work physiology* (3rd ed.). New York: McGraw Hill.

Ayoub, M.M., & Mital, A. (1989). *Manual materials handling.* Philadelphia: Taylor & Francis.

Bigos, S.J., Battie, M.C., Spengler, D.M., Fisher, L.D., Fordyce, W.E., Hansson, T.H., Nachemson, A.L., & Wortley, M.D. (1991). A prospective study of work perceptions and psychosocial factors affecting the report of back injury. *Spine, 16,* 1–6.

Borg, G.V. (1982). Psychophysical bases of perceived exertion. *Medicine and Science in Sports and Exercise, 14,* 377–387.

Borg, G. (1990). Psychophysical scaling with applications in physical work and the perception of exertion. *Scandinavian Journal of Work and Environmental Health, 16,* 55–66.

Burt, S., Hornung, R., Fine, L., Silverstein, B., & Armstrong, T. (1990). *Health hazard evaluation report: Newsday.* U.S. Dept. of Health and Human Services, National Institute for Occupational Safety and Health. HETA 89-250-2046.

Bureau of Labor Statistics. (1991). *Occupational injuries and illnesses in the United States by Industry, 1989. Bulletin 2379.* Washington, DC: U.S. Department of Labor.

Byelle, A., Hagberg, M., & Michaelsson, G. (1979). Clinical and ergonomic factors in prolonged shoulder pain among industrial workers. *Scandinavian Journal of Work, Environment and Health, 5,* 205–210.

Cannon, L., Bernacki, E., & Walter, S. (1981). Personal and occupational factors associated with carpal tunnel syndrome. *Journal of Occupational Medicine, 23,* 255–258.

Chaffin, D.B., & Andersson, G.B.J. (1991). *Occupational biomechanical models.* (2nd ed.). Philadelphia: Wiley Interscience.

Chaffin, D., & Armstrong, T. (1991). *Occupational ergonomics.* University of Michigan, College of Engineering Short Courses, Ann Arbor, Michigan, June 17–21.

Chaffin, D.B., Herrin, G.D., Keyserling, W.M., & Garg, A. (1977). A method for evaluating the biomechanical stresses resulting from manual materials handling jobs. *American Industrial Hygiene Association Journal, 38,* 662–675.

Chaffin, D.B., & Park, K.S. (1973). A longitudinal study of low back pain as associated with occupational weight lifting factors. *American Industrial Hygiene Association Journal, 34,* 513–525.

Christensen, J.M., Topmiller, D.A., & Gill, R.T. (1988). Human factors definitions revisited. *Human Factors Society Bulletin, 31,* 7–8.

Clark, T.S., & Corlett, E.N. (1984). *The ergonomics of workspaces and machines: A design manual.* London: Taylor & Francis.

Corlett, E.N., & Bishop, R.P. (1976). A technique for assessing postural discomfort. *Ergonomics, 19,* 175–182.

Cox, T. (1980). Repetitive work. In C.L. Cooper & R. Payne (Eds.), *Current concerns in occupational stress* (pp. 23–41) Chichester: Wiley.

Deyo, R.A., & Tsui-Wu, Y.J. (1987). Descriptive epidemiology of low back pain and its related medical care in the United States. *Spine, 12,* 264–268.

Drury, C.G. (1987). A biomechanical evaluation of the repetitive motion injury potential of industrial jobs. *Seminars in Occupational Medicine, 2,* 41–49.

Drury, C.G., & Wick, J. (1984). Ergonomic applications in the shoe industry. *Proceeding of the 1984 International Conference on Occupational Ergonomics, 1,* 489–493.

Eastman Kodak Company, Ergonomics Group. (1983). *Ergonomic design for people at work* (Vol. 1). New York: Van Nostrand Reinhold.

Eastman Kodak Company, Ergonomics Group. (1986). *Ergonomic design for people at work* (Vol. 2). New York: Van Nostrand Reinhold.

Feuerstein, M. (1991). A multidisciplinary approach to the prevention, evaluation and management of work disability. *Journal for Occupational Rehabilitation, 1,* 5–12.

Feuerstein, M., & Fitzgerald, T.E. (1992). Biomechanical factors affecting upper extremity cumulative trauma disorders in sign language interpreters. *Journal of Occupational Medicine, 34,* 257–264.

Feuerstein, M., Labbé, E.E., & Kuczmierczyk, A.R. (1986). *Health psychology: A psychobiological perspective.* New York: Plenum.

Feuerstein, M., Sult, S., & Houle, M. (1985). Environmental stressors and chronic low back pain: Life events, family and work environment. *Pain, 22,* 295–307.

Flinn-Wagner, S., Mladonicky, A., & Goodman, G. (1990). Characteristics of workers with upper extremity injuries who make a successful transition to work. *Journal of Hand Therapy, 3,* 51–55.

Frazer, T.M. (1989). *The worker at work.* Philadelphia: Taylor & Francis.

Gallagher, R.M., Rauh, V., Haugh, L.D., Milhous, R., Callas, P.W., Langelier, R., McClallen, J.M., & Frymoyer, J. (1989). Determinants of return to work among low back pain patients. *Pain, 39,* 55–67.

Gamberale, F., Kjellberg, A., Akerstedt, & T., Johansson, G. (1990). Behavioral and psychophysicological effects of the physical work environment. *Scandinavian Journal of Work and Environmental Health, 16,* 5–16.

Grandjean, E. (1988). *Fitting the task to the man: A textbook of occupational ergonomics.* Philadelphia: Taylor & Francis.

Hadler, N.M. (1989). Work related disorders of the upper extremity: Part 1. Cumulative trauma disorders—a critical review. *Occupational Problems in Medical Practice, 4,* 1–8.

Kelsey, J.L., & Golden, A.L. (1987). Occupational and workplace factors associated with low back pain. *Spine: State of the Art Reviews, 2,* 7–16.

Kelsey, J.L., & Hardy, E.J. (1975). Driving of motor vehicles as a risk factor for acute herniated lumbar intervertebral disc. *American Journal of Epidemiology, 102,* 63–73.

Kemmlert, J., & Kilbom, K.K. (1986). *The Nordic Questionnaires.* National Board of Occupational Safety and Health Research Department, Work Physiology Unit, 171 84 Solna Sweden.

Keyserling, W.M. (1986). A computer-aided system to evaluate postural stress in the workplace. *American Industrial Hygiene Association, 47,* 641–649.

Keyserling, W.M., Armstrong, T.J., & Punnett, L. (1991). Ergonomic job analysis: A structured approach for identifying risk factors associated with overexertion injuries and disorders. *Applied Occupational Environmental Hygiene, 6,* 353–363.

Keyserling, W.M., Punnett, L., & Fine, L.J. (1988). Trunk posture and back pain: Identification and control of occupational risk factors. *Applied Industrial Hygiene, 3,* 87–92.

Knapp, D.A., & Koch, H. (1984). *The management of new pain in office-based ambulatory care. National Ambulatory Medical Care Survey, 1980 and 1981.* National Center for Health Statistics. *Advance Data from Vital and Health Statistics*, No. 97, (DHHS Pub. No. PHS 84-1250). Hyattsville, MD: Public Health Service.

Kroemer, K.H.E., Kroemer, H.J., & Kroemer-Elbert, K.E. (1990). *Engineering physiology: Bases of human factors/ergonomics* (2nd ed.). New York: Van Nostrand Reinhold.

Kurppa, K., Warris, P., & Kokkanen, P. (1979). Tennis elbow. *Scandinavian Journal of Work, Environment and Health, 5*, 15–18.

Magora, A. (1972). Investigation of the relationship between low back pain and occupation: III. Physical requirements: Sitting, standing and weight lifting. *Industrial Medicine Surgery.* 4:5–9.

Mayer, T.G., Gatchel, R.J., Mayer, H., Kishino, N.D., Keeley, J., & Mooney, V. (1987). A prospective two-year study of functional restoration in industrial low back injury. *Journal of the American Medical Association, 258*, 1763–1767.

McAtee, F.L. (1987). Reducing repetitive motions injuries in overhead assembly: A case study. *Seminars in Occupational Medicine, 2*, 73–74.

McKenzie, F., Stormet, J., Van Hook, P., & Armstrong, T.J. (1985). A program for control of repetitive trauma disorders associated with hand tool operations in a telecommunications manufacturing facility. *American Industrial Hygiene Association Journal, 46*, 674–678.

Mitchell, R.I., & Carmen, G.M. (1990). Results of a multicenter trial using an intensive active exercise program for the treatment of acute soft tissue and back injuries. *Spine, 15*, 514–521.

Morrissey, P.A. (1991). *A primer for corporate America on civil rights for the disabled.* Horsham, PA: LPR Publications.

National Aeronautics and Space Administration. (1978). *Anthropometry source book.* NASA Reference Publications, 1024.

National Center for Health Statistics, Koch, H. (1986). *The management of chronic pain in office-based ambulatory care: National Ambulatory Medical Care Survey. Advance Data from Vital and Health Statistics*, No. 123, (DHHS Pub. No. PHS 86-1250). Hyattsville, MD: Public Health Service.

National Institute for Occupational Safety and Health (1981). *Work practices guide for manual lifting* (Report No. 81-122). Cincinnati, OH: Author.

National Safety Council (1990). *Accredited standards committee: Control of cumulative trauma disorders ANSI Z365.* Secretariat, National Safety Council. Chicago, IL.

Pope, M.H., Andersson, G.B.H., & Chaffin, D.B. (1991). The workplace. In M.H. Pope, G.B.J. Andersson, J.W. Frymoyer, & D.B. Chaffin, (Eds.), *Occupational low-back pain: assessment, treatment and prevention* (pp. 117–131). St. Louis, MO: Mosby Yearbook.

Pope, M.H., Andersson, G.B.J., Frymoyer, D.B., & Chaffin, D.B. (Eds.)(1991). *Occupational low-back pain: Assessment, treatment and prevention.* St. Louis, MO: Mosby Yearbook.

Putz-Anderson, V. (Ed.). (1988). *Cumulative trauma disorder—A manual for musculoskeletal diseases of the upper limbs.* Philadelphia: Taylor & Francis.

Rodgers, S.H. (1988). Job evaluation in worker fitness determination. *Occupational Medicine: State of the Art Reviews, 3*, 219–239.

Rohmert, W. (1973). Problems in determining rest allowances: Part 1. Use of modern methods to evaluate stress and strain in static muscular work. *Applied Ergonomics, 4*, 91.

Salvendy, G. (Ed.). (1987). *Handbook of human factors.* New York: Wiley-Interscience.

Sandover, J. (1983). Dynamic loading as a possible source of low back disorder. *Spine, 8*, 652–658.

Sauter, S.L., Dainoff, M.J., & Smith, M.J. (Eds.). (1990). *Promoting health and productivity in the computerized office: Models of successful ergonomic interventions.* London: Taylor & Francis.

Schackel, B., Chidsey, K.S., & Shipley,P. (1979). The assessment of chair comfort. *Ergonomics, 12*, 269–306.

Silverstein, B.A., Fine, L.J., & Armstrong, T.J. (1987). Occupational factors and carpal tunnel syndrome. *American Journal of Industrial Medicine, 11*, 343–358.

Snook, S.H. (1978). The design of manual handling tasks. *Ergonomics, 21*, 963–985.

Snook, S.H. (1987). Approaches to the control of back pain in industry: Job design, job placement and education/training. *Spine: State of the Art Reviews, 2*, 45–49.

Spitzer, W.O., LeBlanc, F.E., & Dupuis, M. (1987). Scientific approach to the assessment and management of activity-related spinal disorders. *Spine, 12(7S)*.

Stull, G.A., & Clark, A.H. (1971). Patterns of recovery following isometric and isotonic strength decrement. *Medicine and Science in Sports and Exercise, 3*, 135–139.

Svensson, H.O., & Andersson, G.B.J. (1983). Low back pain in 40–47 year old men: Work history and work environment factors. *Spine, 8*, 272–276.

Ulin, S.S., Armstrong, T.J., & Radwin, R.G. (1990). Use of computer aided drafting for analysis and control of posture in manual work. *Applied Ergonomics, 21*, 143–151.

Ulin, S.S., Ways, C.M., Armstrong, T.J. & Snook, S.H. (1990). Perceived exertion and discomfort versus work height with a pistol-shaped screwdriver. *American Industrial Hygiene Associated Journal, 51*, 588–594.

U.S. Department of Health and Human Services. (1981). *Practices guide for manual lifting* (DHSS NIOSH Publication No. 81-122). Cincinnati, OH: National Institute for Occupational Safety and Health.

U.S. Department of Labor. (1977). *Dictionary of occupational titles* (4th ed.). Washington, DC: Author.

U.S. Department of Labor. (1990). *Ergonomics program management for meat packing plants.* OSHA Publication No. 3123. Washington, DC: Author.

Wick, J.L. (1987). Workplace design changes to reduce repetitive motions injuries in an assembly task: A case study. *Seminars in Occupational Medicine, 2*, 75–77.

Wilson, J.R., & Corlett, E.N. (Eds.). 1990. *Evaluation of human work.* Philadelphia: Taylor & Francis.

World Health Organization (1989). Work with visual display terminals: Psychosocial aspects and health. *Journal of Occupational Medicine, 31*, 957–968.

Chapter 7

Impairment, Disability, and Functional Capacity Assessment

SRIDHAR V. VASUDEVAN, MD

Pain and disability are both complex phenomena that are difficult to define, and pose a formidable task in their assessment. Pain is a ubiquitous symptom and is one of the primary reasons individuals contact health care providers. In the majority of situations, pain is a warning of an underlying pathology that can be identified, and the symptoms resolve after the underlying clinical condition is adequately treated, Thus, in most situations pain serves a biologically useful function, helping the patient seek medical attention, and assisting the physician in making appropriate diagnosis and treatment decisions.

Pain also leads to varying degrees of alteration in function. This could vary from a minor inconvenience, to significant disability, such as the inability to work or participate in enjoyable activities. Just as pain is greatly modified by nonmedical variables, functional capacities and disability are affected by numerous psychosocial and environmental factors.

Elsewhere in this handbook, the various methods of measuring pain including psychological as well as behavioral assessments are addressed. This chapter provides an overview regarding the complexity of both pain and disability, and discusses some of the methods

utilized in the assessment of impairment, disability, and functional capacity.

ACUTE VERSUS CHRONIC PAIN

The past three decades have seen an explosion of research in the understanding of pain mechanisms and management. Despite these advances, management of individuals with persistent pain continues to be a major problem throughout the world and great challenge to the health care industry (Osterweis, Kleinman, & Mechanic, 1987). Several factors affect the understanding, measurement, and management of pain. These include (1) lack of uniform definitions of pain, (2) problems with clear explanations of the pain phenomenon, (3) problems with uniformly accepted objective pain measurement techniques, (4) psychological and environmental variables that relate to pain, and (5) cognitive and individual variability of pain based on ethnocultural background, social structures, and so on. (Osterweis et al., 1987; Vasudevan, 1989).

Acute pain is defined or perceived as a subjective sensation. It can also be defined as a unique complex made of up afferent stimuli

100

interacting with the emotional or affective state of the individual, modified by past experience, and present state of mind (Engelberg, 1988).

The model, where pain is related to nociception, works well to explain the process of pain perception when there is an identifiable noxious stimuli (Report of the Commission on Evaluation of Pain, 1986). However, it is well recognized that there could be injury to bodily tissues without pain, and there are clinical situations in which pain occurs without an identifiable injury or pathology. *Thus, there is no one-to-one relationship between injury and pain.* Therefore, acute pain is generally viewed as a biologically meaningful, useful, and time-limited experience.

In a small but significant portion of individuals, pain may persist despite optimal treatment, may recur, and may become chronic. In any given patient, it is impossible to predict the course of the condition at the first episode of pain. It is estimated that acute and chronic pain requiring treatment affects 45% of Americans annually, and costs the U.S. economy $85–$90 billion annually, with one third of the American population estimated to have "chronic pain" (Osterweis et al., 1987; Report of the Commission on Evaluation of Pain, 1986). It is also estimated that 50 million Americans partially or totally lose their ability to work because of pain, with a loss of 700 million work days every year secondary to pain-related disabilities (Report of the Commission on Evaluation of Pain, 1986). Pain that lasts beyond the "usual healing period" can be considered persistent or chronic pain. Black (1990), in an extensive discussion, proposes the term "chronic pain syndrome" for those patients with significant alteration in lifestyle, in addition to intractable, often multiple pain symptoms, many of which are inappropriate to identifiable physical problems or illness.

Gildenberg and DeVaul (1985) describe the features of the patient with chronic pain. In addition to the predominant symptom of pain, similar to the pain that occurred at the time of an injury or episode, such patients have attempted and have been unsuccessful with various medical, surgical, and physical approaches to treating their pain. They also have significant lifestyle changes including dysfunction, deconditioning, drug misuse, depression, and disability that far exceeds underlying pathology usually manifested by dramatic pain behaviors

(Gildenberg & DeVaul, 1985; Osterweis et al., 1987).

It is important to recognize that there are no objective measures or techniques for the absolute measurement of pain. Thus, it is impossible to either "prove" or "disprove" the existence of pain in any given individual. The Commission on Evaluation of Pain (1986), after an extensive study of this topic, states that "no one can know the pain of another person" (p. 54). It bears emphasis that pain behaviors, not pain itself, are observable to the outsider. Such pain behaviors comprise verbal and nonverbal expression or actions indicating that pain is being experienced. Verbal expressions include moans, gasps, and overt statements of complaints of pain. Facial expressions, guarded movements, limping, use of cane or assistive devices are examples of nonverbal pain behaviors. Other behaviors such as frequent reliance upon the health care system by repeatedly seeking medical and health care consultation, excessive use of nonessential medications, multiple surgeries, therapy, and avoidance of work or pleasurable events, are examples of pain behaviors (Osterweis et al., 1987; see also Keefe & Williams, Chapter 16).

Pain behaviors are influenced by a variety of factors other than the underlying identifiable pathological process. Some of these pain behaviors may be under conscious control of an individual. However, the influence by effects of naturally occurring learning processes, wherein any act that is considered a positive reinforcement by the patient for his or her expression of pain may reinforce a continuing occurrence of pain behaviors, should be recognized.

Loeser (1986) has provided a view of pain with four distinct components. These include (1) nociception, which is the tissue damage and the activation of peripheral nerve fibers, (2) pain, which is an unpleasant sensory or emotional experience associated with actual or potential tissue damage, (3) suffering, which is an emotional response to pain involving higher levels of brain function influenced by fear, isolation, anxiety, and depression, and (4) pain behaviors, which are anything a patient says, does or does not do which would lead one to infer that the individual has pain.

In summary, pain is a highly complex phenomenon that involves an interaction of biochemical, physiological, behavioral, and cognitive factors, and is influenced by socioeconomic factors, belief systems, family dynamics, coping abilities, and compensation.

CONCEPTUAL BASIS OF DISABILITY

Disability is similarly a complex problem. Terms such as "impairment" and "disability" are used in different settings to mean something different. In addition, the different systems of disability define disability in different contexts. Although the Social Security Act defines disability "as an inability to work at any substantial gainful activity," it does not provide for partial disability. Most worker's compensation laws have both temporary and permanent disability, as well as partial and total disability. There is also significant variation from state to state, and between the disability systems, making the evaluation of disability a complex process that cannot be easily condensed into a "formula." Although impairment is an objectively documentable state, disability represents an alteration of an individual's capacity to meet social or occupational demands or to meet the statutory or regulatory requirements (Engelberg, 1988; Report of the Commission on Evaluation of Pain, 1986).

The clinician evaluating disability should possess a conceptual understanding of the terminology and the disability process. The *Guides to the Evaluation of Permanent Impairment* (Engelberg, 1988), defines "impairment" as an alteration in an individual's health status that is *assessed by medical means*, whereas "disability" is *assessed by nonmedical means*. Individuals who are "impaired" are not necessarily "disabled." Impairment gives rise to disability only when the medical condition limits the individual's capacity to meet the demands that pertain to specific activities. Or, an individual may have an impairment that may not affect specific demands for that particular individual, thus not producing disability.

Melvin and Nagi (1970) provide a conceptual basis of disability and discuss it under the following four steps:

1. *Pathology*: This is altered anatomy and/or physiology. Pathology includes the initial injury to the body, either from trauma, infection, metabolic disorder, or etiology, and the body's response to such injury. It also includes

aggravation of a previously present problem, such as cervical osteoarthritis or underlying cardiac problem. Examples of pathology include lumbosacral strain, herniated lumbar disc, diabetic polyneuropathy, and so on.

2. *Impairment*: Impairments are defined as an anatomical, physiological, or psychological abnormality or loss (Melvin, 1966; Osterweis et al., 1987). Impairments may be temporary during active pathology or may become permanent, continuing even after the active pathology is adequately treated and resolved. Examples of impairments include decreased range of motion from lumbosacral strain or herniated lumbar disc, altered reflexes, decreased strength or loss of sensation from radiculopathy, or abnormal electromyographic studies seen in individuals with herniated disc or diabetic polyneuropathy. Anatomical impairments include contractures, loss of limb, deformities, and decreased range of motion. Physiological impairments include decreased cardiac output, decreased pulmonary function, abnormal electrophysiological studies, abnormal blood chemistry, muscle weakness, and so on. Changes in cognition and memory, as seen in individuals with closed head injury, and abnormalities of personality detected on the Minnesota Multiphasic Personality Inventory (MMPI), are objective psychological impairments. Thus, it is important to recognize that impairments are *objective* and are *medically determinable* through clinical and/or laboratory assessments.

3. *Functional limitation*: A restriction or the lack of ability to perform an activity or function in the manner within the range considered normal for that person, that results from an impairment, is described as functional limitation. Examples of functional limitation include the inability in an individual with lumbosacral disc disease and nerve compression to lift over 20 lbs., inability to retain more than two-step direction in an individual with head trauma, inability to do stressful activities such as climbing stairs in a person with severe ischemic heart disease, or inability to function safely in a community in an individual with cognitive and affective changes due to closed head injury. *Thus, functional limitations are manifestations of impairment translated in terms of function.*

4. *Disability*: The inability of the individual to perform his or her usual activities and to assume usual obligations can be viewed as disability. Thus, disability is "task specific."

Permanent disability is presumed to be present if an individual's actual or presumed ability to engage in gainful activity is reduced or absent, due to an impairment, which in turn may or may not be combined with other factors (Engelberg, 1988; Osterweis et al., 1987).

The ability to engage in gainful activity is affected by many factors including the individual's age, sex, education, and economic and social environment, in addition to the medically determinable permanent impairments. Thus, disability is viewed as a condition in a given individual that results from impairment, and the functional limitation that prevents a fulfillment of a role that is normal for that individual.

Examples of disability would include a variety of conditions that limit the fulfilling of a role in life such as a father, mother, student, or worker. Thus, *disability is both "task specific and role specific."*

The conceptual framework described above is very important in the assessment of disability. In addition, such a framework is very useful in developing appropriate treatment for the different stages of the disability process. Recognizing and treating the underlying pathology with appropriate pharmacotherapy, surgical, physical, or psychiatric therapy can lead to no residual impairments, thus preventing disability. Physicians and clinicians are also trained to evaluate impairments that are the objective *signs*. Limitation of function can also be assessed through a variety of objective and observable means.

Assessment of disability however, requires knowledge of the individual's previous education, past work experience, specific demands of a job, and other factors such as age, sex, and economic and social environment. Thus disability determination is an administrative decision with input provided through medical information with regard to impairments, which *only* physicians can provide (Engelberg, 1988).

Disability can also be conceived as a pattern of behavior that evolves when impairments actually do, or are perceived to, impose limitations upon an individual's capacities and performance of his or her usual role and activities (Melvin, 1966; Melvin & Nagi, 1970). These authors suggest that the pattern of disability behavior vary considerably as a result of differences in (1) characteristics of impairments, 2) response to impairments by individuals, and

(3) response to impairments by others including family members, friends, employers, co-workers, physicians, and others. Thus the nature and severity of disability imposed by an impairment vary widely from patient to patient.

THE PAIN–DISABILITY RELATIONSHIP

The above discussion has emphasized that both pain and disability are complex processes affected by many psychological, social, and environmental variables. In the acute phase, alteration of function, due to pain and impairment, can lead to disability for both work-related activities and one's social independence.

Both research and clinical experience have demonstrated, however, *that there is no clear relationship between pain and tissue damage and the degree of functional disability* (Osterweis et al., 1987). In the patient with chronic pain, psychosocial and environment variables become inextricably intertwined with the underlying pathophysiological changes (Osterweis et al., 1987; Report of the Commission on Evaluation of Pain, 1986). The psychological and physical factors are not dichotomous in their effects on maintenance of pain. There is also evidence that the effects of chronic pain and resultant disability can be reversed with comprehensive multidisciplinary treatment that includes rehabilitative, behavioral, and social management (Lynch & Vasudevan, 1988; Osterweis et al., 1987; Vasudevan & Lynch, 1991).

It is estimated that more than 1.5 million people file claims each year for Social Security disability in the United States. Of these 10%, or 150,000 per year, have pain as their primary complaint without clinical findings to fully substantiate their symptom, thus resulting in denial for eligibility of Social Security disability benefits (Osterweis et al., 1987). In response to this significant problem faced by individuals claiming Social Security disability with the predominant symptom of pain, the Secretary of the Department of Health and Human Services appointed a Commission on Evaluation of Pain (Report of the Commission on Evaluation of Pain, 1986). This commission presented its analysis in June 1986 and suggested further study. The Institute of Medicine, after a year of deliberation, produced a monograph titled

Pain and Disability: Clinical, Behavioral and Public Policy Perspective, which provides an excellent review of the relationship between pain and disability (Osterweis et al., 1987). In their analysis (Osterweis et al., 1987) they note that the expenditures for disability payments doubled between 1970 and 1982. Variability in definitions of disability and the complexity of the pain phenomenon were emphasized. It was noted that many individuals have considerable pain in the absence of clinical findings accounting for it, whereas others have clear anatomical abnormalities without pain. Despite advances in the assessment of pain described throughout this volume, there is as yet no uniformly acceptable method to measure the complexity of the biopsychosocial phenomenon of pain.

ASSESSMENT OF IMPAIRMENT AND FUNCTIONAL CAPACITY

The determination of one's functional capacity, on one hand, appears to be a relatively routine and simple matter, especially in those with clearly identifiable pathology with resultant impairments. Thus, in an individual with acute lumbosacral muscular strain caused by a traumatic event, the person would be considered "disabled" for the functional requirements of his or her work during the time of active medical treatment. Such a patient can then be returned to work after the resolution of the underlying muscular strain and elimination of symptoms. In individuals with significant paralysis or loss of vision or hearing, the assessment of disability may be a relatively easy process. However, physicians and clinicians are frequently faced with making determination of disability in individuals who have very minimal to no objective medical findings, thus leading to perplexing and difficult situations with implications for both the individual and society (Vasudevan, 1989; Vasudevan & Monsein, 1992).

Determination of Impairment

Impairment, as evidenced by the previous discussion, is an objectively measurable alteration of anatomical, physiological, or psychological status of the human being. It represents "objective signs" that are used in a typical medical evaluation as those objectively determinable.

This is in contrast to symptoms that are reported by the patient and are inherently subjective.

Depending on the area of the body involved, impairments would take on the appropriate assessment of that bodily process from the anatomical and physiological point of view, as well as psychological function where appropriate.

It is beyond the scope of this chapter to address specific assessment techniques for all impairments. Hoppenfeld (1976) provides a guideline for examination of specific impairments and of function of spine and extremities. This should be part of a routine physical examination by physicians in assessment impairments. Vasudevan (1990) provides an outline of a physical examination of the patient with chronic pain focusing on the musculoskeletal and neurological examination. Similarly Mayer and Gatchel (1988) provide a systematic approach to physical examination focused on assessment of critical parameters including objective evidence corroborating pain symptoms, evidence confirming need for possible invasive treatment such as neurological deficits, evidence of systematic illness, and the evidence of symptom magnification with an emphasis on nonorganic signs (see Polatin & Mayer, Chapter 3).

Each phase of the physical examination for impairments involves inspection, palpation, as well as specific testing. Palpation is crucial to assess "muscle spasm" to specifically assess whether such "muscle guarding" is voluntary or involuntary, as well as its presence. Assessment of range of motion of joints, specific muscle strength testing and neurological examination such as assessment of reflexes, neurotension tests such as straight leg raising and specific sensory abnormalities, should be noted.

Radiographs such as plain x-rays, computerized axial tomography scanning, magnetic resonance imaging, and myelography provide examples of testing that could identify anatomical impairments. Blood tests, electromyography, and assessment of evoked potentials are examples of physiological impairment assessment. For details of some of the psychological impairment assessments, the reader is referred to other chapters in this handbook.

Patients with symptoms of low back pain comprise a significant portion of those with chronic pain reporting significant disability especially as it relates to resuming work and social activities. Measurement of objective spinal and joint function has been fraught with limitations. The American Medical Association *Guides to the Evaluation of Impairments* (Engelberg, 1988) provides an overview of the difficulties in assessing spinal mobility. The simple angular test that has been used historically is not only inaccurate but may have prejudiced the current generation of clinicians (Mayer & Gatchel, 1988). A frequently used clinical assessment is that of a modified Schober Test (Macrae & Wright, 1969). Although it is a simple and rapid method of assessment, it is fraught with inaccuracies and does not accurately reflect spinal function. The inclinometer is a method that has been studies and applied universally to assess sagittal, coronal, and axial plane movements (Keely et al., 1986).

Assessment of muscle strength is a routine part of the physical examination. However, there has been considerable variation in assessment of muscle strength and performance. The term "muscular strength" refers to the capacity of muscle for active development of tension, irrespective of the specific condition under which the tension is measured (Sapega, 1990). There are different types of muscle contraction, as well as different methods of testing of muscular performance. Sapega (1990), in a recent extensive review, discusses the muscle performance evaluation in an orthopedic practice. Objective tests of muscle strength are important, and the availability of computerized dynamometry systems has added to some of the objectivity through these sophisticated devices.

Assessment of strength is another method of assessing an identifiable physiological impairment. There are several trunk strength testing systems including the Cybex®, Isotechnologies®, Kin-com devices®, Biodex®, and Lido®. To more accurately assess relevance to function, mechanisms such as lift tasks analysis and task performance simulation are usually utilized. Again, there is no universally acceptable standardized technique in such functional assessment. However, whenever possible, physical as well as functional assessment techniques should be incorporated in assessing impairment and function. The concept of acceptable maximum effort (AME) has been introduced, which refers to a quantitative method of measuring functional abilities in chronic pain (Khalil et al., 1986). AME is the highest level of *voluntary* effort that a person can achieve without inducing unacceptable pain. Quantitative methods such as the AME can provide clinicians and researchers with a vehicle by which evaluation of functional abilities of pain patients can become more standardized (Khalil et al., 1986). Such functional measures can be used in addition to instrumented testing of the back (Hasson & Wise, 1989).

Determination of Functional Capacity

Functional capacity evaluation is defined as a quantitative measurement, by direct or indirect means, of a dynamic aspect of bodily activity necessary in daily living (Mayer & Gatchel, 1988). Referred to also as functional capacity assessment, performance capacity evaluation, performance capacity estimate, and so on, it involves the examination and assessment of a patient's ability to carry out a series of structured activities. In some situations it may involve a specific assessment of trunk and extremity strength and performance of functional tasks. There is, however, to date, no uniformly acceptable series of activities that can be used to assess functional capacity. Some are highly complex, involving lift task analysis compared to some standardized technique, while others are observation of a series of "work-simulated" activities. However, interindividual comparisons are difficult, and there is no standardization that is universally acceptable.

Despite the limitations noted, functional capacity assessment provides a "snapshot" of an individual's demonstrated activities in a structured setting. It does not necessarily reflect what the patient "should be able to do" but rather "what the patient can do" on a particular day, in a particular time period. Thus, all the other variables such as motivational, cognitive, and behavioral factors that affect pain and disability can significantly affect the outcome of functional capacity assessments. At the minimum, these functional capacity assessments include an evaluation of range of motion of the major joints, dynamic strength testing, including axial strength and lifting assessment, along with the assessment of strength and endurance for specific tasks. Mayer and Gatchel (1989) emphasized some of the pitfalls in functional capacity assessment and raised several pertinent questions. These include the need for critical assessment of the validity/accuracy, relevance, replication/reliability, as well as the lack of "normative database" for many of the assessments.

Assessment of Disability

There is obviously no simple technique or formula to evaluate the various manifestations of disability. Social Security disability, worker's compensation, and civil injury are examples of the three common systems through which clinicians interact. Each views the concept of pain and disability in different ways and requires different data elements (Vasudevan & Monsein, 1992).

A major controversy in the determination of disability is the commonly held assumption that physical examination can provide an "objective and consistent" method of assessing impairment that is "medically determinable." Yet studies have demonstrated great diversity among physicians in their evaluation of patients with back pain, particularly regarding nonneurological findings such as muscle spasm and guarding (Nelson, Allen, Clampe, & De Dombal, 1979; Wadell et al., 1982).

Laboratory and x-ray findings have also been generally considered the sine qua non of objectivity with regard to clinical pain conditions. However, in the case of low back pain there is certainly no clear-cut relationship between the presence of degenerative changes and the patient's symptoms. Powell (Powell, Wilson, Szypryt, Symonds, & Worthington, 1986) reported that a third of 302 asymptomatic women for low back pain seen in a gynecological practice were found to have evidence of degenerative disc disease. Similarly, Wiesel (Wiesel, Tsourmas, Feffer, Citrin, & Patronas, 1984) noted that 50% of asymptomatic individuals over the age of 40 years had abnormal CT scans.

The above information is presented not to deny the importance of objective medical information but *to emphasize the lack of one-to-one correlation between clinical findings and disability.* Through extensive reviews, the study by the Institute of Medicine demonstrated the poor relationship and the lack of correlation between objective identifiable pathology and impairments with an individual's function and disability (Osterweis et al., 1987).

In an effort to solve this dilemma, several authors have suggested measurement tools to assess pain and disability. In a review article Deyo (1988) emphasized the criteria that should be considered in developing an ideal instrument. These include practicality, comprehensiveness, replicability, validity, and responsiveness. In addition, several authors have attempted measurement of pain and the "effects of pain" on one's lifestyle (Osterweis et al., 1987; Turk, Rudy, & Stieg, 1989).

This handbook presents a variety of questionnaires and instruments that are available to provide more objective documentation of a patient's level of functioning and the impact of pain on his or her lifestyle. Many of these instruments provide valid and objective assessment of some of the psychological as well as social impairments and "disability." Information from such instruments is essential to reflect pain-related disability, in addition to the physical examination (Turk et al., 1989; Vasudevan & Monsein, 1992).

However, to date, no instrument has been universally accepted as the "gold standard" to assess pain-related disability. Thus, it is difficult to compare one instrument to the other (Deyo, 1988). Turk et al. (1989) review the utilization of multiaxial pain assessment, which measures the impact of pain on an individual's functioning. This approach, discussed elsewhere in this handbook (see Turk & Rudy, Chapter 23), is a step toward providing an instrument that could be reliable, valid, and helpful in the classification of those individuals who report impairment and disability primarily due to pain. Clark et al. (1988) provide an extensive review of the present disability evaluation schedules for low back pain and note that none of these is scientifically based, producing significant discrepancy and interexaminer differences. They proposed a new impairment schedule based on a comprehensive review of medical literature and collections of opinions of large numbers of back specialists.

Vasudevan and Monsein (1992) emphasize that there are significant limitations in the current assessment of impairment, function, and disability. The clinician involved in such determinations should become cognizant of the conceptual framework of the disability process, should recognize the limitations and requirements of each system, and, having a conceptual framework of the disability process described, should prepare an appropriate report to requesting sources to facilitate "case closure" as well as the rehabilitation of individuals with chronic pain-related disability.

CONCLUSIONS

Physicians and other clinicians involved in managing those with chronic pain are frequently involved in the process of determining and certifying disability and residual function. Evaluating patients with symptoms of pain to determine the extent of disability is not only an immensely complex task, but an impossible one. Despite the long-held view that impairments can be determined objectively through physical examination, radiograph, and laboratory tests, there is a lack of uniformly accepted measures of not only impairments but of function. There is a tenuous relationship between pain pathology, resultant impairment, and effect on function and eventual disability.

Functional capacity assessment, although a step toward more objective assessment, determines only what the patient can (is willing to) or cannot (is unwilling to) do in a given structured situation and at a given time, but does not indicate what the person's function should be. It is, however, a supplement to the patient's report of what he or she can or cannot do. Unidimensional measurement of pain and disability has severe limitations given the pleuridimensional nature of pain. As is evident throughout this handbook, assessment of pain is also a multifaceted process with subjective, behavioral, and psychological variables.

Just as pain is a dynamic process, disability determination is also an evolving and dynamic process. However, using a multidisciplinary approach, physicians are in a much better position to determine impairments and resultant functional limitations as well as those activities the patient should be able to perform safely.

Assisting in the disability determination process is an important and integral function of the physician/clinician's role in those individuals with pain. Only with a clear understanding of the complexities of the disability system and its requirements and viewing pain in a pleuridimensional manner can the physician serve both the patient and society.

REFERENCES

Black, R.G. (1990). Evaluation of the pain patient. *Journal of Disability, 1*, 85–97.

Clark, W.L., Haldeman, S., Johnson, P., Morris, J., Schulenberger, D., Traumer, D., & White, A. (1988). Back impairment and disability determination: Another attempt at objective reliable rating. *Spine, 13*, 332–341.

Deyo, R.A. (1988). Measuring the functional status of patients with low back pain. *Archives of Physical Medicine and Rehabilitation, 69*, 1044–1053.

Engelberg, A.L. (Ed.). (1988). *Guides to the evaluation of permanent impairment* (3rd ed.). Chicago: American Medical Association.

Gildenberg, P.L., & DeVaul, R.A. (1985). *The chronic pain patient: Evaluation and management.* New York: Karger.

Hasson, S.M., & Wise, D.D. (1989). Instrumented testing of the back. *Surgical Rounds for Orthopedics, 3*, 28–31.

Hoppenfeld, S. (1976). *Physical examination of the spine and extremities.* New York: Appleton-Century-Crofts.

Keeley, J., Mayer, T., Cox, R., Gatchel, R., Smith, J., & Mooney, V. (1986). Quantification of lumbar function: Part V. Reliability of range of motion measures in the sagittal plane and in vivo torso rotation measurement technique. *Spine, 11*, 31–35.

Khalil, T.M., Goldberg, M.L., Asfour, S.S., Moty, E.A., Rosomoff, R.S., & Rosomoff, H.L. (1986). Acceptable maximum effort (AME): A psychophysical measure of strength in back pain patients. *Spine, 12*, 372–376.

Loeser, J.D., & Egan, K.J. (1989). History and organization of the University of Washington Pain Center. In J.D. Loeser & K.J. Egan (Eds.), *Managing the chronic pain patient: Theory and practice at the University of Washington multidisciplinary pain center.* New York: Raven Press.

Lynch, N.T., & Vasudevan, S.V. (1988). Perspectives in assessment and treatment of the chronic pain patient. In N.T. Lynch & S.V. Vasudevan (Eds.), *Persistent problematic pain: Psychosocial assessment and intervention.* Boston: Kluwer.

Macrae, I., & Wright, V. (1969). Measurement of lumbar spine motion in population studies. *Annals of Rheumatic Diseases, 38*, 329.

Mayer, T.G., & Gatchel, R.J. (1988). *Functional restoration for spinal disorders: The sports medicine approach.* Philadelphia: Lea & Febiger.

Melvin, J.L. (1966). When is permanent permanent? *Trial techniques: The medical issue.* Columbus: Ohio Legal Center Institute.

Melvin, J.L., & Nagi, S.Z. (1970). Factors in behavioral responses to impairments. *Archives of Physical Medicine and Rehabilitation, 51*, 552–557.

Nelson, M.A., Allen, P., Clampe, S.C. & Dombal, F.T. (1979). Reliability and reproducibility of clinical findings in low back pain. *Spine, 4*, 97–101.

Osterweis, M., Kleinman, A., & Mechanic, D. (Eds.). (1987). *Pain and disability—Clinical behavioral and public policy perspective.* Committee on Pain, Disability and Chronic Illness Behavior. Washington, DC: National Academy Press.

Powell, M.D., Wilson, M., Szypryt,P., Symonds, E.M., & Worthington, S.V. (1986). Prevalence of lumbar disc degeneration observed by magnetic resonance in symptomless women. *Lancet, 2*, 1366–1367.

The Report of the Commission on Evaluation of Pain. (1986). United States Department of Health and Human Services (SSATUB) 64-031. Washington, DC: Government Printing Office.

Sapega, A.A. (1990). Muscle performance evaluation in orthopaedic practice. *Journal of Bone and Joint Surgery,*

72-A, 1562–1574.

Turk, D.C., Rudy, T.E., & Stieg, R.L. (1989). The disability determination dilemma: Toward a multiaxial solution. *Pain, 34*, 217–229.

Vasudevan, S.V. (1989). Clinical perspectives on the relationship between pain and disability. *Neurologic Clinics, 7*, 429–439.

Vasudevan, S.V. (1990). Physical examination of the pain patient. In S.E. Abram (Ed.), *The pain clinic manual* (pp. 57–71). Philadelphia: Lippincott.

Vasudevan, S.V., & Lynch, N.T. (1991). Pain centers: Organization and outcome. *Western Journal of Medicine, 154*, 532–535.

Vasudevan, S.V., & Monsein, M. (1992). Evaluation of function and disability in the patient with chronic pain. In P.P. Raj (Ed.), *Practical management of pain* (2nd ed.). St. Louis, MO: Mosby-Year Book Inc.

Waddell, G., Main, C.J., Morris, E.W.E., Venner, R.M., Rae, P.S., Sharmy, S.H., & Galloway, H. (1982). Normality and reliability in clinical assessment of backache. *British Medical Journal, 284*, 1519–1523.

Wiesel, S.W., Tsourmas, M., Feffer, H.L., Citrin, C.M., & Patronas, N. (1984). A study of computer assisted tomography. The incidence of positive CAT scans in asymptomatic group of patients. *Spine, 9*, 549–551.

II

MEASUREMENT OF PAIN

Chapter 8

Psychophysical Approaches to Pain Measurement and Assessment

DONALD D. PRICE, PhD
STEPHEN W. HARKINS, PhD

Modern methods for measurement of different aspects of pain have historical roots in psychophysics, the branch of psychology concerned with the relationships of physical properties of stimuli to sensory experiences of humans and to behavioral responses of several animal species. Psychophysical studies of pain have provided critical information about fundamental attributes of pain and a means of understanding its neurophysiological mechanisms (Bushnell, Taylor, Duncan, & Dubner, 1983; Price, 1988; Tursky, 1976). By using quantitatively controlled stimuli in paradigms of discrimination, direct scaling, and detection, and by relating the results obtained with those derived from similarly designed neurophysiological studies, it has been possible to directly identify types of peripheral and central neurons and neural pathways that are critical for pain (Bushnell et al., 1983; Mountcastle, 1974; Price, 1988; Price, McHaffie, & Stein 1992). Similarly, psychophysical experiments have provided information about neural mechanisms of pain reduction and the relative efficacies of various pain-reducing treatments (Chapman et al., 1985; Gracely, 1989; Price,

Harkins, Rafii, & Price, 1986; Price, Rafii, Watkins, & Buckingham, 1984; Price, von der Gruen, Miller, Raffi, & Price, 1985). This approach has led to improvements in pain measurement and has raised the possibility of standardized quantitative comparisons of efficacies of different treatments for various types of clinical pain (Gracely, 1989; Melzack, 1984; Price & Harkins, 1987). These comparisons can be made for different groups of patients.

This chapter focuses on these advances in the context of explaining the application of psychophysical methods to measurement of different dimensions of pain (i.e., sensory, affective) and stages of pain processing. Emphasis is placed on direct scaling techniques because we feel they have considerable practical value in clinical pain assessment. The measurement of sensory-discriminative features of pain is discussed first, followed by a consideration of measurement of various stages of pain-related affect or emotional disturbance. The latter is discussed in the context of known interrelationships between sensory, cognitive-evaluative, and affective dimensions of pain.

MEASUREMENT OF SENSORY-DISCRIMINATIVE ASPECTS OF PAIN

An important principle in pain measurement, as in any evaluation of sensory experience, is the fact that the critical observations in pain measurement are made by the person who has the pain. Someone who is having pain is asked to *match* the perceived intensity of that pain to a scale. This is done in a variety of ways. For example, one could match numbers or words to pain intensity or match an intensity of experimental pain to that of clinical pain or use more than one of these procedures. In all such methods, the critical observer is the person who has the pain. Similar to visual tests in optometry, pain measurement is directly dependent on subjective reports. The investigator or clinician also has a crucial role in pain measurement. This person provides the scaling procedures, records the reported values, and considers the reliability and validity of the different methods of measurement.

The person with pain can be asked to notice and make quantitative judgments about different dimensions of the experience. For example the individual can observe and rate the relative intensity of the painful sensation, the degree of its immediate unpleasantness, spatial distribution, and qualities. These separate judgments are by no means exclusive to pain and have a long history in the psychophysics of vision, audition, taste, smell, and somatosensory modalities. One can make separate and exquisitely precise judgments of intensity, pitch, timbre, volume, and density of the same sound stimuli as well as their pleasantness or unpleasantness. However, it is the subjective nature of pain measurement and lack of knowledge about methods of pain measurement that sometimes dissuade health-care providers from making anything other than crude assessments of their patients' pain. This is truly unfortunate because many important subjective phenomena can be assessed and even measured with reasonable accuracy. For example, no one would question the psychophysical measurement of vision by optometrists, despite the fact that their assessments rely almost exclusively on the subjective judgments of their patients. Psychophysical methods help to provide psychometric guidelines for pain measurement as indicated by the several criteria with which to evaluate different pain measurement methods.

Criteria for Pain Measurement

Assessments of human pain have evolved from extensive reliance on threshold and tolerance determination to the use of a wide variety of psychological and physiological methods that explicitly recognize that pain experience and pain-related behavior have multiple dimensions. Despite diversity in approaches, ranging from simple category choices to recordings of reflex and brain activity, all methods share a common goal of accurately representing the human pain experience. Although investigators have different emphases, there is general agreement as to the principal criteria for an ideal pain assessment procedure. The following criteria include those suggested by Gracely and Dubner (1981), and one criterion (#1) we have added. The method would:

1. Have ratio scale properties
2. Be relatively free of biases inherent in different psychophysical methods
3. Provide immediate information about the accuracy and reliability of the subjects performance of the scaling responses
4. Be useful for both experimental and clinical pain and allow for reliable comparison between both types of pain
5. Be reliable and generalizable
6. Be sensitive to changes in pain intensity
7. Be simple to use for pain patients and nonpain patients in both clinical and research settings
8. Separately assess the sensory intensive and affective dimensions of pain

The goal of recent research on human pain measurement has been to establish methods that fulfill all or most of these criteria. Several general approaches to pain measurement are briefly discussed in terms of their historical role and the information they have provided about psychophysical attributes of pain. The ability of each method to fulfill the major criteria listed above is reviewed. Emphasis is placed on direct scaling techniques because we feel that they have considerable practical value in clinical pain assessment.

Attempts to quantify pain in human patients or volunteer subjects have utilized five basic approaches (Chapman et al., 1985): (1) methods that define a threshold for pain and measure changes in threshold, (2) methods that define a tolerance for pain and measure changes in tolerance, (3) the measurement of performance behavior on laboratory tasks, usually to obtain measures of discrimination ability or detection, (4) rating scale methods in which subjects rate pain intensity on scales with clearly defined numerical limits and intervals or on verbal rating scales whose words directly indicate a rank order, and (5) magnitude scaling procedures in which direct judgments of sensation intensity or unpleasantness are made by number assignment or cross-modality matching techniques such as handgrip force or line production.

Alternative Methods of Pain Measurement

Pain Threshold Measurements

Pain threshold methods were used by Hardy, Wolf, and Goodell (1954) and Beecher (1959) following World War II, but they have since diminished in popularity in pain research and in sensory psychophysics in general. There are two general procedures for obtaining threshold—the method of limits and the method of constant stimuli (Guilford, 1954). In the former method, stimulus intensity is increased to a point where the subject perceives each stimulus and then decreased to a point where the subject does not perceive each stimulus. The point midway between these two limits is considered threshold. In the method of constant stimuli, stimulus intensity is increased in steps to a point wherein the subject perceives one-half of the stimuli that are presented (Guilford, 1954). Regardless of the exact procedure employed, subjects are required to identify that point on a continuum of increasing stimulus intensity that distinguishes painful from non-painful experience.

Threshold measures cannot directly provide information about pain intensity or ratios of pain intensity (criterion #1). Moreover, pain threshold can be strongly biased by attentional and motivational factors and heavily influenced by whether the threshold is defined in sensory or affective terms (related to criterion #2).

Pain thresholds can be obtained for experimental pain but cannot be determined for clinical pain under most circumstances (related to criterion #4), mainly because of lack of access to the stimulus causing clinical pain. Given adequate instructions to subjects, pain

thresholds are reliable, generalizable across groups of subjects (criterion #5), and simple to obtain (criterion #7). However, under some experimental conditions, they have been shown to be insensitive to effects of clinical proven analgesic drugs for reasons that are not entirely clear (criterion #6) (Beecher, 1959; Chapman, Dingman, & Ginzberg, 1965). Finally, depending on instructions to subjects, pain thresholds can be obtained separately for sensory discriminative (e.g., pricking pain threshold) or affective (e.g., unpleasantness) dimensions of pain (criterion #8) (Blitz & Dinnerstein, 1968; Price, 1988).

Nominal and Ordinal Rating Scale

Nominal and ordinal rating scales are relatively simple and for that reason are very commonly used in clinical studies of pain and even in many experimental studies. Numbers on ordinal scales refer only to rank ordering and cannot be used to reflect ratios of magnitude (criterion #1). For example, if someone initially rates their pain as 8 and then as 6 after a treatment, one can conclude that the pain has reduced in intensity but not that it has reduced by 25%. One variant of an ordinal rating scale is the category scale, whose categories are designed to imply a rank ordering. For example, the scale designed by Melzack & Torgerson (1971) and later included in the McGill Pain Questionnaire (MPQ) (Melzack, 1975, 1984) has the five categories of mild, discomforting, distressing, horrible, and excruciating. Other rating scales are simple numerical scales (e.g., 1–5 or 1–10) that are sometimes anchored by verbal descriptors indicative of extremes such as no pain and severe pain.

A major advantage of ordinal rating scales, like pain threshold, is their relative simplicity (criterion #7). Their most useful attribute is that they can be used to rapidly ascertain whether pain intensity has increased, decreased, or stayed the same. They are reasonably sensitive to changes in pain intensity (criterion #6). These scales are widely used by health-care professionals in ascertaining pain and effects of pain treatments. Patients and health-care personnel both easily understand and can respond to a 1–5 pain scale where 5 equals the most severe pain imaginable. Ordinal scales can be used for both experimental and clinical pain (criterion #4), are reliable and generalizable (criterion #5), and, similar to visual analog scales, can be adapted to assess both sensory intensive and affective dimensions of pain (criterion #8.)

Unfortunately, for the purposes of pain research, ordinal scales of pain have methodological problems and they are widely misused and misinterpreted in clinical studies. One problem is that when pain experiences are classified into categories in scales, the category boundaries are not known and the approximation of the ranked categories to equal intervals is often assumed without supportive evidence. Many investigators simply assign numbers to the categories that are ranked in magnitude and then erroneously use parametric statistics to analyze their data. The numbers clearly belong on an ordinal scale and should be analyzed using nonparametric statistics. This requirement is especially essential in view of Heft and Parker's (1984) demonstration that

category boundaries of pain category scales are not equally spaced.

Category scales are very sensitive to biases that occur when stimuli are spaced differently (related to criterion #2). For example, when most of the presented stimuli are distributed toward the low end of the stimulus intensity continuum, the shape of the stimulus category scale response function is *negatively* accelerating. Conversely, when the stimuli are concentrated toward the upper end of the stimulus range, the shape of this function is *positively* accelerating as in Figures 8.1 and 8.2 (see also Gracely & Dubner, 1981).

Another problem of interpretation posed by verbal category scales is that they are likely to force patients or subjects into choosing a word that really does not apply to their experience and hence into using words in a semantically artificial manner. For example, a category scale

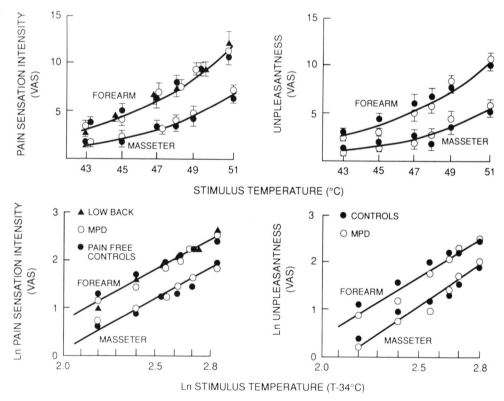

FIGURE 8.1. Temperature–VAS-sensory (*left*) and temperature–VAS affect (*right*) response functions plotted in linear (*top*) and log-log coordinates (*bottom*) for MPD patients (○), low back pain patients (△), and pain-free volunteer subjects (●). The slopes (exponents) of the sensory functions are 2.1 in the log-log coordinates for both masseter and forearm and 2.4 to 2.7 for affect functions. Each point is the group mean response to a given temperature. Note that although there are large differences between VAS ratings of masseter and forearm stimuli, the functions are characterized by the same slope in log-log coordinates, and hence, similar power function exponent. Standard errors are indicated by vertical bars Adapted (redrawn) from Price and Harkins (1987), pages 4–5. Copyright 1987 Raven Press. Adapted by permission.

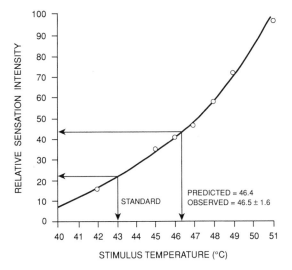

FIGURE 8.2. Strategy used to test whether the VAS-sensory function provides accurate information about ratios of heat-induced pain. The vertical arrows intersecting the function represent the standard temperature (43°C) and the temperature 46.4°C) predicted from the function as twice as intense as the standard (see also horizontal lines). The actual mean temperature chosen by subjects as twice the standard was 46.5°C, a value close to that predicted on the basis of the VAS stimulus–response function. Adapted (redrawn) from Price et al. (1983), page 50. Copyright 1983 Elsevier. Adapted by permission.

used by Melzack and Torgerson (1971) implies that as pain increases beyond a level described as "discomforting," it then becomes replaced by an experience described as "distressing." This is hardly an invariant progression in pain experience. Pain may just as easily become intensely frustrating, depressing, or irritating. The progression from "distressing" to "horrible" is equally questionable. Moreover, these different descriptors refer to qualitatively different human emotions that are unlikely to exist on the same continuum of intensity. Straightforward number scales circumvent this semantic problems to some extent but not the problem of unknown category boundaries.

Finally, a problem with verbal or numerical ordinal scales is the tendency for people to persevere in using words or numbers. For example, patients who have rated their pain as a 3 at 9 A.M. might tend to use the same number 2 hours later simply because of their memory for the previous rating and their desire to remain consistent.

Direct Magnitude Scaling Methods

Direct scaling methods have been critical to the demonstration that sensory intensity-perceived magnitude relationships are power functions and to the development of ratio scales of sensation magnitude. Consequently, direct magnitude scaling techniques have evolved as valuable, accurate methods in psychophysics. These techniques have provided enormous progress in ascertaining the relationships between sensation magnitude and intensity of precisely controlled physical stimuli. Ekman and Sjoberg (1965) summed up this progress as follows:

> After a hundred years of almost general acceptance and practically no experimentation, Fechner's logarithmic law was replaced by the power law.* The amount of experimental work performed in the 1950's on this problem by Stevens and other research workers was enormous. The power law was verified again and again, in literally hundreds of experiments. As an experimental fact, the power law is established beyond any reasonable doubt, possibly more firmly established than anything else in psychology. (p. 455)

Given the firmly ingrained suspiciousness surrounding the measurement of subjective phenomena among many psychological researchers, it is indeed ironic that the most quantitative, precise, and reliable results come from psychophysics, the measurement of subjective responses to physical stimuli.

With the advent of scaling perceived magnitudes by direct scaling methods, ratio scales of perceived sensations were developed (Guilford & Dingman, 1954; Marks, 1974; Stevens, 1975; Stevens & Galanter, 1957; Stevens & Guirao, 1963; A. Teghtsoonian & R. Teghtsoonian, 1965). The procedure for cross-modality matching and generation of a psychophysical scale for a given sense modality is paraphrased below:

Subjects are asked to use a given reference (response continuum) to represent their perceived intensity of a given stimulus. The reference continuum may be a sensory continuum such as intensity of sound or it can be line lengths or numbers. They then match subsequent stimuli along this sensory dimension

---

*The power law of sensory psychophysics is $j = kS^x$, where j is perceived magnitude, k is a constant, S is stimulus magnitude, and x is an exponent that is characteristic for a given sense modality under a standard set of conditions.

accordingly. For example, a subject initially produces a line whose length matches the perceived intensity of a light stimulus. A second light stimulus of a lower or higher intensity is then presented. The subject, remembering his or her response to the first stimulus, now produces a line to the new stimulus in a manner that represents the perceived change in light intensity. Subsequent stimuli are presented until an entire scale is developed, one which constitutes a ratio scale (Stevens, 1975). Considerable practice and numbers of stimuli are sometimes needed to produce precise stimulus–response functions.

With the development of cross-modality matching, it has become apparent that any sensory continuum can be matched to almost any other sensory continuum and to numbers. This potential for matching continua is critical in validating the various power functions that relate perceived magnitudes to stimulus intensity (Guilford & Dingman, 1954; Marks, 1974; Stevens, 1975). Most importantly, these methods are crucial to the development of ratio scales, the types of scale most useful to science. Because measurement on a ratio scale is the first criterion (#1) for ideal pain measurement given above and because direct scaling techniques have the potential for producing ratio scales, the application of direct scaling techniques to pain measurement needs to be discussed in some detail.

Evidence for power functions and ratio scale measurements of pain sensation intensity. Ratio scales differ from ordinal and interval scales in that numbers along a ratio scale serve to reflect actual ratios of magnitude. Thus, conclusions about *how much* more intense one type of pain is compared to another or *how much* pain has reduced (i.e., percentage change) are valid only when ratio scale measurements are made.

Ratio scale methods have been established by psychophysicists for most sensory modalities including taste, temperature, and odor (Marks, 1974; Stevens, 1975). The most convincing demonstrations of ratio scale human judgments are those of common perceptual dimensions with unrestrained or unlimited stimulus magnitude. For example, judgment of length (Stevens & Guirao, 1963; A. Teghtsoonian & R. Teghtsoonian, 1965) is directly proportional to actual length. The ratio properties of judgments also are intimately associated with power law, which states that perceived magnitude is a power function of stimulus magnitude. The power law implies a very simple and parsimonious concept, "that equal stimulus ratios produce equal subjective ratios" (Stevens, 1975, p. 18). A power function whose exponent is 1.0 (i.e., $\psi = kS^{1.0}$) predicts that two stimuli whose ratio of *measured* intensities is 2:1 will result in two *perceived* intensities whose ratio is 2:1. Using this same stimulus ratio (2:1) in the case of a power function whose exponent is 2.0 (i.e., $\psi = kS^{2.0}$), the resulting ratio of *perceived* magnitudes would be 4:1. The relationship of perceived ratios to stimulus ratios would be the same for a given power function, regardless of the units of measurement of stimulus intensity or the stimulus magnitudes used to make up the stimulus intensity ratios. Because accurately perceived ratios are critically necessary for the existence of power functions, the demonstration of a power function is one line of evidence that the response measure used is a ratio scale.

What then is the evidence that direct scaling techniques result in ratio scale measures of pain intensity? Gracely and colleagues had 24 subjects judge the sensation intensity and unpleasantness of electrocutaneous stimuli in several different ways (Gracely, McGrath, & Dubner, 1978). They made handgrip dynomometric responses, time duration responses, and verbal descriptor responses chosen from randomized lists. The verbal descriptor responses were transformed to numerical measures by having the same subjects produce numeric ratings of the perceived magnitudes implied by verbal descriptors. All methods of responding to the electrocutaneous stimuli yielded power functions. The slopes of these functions in log-log coordinates were the power function exponents that were consistent across the different methods of responding. The one exception was that the power function exponents derived on the basis of verbal descriptors were different for affective as compared to sensory-intensive responses to electrocutaneous stimuli (Gracely et al., 1978). The strikingly similar power functions across diverse methods of cross-modality matching (i.e., handgrip, time duration, verbal descriptor) provide an important line of evidence that pain intensity can be measured on a ratio scale.

Evidence for relatively bias-free results (criterion #2). Visual Analogue Scale (VAS) responses to graded nociceptive temperature stimuli likewise have resulted in power functions. It is of considerable significance that simple VAS responses to nociceptive temperatures yield power functions with exponents of 2.1–2.2 for pain sensation and higher exponents for unpleasantness. VAS responses are very easy to obtain from patients and normal volunteers and require little instruction. They fulfill the criterion of simplicity (criterion #7). Thus, the potential use of VAS as a ratio scale and as a means of separately measuring pain sensation and affect has important potential utility (see also Jensen & Karoly, Chapter 9). However, the demonstration of a reliable power function exponent by itself is not sufficient evidence for a ratio scale level of measurement. In addition to this line of evidence, it must be shown that VAS ratings do not produce systematic biases or distortions. Power function exponents can be systematically altered by such factors.

When subjects make marks on VASs without constraints of numerical or verbal categories, they are using perceived length to represent their judgments of relative intensity. This procedure is similar in principle to having subjects produce lines to represent perceived intensity, a procedure that has generally been shown to produce ratio scale judgments (J.C. Stevens & Marks, 1980; S.S. Stevens, 1975; S.S. Stevens & Galanter, 1957; S.S. Stevens & Guiarao, 1963; A. Teghtsoonian & R. Teghtsoonia 1965). One could question whether anchoring VAS by words indicative of extremes produce biases or systematic distortions in rat-

ings. This possibility was examined by comparing results of VAS responses to 43–51°C stimuli with those based on line production responses. As shown in Figure 8.3, both VAS and line production methods produced the same power function exponents for the sensory dimension, thereby demonstrating that using VAS anchored by words does not produce distortions or biases beyond that which might be produced by line production. VAS and verbal descriptor scaling of 43–51°C stimuli likewise produces very similar stimulus–response functions (Duncan, Bushnell, & Levigne, 1986). The lack of bias or distortion in VAS ratings may be partly the result of the facts that, in the studies described, subjects were instructed carefully about how to use the VAS and the entire range of stimulus intensities to be used was gradually presented beforehand.

A critical test of whether VAS or line production measures of pain sensation magnitude are bias-free and reflect true ratios of perceived pain intensity was made by having subjects adjust *stimulus intensities* to indicate different *ratios* of perceived pain sensation intensity (Price et al., 1983). The stimulus intensities chosen by subjects were then compared to those predicted on the basis of the stimulus-VAS sensory response function. The subjects were first presented with a standard stimulus intensity, such as 43°C or 45°C (see Figure 8.2). The stimulus temperature was then slowly increased (0.5°C/sec) to a point where

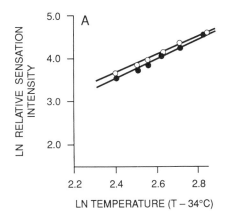
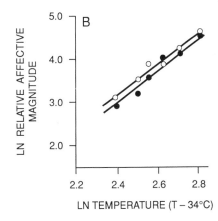

FIGURE 8.3 Mean log relative magnitudes derived from cross-modality matching; VAS (○) and line production (●) of the sensation intensity (A) and the affective magnitude (B) of noxious thermal stimulation are plotted as a function of log stimulus intensity minus baseline skin temperature. Each open circle represents the geometric mean of 40 observations (20 subjects x 2 trials). Each filled circle is the mean response based on line production of 7 trained subjects. Adapted (redrawn) from Price et al. (1983), page 54. Copyright 1983 Elsevier. Adapted by permission.

subjects perceived the stimulus intensity as being twice that of the standard. The average temperatures chosen were precisely consistent with those predicted on the basis of the 43–51°C stimulus-VAS response power functions derived for the same subjects (Figure 8.2). This type of approach demonstrates that VAS pain sensory responses accurately reflect perceived ratios of pain sensation intensity. These results, when combined with the considerable evidence for reliable power function exponents of 2.1–2.2 for pain sensation, simultaneously demonstrate that the scaling methods are relatively bias-free (criterion #2) *and* at least closely approximate a ratio scale level of measurement of pain sensation (criterion #1).

It is important to point out that not all pain VAS are bias-free or are likely to be ratio scales. Studies that have compared the use of different types of VAS have shown that the sensitivity and reliability of VAS are somewhat influenced by the words used to anchor the endpoints, by the length of the VAS, and by other factors (Seymour, Simpson, Charlton, & Phillips, 1985). Those VAS that most clearly delineate extremes (i.e., the worst pain, the most intense pain imaginable) and are 10–15 cm in length have been shown to have the greatest sensitivity and are the least vulnerable to distortions or biases in rating (Scott & Huskisson, 1976; Seymour et al., 1985).

Reliability and generalizability (criterion #5). Contact heat-induced pain also has been consistently demonstrated to follow a positively accelerating power function whose exponent is 2.1–2.2 for the sensory intensity of pain induced by nociceptive (45–51°C) temperatures (Price, Barrell, & Gracely, 1980; Price & Harkins, 1987; Price, McGrath, Rafii, & Buckingham, 1983). Unpleasantness judgments of these same stimulus intensities also were positively accelerating power functions, but with higher and more variable exponents of 2.4–2.7 (Harkins, Price, & Martelli, 1985; Price et al., 1983; Price, von der Gruen, et al., 1985; Price & Harkins, 1987). These results are very consistent across different groups, despite the fact that different types of pain patients and pain-free volunteers participated in the different studies. These similarities are illustrated in Figure 8.1 which compares VAS-sensory and affective responses of myofascial pain dysfunction, low back pain patients, and pain-free

volunteer subjects. This remarkably similar power function for pain sensation intensity obtained at different times for the same subjects and obtained with different groups of subjects fulfills an important criterion that VAS measurements of the sensory-intensive and affective dimensions of pain are both reliable and generalizable (criterion #5).

Internally consistent measures of experimental pain and clinical pain sensation intensity (criteria #3 and #4). The reliability and validity of measures of clinical pain could be at least partly determined by comparing these measures with independent measures of the same experience. For example, an additional measure of clinical pain is obtained if patients match the magnitude of a controllable experimental pain stimulus to the magnitude of their clinical pain. Matching clinical pain to another pain may be easier than matching clinical pain to a word or a line (Gracely, 1989; Heft, Gracely, Dubner, & McGrath, 1980). Matching experimental to clinical pain can then be compared with the same subjects' direct scaling responses to experimental pain and to clinical pain. These comparisons form the basis of a "triangulation validation procedure" devised by Heft et al. (1980) and Gracely (1989).

The triangulation procedure allows assessment of the internal consistency of three types of responses in patients: (1) direct scaling responses to a broad range of experimental pain stimuli, (2) experimental pain intensity matches to clinical pain, and (3) direct scaling responses to clinical pain. The first type of response produces an experimental pain stimulus–response function for which the regression line is plotted on a graph (Figure 8.4). The second type of response, the experimental pain match, can be plotted along the x-axis of this same graph (see vertical dashed-line Figure 8.4). The third type of response, the direct scaling response to clinical pain (dashed-horizontal line, Figure 8.4) is then plotted along the y-axis of this graph. If subjects make all of these responses in an internally consistent manner, then the *intersection* of the experimental pain match (on the x-axis) and direct scaling response to clinical pain (on the y-axis) should lie on or very close to the regression line of the experimental pain stimulus–direct scaling response function. Such a demonstration would show that subjects are making these

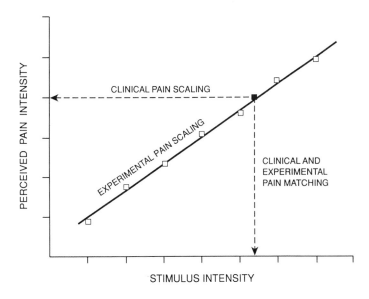

FIGURE 8.4. Hypothetical matching paradigm based on concepts of Heft et al. (1980) and Gracely (1989). Presentation of various intensities of painful stimuli results in a stimulus pain intensity rating function for which a regression line is computed. Subjects choose a stimulus intensity that matches that of their clinical pain (*vertical dashed arrow*). Finally, they rate their level of clinical pain intensity using the same rating procedure previously used to scale experimental pain (*horizontal dashed arrow*). If subjects use these rating and stimulus matching procedures in an internally consistent manner, the intersection of the stimulus matching (vertical arrow) and direct rating (horizontal arrow) of clinical pain should lie on or very close the stimulus pain intensity regression line.

different types of responses in an internally consistent manner and that the same psychological scale applies to both experimental and clinical pain.

Gracely and colleagues (Gracely, 1989; Heft et al., 1980) used the triangulation procedure to show that oral-facial pain patients scaled experimental tooth pulp stimulation pain and their clinical pain in an internally consistent manner. Patients used verbal descriptors of sensory intensity to rate randomly applied electrical tooth pulp stimuli and their own clinical pain. They also determined the intensity of tooth pulp evoked pain (in log mA) that matched the intensity of their clinical pain. The intersection of the experimental pain stimulus match (on the *x*-axis) and verbal descriptor value of their clinical pain (on the *y*-axis) occurred directly on the regression line of the tooth pulp stimulus intensity—verbal descriptor scale response function.

Price (Price & Harkins, 1987; Price et al., 1983) also carried out triangulation validation procedures using 30 chronic low back pain patients and 38 myofascial pain dysfunction (MPD) patients. Their specific methods differed from Gracely (1989) and Heft et al.

(1980) in that they used contact thermal stimuli as their source of experimental pain and VASs. VAS-*sensory* responses to 43–51°C stimuli produced a power function whose exponent was 2.1. Similar to the previous examples (Figure 8.4), the intersection of temperature matches to different levels of clinical pain (on the *y*-axis) occurred directly on the regression lines of the temperature stimulus–VAS response function (Figure 8.5). The consistency of two very different types of responses (VAS and direct temperature match) to clinical pain provides concurrent validation or an accurate check on the patient's performance of the scaling responses. In simple terms, if two quite different ways of scaling clinical pain are in quantitative agreement, one can be more confident in both response measures.

If, as is shown in Figure 8.5, different types of pain patients use VAS in an internally consistent manner to scale clinical and experimental pain and if different types of pain patients and pain-free volunteers have the same temperature–VAS response relationship, then this stimulus–VAS response relationship can serve as a reference standard for pain intensity. Pain sensation intensities of very different types

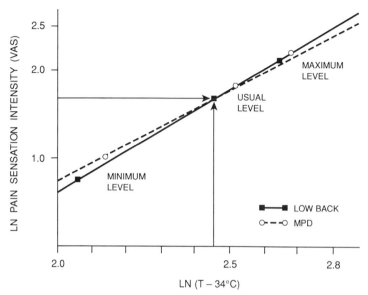

FIGURE 8.5. Nociceptive stimulus temperature–VAS pain sensation functions for 5 seconds of heat stimuli delivered to the forearm and match points (intersection of temperature matches and VAS ratings of clinical pain) derived for 30 low back patients and 38 MPD patients. Regression lines in log-log coordinates are expressed by solid lines for back patients and dashed lines for MPD patients. Match points are indicated by closed circles for back patients and open squares for patients with MPD. Adapted (redrawn) from Price and Harkins (1987), page 6. Copyright 1987 Raven Press. Adapted by permission.

of clinical as well as experimental pain could now be compared along the same psychophysical ratio scale (Figure 8.6). The significance of such a standard is that it could provide a basis for quantitatively comparing effects of different pain-reducing treatments across different groups of pain patients and even across different studies. Comparison of magnitudes of pain reduction from different studies are nearly always difficult to make because different investigations use radically different and usually quite simplistic pain assessment methods such as category scales or simple ordinal scales. This difficulty is increased when only percentage of pain relief measures are used because different groups of pain patients are likely to have different average baseline intensities of pain and effects of treatment are likely to be strongly influenced by baseline pain intensities.

Sensitivity to pain-reducing treatments (criterion #6). The simultaneous direct scaling of experimental and clinical pain also can provide a means of standardized quantitative analysis of relative efficacies of pain-reducing treatments. In a study using this approach, intravenous administration of fentanyl reduced VAS ratings of experimental and clinical pains in an inter-

nally consistent manner as indicated by the result that drug-induced changes in VAS ratings were very similar for both experimental and clinical pain (Price et al., 1986). That low (0.8 μg/kg) to moderate (1.1 μg/kg) doses of fentanyl produced statistically reliable reductions in both experimental and clinical pain provides evidence that this approach to pain measurement is sensitive to changes in pain intensity.

When patients rate a wide range of threshold and suprathreshold nociceptive temperatures, as in the examples above, the antinociceptive effect of a treatment can be measured as a decrease in numerical units on a psychophysical scale (e.g., VAS or verbal descriptor scale) or as an increase in stimulus strength (change in °C) required to produce the same pretreatment level of pain. The latter approach represents what Gracely (1989) refers to as a "stimulus-dependent method."

MEASUREMENT OF AFFECTIVE-MOTIVATIONAL ASPECTS OF PAIN

A final and critical criterion for ideal assessment of pain is the separate measurement of sensory

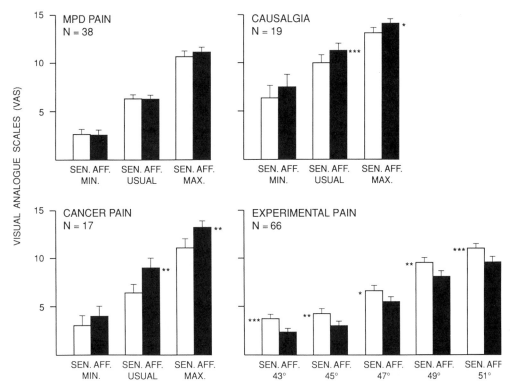

FIGURE 8.6. VAS-sensory (white bars) and VAS-affective (black bars) responses and (and 1 S.E.M.) for three types of clinical pain and for experimental pain. VAS responses related to chronic pain syndromes were obtained at minimum (min.), usual, and maximum (max.) levels experienced during the week prior to their clinical visit. VAS-affective and VAS-sensory responses to pain were compared using paired t tests (* $p < .05$, ** $p < .02$, and *** $p < .001$) (asterisks shown to the right of black bars indicate significantly higher VAS-affective responses than VAS-sensory responses and asterisks to the left of white bars indicate significantly higher VAS-sensory responses than VAS-affective responses). Adapted from Price et al. (1987), page 302. Copyright 1987 Elsevier. Adapted by permission.

discriminative and affective aspects of pain—the two dimensions of pain explicitly recognized by Melzack and Casey (1968) (criterion #8). This brings us to the question of whether and to what extent these two dimensions of pain can be separately measured. Prior to providing evidence for their separate measurement, it is first necessary to consider what constitutes pain-related affect and how it is interrelated with other components of pain.

Emotional Components of Pain—Two Stages of Pain Affect

Pain-related emotions, like emotions in general, depend upon cognitive appraisals (Arnold, 1970). If so, then what cognitive appraisals are associated with the affective dimension of pain? It is apparent from consideration of the experience of pain itself that there are two stages of

pain-related emotional feeling (Figure 8.7). The first is the *immediate affective* stage of pain that is comprised of the moment-by-moment unpleasantness, distress, or annoyance that closely covaries with the intensity of painful sensation and its accompanying arousal. Painful sensations are not only usually intense but are often perceived as spreading, penetrating, and sometimes summating. They are experienced as an intrusion upon both the body and consciousness (Bakan, 1968; Buytendyck, 1961; Price, 1988). Thus, an *immediate* cognitive meaning given to painful sensations is that of *intrusion*, a meaning that requires very little reflection and occurs automatically. It is the meaning conveyed by someone who says, "It bothers me because it hurts!" Thus, similar to states of nausea, intense thirst, hunger, and dizziness, part of the affective dimension of pain is closely linked to nociceptive sensations that are unique to physical pain.

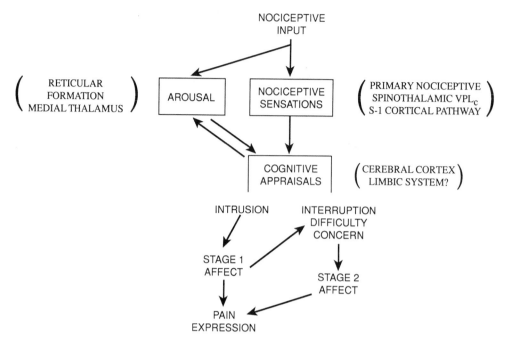

FIGURE 8.7. A schematic used to illustrate interactions between situational factors and nociceptive stimulation, as well as interactions between the various dimension of pain. Variables and factors within experience are shown. From Price (1988), page 227. Copyright 1988 Raven Press. Reprinted by permission.

Nociceptive sensations, then, are one of the direct immediate causes of pain-related emotional disturbance in the same way as sensations of dizziness and nausea are direct causes of unpleasant affective states. Such being the case, both neural and psychological processes related to pain sensation can be conceived as important causal links in the production of pain-related emotional disturbance.

However, a second stage of pain-related affect is based on more reflective cognitive processes (Price, 1988). These involve more elaborate meanings related to the perception of the *implications* of nociceptive sensations. Pain is often experienced not only as an immediate threat to one's body, but also to one's well-being and life in general. It is, then, the cognitions and accompanying negative emotions related to the meanings of how pain influences one's life and activities of daily living that constitute much of the second stage of pain-related affect, a stage that may be thought of as suffering. The second stage of pain affect is heavily dependent on the experienced context of pain, including its perceived implications for future interactions with one's life or intentions, the perceived origin of the pain, and perceived ability to control the pain. One

would expect that the second stage of pain-related affect to be strongly influenced by learning and past experiences and therefore would be related to personality and cultural factors.

It has been suggested that the suffering associated with pain is based on three possible primary meanings (Bakan, 1968; Buytendyck, 1961; Price, 1988). The first is that the intense sensation is *interrupting something*, such as one's thoughts, comfort, well-being, or plans. The second is that the sensation and its accompanying domination of consciousness are a *burden that is difficult to endure over time*. Finally, the nociceptive sensation may mean that *something harmful might happen or has happened*.

In addition to these primary meanings associated with pain, secondary meanings can arise from even more elaborate reflection. For example, one could consider having pain to be unfair and become angry. One could perceive one's pain to be a deserved punishment and feel guilt or remorse. Still further, one could feel jealous of others' good health or alienated from significant relationships (i.e., lonely). Although these emotional reactions may not be considered part of pain itself but as a secondary reaction to pain or as suffering, it is possible that under some circumstances they would covary with the pain sensation itself and would be an integral component of the overall experience of pain. As Buytendyck (1961) has pointed out, pain does indeed evoke reflection and not necessarily that of a constructive variety.

Interrelationships between Cognitive Appraisals and Emotional Reactions during Pain

The meaning of immediate intrusion in stage 1 and those of interruption, enduring a burden over time, and concern for the future in the more reflective second stage, are directed toward the painful sensations, the context in which they occur, and the implications of impending harm. These meanings, in turn, are related to desires and expectations of avoiding both psychological and physical harm. Figure 8.7 summarizes these relevant psychological dimensions and the perceived contextual situational factors that provide the basis for emotions during pain and their possible expression.

It can be discerned from this conceptualization that *different* emotional responses can occur in the same person at different times depending on the meanings experienced, intentions, type of goal, and relative intensities of desire and expectation (Price, 1988; Price & J.J. Barrell, 1980, 1984; Price, J.E. Barrell, & J.J. Barrell, 1985; Price et al., 1980). For example, when a pain patient focuses on the *interruption* related to pain, he or she may feel frustrated, depressed, or angry. When the same patient focuses on avoiding future impairment or deterioration and is uncertain about these consequences, he or she would more likely feel anxious or fearful. When someone in pain focuses on having to endure the burden of pain over time, he or she may feel depressed, frustrated, or anxious depending on whether the focus is on past, present, or future negative consequences, the desire to avoid these consequences, and the level of expectation (Price & J.J. Barrell, 1984; Price, J.E. Barrell, & J.J. Barrell, 1985). There is no unique and invariant emotion associated with the second stage of pain affect. However, the principles that explain the types and intensities of emotions related to this second stage appear to be the same as those that explain emotional states in general (Arnold, 1970; Price, 1988; Price &

Barrell, 1984; Price, J.E. Barrell, & J.J. Barrell, 1985; Price et al., 1980).

Although many different meanings and emotions can coexist in the same patient, there is often one that is salient in influencing the affective dimension of pain. For example, someone who is starting to have pain from cancer may experience the pain as mild in terms of sensation intensity. However, the painful sensation reminds the person of impending deterioration and possible death and is predominantly experienced in terms of a dire threat to health or life. Anxiety and/or fear would most likely be a prominent emotional response of this person. On the other hand, the individual with chronic low back pain is likely to perceive that pain in terms of an intermittent or constant interruption. Pain interrupts activity or comfort, and often comfort and activity are traded off at the expense of the other. Regardless of whether comfort or activity is interrupted, the emotional response associated with this felt sense of interruption is frustration. Depression sets in when one gives up the intention to act in the world and when one has little or no expectation of living an active or fully meaningful life. The depressed pain patient often views his or her condition as an inevitable burden that must be endured over time. In the case of patients with Reflex Sympathetic Dystrophy (RSD) who often have nearly constant unremittant pain, this burden is especially difficult to endure, and many RSD patients suffer with severe depression (Sternbach, 1974).

Thus far, reasons have been given for the multidimensional nature of emotions associated with pain and for the interrelationships between sensory, cognitive, and affective dimensions of pain. Affective responses to pain are a function of the intensities of pain sensation and arousal as well as the kinds of cognitive appraisals that are made of the pain sensations and their implications. Thus, although pain sensation and pain affect covary under many circumstances, there are contextual and psychological factors that can selectively and powerfully alter pain affect. It is therefore extremely important to measure these two dimensions of pain separately in studies of human pain. It has been questioned whether this can be successfully accomplished. The remainder of this chapter provides empirical evidence that the two dimensions of pain can be separately measured in both experimental and clinical settings. The separate assessment of two stages of pain-related affect will then be discussed.

Sensory and Affective Responses during Experimental Pain

As pointed out above, VAS-sensory and VAS-affective responses to nociceptive temperatures (43–51°C) are both positively accelerating power functions. Whereas the exponent of 2.1–2.3 for pain sensation is remarkably consistent across different studies and groups of subjects, that for pain affect varies from 2.4 to 2.7. The two types of VASs differ only in the use of verbal anchor points, for example, "the most intense pain sensation imaginable" and "most unpleasant imaginable" in the case of sensory and affective dimensions respectively. Both VASs are 15 cm in length (Harkins, Price, & Braith, 1989; Price, 1988; Price & Harkins 1987). The generally higher and more variable exponent for pain affect as compared with pain sensation provides one type of evidence for the existence of two measurably separate dimensions of experimental pain. If the stimulus–response functions of pain sensation and pain affect are reliably different, this difference might be interpreted from a psychophysical–neurophysiological perspective, as reflecting different central neural mechanisms. A critical question is what do these differences represent psychologically. That is, what do they tell us about the nature of pain sensation and pain affect and their interrelationships?

The generally higher power function exponent (steeper slope in log-log coordinates) for pain unpleasantness as compared to pain sensation can be mainly accounted for by the fact that unpleasantness ratings were systematically less than sensory ratings when both dimensions of pain were rated on the same length VASs. These lower ratings have the effect of increasing the slope when plotted in logarithmic coordinates. Unpleasantness ratings are, however, subject to a good deal of influence by psychological factors. The lower ratings in this case are due to assurances made to participants that the stimuli will be brief, will not produce tissue damage, and will remain within tolerable limits (Blitz & Dinnerstein, 1968; Chapman et al., 1985; Gracely, 1989; Price, 1988). The sense of impending harm to tissue, health, or life is greatly reduced in experimental pain because subjects of experimental pain studies are given

these assurances. Very different ratings would likely occur if subjects were made anxious about the pain stimuli.

However, the power function exponents for pain affect are not only higher but are more variable than those derived for pain sensation. The reliability of the power function exponent for contact heat-induced pain sensation reflects a principle of stability that is well known for sensory psychophysical relationships in general (Price, Hu, Dubner, & Gracely, 1977; J.C. Stevens & Marks, 1980; S.S. Stevens & Guirao, 1963). This principle is that as long as all other aspects of conditions of physical stimulation are held constant and only stimulus intensity is allowed to vary, the psychophysical stimulus–response relationship will be remarkably reliable across different groups of subjects and experiments. The more *variable* power function exponents for heat-induced pain unpleasantness as compared to heat-induced pain sensation must reflect more than stimulus intensity and stimulus context because the identical stimulus parameters can be shown to give rise to very different stimulus–affect response relationships under different conditions. An explanation has been given that pain-affective responses are associated with the *meanings* of the sensory components of one's experience and of the psychological context in which they occur (Price, 1988). This explanation might partly account for the variability in stimulus–pain affect response relationships. If so, then one should be able to demonstrate that factors related to one's cognitive orientation toward pain selectively influence stimulus intensity–pain affect relationships and that these influences can be reliably assessed.

Several different types of experiments that have used direct scaling techniques have shown that cognitive factors can powerfully and selectively modify the nociceptive stimulus intensity–affect relationship (Gracely, 1989; Gracely et al. 1978, 1979). Using verbal descriptor scaling techniques in combination with cross-modality matching procedures, Gracely et al. (1978) demonstrated that 5 mg diazepam (IV), a common tranquilizer, significantly reduced affective descriptor responses to painful electrocutaneous shock without altering sensory descriptor responses. The reductions were greatest for low intensity noxious stimuli. These results can easily be interpreted in terms of reduction in the anxiety associated with experimental pain because diazepam has been well characterized as an anxiety reducing agent. At least part of the unpleasantness of experimental pain is related to anxiety associated with possible harm to tissue and with other negative consequences. Gracely (1989) used the same verbal descriptor scales and experimental approach to show that affective dimensions of experimental pain could be selectively reduced by saline placebo (Figure 8.8). Similar to diazepam, effects were greater at the low end of the stimulus range (Figure 8.8). Saline placebo effects may have selectively reduced affective ratings by an antianxiety effect.

More direct evidence that cognitive factors can selectively modify affective responses to experimental pain comes from studies in which explicit attempts were made to reduce anxiety or concern by changing instructions or psychological set. In one such study, a psychophysical analysis was made of experiential factors that influence the affective but not sensory-discriminative dimension of heat-induced pain (Price et al., 1980). Seven trained subjects made cross-modality matching responses to both dimensions of pain experience. Nonnoxious (35–42°C) and noxious (45–51°C) skin temperature stimuli were randomly interspersed during each experimental session. Changes in expectation of receiving painful stimulation were induced by preceding one half of all the noxious stimuli by a warning signal.

The average responses of these subjects, shown in Figure 8.9, clearly indicate that 45–51°C noxious temperatures were experienced as less unpleasant when preceded by a warning signal. In contrast, pain sensation magnitudes, evoked by the same stimulus temperatures, were unaffected the warning signal (Figure 8.9). Thus, only the magnitudes of unpleasantness responses were lowered by the warning signal. Interestingly, similar to the effect of saline placebo in Gracely et al.'s study (Figure 8.8), the effects were largest toward the low end of the nociceptive stimulus continuum (Figure 8.9), a result consistent with an anxiety-reducing effect. Apparently, subjects prefer knowing beforehand that the next stimulus will be painful. The uncertainty of knowing whether the next stimulus will be painful is likely to produce anxiety. However, if the intensity of stimulation is high (i.e., 51°C), then it makes little difference whether or not someone is warned (Figure 8.9). Information about the nature of the painful sensations also has been shown to selectively influence pain affect. Johnson (1973) found that subjects who received a description of the sensations produced by ischemia of the forearm had lowered levels of distress compared to subjects who only received a description of the procedure. Pain sensation intensities were unaffected by this difference in description. Combining Johnson's observations with those of Price et al. (1980), it is apparent that advance information about the occurrence and nature of the painful sensations influences the magnitude of affective responses to experimentally induced pain.

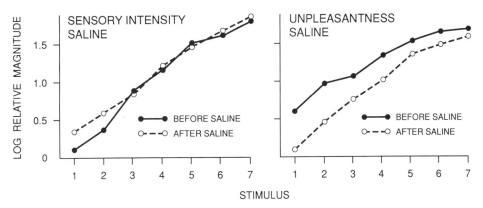

FIGURE 8.8. Sensory intensity and unpleasantness descriptor scales of electrical tooth pulp stimuli before and after the IV administration of saline placebo. Seven tooth pulp stimuli increasing in equal log steps from pain threshold to pain tolerance are shown on the abscissas; log relative magnitude sensory intensity or unpleasantness is shown on the ordinates. Each point is the geometric mean of 60 observations from 10 subjects. The filled circles show the responses before the IV administration of saline, and the open circles show the responses after the IV administration of saline. Adapted (redrawn) from Gracely (1979), page 818. Copyright 1979 Raven Press. Adapted by permission.

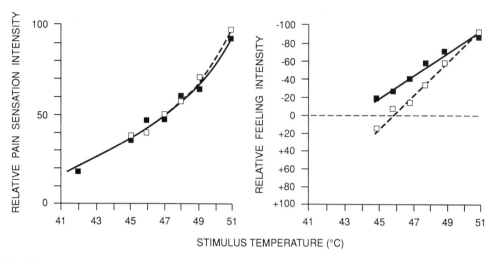

FIGURE 8.9. Selective effect of warning subjects that the stimulus will be intense on affective responses to heat-induced pain. The sensation intensities (left) are unchanged by a warning signal, whereas affective responses (right) to the lower end (45–47°C) of the nociceptive range are more positive (i.e., less unpleasant) as a consequence of the warning signal. Responses to signaled and unsignaled 45–51°C temperatures are designated by solid circles and solid lines and by open circles and dashed lines, respectively. Adapted (redrawn) from Price (1980), pages 142–143. Copyright 1980 Elsevier. Adapted by permission.

Sensory and Affective Responses during Clinical Pain

When separate rating scales for sensation and affect are used in experimental pain studies, the stimulus responses obtained for the two dimensions have different slopes and the affective responses are very sensitive to contextual and cognitive factors. These factors would seem to be even more critical in the case of clinical pain because the implications of clinical pain, in general, are likely to be perceived as more open ended and threatening. Thus, there have been some more attempts to independently assess sensory and affective dimensions of clinical pain in research studies (Harkins et al., 1989; Johnson, 1973; Price et al., 1977; Price et al., 1983; Price et al. 1984; Price, von der Gruen, et al., 1985).

At the same time, there has been considerable doubt whether it is possible or useful to separately measure the sensory and affective dimensions of different types of clinical pain. For example, Turk, Rudy, and Salovey (1985) have reasoned that because affective, sensory, and cognitive responses of the MPQ Pain Rating Index (PRI) are highly intercorrelated, these three components do not have discriminant validity. They conclude that only the total score of the PRI needs to be used to assess pain. Melzack (1985) counters this argument by

citing studies showing that some types of pain patients display greater use of sensory work groups, whereas other types of pain patients display greater use of affective words to describe their pain (Reading, 1982; Reading & Newton, 1977). Nevertheless, a disposition to make predominant use of either sensory or affective words to describe one's own pain may not be necessarily related to experienced magnitudes of unpleasantness as compared to sensation.

Differences in VAS-Sensory and VAS-Affective Ratings among Different Types of Clinical Pain

Thus, it remains to be demonstrated that different types of clinical pain are distinguished by differences in magnitude of pain affect in relation to pain sensation. This deficiency exists despite the claim that there are circumstances under which patients would rate intensities of sensation and magnitudes of unpleasantness quite differently (Gracely, 1989; Price, 1988). For example, patients whose pain is perceived to be associated with a serious threat to health or life might be expected to rate their pain much higher on an affective VAS than patients whose pain is less threatening, even when both types of patients give identical sensory intensity VAS ratings. In a study involving several very different types of clinical and laboratory settings, empirical evidence was provided for this idea by characterizing the relative magnitudes of pain sensation intensities and pain-related emotional feelings experienced by several pain patient populations that had different types of pain (Price, Harkins, & Baker, 1987). The question of main concern was whether different types of clinical pain were characterized by differences in magnitudes of VAS unpleasantness ratings relative to VAS-sensory ratings. Cancer pain patients, chronic pain patients, women with labor pain, and pain-free subjects exposed to experimental pain were compared in terms of their sensory and affective VAS ratings of pain (Figure 8.6). The sensory and affective VASs used were the same as those described earlier in studies of experimental pain.

A salient and distinguishing feature of the types of clinical and experimental pains shown in Figure 8.6, is the difference between affective and sensory VAS ratings. Causalgia and cancer pain patients were distinguished by the fact that affective VAS ratings of pain were significantly greater than sensory VAS ratings

of pain at its usual and maximum intensities. Myofascial pain dysfunction (MPD) patients, in turn, gave nearly equal affective VAS and sensory VAS ratings of their pain. Although sensory VAS ratings of cancer pain patients were very similar to those of MPD patients, cancer pain patients gave affective VAS ratings that were distinctly *greater* than VAS-sensory ratings. In contrast to both cancer and causalgia pain patients, VAS-affective ratings at three of four phases of labor were significantly *less* than VAS-sensory (Figure 8.10). Similarly, pain patients tested for VAS-affective and VAS-sensory ratings of different levels of experimental pain consistently gave lower VAS-affect relative to VAS-sensory ratings of those pains. Therefore, various levels of pain sensation intensity are associated with correspondingly *high* levels of pain unpleasantness in the case of cancer pain and in some types of chronic pain. On the other hand, various levels of pain sensation are associated with relatively *lower* levels of pain unpleasantness in the cases of labor pain and experimental pain (Price, Harkins, & Baker, 1987).

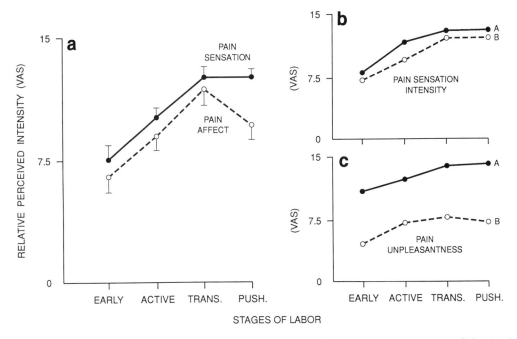

FIGURE 8.10. a: Mean VAS-sensory and VAS-affect ratings of pain of 23 labor patients at various phases of labor (vertical lines are standard errors). **b:** VAS-sensory ratings of women who focused mainly on pain or avoiding pain (group A) compared to women who focused mainly on the impending birth (group B). Note that both groups gave similar VAS-sensory ratings. **c:** VAS-affective ratings of group A and B. Note that VAS-affect ratings of group B are approximately half that of group A. Adapted (redrawn) from Price (1987), page 303. Copyright 1987 Elsevier. Adapted by permission.

Sensory-Affect Relationships in Labor Pain

Figure 8.10 illustrates pain sensation intensity and pain unpleasantness (affective) VAS responses at each stage of labor (Price, Harkins, & Baker, 1987). VAS ratings of pain sensation intensity increased significantly across stages from Early to Active and Active to Transition but not from Transition to Pushing. VAS ratings of pain affect also increased significantly from Early to Active and Active to Transition. However, VAS ratings of pain affect *decreased* significantly between Transition and Pushing. Pain affect VAS responses were consistently lower than pain sensation responses, and this was particularly apparent during pushing (Figure 8.10).

Significant differences in pain VAS-affect ratings were observed as a function of whether the patient was focusing primarily on pain or avoiding pain (Figure 8.10c, A) or on having the baby (Figure 8.10c, B). Patients who focused primarily on having the baby rated the unpleasantness of their pain as approximately half that of patients who focused primarily on pain or avoiding pain. This difference occurred at each stage of labor. In contrast, no significant differences were observed for pain sensation intensity VAS ratings at any stage of labor for women who focused on their pain versus those who were focusing on the impending birth. It is likely that this difference in magnitude of unpleasantness but not sensory intensity was related to difference in cognitive focus rather than differences in peripheral source of pain because this difference in pain unpleasantness persisted across all four phases of labor in the face of major differences in reported intensity of pain, frequency of contractions, and physiological source of nociceptive input (Bonica, 1984).

These different relationships provide evidence consistent with the hypothesis that cognitive and contextual factors selectively influence the affective-motivational dimension of pain. Such potential factors include perceived ability to control the pain, the implications of the pain for the future, and the perception of pain as an interruption. The results illustrated in Figures 8.6 and 8.10 provide evidence in support of the hypothesis that fear and perception of possible life- or health-threatening factors selectively increase the affective over the sensory dimension of pain, as in the case of cancer pain and some types of chronic pain (Price, Harkins, & Baker, 1987). That the affective dimension of pain can be selectively reduced when there is no threat to health or life, as in the case of brief experimental pain (Figures 8.8 and 8.9), or when the pain can be associated with a positive event, as in the case of labor pain (Figure 8.10), is also consistent with this hypothesis.

Assessing Different Stages of Pain-Related Emotional Disturbance

The studies described thus far have demonstrated the importance of separate assessment of sensory and affective components of pain. Most of the examples given so far, however, have emphasized the first stage of pain-related affect that is closely linked to nociceptive events. The second stage of pain-related affect, which is based on cognitive–evaluative processes, is of considerable importance in chronic pain and cancer pain. Just as there are pharmacological, physiological, and psychological factors that can selectively influence pain related affect, so also there may be selective influences on different stages of pain-related emotional disturbance.

Effects of Personality Traits

A study by Harkins et al. (1989) that illustrates and supports this point is that which examined effects of personality dimensions on sensory and affective dimensions of experimental pain and clinical pain as well as on pain-related emotions. The effects of two personality traits, extraversion and neuroticism, on these aspects of pain and pain-related behavior were examined in a group of MPD patients.

First, the personality traits of extraversion and neuroticism had no influence on VAS *sensory* ratings of experimental heat pain, as shown in Figure 8.11. Patients with high and low scores on these two personality dimensions (Eysenck personality inventory) had very similar nociceptive temperature–VAS response curves (Figure 8.11). These high and low score groups of patients also did not significantly differ with respect to their VAS-*sensory* ratings of their clinical pain. Therefore, these personality traits do not appear to influence sensory-intensive judgments reflective of nociceptive processing.

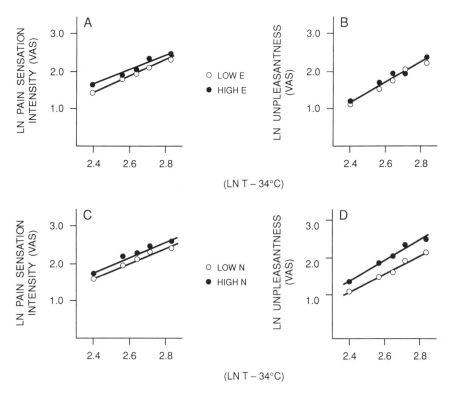

FIGURE 8.11. Relative VAS responses of intensity and unpleasantness of experimental pain in low versus high extraversion (A,B) and on low versus high neuroticism (C,D) pain patients. Significant group differences were observed only for the high N score patients (solid triangles) versus low N score patients (open triangles) for the affective dimension of experimental pain (D). Adapted (redrawn) from Harkins et al. (1989), page 212. Copyright 1989 Elsevier. Adapted by permission.

Second, although extraverts did not differ from intraverts in their VAS-*affective* ratings of these same nociceptive temperature stimuli, high neurotic score patients gave marginally higher VAS-*affective* ratings to these stimuli as compared to low neurotic score patients (Figure 8.11). This pattern of response differences also was obtained for VAS ratings of *clinical pain* (Figure 8.12). As with experimental pain, extraverts and intraverts did not differ in VAS-affective ratings, whereas high neurotic score patients gave somewhat higher VAS-affective ratings of clinical pain than did low neurotic score patients (Figure 8.12). These results indicate a modest but significant effect of neuroticism on early stages of pain-related affect (i.e., stage 1).

Finally, it was at the level of emotions related to suffering (stage 2) that the personality traits of neuroticism but not extraversion appeared to exert large influences. As hypothesized, high neurotic score patients gave higher VAS ratings of emotions related to suffering (i.e., depression, frustration, anxiety, etc.) as compared to low neurotic score patients (Figure 8.13). Extraverts and introverts did not differ in their ratings of these emotions. Neurotic patients also had much greater hypochondriasis, irritability, and emotional disturbance, as measured by the Pilowsky Illness Behavior Questionnaire. Overall, this type of analysis indicates that personality traits, such as neuroticism, exert their largest influence *not* on sensory mechanisms of nociceptive processing or even on early stages of pain-related affect, but on cognitive processes related to the ways people constitute the meanings and implications that pain holds for their life in general.

The results of this analysis have implications for how psychological interventions on chronic pain can be assessed. Just as at least some personality dimensions strongly influence emotional disturbance and pain behavior, so might some psychological interventions also exert

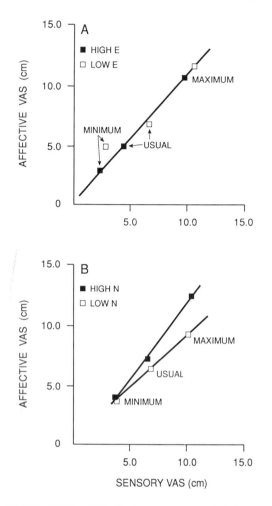

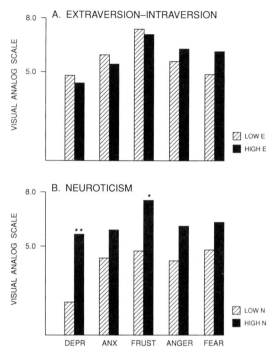

FIGURE 8.13. Mean emotion visual analogue responses of MPD patients' to their clinical pain. Note similarities of VAS ratings of high and low extraversion groups and higher VAS ratings of high as compared to low neuroticism groups (**$p < .01$; *$p < .05$; 1-tailed; Depr. = depression; Anx. = anxiety; Frust. = frustration). Adapted (redrawn) from Harkins et al. (1989), page 215. Copyright 1989 Elsevier. Adapted by permission.

FIGURE 8.12. VAS-affective responses to clinical pain plotted as a function of VAS-sensory responses to clinical pain for MPD pain patients with high (●) and low (○) extraversion scores (A) and for pain patients with high (●) and low (○) neuroticism scores (B). Sensory-affective functions are similar for extraversion groups while the affective response of high neuroticism (N) scorers is greater than low N scorers for equivalent VAS sensory intensity ratings. Adapted (redrawn) from Harkins et al. (1989), page 214. Copyright 1989 Elsevier. Adapted by permission.

their greatest influence at this level. The differential analysis of how treatments affect different stages and dimensions of pain is both logical and compelling. If chronic pain is multidimensional and multiple treatments are used in its management, then its assessment likewise needs separate measures of nociception, immediate pain-related affective disturbance, affective dimensions related to suffering, and pain-related behavior.

The separate assessment of different stages and dimensions of pain would benefit from an approach that assesses different emotions associated with chronic pain As discussed above, chronic pain can be accompanied by a variety of disturbing emotions. In the study by Harkins et al., just described, five separate emotion VASs were used to assess effects of personality traits on pain-related emotional disturbance. Although composite ratings of these five VASs were augmented by neuroticism, examination of patients' VAS ratings revealed considerable variabilities in the ratings of specific types of emotions indicating considerable heterogeneity in the types and magnitudes of emotions felt by chronic pain patients. Thus, the possible differential assessment of specific pain-related emotions among individual chronic pain patients remains an intriguing possibility.

Assessing Individual Pain-Related Emotions

An emotional component analysis of these emotion VASs and their association with Beck Depression Inventory (BDI) and MMPI demonstrated that the five VASs were reliable and valid instruments for assessing specific pain-related emotions (Wade, Price, Hamer, Schwartz, & Hart, 1990). First, the test–retest reliabilities of these VAS were at acceptable levels (r = .67 – .94). Second, analyses relating this negative feeling VAS to VAS ratings of pain unpleasantness and to depression indices from the MMPI (scale 2) and BDI (sum score) yielded significant canonical correlations. Third, multiple regression further clarified the relationships between specific emotion VAS and indices of depression (MMPI and BDI) and between emotion VAS and pain unpleasantness ratings. These associations were determined after statistically controlling for pain sensation intensity. Both anxiety and frustration VAS ratings but not depression or fear ratings significantly predicted pain unpleasantness VAS ratings. Both depression and anger VAS but not frustration or fear VAS predicted BDI and MMPI depression scores. Finally, these chronic pain patients rated frustration the highest of the five negative emotional feelings, as shown in Figure 8.14 . In contrast, and as

might be expected, women with labor pain rated frustration the lowest and fear and anxiety the highest among the five emotions (Figure 8.14). This combination of results indicate that each emotion VAS makes a unique contribution to the overall magnitude of pain-related emotional unpleasantness and that patients appear to be responding to these VASs in a manner consistent with the meanings directly implied by the verbal descriptors (i.e., depression, anxiety, frustration, anger, and fear).

Thus, the composite of the five emotion VASs can be construed as a general measure of pain-related emotional disturbance, whereas each individual emotion VAS separately assesses the contribution of specific emotional feelings to pain-related emotional unpleasantness. This separate assessment is important because psychological approaches to pain management need to target specific emotions that comprise each patient's emotional disturbance. Psychological approaches to pain treatment frequently focus on reducing symptoms of depression by antidepressant medication and on reducing anxiety with biofeedback and relaxation techniques (Sternbach, 1974). However, frustration represents a unique emotion that is distinct from depression and represents a large component of suffering among chronic pain patients (Wade et al., 1990). Therefore,

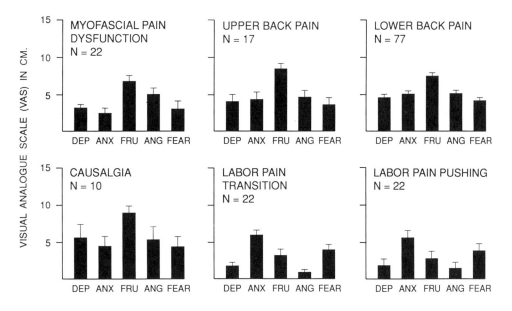

FIGURE 8.14. Profiles of VAS ratings of five distinct types of emotional feelings during different types of clinical pain. Adapted from Price (1988), page 59. Copyright 1988 Raven Press. Adapted by permission.

this emotion needs to be recognized among those who psychologically assess chronic pain patients, and specific thereapeutic approaches need to be used to deal with frustration. Similarly, treatments directed specifically toward anger and fear also need to be designed.

Conclusions about Different Methods of Pain Measurement

Single-dimensional pain measures such as pain threshold and tolerance are simple to use but are limited by their inability to directly assess the magnitudes of different types of pain. Category scales also are simple to use and can quickly provide assessments of *changes* in pain intensity. However, there is now considerable evidence that some forms of simple direct magnitude scaling techniques, such as some types of VASs and verbal descriptor techniques, fulfill all or most of the criteria for an ideal method of pain measurement. They have been shown to yield judgments of sensory intensity that at least approximate a ratio scale level of measurement and can provide a check on the scaling behavior of subjects. For example, subjects' VAS and verbal descriptor scale responses can be compared for internal consistency. They can separately assess two distinct dimensions of pain experience, sensation intensity, and unpleasantness. These separate measures are critically important in distinguishing whether treatments have antinociceptive affects and/or alter the affective dimension of pain through psychological factors. The nociceptive temperature–pain sensation intensity function is fairly stable and directly parallels the stimulus–impulse frequency response functions of nociceptive neurons throughout the peripheral and central nervous sytem (Price, 1988; Price et al., 1992). It can be interpreted as an index of nociceptive sensory processing and reductions in this sensory response function can be at least generally interpreted as resulting from antinociceptive effects. The nociceptive temperature–pain *affective intensity* function, although normally dependent on the sensory intensity function, additionally reflects the cognitive mediating processes that occur during pain experience. Thus, alterations in the meanings of the nociceptive sensation and in one's overall context can sometimes alter the affective response, as in the case of cognitive focus during labor pain or in the case of placebo responses.

The common measurement of pain, as if it were a single simple dimension, can totally obscure the distinction between antinociceptive effects versus selective effects on the emotional feeling component. For example, if only a single measure of pain intensity had been used in the labor pain study described above, changes in pain experience that occurred between transition and pushing phases would not likely have been detected (cf. Figure 8.10). Likewise, the effects of anxiety reducing factors, such as placebo and diazepam, would easily be obscured in studies using a unitary pain intensity measure. Although pain sensation and affect may closely covary under many circumstances, as in the case of many types of experimental pain, there are factors and circumstances that can selectively and powerfully influence the affective dimension of pain, particularly the second stage. Simple, direct scaling measures of pain sensation, immediate pain-related affect, and longer term pain-related emotional feelings may be extremely helpful in identifying these factors in individual patients and within specific types of treatments.*

In the case of chronic pain, the separate measurement of pain sensation intensity and pain affect, although very critical, is itself too simplistic because chronic pain can be accompanied by a variety of disturbing emotions. As explained above, pain is not necessarily associated with one particular emotion, such as depression, but also may be accompanied by anxiety, frustration, anger, or fear depending on a variety of circumstances.

REFERENCES

Arnold, M.B. (1970). *Feelings and emotions*. New York: Academic Press.

Bakan, D. (1968). *Disease, pain and sacrifice*. Chicago: University of Chicago Press.

Beecher, H.K. (1959). *Measurement of subjective responses: Quantitative effects of drugs*. New York: Oxford University Press.

Blitz, B. & Dinnerstein, A.J. (1968). Effects of different types of instructions on pain parameters. *Journal of Abnormal Psychology, 73*, 276–280.

Bonica, J.J. (1984). Labour pain. In P.D. Wall & R.

---

*Mechanical VASs have been designed for assessment of these dimensions of pain. They provide a simple and rapid method of assessment of pain sensation intensity, unpleasantness, and pain-related emotions by means of sliding plastic scales whose numbers can be immediately read on the back. For more information, write to Algometrics, Inc., PO Box 17244, Richmond, VA 23226-7244.

Melzack (Eds.), *Textbook of pain* (pp. 377–392). Edinburgh: Churchill-Livingstone.

Bushnell, M.C., Taylor, M.B., Duncan, G.H., & Dubner, R. (1983). Discrimination of innocuous and noxious thermal stimuli applied to the face in human and monkey. *Somatosensory Research*, 1, 119–129.

Buytendyck, F.J.J. (1961). *Pain.* London: Hutchinson.

Chapman, C.R., Casey, K.L., Dubner, R., Folley, K.M., Gracely, R.H., & Reading, A.E. (1985). Pain measurement: An overview. *Pain*, 22, 1–31.

Chapman, L.F., Dingman, H.F., & Ginzberg, S.P. (1965). Failure of systemic analgesic agents to alter the absolute sensory threshold for the simple detection of pain. *Brain*, 88, 1011–1022.

Duncan, G., Bushnell, C., & Levigne, G. (1986). Comparison of verbal and visual analogue scales for measuring experimental pain. *Journal of Dental Research*, 65 (special issue), 1239.

Ekman, G. & Sjoberg, L. (1965). Scaling. *Annual Review of Psychology*, 16, 451–474.

Gracely, R.H. (1979). Psychophysical assessment of human pain. In J.J. Bonica et al. (Eds.), *Advances in pain research and therapy* (Vol. 3, p. 818). New York: Raven Press.

Gracely, R.H. (1989). Pain psychophysics. In C.R. Chapman & J.D. Loeser (Eds.), *Advances in pain research and therapy* (Vol. 12, pp. 211–229). New York: Raven Press.

Gracely, R.H., & Dubner, R. (1981). Pain assessment in humans—a reply to Hall. *Pain*, 11, 109–120.

Gracely, R.H., McGrath, P., & Dubner, R. (1978). Ratio scales of sensory and affective verbal pain descriptors. *Pain*, 5, 5–18.

Gracely, R.H., McGrath, P., & Dubner, R. (1979). Narcotic analgesia: Fentanyl reduces the intensity but not the unpleasantness of painful tooth pulp sensations. *Science*, 203, 1261–1263.

Guilford, J.P. (1954). *Psychometric methods* (p. 597). New York: McGraw-Hill.

Guilford, J.P. & Dingman, H.F. (1954). A validation study of ratio-judgment methods. *American Journal of Psychology*, 67, 395–410.

Hardy, J.D., Wolff, H.G., & Goodell, H. (1954). *Pain sensation and reactions.* Baltimore: Williams & Wilkins.

Harkins, S.W., Price, D.D., & Braith, J. (1989). Effects of extraversion and neuroticism on experimental pain, clinical pain, and illness behavior. *Pain*, 36, 209–318.

Harkins, S.W., Price, D.D., & Martelli, M. (1985). Effects of age on pain perception: Thermonociception. *Journal of Gerontology*, 41, 58–63.

Heft, M.W., & Parker, S.R. (1984). An experimental basis for revising the graphic rating scale for pain. *Pain*, 19, 153–161.

Heft, M.W., Gracely, R.H., Dubner, R., & McGrath, P.A. (1980). A validation model for verbal descriptor scaling of human clinical pain. *Pain*, 9, 363–373.

Johnson, J.E. (1973). Effects of accurate expectations about sensations on the sensory and distress components of pain. *Journal of Personality and Social Psychology*, 27, 261–275.

Marks, L.E. (1974). Sensory processes. *The new psychophysics* (p. 334). New York: Academic Press.

Melzack, R. (1975). The McGill Pain Questionnaire: Major properties and scoring methods. *Pain*, 1, 277–299.

Melzack, R. (1984). Neuropsychological basis of pain

measurement. In L. Knuger & J.C. Liebeskind (Eds.), *Advances in pain research and therapy* (Vol. 6, pp. 322–339). New York: Raven Press.

Melzack, R. (1985). Letter to the editor. *Pain*, 23, 201–203.

Melzack, R., & Casey, K.L. (1968). Sensory, motivational and central control of determinants of pain. In Kenshalo (Ed.), *The skin senses* (pp. 423–439). Springfield, IL: Chas C. Thomas.

Melzack, R., & Torgerson, W.S. (1971). On the language of pain. *Anesthesiology*, 34, 50–59.

Mountcastle, V.B. (1974). Pain and temperature sensibilities. In V.B. Mountcastle (Ed.), *Medical physiology* (13th ed., Vol. 1, pp. 348–381). Saint Louis: Mosby.

Price, D.D. (1988). *Psychological and neural mechanisms of pain.* New York: Raven Press.

Price, D.D., Barrell, J.E., & Barrell, J.J. (1985). A quantitative-experiential analysis of human emotions. *Motivation and Emotions*, 9, 19–38.

Price, D.D., & Barrell, J.J. (1980). An experiential approach with quantitative methods: A research paradigm. *Journal of Human Psychology*, 20, 75–95.

Price, D.D., & Barrell, J.J. (1984). Some general laws of human emotion: Interrelationships between intensities of desire, expectation, and emotional feeling. *Journal of Personality*, 52, 389–409.

Price, D.D., Barrell, J.J., & Gracely, R.H. (1980). A psychophysical analysis of experiential factors that selectively influence the affective dimension of pain. *Pain*, 8, 137–179.

Price, D.D., & Harkins, S.W. (1987). The combined use of visual analogue scales and experimental pain in proving standardized assessment of clinical pain. *Clinical Journal of Pain*, 3, 1–8.

Price, D.D., Harkins, S.W., & Baker, C. (1987). Sensory-affective relationships among different types of clinical and experimental pain. *Pain*, 28, 291–299.

Price, D.D., Harkins, S.W., Rafii, A., & Price, C. (1986). A simultaneous comparison of fentanyl's analgesic effects on experimental and clinical pain. *Pain*, 24, 197–203.

Price, D.D., Hu, J.W., Dubner, R., & Gracely, R.H. (1977). Peripheral suppression of first pain and central summation of second pain evoked by noxious heat pulses. *Pain*, 3, 57–68.

Price, D.D., McGrath, P.A., Rafii, A., & Buckingham, B. (1983). The validation of visual analogue scales as ratio scale measures for chronic and experimental pain. *Pain*, 17, 45–56.

Price, D.D., McHaffie, J.G., & Stein, B.E. (1992). The psychophysical attributes of heat-induced pain and their relationships to neural mechanisms. *Journal of Cognitive Neuroscience*, 4, 1–14.

Price, D.D., Rafii, A., Watkins, L.R., & Buckingham, B. (1984). A psychophysical analysis of acupuncture analgesia. *Pain*, 19, 27–42.

Price, D.D., von der Gruen, A., Miller, J., Rafii, A., & Price, C. (1985). A psychophysical analysis of morphine analgesia. *Pain*, 22, 261–269.

Reading, A.E. (1982). An analysis of the language of pain in chronic and acute patient groups. *Pain*, 13, 185–192.

Reading, A.E., & Newton, J.R. (1977). On a comparison of dysmenorrhea and intrauterine device related to pain. *Pain*, 3, 265–276.

Scott, J., & Huskisson, E.C. (1976). Graphic representation of pain. *Pain, 2*, 175–184.

Seymour, R.A., Simpson, J.M., Charlton, J.E., & Phillips M.E. (1985). An evaluation of length and end-phrase of visual analogue scales in dental pain. *Pain, 21*, 177–186.

Sternbach, R.A. (1974). *Pain patients: Traits and treatment.* New York: Academic Press.

Stevens, J.C., & Marks, L.C. (1980). Cross-modality matching functions generated by magnitude estimation. *Perception and Psychophysics, 12*, 417–434.

Stevens, S.S. (1975). *Psychophysics: Introduction to its perceptual, neural and social prospects* (p. 329). New York: Wiley.

Stevens, S.S., & Galanter, E.G. (1957). Ratio scales and category scales for a dozen perceptual continua. *Journal of Experimental Pscyhology, 54*, 377–411.

Stevens, S.S., & Guirao, M. (1963). Subjective scaling of length and area and the matching of length to loudness and brightness. *Journal of Experimental Psychology, 66*, 177–186.

Teghtsoonian, A., & Teghtsoonian, R. (1965). Seen and felt length. *Psychology of Science, 3*, 465–466.

Turk, D.C., Rudy, T.E., & Salovey, P. (1985). The McGill Pain Questionnaire reconsidered: Confirming the factor structure and examining appropriate uses. *Pain, 21*, 385–397.

Tursky, B. (1976). The development of pain perception profile: A psychophysical approach. In M. Weisenberg & B. Tursky (Eds.), *Pain: New perspectives in therapy and research* (pp. 171–194). New York: Plenum Press.

Wade, J.B., Price, D.D., Hamer, R.M., Schwartz, S.M., & Hart, R.P. (1990). An emotional component analysis of chronic pain. *Pain, 40*, 303–310.

Chapter 9

Self-Report Scales and Procedures for Assessing Pain in Adults

MARK P. JENSEN, PhD
PAUL KAROLY, PhD

Pain and suffering are private, internal events that cannot be directly observed by clinicians or assessed via bioassays. Assessment of the pain experience is, therefore, frequently built upon the use of patient self-report. The purpose of this chapter is to critically evaluate the available self-report measures of pain. Our hope is that the chapter will assist clinicians and researchers to select the procedures that best serve their purposes. We begin with a brief discussion of issues relevant to the use of self-report pain scales. We then describe and critique the methods currently available for assessing three dimensions of the pain experience: pain intensity, pain affect, and pain location.

THEORETICAL AND ASSESSMENT MODEL

Because decisions about the choice of pain assessment procedures are (ideally, but not always) based on one's model or conceptualization of pain, it is important to make explicit the theoretical and assessment model that we use to guide our understanding of pain. We

label our assumptive framework the Pain Context Model (Karoly, 1985, 1991; Karoly & Jensen, 1987). Like that of others (see Flor, Birbaumer, & Turk, 1990), our model is based on the assumption that the pain experience can be examined at several levels, and that the data obtained can be influenced by numerous psychological, medical, and social factors (see also Kerns & Jacob, Chapter 14).

In the Pain Context Model, *pain* is considered to be a construct (see Cleeland, 1986; 1989; Rudy, 1989; Turk, 1989). A construct is a label for categorizing a related group of observations. Pain is similar to other constructs, such as depression, anxiety, and intelligence, in that it is not directly observable, but rather is inferred from varied observations.

Even the best measures or indicants of a construct are not always closely related to one another (Cleeland, 1986). This is because the different observations or components that make up a construct do not always co-occur in time or in the same configuration in all people. For example, even though the pain construct consists of such dimensions as pain behavior and self-reported pain, one person may display nonverbal pain behaviors without complaining of pain, another may complain bitterly of pain and yet display no nonverbal pain activities, and a third person may display pain behaviors *and* report intense pain and suffering (see Keefe & Williams, Chapter 16). Because of the multidimensionality of pain, no single measure can adequately assess the construct. An important, preliminary task in pain assessment is therefore to define the dimensions of pain relevant to one's purposes, and to demonstrate that the selected dimensions are conceptually related to pain and distinct from one another.

A considerable amount of work has already gone into defining the dimensions of subjective pain. Although there is more work to be done, at this point in time there appears to be at least three distinct dimensions of the pain experience that can be assessed in nearly all pain patient populations: pain intensity, pain affect, and pain location (see also Price & Harkins, Chapter 8). Pain intensity may be defined as *how much* a person hurts. Patients are usually able to provide pain intensity estimates relatively quickly, and all measures of pain intensity tend to be closely related to one another statistically (Jensen, Karoly, & Braver, 1986; Jensen, Karoly, O'Riordan, Bland, & Burns, 1989). These findings suggest that pain intensity is a fairly homogeneous dimension, and one that is relatively easy for people to identify and gauge.

Pain affect, on the other hand, appears to be more complex than pain intensity. We define pain affect as the degree of activation or changes in action readiness caused by the sensory experience of pain. This arousal is often felt as distressing or frightening, and can lead to interference in daily activities and habitual modes of response. In chronic pain, the emotional aspects can come to dominate the clinical picture.

Measures of pain affect have been shown to be statistically distinct from measures of pain intensity (Jensen et al., 1989). Furthermore, measures of pain affect do not appear to be as homogeneous as measures of pain intensity— they are less likely than measures of pain intensity to be strongly related to one another. This finding suggests that the affective component of pain may consist of a variety of emotive reactions (Morley, 1989). Perhaps pain is similar to other sensory-perceptual experiences, such as those involved in the perception of light and sound. Like perceived pain intensity, the color intensity or brightness reflecting off of

a painting might be relatively easy to rate, whereas judgments regarding how that color makes one feel might require considerably more reflection. Such affective responses may also require more than a single word or number to adequately describe.

Pain location can be defined as the perceived location(s) of pain that patients experience on or in their bodies. Clinicians have learned to pay attention to several aspects of patient descriptions of pain location. *Where* patients describe pain, the *number of locations* indicated and the way in which patients describe the location(s) of their pain all appear to be related to physical and psychosocial functioning.

On the Multiple Contexts of Pain Measurement

The Pain Context Model directs one's attention to (among other things) the degree to which the pain experience is embedded in its surroundings. Pain is a dynamic, developmental process, not a single event or simple countable product. Thus, when we and others talk of "objective" measures or "quantifiable" indices, the reader should understand that we do not intend to depict pain as a static, all-or-none, unidimensional, body-centered occurrence that exists somehow independent of time, place, the patient's cognition, or the observer's presuppositions. As we have elsewhere noted:

> As pain assessors, we are coparticipants, not merely observers and, therefore, although there is no single best way to interpret pain, we can probably serve our patients better if we acknowledge that we are jointly engaged in creating the pain dimensions we seek to measure. (Karoly & Jensen, 1987, p. 7)

Language habits and cultural conventions force us to further decontextualize the pain experience by addressing separately an individual's awareness of pain (e.g., "my arm hurts"), emotional reactivity (e.g., "the pain in my arm is killing me"), and behavioral (motor) responses (e.g., the tendency to use the other arm, to keep the arm in a sling, etc.). However, it is critical to remember that thought, action, and emotion are inextricably bound together in the sentient organism — and they are separable only for the sake of convenience.

Research from a number of sources and with

different populations provides strong evidence that many factors influence communication about pain. A brief review of this research will help to illustrate this important pain.

Levine and De Simone (1991) assigned college students to be in the presence of an attractive male or female while holding their hand in ice water and rating pain. Based on gender role expectations, Levine and De Simone (1991) predicted that males would report less pain in the presence of the female as opposed to the male experimenter. This is exactly what they found. Female students, on the other hand, were not significantly influenced by the gender of the experimenter. In another study, Craig and Weiss (1971) found that modeling of pain tolerance impacts the report of pain. Subjects who observed people modeling high pain tolerance reported higher pain tolerance (in response to electric shock) than subjects who observed people modeling low pain tolerance. Finally, Dworkin and Chen (1982) showed that changing the environment influenced pain report. Their subjects reported that tooth pulp stimulation hurt more when they were administered in a dental clinic than when they were administered in a research laboratory setting.

Research also indicates that the time of day is related to pain intensity ratings. Folkard, Glynn, and Lloyd (1976) asked chronic pain patients to rate their pain intensity every 2 hours from 8:00 A.M. to 10:00 P.M. On average, reported pain demonstrated an increase over the course of a day, with "peaks" occurring at 12:00 noon and 6:00 P.M. However, there was much individual variation between patients regarding their diurnal variation in pain report. Similarly, Jamison and Brown (1991) found that pain intensity reports changed in a predictable pattern throughout the course of a day for the majority of chronic pain patients, although the specific temporal pattern varied from individual to individual.

There are two implications of the above findings for assessing and interpreting self-report pain data. First, the findings illustrate that self-reports of pain do not stand in a one-to-one relationship to nociception. (Nociception is the activation of sensory transduction in nerves that convey information about tissue damage.) Although it is likely that people attempt to honestly report their subjective pain experience in most situations, there are no guarantees that what people tell us about pain

experience accurately reflects their pain experience. These considerations have caused some clinicians and investigators to advocate the elimination of self-report data. Although we do not agree with this extreme position, we strongly advise that clinicians and researchers be wary of relying solely on decontextualized subjective pain reports when attempting to understand an individual's life circumstances.

A second implication of this body of research is that clinicians and researchers should take the factors known to influence self-report into account when assessing pain. *The conditions under which the self-report of pain are made should be as similar as possible between comparison groups or between assessment periods.* Attempts should be made, for example, to have patients rate their pain at the same time of day, in the same place, and in the presence of the same people at each assessment period. Aggregating multiple measures (e.g., taking the average of several pain measures) may help to minimize the influence of extraneous or irrelevant contextual factors. In support of this practice, aggregated pain measures have been shown to be more sensitive to treatment effects than single measures (Max, 1991).

We have briefly discussed some theoretical and practical issues related to the assessment of the subjective experience of pain in order to provide the reader with a context within which to use and understand self-report data. Given this background, we are now ready to describe and critique the available self-report measures of pain experience. The next three sections discuss the procedures that may be used to assess the three dimensions of pain experience introduced above: pain intensity, pain affect, and pain location.

ASSESSING PAIN INTENSITY

Pain intensity is a quantitative estimate of the severity of felt pain. The three most commonly used methods to assess pain intensity are the Verbal Rating Scale, the Visual Analog Scale, and the Numerical Rating Scale. Less common measures include the Behavior Rating Scale, the Picture Scale, the Box Scale, and the Descriptor Differential Scale.

Verbal Rating Scales

A Verbal Rating Scale (VRS) consists of a list of adjectives describing different levels of pain intensity. An adequate VRS of pain intensity should include adjectives that reflect the extremes of this dimension (e.g., from *no pain* to *extremely intense pain*) and sufficient additional adjectives to capture the gradations of pain intensity that may be experienced. Patients are asked to read over the list of adjectives, and select the word or phrase that best describes their level of pain. Many different VRS lists have been created (Frank, Moll, & Hort, 1982; Gracely, McGrath, & Dubner, 1978a; Joyce, Zutshi, Hrubes, & Mason, 1975; Kremer, Atkinson, & Ignelzi, 1981; Seymour, 1982; Tursky, Jamner, & Friedman, 1982) and two examples are presented in Table 9.1. As can be seen, the number of pain intensity levels represented in these VRSs varies considerably from scale to scale.

VRSs are usually scored by listing the adjectives in order of pain severity, and assigning each one a score as a function of its rank. In the 4-point VRS used by Seymour (1982), for example, *no pain* would be given a score of 0, *mild pain* a score of 1, *moderate pain* a score of 2, and *severe pain* a score of 3. The number associated with the adjective chosen by the patient would constitute his or her pain intensity score.

A criticism frequently raised with respect to the rank scoring method is that it assumes

TABLE 9.1. Verbal Rating Scales of Pain Intensity

5-Point Scale[a]	15-Point Scale[b]
None	Extremely weak
Mild	Very weak
Moderate	Weak
Severe	Very mild
Very severe	Mild
	Very moderate
	Slightly moderate
	Moderate
	Barely strong
	Slightly intense
	Strong
	Intense
	Very strong
	Very intense
	Extremely intense

[a]From Frank, Moll, and Hart (1982), page 211. Copyright 1982 British Association of Rheumatology and Rehabilitation. Reprinted by permission.
[b]From Gracely, McGrath, and Dubner (1978a). Copyright 1978 Elsevier Science Publishers. Reprinted by permission.

equal intervals between the adjectives, even though it is extremely unlikely that equal intervals exist. That is, the interval between *no pain* and *mild pain* may be much smaller than that between *moderate pain* and *severe pain*, yet each interval is scored as if the difference were the same. This characteristic of rank scoring procedures can pose several problems when interpreting VRS data. For example, rank scores do not allow for adequate interpretations of the magnitude of any differences found. A change from 3 to 2 (on a 4-point scale) might represent a 10% change in perceived pain or a 50% change, depending on the perceived interval represented by the words on the list. A second problem is that VRSs represent *ordinal* (ranked) scaling data; yet VRS scores are often treated as if they were *interval* (such that the difference between a 1 and a 2 is viewed as the same as that between a 2 and a 3) or *ratio* (interval data with a true zero point) data, and subsequently analyzed using parametric statistical procedures (procedures reserved for interval and ratio scaling) rather than appropriate nonparametric procedures. The statistical results obtained by treating ordinal data as if they were interval or ratio are suspect, although less so if the number of categories on the scale is five or more (Cicchetti, Showalter, & Tyrer, 1985; see also Rasmussen, 1989).

Cross-modality matching procedures have been used as a means of transforming VRS ratings to scales that are more likely to have ratio properties (Gracely, McGrath, & Dubner, 1978a, 1978b; see also Price & Harkins, Chapter 8). This procedure involves asking each patient to indicate the severity that each word represents in reference to one or more other modalities (such as the loudness of a tone, the length of a line, or handgrip force). The rating that the patient gives to a particular word (or the average of several if the patient rates each word more than once) is then used as the score for that word. Because the modalities used by patients to match pain descriptors can themselves be indexed using ratio scales, the numbers or scores derived from these procedures are more likely to have ratio properties and to reflect actual perceived differences in magnitudes.

There are two major limitations of cross-modality procedures. First, the procedure is time-consuming and can be tedious, which can make compliance difficult (Ahles, Ruckdeschel, & Blanchard, 1984). One way around this problem is to assign standardized scores for each word based on data from groups of previously tested individuals (for standardized scores for specific words, see Gracely et al., 1978a; Tursky, Jamner, & Friedman, 1982; Urban, Keefe, & France, 1984). However, most of the standardized scores have been developed using nonpatients in response to experimental pain, and there is evidence that chronic pain patients may rate the intensity of pain words differently from the way acute (i.e., postoperative) pain patients do (Wallenstein, Heidrich, Kaiko, & Houde, 1980). Even within diagnostic subgroups, the score given a word by one patient has been shown to vary from that given by other patients, indicating that standardized scores for VRS adjectives may be less reliable than originally hoped (Urban et al., 1984).

Moreover, VRS scores obtained through cross-modality procedures may correlate so highly with those obtained by using the ranking method that they contain essentially the same degree of useful information (Hall, 1981; Levine & De Simone, 1991). Similarly, VRS scores created by either of the two methods show the same patterns of associations to other pain measures, again suggesting that the information contained in the scores derived from the two methods are comparable (Jensen et al., 1989). Therefore, we recommend that the simpler ranking method may be used when relationships between pain intensity and other factors are examined. The more sophisticated cross-modality matching procedures should be used when ratio-like scaling is desired (i.e., when one wishes to compare pain ratings across time or between groups).

The strengths of VRSs include the ease with which they can be administered and scored, provided that scores are calculated using the ranking method or from data developed from previous cross-modality matching experiments. Because they are generally easy to comprehend, compliance rates for VRSs are as good or better than those for other measures of pain intensity under most conditions (Jensen et al., 1986; Jensen et al., 1989). Also, VRSs have consistently demonstrated their validity as indicants of pain intensity. They are related positively and significantly to other measures of pain intensity (Ahles et al., 1984; Downie et al., 1978; Jensen et al., 1986; Jensen et al., 1989; Kremer, Atkinson, & Ignelzi, 1981; Littman, Walker, & Schneider, 1985; Ohnhaus & Adler, 1975; Woodforde & Merskey, 1972). VRSs also consistently demonstrate sensitivity to

treatments that are known to impact pain intensity (Fox & Melzack, 1976; Ohnhaus & Adler, 1975; Rybstein-Blinchik, 1979).

Despite these strengths, we hesitate to recommend VRSs as the method of choice if only one index is employed. One of their weaknesses is that patients need to read over, or be familiar with, the entire list of pain adjectives before they can select the one that most closely describes their pain. For longer lists (e.g., 15 or more items), this can make the task time-consuming. Also, because VRSs require patients to select from a finite number of descriptors, they may be unable to find one that accurately describes their perceived pain intensity (Joyce, Zutshi, Hrubes, & Mason, 1975). Among illiterate patients, VRSs are less reliable than other pain intensity measures (Ferraz et al., 1990). Finally, a clinician or researcher using a VRS must select a scoring procedure; and, as already discussed, each scoring method has its drawbacks.

Visual Analogue Scales and Graphic Rating Scales

The VAS consists of a line, usually 10 cm long, whose ends are labeled as the extremes of pain (e.g., *no pain* to *pain as bad as it could be*). A VAS may have specific points along the line that are labeled with intensity-denoting adjectives or numbers. Such scales are called Graphic Rating Scales (GRSs). Patients are asked to indicate which point along the line best represents their pain intensity. The distance from the *no pain* end to the mark made by the patient is that patients' pain intensity score. Figure 9.1 illustrates a VAS and two Graphic Rating Scales.

Like VRSs, there is much evidence supporting the validity of VASs of pain intensity. Such scales demonstrate positive relations to other self-report measures of pain intensity (Downie et al., 1978; Elton, Burrows, & Stanley, 1979; Jensen et al., 1986; Jensen et al., 1989; Kremer et al., 1981; Littman et al., 1985; Ohnhaus & Adler, 1975; Seymour, 1982; Woodforde & Merskey, 1972) as well as to observed pain behavior (Teske, Daut, & Cleeland, 1983). They are sensitive to treatment effects (Joyce et al., 1975; Schachtel, Fillingim, Thoden, Lane, & Baybutt, 1988; Seymour, 1982; Turner, 1982) and are distinct from measures of other subjective components of pain (Ahles et al., 1984). The scores from VASs appear to have the qualities of ratio data,

VISUAL ANALOGUE SCALE

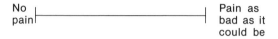

VERBAL GRAPHIC RATING SCALE

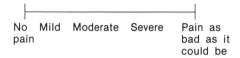

NUMERICAL GRAPHIC RATING SCALE

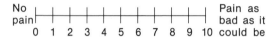

FIGURE 9.1. The Visual Analogue Scale and two Graphic Rating Scales of pain intensity.

and so may be treated as such statistically (Price & Harkins, 1987; Price, McGrath, Rafii, & Buckingham, 1983). VASs also have a high number of response categories. Because they are usually measured in millimeters, the scale can be considered as having 101 points. This high number of response categories makes the VAS, potentially, more sensitive to changes in pain intensity than measures with limited numbers of response categories.* Research indicates that VASs of pain intensity are usually (but not always) more sensitive to treatment change than VRSs (see Joyce et al., 1975; Littman et al., 1985; Machin, Lewith, & Wylson, 1988; Max, Schafer, Culnane, Dubner, & Gracely, 1987; Ohnhaus & Adler, 1975; Seymour, 1982; Sriwatanskul et al., 1983; Stambaugh & McAdams, 1984; Turner, 1982; Wallenstein et al., 1980).

Two problems limit the use of VASs. First, although they are easy to administer, scoring the VAS is more time-consuming and involves

*There is probably an upper limit to the number of response categories necessary to fully characterize different levels of perceived pain intensity. For example, 1,000,001 categories (i.e., "choose a number between 0 and 1,000,000 that best represents your pain intensity") is unlikely to be more sensitive than 101 response categories. Laboratory research indicates that people are unable to identify more than 21 noticeable differences between weak and intolerable experimental pain (Hardy, Wolff, & Goodell, 1952). Based on these findings, scale sensitivity is likely to be maximal if a measure has at least 22 levels.

more steps (and therefore more opportunity for error) than the other measures of pain intensity. Also, some patients have difficulty understanding and using VAS measures (Jensen et al., 1986; Kremer et al., 1981; Littman et al., 1985; Walsh, 1984; however, see Price & Harkins, Chapter 8). The second problem is of particular concern, especially when considered in light of the existence of other measures (e.g., the Numerical Rating Scale, NRS, and the Box Scale) that appear to be easier for people to understand and use. Thus, unless a particular clinician or researcher has a very strong rationale for using a VAS over other scales, we recommend against using the VAS as a *primary* (or sole) measure of pain intensity in adult clinical populations. If an investigator plans to use VAS measures, careful explanation and patient practice with the scale may decrease the failure rate (Scott & Huskisson, 1976), although high failure rates can still occur despite careful explanations (Walsh, 1984).

Numerical Rating Scales

An NRS involves asking patients to rate their pain from 0 to 10 (11-point scale) or 0 to 100 (101-point scale), with the understanding that the 0 represents one end of the pain intensity continuum (i.e., *no pain*) and the 10 or 100 represents the other extreme of pain intensity (e.g., *pain as bad as it could be*). The number that the patient states represents his or her pain intensity score.

The validity of NRSs has been well documented. They demonstrate positive and significant correlations with other measures of pain intensity (Downie et al., 1978; Jensen et al., 1986; 1989; Kremer et al., 1981; Seymour, 1982; Wallenstein et al., 1980). They have also demonstrated sensitivity to treatments that are expected to impact pain intensity (Chesney & Shelton, 1976; Kaplan, Metzger, & Jablecki, 1983; Keefe, Schapira, Williams, Brown, & Surwit, 1981; Seymour, 1982; Stenn, Mothersill, & Brooke, 1979). NRSs are likewise extremely easy to administer and score, so they can be used with a greater variety of patients (e.g., geriatric patients) than is possible with the VAS. The simplicity of the measure may be one of the reasons for the high rate of comparative compliance with the measurement task (Jensen et al., 1986). NRS scores may be treated as ratio data. Also, if an investigator chooses to use the 101-point NRS, then the instrument can be considered to have a large number of response categories (like the VAS), and thus may be more sensitive to small changes than those measures with fewer response categories.

The primary weakness of the NRSs is the lack of research comparing their sensitivity to that of other measures, particularly the VAS. One study found that VAS was more sensitive to the effects of cognitive-behavioral treatment than an 11-point NRS (Turner, 1982). Until further research comparing the treatment sensitivity of NRSs (especially NRS-101s) to VASs is performed, it is difficult to give an unqualified recommendation for the use of NRSs over VASs. Also, when using the NRS-101, instructions should clearly state that the upper limit of the scale is 100, as some patients may treat the measure as an NRS-11 (i.e., 0 to 10 scale) because the later scale is used so frequently by clinicians.

Other Intensity Measures

Behavior Rating Scale

The Behavior Rating Scale (BRS) was developed to provide patients with a behaviorally based means of assessing pain intensity (Budzynski, Stoyva, Adler, & Mullaney, 1973). Patients are asked to indicate the severity of their pain in terms of the degree to which it interferes with concentration and everyday tasks. Thus, it can be seen as a measure that combines patients' ratings of subjective pain and the effects of that pain. An adaptation of this scale is presented in Table 9.2.

Empirical evidence provides some (albeit limited) support for the validity of the BRS as a measure of pain intensity. It correlates in expected directions with other measures of pain intensity, and demonstrates weaker correlations with measures of other subjective components of pain (Andrasik, Blanchard, Ahles, Pallmeyer, & Barron, 1981; Jensen et al., 1986; Jensen et al, 1989). It has also demonstrated sensitivity to treatment effects (Budzynski et al., 1973). The BRS is very easy to administer and to score. Because it provides behavioral markers with which to judge pain, it may be more meaningful to some patients

TABLE 9.2. Behavior Rating Scale of Pain Intensity

No pain
Low level pain that enters awareness only when I pay attention to it
Pain exists, but can be ignored at times
Pain exists, but I can continue performing all the tasks I normally would
Very severe pain that makes concentration difficult, but allows me to perform tasks of an undemanding nature
Intense, incapacitating pain.

Note: Adapted from Budzynski, Stoyva, Adler, and Mullaney (1973), page 485. Copyright 1973 Elsevier Science Publishers. Adapted by permission.

(Collins & Thompson, 1979). However, because the BRS assesses pain intensity in terms of its effects, it may confound pain intensity with pain interference, and thus should be considered, at best, an indirect measure of subjective experience. This conclusion is supported empirically by the finding that the BRS demonstrates a weaker relationship to a composite measure of pain intensity when compared with other pain intensity measures (Jensen et al., 1986; Jensen et al., 1989).

Picture Scale

The Picture Scale (PS) employs eight line drawings that illustrate facial expressions of persons experiencing different levels of pain intensity (Frank, Moll, & Hort, 1982). Patients are asked to indicate which one of the eight expressions best represents his or her pain experience. The pictures are presented to the patient in a random order. Each one has a number (from 0 to 7) representing the rank order of pain illustrated, and the number associated with the picture chosen by the patient represents that individual's pain intensity score. Figure 9.2 illustrates the facial expression used in the PS.

The PS has yielded some, but as yet, limited, empirical evidence for its validity (Frank et al., 1982; Mann et al., 1984). The PS does not require the patient to be literate, and thus provides an option for individuals who have difficulty with written language. However, the scale has yet to gain wide use among researchers and clinicians. The expressions illustrated on the measure appear to be highly affect laden, so the scale may be closely associated with the affective component of pain. Additional re-

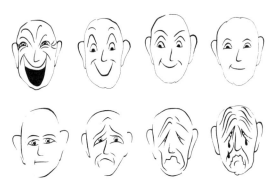

FIGURE 9.2. The facial expressions of the Picture Scale. From Frank, Moll, and Hurt, (1982), page 212. Copyright 1982 British Association of Rheumatology and Rehabilitation. Illustrations by J. M. H. Moll. Reprinted by permission.

search with the PS is needed before it can be recommended as a measure of pain intensity.

Box Scale

The Box Scale can be considered as a combination of an 11-point NRS and a VAS (see Figure 9.3). It consists of 11 numbers (0 through 10) presented in ascending order and surrounded by boxes (Downie et al., 1978). Patients are told that the 0 represents one extreme of pain intensity (*no pain*), and the 10 represents the other extreme (e.g., *pain as bad as it could be*). Patients are asked to place an "X" through the number representing his or her pain level. Perhaps because of the inclusion of the numbers, older patients do not appear to have as much difficulty with this measure as they do with the traditional VAS (Jensen et al., 1986).

Like the PS, the Box Scale has not yet been widely adopted among clinicians and researchers. However, preliminary empirical evidence supports the validity of the measure. It demonstrates a strong relationship to a composite measure of pain intensity, and an appropriately weak relationship to pain affect (Jensen et al., 1986; Jensen et al., 1989). The measure is

If a zero means "no pain" and a ten means "pain as bad as it could be," on this scale of 0 to 10, what is your level of pain? Put an "X" through that number.

0	1	2	3	4	5	6	7	8	9	10

FIGURE 9.3. The Box Scale of pain intensity.

extremely easy to administer and to score, and demonstrates high compliance rates. Unfortunately, the measure's relative sensitivity to treatment effects has not yet been examined empirically.

Descriptor Differential Scale

The Descriptor Differential Scale (DDS) is a relatively new measure of pain intensity (Gracely & Kwilosz, 1988). It consists of a list of adjectives describing different levels of pain intensity. Patients are asked to rate the intensity of their pain as being more or less than each word on the list (see Table 9.3). If their experienced pain is greater than that described by the word, they place a check mark to the right of the word in proportion to how much greater their pain is. If their pain is less than that described by the word, they place a check mark to the left of the word. If the word exactly describes their pain level, they place a check mark directly below the descriptor. There are 10 points along which patients can rate their pain intensity to the right and left of each word, so pain is rated along a 21-point scale for each word. Pain intensity is defined as the mean of *each* rating, and so can range from 0 to 20.

The scale has many strengths. Because it is a multiple-item measure, it is possible to assess the internal consistency of the scale, and its internal consistency appears to be very high (Gracely & Kwilosz, 1988). Test–retest stability has also been shown to be very high (Gracely & Kwilosz, 1988). Another advantage of the scale is that the consistency with which individuals use the scale (compared to themselves on different occasions or compared to other individuals) can be assessed. Patients who are using the measure in an inconsistent fashion can be eliminated from study trials, therefore increasing the potential power of controlled treatment outcome studies.

The major weaknesses of the scale are related to its youth. Much about the scale's properties has not yet been explored. Thus, the utility of the measure with different patient populations (e.g., older patients) is not known.* Relative sensitivity of the measure to treatment (com-

---

*Preliminary research suggests that the DDS may be difficult for naive chronic pain patients to complete, but that patients can learn to use the measure with minimal training (Good, Slater, & Doctor, 1991).

TABLE 9.3. Descriptor Differential Scale of Pain Intensity[a]

Instructions: Each word represents an amount of sensation. Rate your sensation in relation to each word with a check mark.

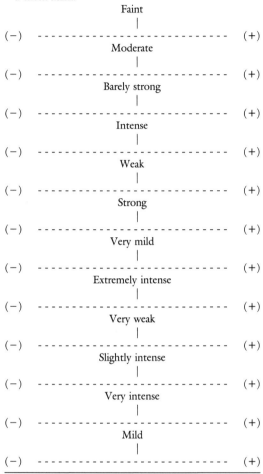

Faint

(−) ------------------------------ (+)

Moderate

(−) ------------------------------ (+)

Barely strong

(−) ------------------------------ (+)

Intense

(−) ------------------------------ (+)

Weak

(−) ------------------------------ (+)

Strong

(−) ------------------------------ (+)

Very mild

(−) ------------------------------ (+)

Extremely intense

(−) ------------------------------ (+)

Very weak

(−) ------------------------------ (+)

Slightly intense

(−) ------------------------------ (+)

Very intense

(−) ------------------------------ (+)

Mild

(−) ------------------------------ (+)

[a]From Gracely & Kwilosz (1988), page 280. Copyright by Elsevier Science Publishers. Reprinted by permission.

pared to other pain intensity measures) has likewise not yet been examined. Finally, the scale may require more time to complete than other pain intensity measures. Perhaps the scale's greatest utility will be found in the version created to assess pain affect, where multiple-item measures may prove to be most useful (see below).

Summary and Recommendations Regarding Pain Intensity Measures

A summary of the strengths and weaknesses of the seven measures of pain intensity described

is presented in Table 9.4. Because pain intensity is a relatively easy dimension of pain experience for patients to report, most self-report measures of pain intensity are strongly related to one another, and so can probably be used interchangeably in many situations. However, each procedure has its particular strengths and weaknesses (as outlined in Table 9.4), and these should be considered when choosing among measures.

ASSESSING PAIN AFFECT

There is evidence for an affective component of pain that is conceptually and empirically distinct from pain intensity (Gracely et al., 1978a, 1978b; Jensen et al., 1989; Jensen, Karoly, & Harris, 1991; Melzack & Wall, 1983; Tursky, 1976). Where pain intensity may be defined as how much a person hurts, pain affect may be defined as the emotional arousal and disruption engendered by the pain experience. Because people's feelings about events can be mixed, it is likely that the domain of pain affect consists of multiple dimensions, which may be closely related to one another (Morley, 1989). However, it is still unclear whether pain affect is best assessed as a single domain, multiple dimensions, or may be reliably assessed as both a global construct *and* a set of related dimensions. The complex nature of pain affect suggests that single-item measures may be less comprehensive and less reliable than multiple-item measures. However, depending on the specific items included in a scale, even multiple-item measures may assess only a limited number of the dimensions associated with pain affect.

By far the most widely used measure of pain affect is the Affective subscale of the McGill Pain Questionnaire (MPQ) (Melzack, 1975a, 1975b). This subscale, along with the other subscales of the MPQ, is described in detail in Chapter 10 of this volume, and will not be discussed in detail here. Four additional methods of assessing pain affect are VRSs, VASs, the DDS, and the Pain Discomfort Scale.

Verbal Rating Scales

Two VRSs have been developed to assess the suffering component of pain (Tursky et al., 1982; Gracely et al., 1978a), and one of these

TABLE 9.4. The Strengths and Weaknesses of Seven Measures of Pain Intensity

Scale	Strengths	Weaknesses
Verbal Rating Scale	Easy to administer Easy to score Good evidence for construct validity Compliance with measurement task is high May approximate ratio scaling if cross modality matching methods (or scores developed from cross modality matching methods) are used	Can be difficult for persons with limited vocabulary Relatively few response categories compared to the VAS or NRS-101[a] If scored using the ranking method, the scores represent ordinal data and should be treated as such statistically People forced to choose one word, even if no word on the scale adequately describes their pain intensity
Visual Analogue Scale	Easy to administer Many ("infinite") response categories Scores can be treated as ratio data Good evidence for construct validity	Extra step in scoring the measure can take more time and adds an additional source of error Some people, especially older people, have difficulty using VASs
Numerical Rating Scale	Easy to administer Many response categories if NRS-101 chosen Easy to score Compliance with measurement task is high Good evidence for construct validity Scores can be treated as ratio data	No evidence regarding relative treatment sensitivity of the NRS-101 compared to other measures Limited number of response categories if the NRS-11 is used NRS-11 may be less sensitive to treatment effects than VASs
Behavior Rating Scale	Easy to administer Easy to score Limited evidence for construct validity	No evidence regarding relative compliance rates Limited number of response categories No evidence regarding relative treatment sensitivity Scores need to be treated as ordinal data statistically May confound pain intensity with pain interference
Picture Scale	Easy to administer Easy to score Limited number of response categories	No evidence regarding relative compliance rates Limited evidence for construct validity No evidence regarding the relative treatment sensitivity compared to other measures Scores need to be treated as ordinal data statistically
Box Scale	Easy to administer Easy to score Good evidence for construct validity Compliance rate with the measure is high Scores can be treated as ratio data	No evidence regarding relative treatment sensitivity compared to other measures Limited response categories
Descriptor Differential Scale	Because the scale has several items, it may be more reliable Allows for estimates of the consistency with which people complete the measure	Some patients may have difficulty comprehending the measure Limited research on the validity and sensitivity of the measure Completion of the scale takes more time than other measures

[a]There is no evidence that VRSs with 15 or more items are less sensitive to treatment effects than VASs or NRSs, but evidence does suggest that VRSs with 5 or fewer categories may be less sensitive in some situations.

is illustrated in Table 9.5. Similar to VRSs of pain intensity, affect VRSs consist of adjectives describing increasing amounts of discomfort and/or suffering. Respondents select a single word from the list that best describes the degree of unpleasantness of their pain. Like VRS-intensity measures, VRS-affect scales may be scored in three ways: (1) the ranking method, (2) the cross-modality matching method, or (3) the standardized score method (using scores developed from cross-modality matching procedures with a standardization group). The advantages and disadvantages of these methods were already discussed with respect to VRSs of pain intensity, and therefore we make the same recommendations here. That is, we recommend the simpler ranking method if the investigator wishes to examine the relation between pain intensity and other constructs, and the use of standardized scores developed from cross-modality matching procedures if the investigator requires a measure more likely to have ratio properties.

Evidence for the validity of VRSs of pain affect is mixed. On the positive side, VRSs of pain affect appear to be more sensitive than measures of pain intensity to treatments designed to impact the emotional component of pain (Gracely, Dubner, & McGrath, 1979; Gracely et al., 1978a; 1978b; Heft, Gracely, & Dubner, 1984). On the other hand, recent factor analytic and correlational investigations among chronic pain patients, postoperative pain patients, and laboratory volunteers indicate that VRSs designed to measure pain affect are not always distinct from measures of pain intensity (Jensen et al., 1989; Jensen & Karoly, 1987; Levine & De Simone, 1991). This pattern may have something to do with the relatively low level of reliability of single-item

measures. Another drawback to VRS measures of pain affect is that they allow respondents to choose only one descriptor, even when none of the available descriptors (or more than one of the available descriptors) captures their affective response to pain.

Visual Analogue Scale

VASs for pain affect are very similar to VASs for pain intensity. Only the end-point descriptors are different. Examples of the extremes used in VAS-affect scales are "not bad at all" and "the most unpleasant feeling possible for me" (Price, Harkins, & Baker, 1987). A great deal of evidence supports the validity of VAS-affect measures. They are more sensitive than VAS intensity measures to treatments that should influence pain affect more than pain intensity (Price, Barrell, & Gracely, 1980; Price et al., 1987). They appear to have the qualities of ratio scales (Price & Harkins, 1987; Price et al., 1983). Also, they are sensitive to treatment effects (Price & Barber, 1987; Price, Harkins, Rafii, & Price, 1986; Price, Von der Gruen, Miller, Rafii, & Price, 1985).

The weaknesses of VAS-affect measures are likely to be similar to those of VAS-intensity measures. Most research using these measures have used young or middle-aged subjects. The utility of such measures in geriatric (i.e., over 80 years old) populations has not yet been examined, and it may be that older people have difficulty with VAS-affect scales as they do with VAS-intensity scales (see Harkins & Price, Chapter 18). Because VAS-affect measures are single-item scales, they may be less reliable and less valid for examining the full spectrum of affective responses relative to multiple-item measures, described below. Also, there is limited research comparing VAS-affect measures to other measures of pain affect. A single experiment suggests that VAS-affect measures may be less able to discriminate between pain intensity and pain affect measures than VRS-affect measures (Duncan, Bushnell, & Lavigne, 1989).

Descriptor Differential Scale

The DDS for pain affect is similar to the DDS for pain intensity, but uses different descriptors (see Table 9.6). Although the scale is new, and has yet to demonstrate validity and reliability across patient populations, it shares the advan-

TABLE 9.5. Verbal Rating Scales of Pain Affect

15-Point Scale[a]	
Bearable	Frightful
Distracting	Dreadful
Unpleasant	Horrible
Uncomfortable	Agonizing
Distressing	Unbearable
Oppressive	Intolerable
Miserable	Excruciating
Awful	

[a]From Gracely, McGrath, and Dubner (1978a), page 11. Copyright 1978 by Elsevier Science Publishers. Reprinted by permission.

TABLE 9.6. Descriptor Differential Scale of Pain Affect[a]

Instructions: Each word represents an amount of sensation. Rate your sensation in relation to each word with a check mark.

Slightly unpleasant
|
(−) - (+)

Slightly annoying
|
(−) - (+)

Unpleasant
|
(−) - (+)

Annoying
|
(−) - (+)

Slightly Distressing
|
(−) - (+)

Very Unpleasant
|
(−) - (+)

Distressing
|
(−) - (+)

Very annoying
|
(−) - (+)

Slightly intolerable
|
(−) - (+)

Very distressing
|
(−) - (+)

Intolerable
|
(−) - (+)

Very intolerable
|
(−) - (+)

[a]From Gracely and Kwilosz (1988), page 282. Copyright 1988 by Elsevier Science Publishers. Reprinted by permission.

tages of the DDS for pain intensity. It is a multiple-item measure, and so may provide more reliable and valid assessments of pain affect than single-item scales. It demonstrates excellent test–retest stability and internal consistency (Gracely & Kwilosz, 1988). Also, investigators may compare an individual's response at one time to his or her response at another time (or to group responses), in order to assess how consistently a particular person is performing on the assessment task.

Pain Discomfort Scale

The PDS is designed to assess negative affect that patients attribute to their pain and pain problem (see Table 9.7). It consists of ten items affirming (or denying) different affective responses to pain (Jensen et al., 1991). Patients are asked to indicate their level of agreement (on 5-point Likert scales) to each affective response. Scale development data indicate a high degree of internal consistency and test–retest stability for the measure (Jensen et al., 1991). Construct validity was also supported, in that the PDS correlated significantly and positively with other measures of affective responding, and nonsignificantly with measures of pain intensity.

The results of an exploratory factor analysis of the PDS, performed on the same subjects used in the Jensen et al. (1991) article, yielded four factors. The first was made up of the items referring to the extent to which pain is unbearable, torturing, and tolerable (the last reverse scored), and might be labeled a "pain is intolerable" factor. The second consisted of the items referring to the denial of distress (items 7 and 8 on Table 9.7), and may be labeled a "distress denial" factor. The items loading on

TABLE 9.7. The Pain Discomfort Scale

Instructions: Please indicate by circling the appropriate number whether each of the statements below is more true or false for you. Please answer every question and circle only one number per question. Answer by circling the appropriate number (0 through 4) according to the following scale:

    0 = This is very untrue for me.
    1 = This is somewhat untrue for me.
    2 = This is neither true nor untrue for me (or it does not apply to me).
    3 = This is somewhat true for me.
    4 = This is very true for me.

1. I am scared about the pain I feel.	0 1 2 3 4
2. The pain I experience is unbearable.	0 1 2 3 4
3. The pain I feel is torturing me.	0 1 2 3 4
4. My pain does not stop me from enjoying life.[a]	0 1 2 3 4
5. I have learned to tolerate the pain I feel.[a]	0 1 2 3 4
6. I feel helpless about my pain.	0 1 2 3 4
7. My pain is a minor annoyance to me.[a]	0 1 2 3 4
8. When I feel pain I am hurting, but I am not distressed.[a]	0 1 2 3 4
9. I never let the pain in my body affect my outlook on life.[a]	0 1 2 3 4
10. When I am in pain, I become almost a different person.	0 1 2 3 4

Note: From Jensen, Karoly, and Harris (1991), page 151. Copyright 1990 M. P. Jensen & P. Karoly. Reprinted by permission.

[a]These items are reverse scored.

the third factor were those relating to the extent to which pain does not affect one's outlook, does not stop one from enjoying life, and makes one a different person (the last reverse scored). This could be labeled a "denial of impact" factor. The final factor was made up of the items referring to feeling helpless and scared because of pain, and may be labeled an "emotional distress" factor. Although these specific factors may not emerge in future factor analyses of the PDS, the fact that several factors emerged in an exploratory analysis provides additional evidence that the affective component of pain is multidimensional.

The PDS has several drawbacks in its present form. First, because the measure is new, its internal structure has not yet been cross validated. Furthermore, unlike other more established measures (VRS-affect, VAS-affect, and MPQ-affect) there is not yet a large database supporting its validity. Finally, the PDS was developed (and validated) for use with chronic pain populations only. Many of the items are not appropriate for individuals suffering from acute pain. Additional research and clinical experience with the measure will be necessary before its strengths and limitations are more fully understood.

Summary and Recommendations for Assessing Pain Affect

Pain affect is more complex than pain intensity, and there are fewer measures available to assess this construct. Also, there are several unresolved questions regarding the dimension of pain affect: Is pain affect best thought of as a single dimension or as several distinct dimensions? Even if pain affect is best conceptualized as reflecting several related dimensions, is it still reasonable to use a global measure of the distress associated with pain, or is there a need for separate indices that assess distinct dimensions? Are single-item measures of pain affect less reliable than multiple-item measures, as would be suggested given the complexity of pain affect? These and other basic questions will need to be addressed in future research.

In the meantime, investigators have several options for the assessment of pain affect. Among the single-item measures are VRS-affect and VAS-affect scales. Both of these procedures have demonstrated discriminant validity (from pain intensity) in some treatment outcome studies. However, both also appear closely related to single-item measures of pain intensity

in other situations. A multiple-item scale, the DDS of pain affect, shows great promise. Unfortunately, because the scale is relatively new, there is little empirical support for the measure at this time. The PDS is another promising measure of pain affect in chronic pain patients. However, it is also too new to have a large database supporting its reliability and validity. Investigators may choose to use *both* a single-item measure as well as a multiple-item measure (such as the DDS, the PDS, or the Affective subscale of the MPQ) to determine which measure best discriminates pain affect from pain intensity in their setting.

ASSESSING PAIN LOCATION

A third dimension of subjective experience is the location of pain. The instrument most commonly used to assess pain location is the pain drawing. This procedure usually involves a line drawing of the front and back of the human body. Sometimes, line drawings of the face, head, and neck are also presented for patients experiencing localized pain. Patients are asked to indicate the location of their pain on the surface of the drawings. It is possible to vary the instructions regarding how patients are to indicate their pain to suit the purposes of the investigator. Patients may be asked to distinguish between various sensations of their pain experience and to indicate the location of these sensations by means of different symbols. For example, the letters "E" and "I" have been used for external (surface) and internal (deep somatic) pain, respectively (Melzack, 1975b). Similarly, "–" has been used for numbness, "oo" for pins and needles, "xx" for burning, and "//" for stabbing pain (Ransford, Cairns, & Mooney, 1976). The most common procedure is to ask patients to simply shade in the areas of their body that are "in pain."

Toomey, Gover, and Jones (1983) divided line drawings of the human body into 32 regions, and gave their patients a score equal to the number of regions that were shaded (see Figure 9.4 for an example of a pain drawing scoring template). This score was found to be related to many important pain-related constructs such as dimensions of the MPQ (Number of Words Chosen, MPQ-Sensory and MPQ-Total subscale scores); self-report of time spent reclining; interference of pain with basic activities such as walking, working, socializing, and recreation; number of health-care profes-

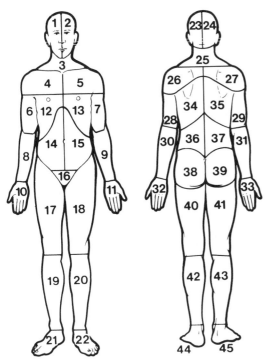

FIGURE 9.4. Scoring template for a pain drawing. From Margolis, Tait, and Krause, (1986), page 60. Copyright 1986 Elsevier Science Publishers, B. V. Reprinted by permission.

sionals consulted; and medication use. Interestingly, the number of pain sites shaded was unrelated to pain intensity, duration of the pain problem, and pain affect (see also Hildebrandt, Franz, Choroba-Mehnen, & Temme, 1988). These findings provide further evidence that the total body area in pain is a distinct dimension and an important one to consider apart from pain intensity or affect. Evidence for the predictive validity of pain site was found by Toomey, Gover, and Jones (1984), who demonstrated that patients with low back pain (or low back pain plus head and neck pain) were more likely than other patients to report interference of pain with life's activities. The reliability of pain-drawing data has also been established. Test–retest stability is high and does not appear to decrease even after three months (Margolis, Chibnall, & Tait, 1988). Scoring for "inappropriate" drawings (see below) as well as for total body area in pain appears to be extremely reliable from person to person (Udén, Åström, & Bergenudd, 1988; Margolis, Tait, & Krause, 1986).

Some clinicians have suggested that information regarding psychopathology may be contained in the manner by which patients complete pain drawings. To examine this hypothesis, Ransford et al. (1976) developed a system for rating the normality/abnormality of pain drawings. These investigators found patients with abnormal drawings to have higher Hysteria (Hs) and Hypochondriasis (Hy) scale scores on the Minnesota Multiphasic Personality Inventory (MMPI), suggesting that exaggerated pain drawing may reflect a tendency toward somatic preoccupation. Although the relationship between abnormal pain drawings and various measures of psychopathology has continued to be positive in subsequent research, this relationship has been shown to be quite weak (Ginzburg, Merskey, & Lau, 1988; Schwartz & DeGood, 1984; Tait, Chibnall, & Margolis, 1990; Von Baeyer, Bergstrom, Brodwin, & Brodwin, 1983). Therefore, we do not recommend that pain drawings be relied upon as a proxy measure of psychopathology. Although drawings that appear overly detailed or exaggerated may cause a clinician to look more carefully for hypochondriacal tendencies, it is possible that a detailed drawing may reflect a person's wish to be extremely thorough in providing data. Caution should be extended in any attempt to overinterpret pain-drawing data. Pain drawings should be relied on to assess what they measure well—the patient's report of the sensory distribution of pain.

SUMMARY AND CONCLUSION

The assessment of pain intensity, pain affect, and pain location continues to be important to clinicians and researchers alike. Self-report is the most direct way to access these dimensions. Although more research is needed to answer important questions regarding the nature and dimensionality of pain experience, most of the measures that are now available have demonstrated adequate to excellent reliability and validity. Clinicians and researchers should select measures with full knowledge of their psychometric strengths and weaknesses, as well as in keeping with their explicit conceptual model(s) of pain. In this chapter, we have attempted to provide the investigator with some of the information necessary to make informed decisions regarding the use of self-report measures of pain in adults.

REFERENCES

Ahles, T. A., Ruckdeschel, J. C., & Blanchard, E. B. (1984). Cancer-related pain: II. Assessment with visual analogue scales. *Journal of Psychosomatic Research*, 28, 121–124.

Andrasik, F., Blanchard, E. B., Ahles, T., Pallmeyer, T., & Barron, K. D. (1981). Assessing the reactive as well as the sensory component of headache pain. *Headache*, 21, 218–221.

Budzynski, T. H., Stoyva, J. M., Adler, C. S., & Mullaney, D. J. (1973). EMG biofeedback and tension headache: A controlled outcome study. *Psychosomatic Medicine*, 35, 484–496.

Chesney, M. A., & Shelton, J. L. (1976). A comparison of muscle relaxation and electromyogram biofeedback treatments for muscle contraction headache. *Journal of Behavior Therapy and Experimental Psychiatry*, 7, 221–225.

Cicchetti, D. V., Showalter, D., & Tyrer, P. J. (1985). The effect of number of rating scale categories on levels of interrater reliability: A Monte Carlo investigation. *Applied Psychological Measurement*, 9, 31–36.

Cleeland, C. S. (1986). How to treat a "construct." *Journal of Pain and Symptom Management*, 1, 161–162.

Cleeland, C. S. (1989). Measurement of pain by subjective report. In C. R. Chapman & J. D. Loeser (Eds.), *Advances in pain research and therapy* (Vol. 12, pp. 391–403). New York: Raven Press.

Collins, F. L., & Thompson, J. K. (1979). Reliability and standardization in the assessment of self-reported headache pain. *Journal of Behavioral Assessment*, 1, 73–86.

Craig, K. D., & Weiss, S. M. (1971). Vicarious influences on pain-threshold determinations. *Journal of Personality and Social Psychology*, 19, 53–59.

Downie, W. W., Leatham, P. A., Rhind, V. M., Wright, V., Branco, J. A., & Anderson, J. A. (1978). Studies with pain rating scales. *Annals of the Rheumatic Diseases*, 37, 378–381.

Duncan, G. H., Bushnell, M. C., & Lavigne, G. J. (1989). Comparison of Verbal and Visual Analogue Scales for measuring the intensity and unpleasantness of experimental pain. *Pain*, 37, 295–303.

Dworkin, S. F., & Chen, A. C. N. (1982). Pain in clinical and laboratory contexts. *Journal of Dental Research*, 6, 772–774.

Elton, D., Burrows, G. D., & Stanley, G. V. (1979). Clinical measurement of pain. *Medical Journal of Australia*, 1, 109–111.

Ferraz, M. B., Quaresma, M. R., Aquino, L. R. L., Atra, E., Tugwell, P., & Goldsmith, C. H. (1990). Reliability of pain scales in the assessment of literate and illiterate patients with rheumatoid arthritis. *Journal of Rheumatology*, 17, 1022–1024.

Flor, H., Birbaumer, N., & Turk, D. C. (1990). The psychobiology of chronic pain. *Advances in Behaviour Research and Therapy*, 12, 47–84.

Folkard, S., Glynn, C. J., & Lloyd, J. W. (1976). Diurnal variation and individual differences in the perception of intractable pain. *Journal of Psychosomatic Research*, 20, 289–301.

Fordyce, W. E. (1976). *Behavioral methods for chronic pain and illness*. St. Louis: Mosby.

Fox, E. J., & Melzack, R. (1976). Trancutaneous electrical stimulation and acupuncture: Comparison of treatment for low-back pain, *Pain*, 2, 141–148.

Frank, A. J. M., Moll, J. M. H., & Hort, J. F. (1982). A comparison of three ways of measuring pain. *Rheumatology and Rehabilitation*, 21, 211–217.

Good, A. B., Slater, M. A., & Doctor, J. (1991, November). *Validation of the Descriptor Differential Scale for Pain Measurement*. Poster presented at the 10th Annual Meeting of the American Pain Society, New Orleans, LA.

Ginzburg, B. M., Merskey, H., & Lau, C. L. (1988). The relationship between pain drawings and the psychological state. *Pain*, 35, 141–146.

Gracely, R. H., Dubner, R., & McGrath, P. A. (1979). Narcotic analgesia: Fentanyl reduces the intensity but not the unpleasantness of painful tooth pulp sensations. *Science*, 203, 1261–1263.

Gracely, R. H., McGrath, P., & Dubner, R. (1978a). Ratio scales of sensory and affective verbal pain descriptors. *Pain*, 5, 5–18.

Gracely, R. H., McGrath, P., & Dubner, R. (1978b). Validity and sensitivity of ratio scales of sensory and affective verbal pain descriptors: Manipulation of affect by diazepam. *Pain*, 5, 19–29.

Gracely, R. H., & Kwilosz, D. M. (1988). The Descriptor Differential Scale: Applying psychophysical principles to clinical pain assessment. *Pain*, 35, 279–288.

Hall, W. (1981). On "ratio scales of sensory and affective verbal pain descriptors." *Pain*, 4, 101–107.

Hardy, J. D., Wolff, H. G., & Goodell, H. (1952). *Pain sensations and reactions*. Baltimore: Williams & Wilkins.

Heft, M. W., Gracely, R. H., & Dubner, R. (1984). Nitrous oxide analgesia: A psychophysical evaluation using verbal descriptor scaling. *Journal of Dental Research*, 63, 129–132.

Hildebrandt, J., Franz, C. E., Choroba-Mehnen, B., & Temme, M. (1988). The use of pain drawings in screening for psychological involvement in complaints of low-back pain. *Spine*, 13, 681–685.

Jamison, R. N., & Brown, G. K. (1991). Validation of hourly pain intensity profiles with chronic pain patients. *Pain*, 45, 123–128.

Jensen, M. P., & Karoly, P. (1987). *Assessing the subjective experience of pain: What do the scale scores of the McGill Pain Questionnaire measure?* Poster presented at the eighth annual scientific sessions of the Society of Behavioral Medicine, Washington, DC

Jensen, M. P., Karoly, P., & Braver, S. (1986). The measurement of clinical pain intensity: A comparison of six methods. *Pain*, 27, 117–126.

Jensen, M. P., Karoly, P., & Harris, P. (1991). Assessing the affective component of chronic pain: Development of the Pain Discomfort Scale. *Journal of Psychosomatic Research*, 35, 149–154.

Jensen, M. P., Karoly, P., O'Riordan, E. F., Bland, F., Jr., & Burns, R. S. (1989). The subjective experience of acute pain: An assessment of the utility of 10 indices. *Clinical Journal of Pain*, 5, 153–159.

Joyce, C. R. B., Zutshi, D. W., Hrubes, V., & Mason, R. M. (1975). Comparison of fixed interval and Visual Analogue Scales for rating chronic pain. *European Journal of Clinical Pharmacology*, 8, 415–420.

Kaplan, R. M., Metzger, G., & Jablecki, C. (1983). Brief cognitive and relaxation training increases tolerance for a painful clinical electromyographic examination. *Psychosomatic Medicine*, 45, 155–162.

Karoly, P. (1985). The assessment of pain: Concepts and issues. In P. Karoly (Ed.), *Measurement strategies in health psychology* (pp. 1–43). New York: Wiley.

Karoly, P. (1991). Assessment of pediatric pain. In J. P. Bush & S. W. Harkins (Eds.), *Children in pain: Clinical and research issues from a developmental perspective* (pp. 59–82). New York: Springer-Verlag.

Karoly, P., & Jensen M. P. (1987). *Multimethod assessment of chronic pain*. New York: Pergamon.

Keefe, F. J., Schapira, B., Williams, R. B., Brown, C., & Surwit, R. S. (1981). EMG-assisted relaxation training in the management of chronic low back pain. *American Journal of Clinical Biofeedback*, 4, 93–103.

Kremer, E., Atkinson, J. H., & Ignelzi, R. J. (1981). Measurement of pain: Patient preference does not confound pain measurement. *Pain*, 10, 241–248.

Levine, F. M., & De Simone, L. L. (1991). The effects of experimenter gender on pain report in male and female subjects. *Pain*, 44, 69–72.

Littman, G. S., Walker, B. R., & Schneider, B. E. (1985). Reassessment of verbal and visual analog ratings in analgesic studies. *Clinical Pharmacology and Therapeutics*, 38, 16–23.

Machin, D., Lewith, G. T., & Wylson, S. (1988). Pain measurement in randomized clinical trials. *Clinical Journal of Pain*, 4, 161–168.

Mann, S. G., Kimber, G., Diggins, J. B., Jenkins, R., Vandenburg, M. J., & Currie, W. J. C. (1984). Methods of assessing pain in clinical trials. *Clinical Science*, 66, 78.

Margolis, R. B., Chibnall, J. T., & Tait, R. C. (1988). Test–retest reliability of the pain drawing instrument. *Pain*, 33, 49–51.

Margolis, R. B., Tait, R. C., & Krause, S. J. (1986). A rating system for use with patient pain drawings. *Pain*, 24, 57–65.

Max, M. B. (1991). Neuropathic pain syndromes. In M. Max, R. Portenoy, & E. Laska (Eds.), *Advances in pain research and therapy* (Vol. 18, pp. 193–219). New York: Springer.

Max, M. B., Schafer, S. C., Culnane, M., Dubner, R., & Gracely, R. H. (1987). Association of pain relief with drug side effects in postherpetic neuralgia: A single-dose study of clonidine, codeine, ibuprofen, and placebo. *Clinical Pharmacology and Therapeutics*, 43, 363–371.

Melzack, R. (1975a). The McGill Pain Questionnaire. In R. Melzack (Ed.), *Pain measurement and assessment* (pp. 41–47). New York: Raven Press.

Melzack, R. (1975b). The McGill Pain Questionnaire: Major properties and scoring methods. *Pain*, 1, 277–299.

Melzack, R., & Wall, P. D. (1983). *The challenge of pain*. New York: Basic Books.

Morley, S. (1989). The dimensionality of verbal descriptors in Tursky's pain perception profile. *Pain*, 37, 41–49.

Ohnhaus, E. E., & Adler, R. (1975). Methodological problems in the measurement of pain: A comparison between the Verbal Rating Scale and the Visual Analogue Scale. *Pain*, 1, 379–384.

Price, D. D., & Barber, J. (1987). An analysis of factors that contribute to the efficacy of hypnotic analgesia. *Journal of Abnormal Psychology*, 96, 46–51.

Price, D. D., Barrell, J. J., & Gracely, R. H. (1980). A psychophysical analysis of experiential factors that selectively influence the affective dimension of pain. *Pain*, 8, 137–149.

Price, D. D., & Harkins, S. W. (1987). Combined use of experimental pain and Visual Analogue Scales in providing standardized measurement of clinical pain. *Clinical Journal of Pain*, 3, 1–8.

Price, D. D., Harkins, S. W., & Baker, C. (1987). Sensory-affective relationships among different types of clinical and experimental pain. *Pain*, 28, 297–307.

Price, D. D., Harkins, S. W., Rafii, A., & Price, C. (1986). A simultaneous comparison of fentanyl's analgesic effects on experimental and clinical pain. *Pain*, 24, 197–203.

Price, D. D., McGrath, P. A., Rafii, A., & Buckingham, B. (1983). The validation of Visual Analogue Scales as ratio scale measures for chronic and experimental pain. *Pain*, 17, 45–56.

Price, D. D., Von der Gruen, A., Miller, J., Rafii, A., & Price, C. (1985). A psychophysical analysis of morphine analgesia. *Pain*, 22, 261–269.

Ransford, A. O., Cairns, D., & Mooney, V. (1976). The pain drawing as an aid to the psychologic evaluation of patients with low-back pain. *Spine*, 1, 127–134.

Rasmussen, J. L. (1989). Analysis of Likert-Scale data: A reinterpretation of Gregoire and Driver. *Psychological Bulletin*, 105, 167–170.

Rudy, T. E. (1989). Innovations in pain psychometrics. In C. R. Chapman & J. D. Loeser (Eds.), *Advances in pain research and therapy* (Vol. 12, pp. 51–61). New York: Raven Press.

Rybstein-Blinchik, E. (1979). Effects of different cognitive strategies on chronic pain experience. *Journal of Behavioral Medicine*, 2, 93–101.

Schachtel, B. P., Fillingim, J. M., Thoden, W. R., Lane, A. C., & Baybutt, R. I. (1988). Sore throat pain in the evaluation of mild analgesics. *Clinical Pharmacology and Therapeutics*, 44, 704–711.

Schwartz, D. P., & DeGood, D. E. (1984). Global appropriateness of pain drawings: Blind ratings predict patterns of psychological distress and litigation status. *Pain*, 19, 383–388.

Scott, J., & Huskisson, E. C. (1976). Graphic representation of pain. *Pain*, 2, 175–184.

Seymour, R. A. (1982). The use of pain scales in assessing the efficacy of analgesics in post-operative dental pain. *European Journal of Clinical Pharmacology*, 23, 441–444.

Sriwatanskul, K., Kelvie, W., Lasagne, L., Calimlim, J. F., Weis, O. F., & Mehta, G. (1983). Studies with different types of visual analog scales for measurement of pain. *Clinical Pharmacology and Therapeutics*, 34, 235–239.

Stambaugh, J. E., Jr., & McAdams, J. (1984). Comparison of verbal and visual analogue scriptors of analgesic efficacy of parenteral dezocine (Dalgan) to butorphanol and placebo in patients with chronic cancer pain. *Journal of Clinical Pharmacology*, 24, 398.

Stenn, P. G., Mothersill, K. J., & Brooke, R. I. (1979). Biofeedback and a cognitive behavioral approach to treatment of myofascial pain dysfunction syndrome. *Behavior Therapy*, 10, 29–36.

Tait, R. C., Chibnall, J. T., & Margolis, R. B. (1990). Pain extent: Relations with psychological state, pain severity, pain history, and disability. *Pain*, 41, 295–301.

Teske, K., Daut, R. L., & Cleeland, C. S. (1983). Relationships between nurses' observations and patients' self-reports of pain. *Pain*, 16, 289–296.

Toomey, T. C., Gover, V. F., & Jones, B. N. (1983). Spatial distribution of pain: A descriptive characteristic of chronic pain. *Pain*, 17, 289–300.

Toomey, T. C., Gover, V. F., & Jones, B. N. (1984). Site of pain: Relationship to measures of pain description, behavior and personality. *Pain*, 19, 389–397.

Turk, D. C. (1989). Assessment of pain: The elusiveness of latent constructs. In C. R. Chapman & J. D. Loeser (Eds.), *Advances in pain research and therapy* (Vol. 12, pp. 267–279). New York: Raven Press.

Turner, J. A. (1982). Comparison of group progressive-relaxation training and cognitive-behavioral group therapy for chronic low back pain. *Journal of Consulting and Clinical Psychology, 50,* 757–765.

Tursky, B. (1976). The development of a pain perception profile: A psychophysical approach. In M. Weisenberg & B. Tursky (Eds.), *Pain: New perspectives in therapy and research* (pp. 171–194). New York: Plenum Press.

Tursky, B., Jamner, L. D., & Friedman, R. (1982). The pain perception profile: A psychophysical approach to the assessment of pain report. *Behavior Therapy, 13,* 376–394.

Udén, A., Åström, M., & Bergenudd, H. (1988). Pain drawings in chronic back pain. *Spine, 13,* 389–392.

Urban, B. J., Keefe, F. J., & France, R. D. (1984). A study of psychophysical scaling in chronic pain patients. *Pain, 20,* 157–168.

Von Baeyer, C. L., Bergstrom, K. J., Brodwin, M. G., & Brodwin, S. K. (1983). Invalid use of pain drawings in psychological screening of back pain patients. *Pain, 16,* 103–107.

Wallenstein, S. L., Heidrich, G., III, Kaiko, R., & Houde, R. W. (1980). Clinical evaluation of mild analgesics: The measurement of clinical pain. *British Journal of Clinical Pharmacology, 10,* 319S–327S.

Walsh, T. D. (1984). Practical problems in pain measurement. *Pain, 19,* 96–98.

Woodforde, J. M., & Merskey, H. (1972). Some relationships between subjective measures of pain. *Journal of Psychosomatic Research, 16,* 173–178.

Chapter 10

The McGill Pain Questionnaire: Appraisal and Current Status

RONALD MELZACK, PhD
JOEL KATZ, PhD

Pain is a personal, subjective experience influenced by cultural learning, the meaning of the situation, attention, and other psychological variables (Melzack & Wall, 1988). Pain processes do not begin with the stimulation of receptors. Rather, injury or disease produces neural signals that enter an active nervous system that is the substrate of past experience, culture, anxiety, and depression. These brain processes actively participate in the selection, abstraction, and synthesis of information from the total sensory input. Pain, then, is not simply the end product of a linear sensory transmission system; rather, it is a dynamic process that involves continuous interactions among complex ascending and descending systems.

DIMENSIONS OF PAIN EXPERIENCE

Research on pain, since the beginning of this century, has been dominated by the concept that pain is purely a sensory experience. Yet pain also has a distinctly unpleasant, affective quality. It becomes overwhelming, demands immediate attention, and disrupts ongoing behavior and thought. It motivates or drives the organism into activity aimed at stopping the pain as quickly as possible. To consider only the sensory features of pain and ignore its motivational-affective properties is to look at only part of the problem. Even the concept of pain as a perception, with full recognition of past experience, attention, and other cognitive influences, still neglects the crucial motivational dimension.

These considerations led Melzack and Casey (1968) to suggest that there are three major psychological dimensions of pain: sensory-discriminative, motivational-affective, and cognitive-evaluative. They proposed, moreover, that these dimensions of pain experience are subserved by physiologically specialized systems in the brain: the sensory discriminative dimension of pain is influenced primarily by the rapidly conducting spinal systems; the powerful motivational drive and unpleasant affect characteristic of pain are subserved by activities in reticular and limbic structures that are influenced primarily by the slowly conducting spinal systems; neocortical or higher central nervous system processes, such as evaluation of the input in terms of past experience, exert control over activity in both the discriminative and motivational systems.

It is assumed that these three categories of activity interact with one another to provide *perceptual information* on the location, magnitude, and spatiotemporal properties of the noxious stimuli, *motivational tendency* toward escape or attack, and *cognitive information* based on past experience and probability of outcome of different response strategies (Melzack & Casey, 1968). All three forms of activity could then influence motor mechanisms responsible for the complex pattern of overt responses that characterize pain.

THE LANGUAGE OF PAIN

Clinical investigators have long recognized the varieties of pain experience. Descriptions of the burning qualities of pain after peripheral nerve injury, or the stabbing, cramping qualities of visceral pains, frequently provide the key to diagnosis and may even suggest the course of therapy. Despite the frequency of such descriptions, and the seemingly high agreement that they are valid descriptive words, studies of their use and meaning are relatively recent.

Anyone who has suffered severe pain and tried to describe the experience to a friend or to the doctor often finds himself at a loss for words. The reason for this difficulty in expressing pain experience, actually, is not because the words do not exist. As we shall soon see, there is an abundance of appropriate words. Rather, the main reason is that, fortunately, they are not words that we have occasion to use often. Another reason is that the words may seem absurd. We may use descriptors such as splitting, shooting, gnawing, wrenching, or stinging, but there are no external objective references for these words. If we talk about a blue pen or a yellow pencil we can point to an object and say, "That is what I mean by yellow," or "This color of the pen is blue." But what can we point to to tell another person precisely what we mean by smarting, tingling, or rasping? A person who suffers terrible pain may say that the pain is burning and add, "It feels as if someone is shoving a red-hot poker through my toes and slowly twisting it around." These "as if" statements are often essential to convey the qualities of the experience.

If the study of pain in people is to have a scientific foundation, it is essential to measure it. If we want to know how effective a new drug is, we need numbers to say that the pain decreased by some amount. Yet, although overall intensity is important information, we also want to know whether the drug specifically decreased the burning quality of the pain, or if the especially miserable, tight, cramping feeling is gone.

TRADITIONAL MEASURES OF PAIN INTENSITY

Until recently, the methods that were used for pain measurement treated pain as though it were a single, unique quality that varies only in intensity (Beecher, 1959). These methods include the use of verbal rating scales (e.g., mild, moderate, severe), numerical rating scales (1–100), and visual analogue scales (Huskisson, 1974; Joyce, Zutshi, Hrubes, & Mason, 1975). These simple methods have all been used effectively in hospital clinics, and have provided valuable information about pain and analgesia.

Visual analog scales (VASs) provide simple, efficient, and minimally intrusive measures of pain intensity that have been used widely in clinical and research settings where a quick index of pain is required and to which a numerical value can be assigned. The VAS consists of a 10-cm horizontal (Huskisson, 1983) or vertical (Sriwatanakul et al., 1983) line with the two endpoints labeled "no pain" and "worst pain ever" (or a similar verbal descriptor representing the upper pole). The patient is required to place a mark on the 10-cm line at a point that corresponds to the level of pain intensity he or she presently feels. The distance in centimeters from the low end of the VAS to the patient's mark is used as a numerical index of the severity of pain. The VAS is sensitive to pharmacologic and non-pharmacologic procedures that alter the experience of pain (Bélanger, Melzack, & Lauzon, 1989; Choiniére, Melzack, Girard, Rondeau, & Paquin, 1990) and correlates highly with pain measured on verbal and numerical rating scales (Ekblom & Hansson, 1988; Kremer & Atkinson, 1983; Ohnhaus & Adler, 1975).

A major advantage of the VAS as a measure of sensory pain intensity is its ratio scale properties (Price, 1988; Price, McGrath, Rafii, & Buckingham, 1983). In contrast to many other pain measurement tools, equality of ratios is implied, making it appropriate to speak meaningfully about percentage differences between VAS measurements obtained either at multiple points in time or from independent samples of subjects. Other advantages of the VAS include (1) its ease and brevity of administration and scoring (Jensen, Koroly, & Braver, 1986), (2) minimal intrusiveness, and (3) its conceptual simplicity, providing that adequately clear instructions are given to the patient (Chapman et al., 1985; Huskisson, 1983).

The major disadvantage of the VAS is its assumption that pain is a unidimensional experience (Melzack, 1975). Although intensity is, without a doubt, a salient dimension of pain, it is clear that the word "pain" refers to an endless variety of qualities that are categorized under a single linguistic label, not to a specific, single sensation that varies only in intensity. Each pain has unique qualities. The pain of a toothache is obviously different from that of a pin prick, just as the pain of a coronary occlusion is uniquely different from the pain of a broken leg. To describe pain solely in terms of intensity is like specifying the visual world only in terms of light flux without regard to pattern, color, texture, and the many other dimensions of visual experience.

THE McGILL PAIN QUESTIONNAIRE

Development and Description

Melzack and Torgerson (1971) have made a start toward specifying the qualities of pain. In the first part of their study, they asked physicians and other university graduates to classify 102 words, obtained from the clinical literature, into small groups that describe distinctly different aspects of the experience of pain. On the basis of the data, the words were categorized into three major classes and 16 subclasses (Figure 10.1). The classes are (1) words that describe the sensory qualities of the experience in terms of temporal, spatial, pressure, thermal, and other properties; (2) words that describe affective qualities in terms of tension, fear, and autonomic properties that are part of the pain experience; and (3) evaluative words that describe the subjective overall intensity of the total pain experience. Each subclass, which was given a descriptive label, consists of a group of words that were considered by most subjects to be qualitatively similar. Some of these words are undoubtedly synonyms, others seem to be synonymous but vary in intensity, and many provide subtle differences or nuances (despite their similarities) that may be of importance to a patient who is trying desperately to communicate to a physician.

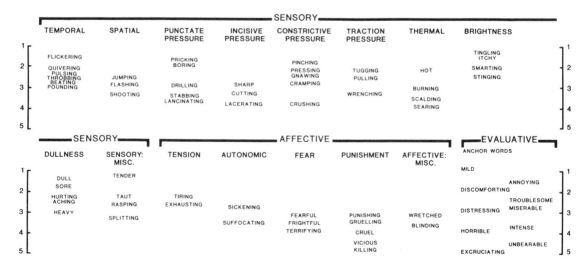

FIGURE 10.1. Spatial display of pain descriptors based on intensity ratings by patients. The intensity scale values range from 1 (mild) to 5 (excruciating). Copyright 1971 Ronald Melzack and Warren S. Torgerson.

The second part of the Melzack and Torgerson (1971) study was an attempt to determine the pain intensities implied by the words within each subclass. Groups of physicians, patients, and students were asked to assign an intensity value to each word, using a numerical scale ranging from least (or mild) pain to worst (or excruciating) pain. When this was done, it was apparent that several words within each subclass had the same relative intensity relationships in all three sets. For example, in the spatial subclass, "shooting" was found to represent more pain than "flashing," which in turn implied more pain than "jumping." Although the precise intensity scale values differed for the three groups, all three agreed on the positions of the words relative to one another. The scale values of the words for patients, based on the precise numerical values listed in Melzack and Torgerson (1971), are shown in Figure 10.1.

Because of the high degree of agreement on the intensity relationships among pain descriptors by subjects who have different cultural, socioeconomic, and educational backgrounds, a pain questionnaire (Figure 10.2) was developed as an experimental tool for studies of the effects of various methods of pain management. In addition to the list of pain descriptors, the questionnaire contains line drawings of the body to show the spatial distribution of the pain, words that describe temporal properties of pain, and descriptors of the overall present pain intensity (PPI). The PPI is recorded as a number from 1 to 5, in which each number is associated with the following words: 1, mild; 2, discomforting; 3, distressing; 4, horrible; 5, excruciating. The mean scale values of these words, which were chosen from the evaluative category, are approximately equally far apart (Melzack & Torgerson, 1971), so that they represent equal scale intervals and thereby provide "anchors" for the specification of the overall pain intensity.

In a preliminary study, the pain questionnaire consisted of the 16 subclasses of descriptors shown in Figure 10.1, as well as the additional information deemed necessary for the evaluation of pain. It soon became clear, however, that many of the patients found certain key words to be absent. These words were then selected from the original word list used by Melzack and Torgerson (1971), categorized appropriately, and ranked according to their mean scale values. A further set of words—cool, cold, freezing—was used by patients on rare occasions but was indicated to be essential for an adequate description of some types of pain. Thus, four supplementary—or "miscellaneous"—subclasses were added to the word lists of the questionnaire (Figure 10.2). The final classification, then, appeared to represent the most parsimonious and meaningful set of subclasses without at the same time losing subclasses that represent important qualitative properties. A description of the properties and scoring methods of the questionnaire, which is referred to as the McGill Pain Questionnaire (MPQ) has been published (Melzack, 1975), and it has become a widely used clinical and research tool (Melzack, 1983; Reading, 1989; Wilke, Savedra, Holzemer, Tesler, & Paul, 1990).

Measures of Pain Experience

The descriptor lists of the MPQ are read to a patient with the explicit instruction that he or she choose only those words that describe his or her feelings and sensations at that moment. Three major indices are obtained:

1. The pain rating index (PRI) based on the rank values of the words. In this scoring system, the word in each subclass implying the least pain is given a value of 1, the next word is given a value of 2, and so on. The rank values of the words chosen by a patient are summed to obtain a score separately for the sensory (subclasses 1–10), affective (subclasses 11–15), evaluative (subclass 16), and miscellaneous (subclasses 17–20) words, in addition to providing a total score (subclasses 1–20). Figure 10.3 shows MPQ scores (total score from subclasses 1–20) obtained by patients with a variety of acute and chronic pains.

2. The number of words chosen (NWC).

3. The PPI, the number-word combination chosen as the indicator of overall pain intensity at the time of administration of the questionnaire.

Recently several additional scoring procedures have been suggested. Hartman and Ainsworth (1980) have proposed transforming the data into a pain ratio or fraction: The "pain

McGill Pain Questionnaire

Patient's Name _____ Date _____ Time_____am/pm

PRI: S_____ A _____ E_____ M_____ PRI(T)_____ PPI____
       (1–10)   (11–15)   (16)   (17–20)   (1–20)

1 FLICKERING __ QUIVERING __ PULSING __ THROBBING __ BEATING __ POUNDING __	11 TIRING __ EXHAUSTING __ 12 SICKENING __ SUFFOCATING __
2 JUMPING __ FLASHING __ SHOOTING __	13 FEARFUL __ FRIGHTFUL __ TERRIFYING __
3 PRICKING __ BORING __ DRILLING __ STABBING __ LANCINATING __	14 PUNISHING __ GRUELLING __ CRUEL __ VICIOUS __ KILLING __
4 SHARP __ CUTTING __ LACERATING __	15 WRETCHED __ BLINDING __
5 PINCHING __ PRESSING __ GNAWING __ CRAMPING __ CRUSHING __	16 ANNOYING __ TROUBLESOME __ MISERABLE __ INTENSE __ UNBEARABLE __
6 TUGGING __ PULLING __ WRENCHING __	17 SPREADING __ RADIATING __ PENETRATING __ PIERCING __
7 HOT __ BURNING __ SCALDING __ SEARING __	18 TIGHT __ NUMB __ DRAWING __ SQUEEZING __ TEARING __
8 TINGLING __ ITCHY __ SMARTING __ STINGING __	19 COOL __ COLD __ FREEZING __
9 DULL __ SORE __ HURTING __ ACHING __ HEAVY __	20 NAGGING __ NAUSEATING __ AGONIZING __ DREADFUL __ TORTURING __
10 TENDER __ TAUT __ RASPING __ SPLITTING __	PPI 0 NO PAIN __ 1 MILD __ 2 DISCOMFORTING __ 3 DISTRESSING __ 4 HORRIBLE __ 5 EXCRUCIATING __

BRIEF __	RHYTHMIC __	CONTINUOUS __
MOMENTARY __	PERIODIC __	STEADY __
TRANSIENT __	INTERMITTENT __	CONSTANT __

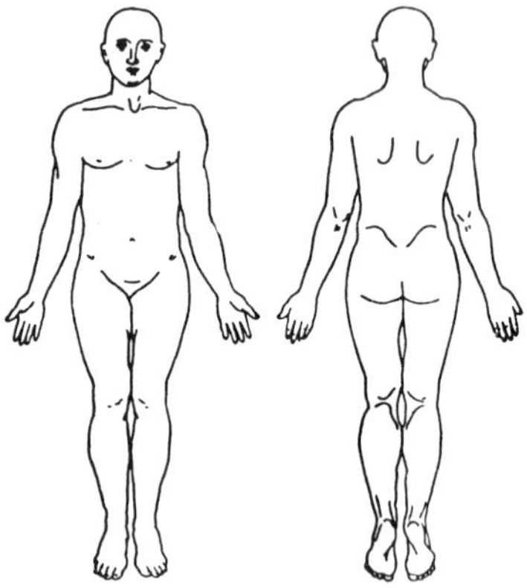

E = EXTERNAL
I = INTERNAL

COMMENTS:

FIGURE 10.2. McGill Pain Questionnaire. The descriptors fall into four major groups: sensory, 1 to 10; affective, 11–15; evaluative, 16; and miscellaneous, 17–20. The rank value for each descriptor is based on its position in the word set. The sum of the rank values is the pain rating index (PRI). The present pain intensity (PPI) is based on a scale of 0 to 5. Copyright 1975 Ronald Melzack.

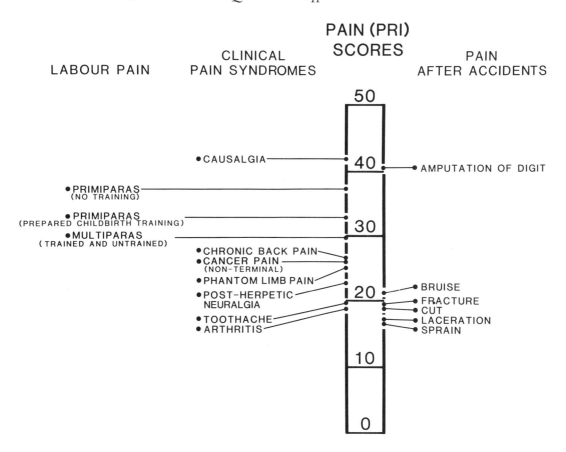

FIGURE 10.3. Comparison of pain scores using the McGill Pain Questionnaire, obtained from women during labor (Melzack et al., 1981), and from patients in a general hospital pain clinic (Melzack, 1975) and an emergency department (Melzack et al., 1982). The pain score for causalgic pain is reported by Tahmoush (1981). Copyright 1975, 1981, 1982 Ronald Melzack.

ratio was calculated for each session by dividing the postsession rating by the sum of the pre- and postsession ratings" (p. 40). Kremer, Atkinson, and Ignelzi (1982) suggested dividing the sum of the obtained ranks within each dimension by the total possible score for a particular dimension, thus making differences between the sensory, affective, evaluative, and miscellaneous dimensions more interpretable.

A final form of computation (Melzack, Katz, & Jeans, 1985) may be useful because it has been argued (Charter & Nehemkis, 1983) that the MPQ fails to take into account the true relative intensity of verbal descriptors since the rank-order scoring system loses the precise intensity of the scale values obtained by Melzack and Torgerson (1971). For example, Figure 10.1 shows that the affective descriptors generally have higher scale values than the sensory words. This is clear when we consider the fact

that the words "throbbing" and "vicious" receive a rank value of 4, but have scale values of 2.68 and 4.26, respectively, indicating that the latter descriptor implies considerably more pain intensity than the former. A simple technique was developed (Melzack et al., 1985) to convert rank values to weighted rank values that more closely approximate the original scale values obtained by Melzack and Torgerson (1971). Use of this procedure may provide enhanced sensitivity in some statistical analyses (Melzack et al., 1985). The weights for each descriptor category are presented in Appendix 10.A.

Usefulness of the McGill Pain Questionnaire

The most important requirement of a measure is that it be valid, reliable, consistent, and above all useful. The MPQ appears to meet all of these requirements (Chapman et al., 1985; Melzack, 1983; Reading, 1989; Wilke et al., 1990) and provides a relatively rapid way of measuring subjective pain experience (Melzack, 1975). When administered to a patient by reading each subclass, it can be completed in about 5 minutes. It can also be filled out by the patient in a more leisurely way as a paper-and-pencil test, although the scores are somewhat different (Klepac, Dowling, Rokke, Dodge, & Schafer, 1981).

Since its introduction in 1975, the MPQ has been used in over 100 studies of acute, chronic, and laboratory-produced pains. It has been translated into several languages and has also spawned the development of similar pain questionnaires in other languages (Table 10.1).

Because pain is a private, personal experience, it is impossible for us to know precisely what someone else's pain feels like. No man can possibly know what it is like to have menstrual cramps or labor pain. Nor can a psychologically healthy person know what a psychotic patient is feeling when he or she complains of excruciating pain (Veilleux & Melzack, 1976). But the MPQ provides us with an insight into the qualities that are experienced. Recent studies indicate that each kind of pain is characterized by a distinctive constellation of words. There is a remarkable consistency in the choice of words by patients suffering the same or similar pain syndromes (Graham, Bond, Gerkovich, & Cook, 1980; Grushka, Sessle, & Miller, 1984; Katz & Melzack, 1991; Melzack, Taenzer, Feldman, & Kinch, 1981; Van Buren & Kleinknecht, 1979).

Reliability and Validity of the McGill Pain Questionnaire

Reading, Everitt, and Sledmere (1982) investigated the reliability of the groupings of adjectives in the MPQ by using different methodological and statistical approaches. Subjects sorted each of the 78 words of the MPQ into groups that described similar pain qualities. The mean number of groups was 19 (with a range of 7 to 31), which is remarkably close to the MPQ's 20 groups. Moreover, there were distinct subgroups for sensory and affective-evaluative words. Because the cultural backgrounds of subjects in this study and in Melzack and Torgerson's (1971) were different, and the methodology and data analysis were dissimilar, the degree of correspondence is impressive. Nevertheless, interesting differences between the studies were found that suggest alternative approaches for future revisions of the MPQ.

Evidence for the stability of the MPQ was recently provided by Love, Leboeuf, and Crisp (1989), who administered the MPQ to patients with chronic low back pain on two occasions (separated by several days) prior to receiving treatment. Their results show very strong test–retest reliability coefficients for the MPQ pain rating indexes as well as for some of the 20 categories. The lower coefficients for the 20 categories may be explained by the suggestion that many clinical pains show fluctuations in quality over time, yet they still represent the "same" pain to the person who experiences it.

Studies of the validity of the 3-dimensional framework of the MPQ are numerous, and have recently been reviewed by Reading (1989). Generally, the distinction between sensory and affective dimensions has held up extremely well, but there is still considerable debate on the separation of the affective and evaluative dimensions. Nevertheless, several excellent studies (Reading, 1979; McCreary, Turner, & Dawson, 1981; Prieto et al., 1980) have reported a discrete evaluative factor. The

TABLE 10.1. Pain Questionnaires in Different Languages Based on the McGill Pain Questionnaire

Language	Authors
Arabic	Harrison (1988)
Chinese	Hui & Chen (1989)
Dutch (Flemish)	Vanderiet et al. (1987)
	Verkes et al. (1989)
Finnish	Ketovuori, & Pöntinen (1981)
French	Boureau et al. (1984)
German	Kiss et al. (1987)
	Radvila et al. (1987)
	Stein & Mendl (1988)
Italian	De Benedittis et al. (1988)
	Ferracuti et al. (1990)
	Maiani & Sanavio (1985)
Japanese	Satow et al. (1990)
Norwegian	Strand & Wisnes (1991)
Polish	Sedlak (1990)
Slovak	Bartko et al. (1984)
Spanish	Bejarano et al. (1985)
	Laheurta et al. (1982)

different factor-analytic procedures that were used undoubtedly account for the reports of 4 factors (Reading, 1979), 5 factors (Crockett, Prkachin, & Craig, 1977), or 7 factors (Leavitt, Garron, Whisler, & Sheinkop, 1978). The major source of disagreement, however, seems to us to be the different patient populations that are used to obtain data for factor analyses. The range includes brief laboratory pains, dysmenorrhea, back pain, and cancer pain. In some studies, relatively few words are chosen, while large numbers are selected in others. It is not surprising, then, that factor-analytic studies based on such diverse populations have confused rather than clarified some of the issues.

A recent study by Turk, Rudy, and Salovey (1985) studied the internal structure of the MPQ by using techniques that avoided the problems of most earlier studies and confirmed the three sensory, affective, and evaluative dimensions. Still more recently, Lowe, Walker, and McCallum (1991) again confirmed the 3-factor structure of the MPQ, using elegant statistical procedures and a large number of subjects. Finally, a recent paper by Chen, Dworkin, Haug, and Gerhig (1989) presents data on the remarkable consistency of the MPQ across five studies using the cold pressor task, and Pearce and Morley (1989) provided further confirmation of the construct validity of the MPQ using the Stroop color naming task with chronic pain patients.

Discriminative Capacity of the McGill Pain Questionnaire

One of the most exciting features of the MPQ is its potential value as an aid in the differential diagnosis between various pain syndromes. The first study to demonstrate the discriminative capacity of the MPQ was carried out by Dubuisson and Melzack (1976), who administered the questionnaire to 95 patients suffering from one of eight known pain syndromes: postherpetic neuralgia, phantom limb pain, metastatic carcinoma, toothache, degenerative disc disease, rheumatoid arthritis or osteoarthritis, labor pain, and menstrual pain. A multiple group discriminant analysis revealed that each type of pain is characterized by a distinctive constellation of verbal descriptors (Figure 10.4). Further, when the descriptor set for each patient was classified into one of the eight

diagnostic categories, a correct classification was made in 77% of cases. Table 10.2 shows the pain descriptors that are most characteristic of the eight clinical pain syndromes in the Dubuisson and Melzack study.

Descriptor patterns can also provide the basis for discriminating between two major types of low back pain. Some patients have clear physical causes such as degenerative disc disease, whereas others suffer low back pain even though no physical causes can be found. Using a modified version of the MPQ, Leavitt and Garron (1980) found that patients with physical—"organic"—causes use distinctly different patterns of words from patients whose pain has no detectable cause and is labeled as "functional." A concordance of 87% was found between established medical diagnosis and classification based upon the patients' choice of word patterns from the MPQ. Specific verbal descriptors of the MPQ have also been shown recently to discriminate between reversible and irreversible damage of the nerve fibers in a tooth (Grushka & Sessle, 1984), and between leg pain caused by diabetic neuropathy and leg pain arising from other causes (Masson, Hunt, Gem, & Boulton, 1989).

More recently, Melzack, Terrence, Fromm, and Amsel (1986) provided further evidence of the discriminative capacity of the MPQ to differentiate between trigeminal neuralgia and atypical facial pain. Fifty-three patients were given a thorough neurological examination which led to a diagnosis of either trigeminal neuralgia or atypical facial pain. Each patient rated his or her pain using the MPQ, and the scores were submitted to a discriminant analysis. Ninety-one percent of the patients were correctly classified using seven key descriptors. To determine how well the key descriptors were able to predict either diagnosis, the discriminant function derived from the 53 patients was applied to MPQ scores obtained from a second, independent validation sample of patients with trigeminal neuralgia or atypical facial pain. The results showed a correct prediction for 90% of the patients.

It is evident, however, that the discriminative capacity of the MPQ has limits. High levels of anxiety and other psychological disturbance, which may produce high affective scores, may obscure the discriminative capacity (Kremer & Atkinson, 1983). Moreover, certain key words that discriminate among specific syndromes

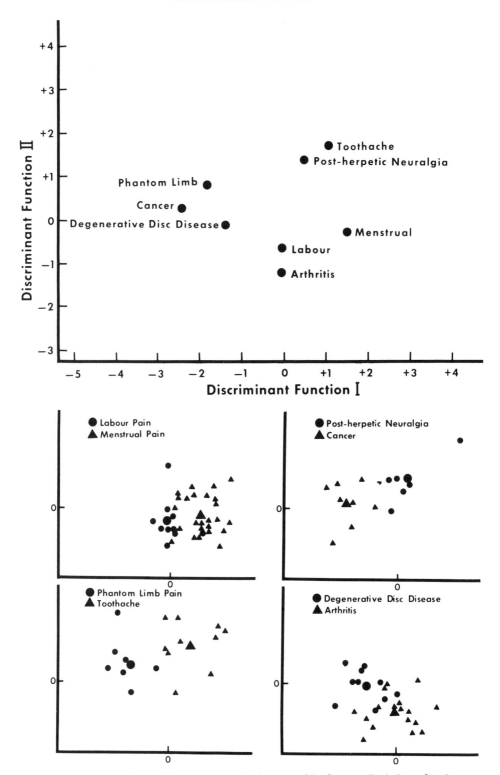

FIGURE 10.4. *Top*: Centroids of eight diagnostic groups in the space of the first two discriminant functions reported by Dubuisson and Melzack (1976). *Bottom*: Individual patients' scores on the first two discriminant functions, for each diagnostic group. Large circle or triangle represents group centroid; small circles and triangles represent individual scores. Copyright 1976 Ronald Melzack.

TABLE 10.2. Descriptions Characteristic of Clinical Pain Syndromes[a]

Menstrual pain (n = 25)	Arthritic pain (n = 16)	Labour pain (n = 11)	Disc disease pain (n = 10)	Toothache (n = 10)	Cancer pain (n = 8)	Phantom limb pain (n = 8)	Postherpetic pain (n = 6)
Sensory							
Cramping (44%)	Gnawing (38%)	Pounding (37%)	Throbbing (40%)	Throbbing (50%)	Shooting (50%)	Throbbing (38%)	Sharp (84%)
Aching (44%)	Aching (50%)	Shooting (46%)	Shooting (50%)	Boring (40%)	Sharp (50%)	Stabbing (50%)	Pulling (67%)
		Stabbing (37%)	Stabbing (40%)	Sharp (50%)	Gnawing (50%)	Sharp (38%)	Aching (50%)
		Sharp (64%)	Sharp (60%)		Burning (50%)	Cramping (50%)	Tender (83%)
		Cramping (82%)	Cramping (40%)		Heavy (50%)	Burning (50%)	
		Aching (46%)	Aching (40%)			Aching (38%)	
			Heavy (40%)				
			Tender (50%)				
Affective							
Tiring (44%)	Exhausting (50%)	Tiring (37%)	Tiring (46%)	Sickening (40%)	Exhausting (50%)	Tiring (50%)	Exhausting (50%)
Sickening (56%)		Exhausting (46%)	Exhausting (40%)			Exhausting (38%)	
		Fearful (36%)				Cruel (38%)	
Evaluative							
	Annoying (38%)	Intense (46%)	Unbearable (40%)	Annoying (50%)	Unbearable (50%)		
Temporal							
Constant (56%)	Constant (44%)	Rhythmic (91%)	Constant (80%)	Constant (60%)	Constant (100%)	Constant (88%)	Constant (50%)
	Rhythmic (56%)		Rhythmic (70%)	Rhythmic (40%)	Rhythmic (88%)	Rhythmic (63%)	Rhythmic (50%)

[a]Only those words chosen by more than one-third of the patients are listed, and the percentages of patients who chose each word are shown below the word.

may be absent (Reading, 1982). Nevertheless, it is clear that there are appreciable and quantifiable differences in the way various types of pain are described, and that patients with the same disease or pain syndrome tend to use remarkably similar words to communicate what they feel.

THE SHORT-FORM McGILL PAIN QUESTIONNAIRE

The short-form McGill Pain Questionnaire (SF-MPQ) (Melzack, 1987; Figure 10.5) was developed for use in specific research settings when the time to obtain information from patients is limited and when more information is desired than that provided by intensity measures such as the VAS or PPI. The SF-MPQ consists of 15 representative words from the sensory (n = 11) and affective (n = 4) categories of the standard, long-form (LF-MPQ). The PPI and a VAS are included to provide indices of overall pain intensity. The 15 descriptors making up the SF-MPQ were selected on the basis of their frequency of endorsement by patients with a variety of acute, intermittent, and chronic pains. An additional word—split

SHORT-FORM McGILL PAIN QUESTIONNAIRE
RONALD MELZACK

PATIENT'S NAME: _____   DATE: _____

	NONE	MILD	MODERATE	SEVERE
THROBBING	0) _____	1) _____	2) _____	3) _____
SHOOTING	0) _____	1) _____	2) _____	3) _____
STABBING	0) _____	1) _____	2) _____	3) _____
SHARP	0) _____	1) _____	2) _____	3) _____
CRAMPING	0) _____	1) _____	2) _____	3) _____
GNAWING	0) _____	1) _____	2) _____	3) _____
HOT-BURNING	0) _____	1) _____	2) _____	3) _____
ACHING	0) _____	1) _____	2) _____	3) _____
HEAVY	0) _____	1) _____	2) _____	3) _____
TENDER	0) _____	1) _____	2) _____	3) _____
SPLITTING	0) _____	1) _____	2) _____	3) _____
TIRING-EXHAUSTING	0) _____	1) _____	2) _____	3) _____
SICKENING	0) _____	1) _____	2) _____	3) _____
FEARFUL	0) _____	1) _____	2) _____	3) _____
PUNISHING-CRUEL	0) _____	1) _____	2) _____	3) _____

NO PAIN |—————————————————————————————| WORST POSSIBLE PAIN

PPI

0	NO PAIN	_____
1	MILD	_____
2	DISCOMFORTING	_____
3	DISTRESSING	_____
4	HORRIBLE	_____
5	EXCRUCIATING	_____

FIGURE 10.5. The short-form McGill Pain Questionnaire. Descriptors 1–11 represent the sensory dimension of pain experience and 12–15 represent the affective dimension. Each descriptor is ranked on an intensity scale of 0 = none, 1 = mild, 2 = moderate, 3 = severe. The Present Pain Intensity (PPI) of the standard long-form MPQ and the Visual Analogue Scale are also included to provide overall pain intensity scores. Copyright 1984 Ronald Melzack.

ting—was added because it was reported to be a key discriminative word for dental pain (Grushka & Sessle, 1984). Each descriptor is ranked by the patient on an intensity scale of 0 = none, 1 = mild, 2 = moderate, 3 = severe.

The SF-MPQ correlates very highly with the major PRI indices (sensory, affective, and total) of the LF-MPQ and is sensitive to traditional clinical therapies—analgesic drugs, epidural blocks, and transcutaneous electrical nerve stimulation (TENS) (Melzack, 1987). Preliminary results from a study designed to examine the qualities of pain experienced by patients in a physical rehabilitation hospital indicate that the sensory dimension of the SF-MPQ correlates highly with analgesic use among a subgroup of patients with high pain scores (Katz & Vadnais, 1990). The SF-MPQ has also recently been used in studies of chronic pain of diverse etiology (Grönblad, Lukinmaa, & Konttinen, 1990; Guieu, Tardy-Gervet, & Roll, 1991). Furthermore, initial data (Melzack, 1987) suggest that the SF-MPQ may be capable of discriminating among different pain syndromes, which is an important property of the long form. A Czech version of the SF-MPQ has been recently developed (Solcovä, Jakoubek, Sÿkora, & Hnïk, 1990).

MULTIDIMENSIONAL PAIN EXPERIENCE

Recently, Turk et al. (1985) evaluated the theoretical structure of the MPQ using new methods to analyze their data. They concluded that the 3-factor structure of the MPQ—sensory, affective, and evaluative—is strongly supported by the analyses. In addition, like most others who have used the MPQ, they find high intercorrelations (.64−.81) among the 3 factors. However, Turk et al. then argue that because the 3 factors measured by the MPQ are highly intercorrelated, they are therefore not distinct. They conclude that the MPQ does not discriminate among the 3 factors and only the PRI-Total should be used. We believe that their argument is fallacious. There is, in fact, considerable evidence that the MPQ is effective in discriminating among the 3 factors.

First, a high correlation among variables does

not necessarily imply a lack of discriminant capacity. Traditional psychophysics has shown repeatedly that, in the case of vision, increasing the intensity of light produces increased capacity to discriminate color, contours, texture, and distance (Kling & Riggs, 1971). Similarly, in the case of hearing, increases in volume lead to increased discrimination of timbre, pitch, and spatial location (Kling and Riggs, 1971). In these cases, there are clearly very high intercorrelations among the variables in each modality. But this does not mean that we should forget about the differences between color and texture, or between timbre and pitch, just because they intercorrelate highly. This approach would lead to the loss of valuable, meaningful data.

Second, many papers have demonstrated the discriminant validity of the MPQ. Reading and Newton (1977) showed, in a comparison of primary dysmenorrhea and intrauterine device (IUD) related pain, that the "pain intensity scores were reflected in a larger sensory component with IUD users, whereas with dysmenorrhea the affective component predominated." In a later study, Reading (1982) compared MPQ profiles of women experiencing chronic pelvic pain and postepisiotomy pain, and showed that "acute-pain patients displayed greater use of sensory word groups, testifying to the pronounced sensory input from the damaged perinium. Chronic pain patients used affective and reaction subgroups with greater frequency."

In a study of hypnosis and biofeedback, Melzack and Perry (1975) found that "there were significant decreases in both the sensory and affective dimensions, as well as the overall PRI, but that the affective dimension shows the largest decrease." In studies on labor pain, Melzack and his colleagues (Melzack, Kinch, Dobkin, Lebrun, & Taenzer, 1984; Melzack et al., 1981) found that distinctly different variables correlated with the sensory, affective, and evaluative dimensions. Prepared childbirth practice, for example, correlated significantly with the sensory and affective dimensions but not the evaluative one. Menstrual difficulties correlated with the affective but neither the sensory nor evaluative dimension. Physical factors, such as mother's and infant's weight, also correlate selectively with one or another dimension.

Similarly, a study of acute pain in emergency

ward patients (Melzack, Wall, & Ty, 1982) has "revealed a normal distribution of sensory scores but very low affective scores compared to patients with chronic pain." Finally, Chen et al. (1989) have consistently identified a group of pain-sensitive and pain-tolerant subjects in five laboratory studies of tonic (prolonged) pain. Compared with pain-tolerant subjects, pain-sensitive subjects show significantly higher scores on all PRIs except the sensory dimension. Atkinson, Kremer, and Ignelzi (1982) are undoubtedly right that high affect scores tend to diminish the discriminant capacity of the MPQ so that, at high levels of anxiety and depression, some discriminant capacity is lost. However, the MPQ still retains good discriminant function even at high levels of anxiety.

A recent study is of particular interest because it examines laboratory models of phasic (brief) and tonic (prolonged) pain and compares them by using the MPQ. Chen and Treede (1985) found a very high sensory loading for phasic pain and relatively few choices of affective and evaluative words. In contrast, tonic pain was characterized by much higher scores in the affective and evaluative dimensions. Furthermore, they found that when tonic pain is used to inhibit the phasic pain, "the sensory component is reduced by 32%, whereas the affective component vanishes almost completely."

In summary, we believe that (1) high intercorrelations among psychological variables do not mean that they are all alike and can therefore be lumped into a single variable such as intensity; rather, certain biological and psychological variables can co-vary to a high degree yet represent distinct, discriminable entities; and (2) the MPQ has been shown in many studies to be capable of discriminating among the 3 component factors.

SUMMARY

Pain is a personal, subjective experience influenced by cultural learning, the meaning of the situation, attention, and other psychological variables. Approaches to the measurement of pain include verbal and numeric self-rating scales, behavioral observation scales, and physiological responses. The complex nature of the experience of pain suggests that measurements from these domains may not always show high concordance. But because pain is subjective, the patient's self-report provides the most valid measure of the experience. The visual analog scale and the McGill Pain Questionnaire are probably the most frequently used self-rating instruments for the measurement of pain in clinical and research settings. The McGill Pain Questionnaire is designed to assess the multi-dimensional nature of pain experience and has been demonstrated to be a reliable, valid, and consistent measurement tool. A short-form McGill Pain Questionnaire is available for use in specific research settings when the time to obtain information from patients is limited and when more information than simply the intensity of pain is desired. Further development and refinement of pain measurement techniques will lead to increasingly accurate tools with greater predictive powers.

Acknowledgments. Supported by Grant A7891 from the Natural Sciences and Engineering Research Council of Canada (RM), and Fellowships from the Health Research Personnel Development Program of the Ontario Ministry of Health and the Medical Research Council of Canada (JK). The results and conclusions derived herein are those of the authors, and no official endorsement by the Ontario Ministry of Health is intended or should be inferred.

APPENDIX 10.A
Conversion Values for Weighted Ranks

To correct for the loss of information that results from using the rank rather than scale values to score the MPQ, Melzack et al. (1985) have developed an alternate weighted-rank method. The rank scores are rescaled by multiplying the rank of each descriptor within a category by one of 20 weights. The 20 weights were derived by the following formula:

$$W_i = \sum_{j=1}^{n} S_{ij} \Big/ \sum_{j=1}^{n} R_{ij}$$

where W_i is the weighted correction factor for category i (i ranges from 1 to 20), S_{ij} is the mean intensity scale value of the doctors' and patients' ratings of the jth descriptor in category i, and R_{ij} is the corresponding rank of the jth descriptor in category i. For category 1, the formula yields

$$W_1 = (1.65 + 2.05 + 2.43 + 2.62 \\ + 2.73 + 2.98)/(1 + 2 + 3 \\ + 4 + 5 + 6) = 0.69.$$

The weights for the 20 categories are presented in Table 10A.1, along with sample MPQ choices and a demonstration of the weighted-rank scoring method. Category 19 does not appear in the Melzack and Torgerson (1971) paper and was therefore given a weight of 1.0.

Melzack et al. (1985) used the MPQ pain scores of two groups of patients to assess how well the weighted rank and rank values of the MPQ descriptors approximate their original intensity scale values (Melzack & Torgerson, 1971). MPQ pain scores from 81 chronic low back pain patients and 64 patients with musculoskeletal pain were submitted to one-way, repeated measurements multivariate analyses of variance using the three scoring methods (scale, weighted-rank, and rank) as the repeated measurements factor, and the four pain rating indexes (PRI-Sensory, PRI-Affective, PRI-Evaluative, and PRI-Miscellaneous) as the dependent variables. Separate univariate ANOVAs were then computed, and for each of the four dependent variables, two orthogonal null contrasts (the linear and quadratic components) were evaluated across the cell means of the three MPQ scoring methods. The MPQ total pain rating index (PRI-T) was not included in the multivariate ANOVA because of its linear dependence on the other PRIs (i.e., PRI-S + PRI-A + PRI-E + PRI-M = PRI-T), and instead was submitted to a univariate, one-way ANOVA using the three scoring methods as the repeated measures factor, and the linear and quadratic components across the cell means were then evaluated.

The linear component describes a statistical comparison between the mean scale value and the mean weighted-rank value. The quadratic component contrasts the sum of the mean scale and mean weighted-rank values with twice the mean rank value. A statistically nonsignificant linear component would demonstrate that the weighted-rank method provides an equivalent alternative measure to the scale values, and a significant quadratic component would indicate that the rank approximation to the scale values results in a PRI that is either too large or too small. This pattern of findings would clearly favor the use of the weighted-rank method of scoring the MPQ over the rank method for a more accurate quantitative assessment of a patient's pain.

Table 10A.2 contains the mean scale, weighted-rank, and rank values of the PRI-S, -A, -E, -M, and -T for the two diagnostic groups. Also shown are the results of the linear and quadratic contrasts that compare the three scoring methods. It can be seen that the pattern of results is the same for patients with low-back and musculoskeletal pain. The multivariate test of Wilks' lambda by Rao's approximate F was highly significant for both groups ($F(8, 73) = 106.94$, $p < .00001$; $F(8, 56) = 75.86$, $p < .00001$, respectively). Nonsignificant linear components and significant quadratic components were found for the PRI-S, -A, and -M. The same pattern was found for the PRI-T scores following the univariate ANOVA (Table 10A.2). These findings indicate that, for the PRI-S, -A, -M, and -T, the weighted-rank method produces values that are statistically equivalent to the scale values and hence preferable to the rank approximations that depart in either direction from the scale values. An examination of the statistical contrasts across the means of the PRI-E for both patient groups yielded nonsignificant linear and quadratic components. Thus, for the PRI-E, the rank and weighted-rank scoring methods approximate the intensity scale values equally well.

In general, the rank-value scoring system has been sufficiently sensitive to evaluate the effectiveness of a variety of pain-relieving procedures as well as to discriminate among different pain syndromes. The correction by weighted ranks may not be necessary for most research studies but can be valuable when results are statistically marginal by maximizing the sensitivity of the MPQ.

TABLE 10A.1. Sample MPQ Responses and Scoring Using the Weighted-Rank Method[a]

MPQ category	Weight (W_i)	Descriptor chosen	Rank score	Weighted-rank score
1	0.69	Pulsing	3	2.07
2	1.38	—	0	0.00
3	0.93	Stabbing	4	3.72
4	1.59	Sharp	1	1.59
5	0.81	—	0	0.00
6	1.19	Wrenching	3	3.57
7	1.28	Hot	1	1.28
8	0.70	Smarting	3	2.1
9	0.72	Aching	4	2.88
10	0.95	Tender	1	0.95
			PRI-S = 20	18.16
11	1.74	Exhausting	2	3.48
12	2.22	Sickening	1	2.22
13	1.87	Frightful	2	3.74
14	1.32	Vicious	4	5.28
15	2.33	Wretched	1	2.33
			PRI-A = 10	17.05
16	1.01	Intense	4	4.04
			PRI-E = 4	4.04
17	1.22	—	0	0.00
18	0.82	Numb	2	1.64
19	1.0	Cool	1	1.0
20	1.15	Agonizing	3	3.54
			PRI-M = 6	6.09
			PRI-T = 40	45.34

[a]The rank score of each descriptor chosen by the patient is multiplied by the weight (Wi) for that category to obtain the corresponding weighted rank score. These scores are summed as usual to form the MPQ PRIs.

TABLE 10A.2. Mean Scale, Weighted-Rank, and Rank Values of the Pain Rating Indexes (PRI) for Patients with Low-Back Pain and Musculoskeletal Pain[a]

	Mean scale values	Mean weighted-rank values	Mean rank values	F_{lin}	p	F_{quad}	p
Low-back pain ($n = 81$)							
PRI-S	16.9	17.0	18.2	0.14	NS	55.26	0.00001
PRI-A	7.9	7.6	4.4	2.00	NS	163.97	0.00001
PRI-E	2.9	3.0	2.9	0.90	NS	0.09	NS
PRI-M	6.7	6.5	6.1	1.96	NS	55.09	0.00001
PRI-T	34.4	34.1	31.6	0.93	NS	74.61	0.00001
Musculoskeletal pain ($n = 64$)							
PRI-S	16.5	16.2	17.4	2.29	NS	32.16	0.00001
PRI-A	6.3	6.3	3.7	0.01	NS	99.44	0.00001
PRI-E	2.9	2.9	2.9	0.01	NS	1.16	NS
PRI-M	6.5	6.7	6.2	1.32	NS	27.10	0.00001
PRI-T	32.2	32.1	30.2	0.16	NS	42.03	0.00001

[a]The major PRI classes are sensory (S), affective (A), evaluative (E), miscellaneous (M), and Total (T).

REFERENCES

Atkinson, J.H., Kremer, E.F., & Ignelzi, R.J. (1982). Diffusion of pain language with affective disturbance confounds differential diagnosis. *Pain, 12,* 375–384.

Bartko, D., Kondas, M., & Jansco, S. (1984). Quantifica-

tion of pain in neurology. Slovak version of the McGill-Melzack's Questionnaire on pain. *Ceskoslovenska Neurologie a Neurochirurgie, 47,* 113–121.

Beecher, H.K. (1959). *Measurement of subjective responses.* New York: Oxford University Press.

Bejarano, P.F., Noriego, R.D., Rodriquez, M.L. & Berrio, G.M. (1985). Evaluación del dolor: Adaptación del cuestionario de McGill [Evaluation of pain: Adaptation of the McGill Pain Questionnaire]. *Revista Columbia Anestesia, 13,* 321–351.

Bélanger, E., Melzack, R., & Lauzon, P. (1989). Pain of first-trimester abortion: A study of psychosocial and medical predictors. *Pain, 36,* 339–350.

Boureau, F., Luu, M., Doubrère, J.F., & Gay, C. (1984). Elaboration d'un questionnaire d'auto-évaluation de la douleur par liste de qualicatifs [Development of a self-evaluation questionnaire comprising pain descriptors.]. *Thérapie, 39,* 119–129.

Chapman, C.R., Casey, K.L., Dubner, R., Foley, K.M., Gracely, R.H., & Reading, A.E. (1985). Pain measurement: An overview. *Pain, 22,* 1–31.

Charter, R.A., & Nehemkis, A.M. (1983). The language of pain intensity and complexity: New methods of scoring the McGill Pain Questionnaire. *Perceptual and Motor Skills, 56,* 519–537.

Chen, A.C.N., Dworkin, S.F., Haug, J., & Gerhig, J. (1989). Human pain responsivity in a tonic pain model: Psychological determinants. *Pain, 37,* 143–160.

Chen, A.C.N., & Treede, R.D. (1985). McGill Pain Questionnaire in assessing the differentiation of phasic and tonic pain: Behavioral evaluation of the "pain inhibiting pain" effect. *Pain, 22,* 67–79.

Choinière, M., Melzack, R., Girard, N., Rondeau, J., & Paquin, M.J. (1990). Comparisons between patients' and nurses' assessments of pain and medication efficacy in severe burn injuries. *Pain, 40,* 143–153.

Crockett, D.J., Prkachin, K.M., & Craig, K.D. (1977). Factors of the language of pain in patients and normal volunteer groups. *Pain, 4,* 175–182.

De Benedittis, G., Massei, R., Nobili, R., & Pieri, A. (1988). The Italian pain questionnaire. *Pain, 33,* 53–62.

Dubuisson, D., & Melzack, R. (1976). Classification of clinical pain descriptions by multiple group discriminant analysis. *Experimental Neurology, 51,* 480–487.

Ekblom, A., & Hansson, P. (1988). Pain intensity measurements in patients with acute pain receiving afferent stimulation. *Journal of Neurology, Neurosurgery and Psychiatry, 51,* 481–486.

Ferracuti, S., Romeo, G., Leardi, M.G., Cruccu, G., & Lazzari, R. (1990). New Italian adaptation and standardization of the McGill Pain Questionnaire. *Pain (Suppl. 5),* S300.

Graham, C., Bond, S.S., Gerkovich, M.M., & Cook, M.R. (1980). Use of the McGill Pain Questionnaire in the assessment of cancer pain: Replicability and consistency. *Pain, 8,* 377–387.

Grönblad, M., Lukinmaa, A., & Konttinen, Y.T. (1990). Chronic low-back pain: Intercorrelation of repeated measures for pain and disability. *Scandinavian Journal of Rehabilitation Medicine, 22,* 73–77.

Grushka, M., & Sessle, B.J. (1984). Applicability of the McGill Pain Questionnaire to the differentiation of "toothache" pain. *Pain, 19,* 49–57.

Grushka, M., Sessle, B.J., & Miller, R. (1987). Pain and personality profiles in burning mouth syndrome. *Pain, 28,* 155–167.

Guieu, R., Tardy-Gervet, M.F., & Roll, J.P. (1991). Analgesic effects of vibration and transcutaneous electrical nerve stimulation applied separately and simultaneously to patients with chronic pain. *Canadian Journal of Neurological Sciences, 18,* 113–119.

Harrison, A. (1988). Arabic pain words. *Pain, 32,* 239–250.

Hartman, L.M., & Ainsworth, K.D. (1980). Self-regulation of chronic pain. *Canadian Journal of Psychiatry, 25,* 38–43.

Hui, Y.L., & Chen, A.C. (1989). Analysis of headache in a Chinese patient population. *Ma Tsui Hsueh Tsa Chi, 27,* 13–18.

Huskisson, E.C. (1974). Measurement of pain. *Lancet, 2,* 1127–1131.

Huskisson, E.C. (1983). Visual Analogue Scales. In R. Melzack (Ed.), *Pain measurement and assessment* (pp. 33–37). New York: Raven Press.

Jensen, D.M., Karoly, P., & Braver. S. (1986). The measurement of clinical pain intensity: A comparison of six methods. *Pain, 27,* 117–126.

Joyce, C.R.B., Zutshi, D.W., Hrubes, V., & Mason, R.M. (1975). Comparison of fixed interval and Visual Analogue Scales for rating chronic pain. *European Journal of Clinical Pharmacology, 8,* 415–420.

Katz, J., & Melzack, R. (1991). Auricular transcutaneous electrical nerve stimulation (TENS) reduces phantom limb pain. *Journal of Pain & Symptom Management, 6,* 73–83.

Katz, J., & Vadnais, M. (1990). A survey of pain and analgesic use in a physical rehabilitation hospital. *Canadian Pain Society Abstracts,* p. 30.

Ketovuori, H., & Pöntinen, P.J, (1981). A pain vocabulary in Finnish—the Finnish pain questionnaire. *Pain, 11,* 247–253.

Kiss, I., Müller, H., & Abel, M. (1987). The McGill Pain Questionnaire—German version. A study on cancer pain. *Pain, 29,* 195–207.

Klepac, R.K., Dowling, J., Rokke, P., Dodge, L., & Schafer, L. (1981). Interview vs. paper-and-pencil administration of the McGill Pain Questionnaire. *Pain, 11,* 241–246.

Kling, J.W., & Riggs, L.A. (1971). *Experimental psychology.* New York: Holt, Rinehart, & Winston.

Kremer, E., & Atkinson, J.H. (1983). Pain language as a measure of affect in chronic pain patients. In R. Melzack (Ed.), *Pain measurement and assessment* (pp. 119–127) New York: Raven Press.

Kremer, E., Atkinson, J.H., & Ignelzi, R.J. (1982). Pain measurement: The affective dimensional measure of the McGill Pain Questionnaire with a cancer pain population. *Pain, 12,* 153–163.

Laheurta, J., Smith, B.A., & Martinez-Lage, J.L. (1982). An adaptation of the McGill Pain Questionnaire to the Spanish language. *Schmerz, 3,* 132–134.

Leavitt, F., & Garron, D.C. (1980). Validity of a back pain classification scale for detecting psychological disturbance as measured by the MMPI. *Journal of Clinical Psychology, 36,* 186–189.

Leavitt, F., Garron, D.C., Whisler, W.W., & Sheinkop, M.B. (1978). Affective and sensory dimensions of pain. *Pain, 4,* 273–281.

Love, A., Loeboeuf, D.C., & Crisp, T.C. (1989). Chiropractic chronic low back pain sufferers and self-report assessment methods. Part 1. A reliability study of the Visual Analogue Scale, the pain drawing and the McGill Pain Questionnaire. *Journal of Manipulative and Physiological Therapeutics, 12,* 21–25.

Lowe, N.K., Walker, S.N., & McCallum, R.C. (1991). Confirming the theoretical structure of the McGill Pain Questionnaire in acute clinical pain. *Pain, 46,* 53–60.

Maiani, G., & Sanavio, E. (1985). Semantics of pain in Italy: The Italian version of the McGill Pain Questionnaire. *Pain, 22,* 399–405.

Masson, E.A., Hunt, L., Gem., J.M., & Boulton, A.J.M. (1989). A novel approach to the diagnosis and assessment of symptomatic diabetic neuropathy. *Pain, 38,* 25–28.

McCreary, C., Turner, J., & Dawson, E. (1981). Principal dimensions of the pain experience and psychological disturbance in chronic low back pain patients. *Pain, 11,* 85–92.

Melzack, R. (1975). The McGill Pain Questionnaire: Major properties and scoring methods. *Pain, 1,* 277–299.

Melzack, R. (Ed.). (1983). *Pain measurement and assessment.* New York: Raven Press.

Melzack, R. (1987). The short-form McGill Pain Questionnaire. *Pain, 30,* 191–197.

Melzack, R., & Casey, K.L. (1968). Sensory, motivational, and central control determinants of pain: A new conceptual model. In D. Kenshalo (Ed.), *The skin senses* (pp. 423–439). Springfield, IL: Chas C. Thomas.

Melzack, R., Katz, J., & Jeans, M.E. (1985). The role of compensation in chronic pain: Analysis using a new method of scoring the McGill Pain Questionnaire. *Pain, 23,* 101–112.

Melzack, R., Kinch, R., Dobkin, P., Lebrun, M., & Taenzer, P. (1984). Severity of labour pain: Influence of physical as well as psychologic variables. *Canadian Medical Association Journal, 130,* 579–584.

Melzack, R., & Perry, C. (1975). Self-regulation of pain: The use of alpha-feedback and hypnotic training for the control of chronic pain. *Experimental Neurology, 46,* 452–469.

Melzack, R., Taenzer, P., Feldman, P., & Kinch, R.A. (1981). Labour is still painful after prepared childbirth training. *Canadian Medical Association Journal, 125,* 357–363.

Melzack, R., Terrence, C., Fromm, G., & Amsel, R. (1986). Trigeminal neuralgia and atypical facial pain: Use of the McGill Pain Questionnaire for discrimination and diagnosis. *Pain, 27,* 297–302.

Melzack, R., & Torgerson, W.S. (1971). On the language of pain. *Anesthesiology, 34,* 50–59.

Melzack, R., & Wall, P.D. (1988). *The challenge of pain* (2nd ed.). London: Penguin Books.

Melzack, R., Wall, P.D., & Ty, T.C. (1982). Acute pain in an emergency clinic: Latency of onset and description patterns related to different injuries. *Pain, 14,* 33–43.

Ohnhaus, E.E., & Adler, R. (1975). Methodological problems in the measurement of pain: A comparison between the Verbal Rating Scale and the Visual Analogue Scale. *Pain, 1,* 374–384.

Pearce, J., & Morley, S. (1989). An experimental investigation of the construct validity of the McGill Pain Questionnaire. *Pain, 39,* 115–121.

Price, D.D. (1988). *Psychological and neural mechanisms of pain.* New York: Raven Press.

Price, D.D., McGrath, P.A., Rafii, A., & Buckingham, B. (1983). The validation of visual analogue scales as ratio scale measures for chronic and experimental pain. *Pain, 17,* 45–56.

Prieto, E.J., Hopson, L., Bradley, L.A., Byrne, M., Geisinger, K.F., Midax, D., & Marchisello, P.J. (1980). The language of low back pain: Factor structure of the McGill Pain Questionnaire. *Pain, 8,* 11–19.

Radvila, A., Adler, R.H., Galeazzi, R.L., & Vorkauf, H. (1987). The development of a German language (Berne) pain questionnaire and its application in a situation causing acute pain. *Pain, 28,* 185–195.

Reading, A.E. (1979). The internal structure of the McGill Pain Questionnaire in dysmenorrhea patients. *Pain, 7,* 353–358.

Reading, A.E. (1982). An analysis of the language of pain in chronic and acute patient groups. *Pain, 13,* 185–192.

Reading, A.E. (1989). Testing pain mechanisms in persons in pain. In P.D. Wall & R. Melzack (Eds.), *The textbook of pain* (2nd ed., pp. 269–280). Edinburgh: Livingstone Churchill.

Reading, A.E., Everitt, B.S., & Sledmere, C.M. (1982). The McGill Pain Questionnaire: A replication of its construction. *British Journal of Clinical Psychology, 21,* 339–349.

Reading, A.E., & Newton, J.R. (1977). On a comparison of dysmenorrhea and intrauterine device related pain. *Pain, 3,* 265–276.

Satow, A., Nakatani, K., Taniguchi, S., & Higashiyama, A. (1990). Perceptual characteristics of electrocutaneous pain estimated by the 30-word list and Visual Analog Scale. *Japanese Psychological Review, 32,* 155–164.

Sedlak, K. (1990). A Polish version of the McGill Pain Questionnaire. *Pain (Suppl. 5),* S308.

Solcová, I., Jakoubek, B., Sýkora, J., & Hnïk, P. (1990). Characterization of vertebrogenic pain using the short form of the McGill Pain Questionnaire. *Casopis Lekaru Ceskych, 129,* 1611–1614.

Sriwatanakul, K., Kelvie, W., Lasagna, L., Calimlin, J.F., Weis, O.F., & Mehta, G. (1983). Studies with different types of Visual Analog Scales for measurement of pain. *Clinical Pharmacology and Therapeutics, 34,* 234–239.

Stein, C., & Mendl, G. (1988). The German counterpart to McGill Pain Questionnaire. *Pain, 32,* 251–255.

Strand, L.I., & Wisnes, A.R. (1991). The development of a Norwegian pain questionnaire. *Pain, 46,* 61–66.

Tahmoush, A.J. (1981). Causalgia: Redefinition as a clinical pain syndrome. *Pain, 10,* 187–197.

Turk, D.C., Rudy, T.E., & Salovey, P. (1985). The McGill Pain Questionnaire reconsidered: Confirming the factor structures and examining appropriate uses. *Pain, 21,* 385–397.

Van Buren, J., & Kleinknecht, R. (1979). An evaluation of the McGill Pain Questionnaire for use in dental pain assessment. *Pain, 6,* 23–33.

Vanderiet, K., Adriaensen, H., Carton, H., & Vertommen, H. (1987). The McGill Pain Questionnaire constructed for the Dutch language (MPQ-DV). Preliminary data concerning reliability and validity. *Pain, 30,* 395–408.

Veilleux, S., & Melzack, R. (1976). Pain in psychotic patients. *Experimental Neurology, 52,* 535–563.

Verkes, R.J., Van der Kloot, W.A., & Van der Meij, J. (1989). The perceived structure of 176 pain descriptive words. *Pain, 38,* 219–229.

Wilke, D.J., Savedra, M.C., Holzemer, W.L., Tesler, M.D., & Paul, S.M. (1990). Use of the McGill Pain Questionnaire to measure pain: A meta-analysis. *Nursing Research, 39,* 36–41.

Chapter 11

Psychophysiological Recording Methods

HERTA FLOR, PhD
WOLFGANG MILTNER, PhD
NIELS BIRBAUMER, PhD

In the past decades, psychophysiological assessment methods have gained importance for both somatic and psychological disorders (Turpin, 1989). They are primarily used as a tool to determine the influence of psychological factors on bodily functioning, and specifically, to assess their contribution to the initiation and maintenance of symptoms. In many chronic pain syndromes as well as in acute pain states psychophysiological factors play a major role in the development and/or maintenance of the problem (e.g., Flor, 1991, in press; Flor, Birbaumer, & Turk, 1990; Miltner, Birbaumer, & Gerber, 1986). This chapter provides an overview of the role of psychophysiological assessments in both clinical and laboratory pain and suggests a framework for the integration of psychophysiological assessment data within the comprehensive interdisciplinary assessment and treatment of pain. The chapter is divided into two parts: the first discusses peripheral psychophysiological measures that are of primary importance in the assessment of chronic pain syndromes, while the second focuses on central psychophysiological measures that are primarily used in laboratory pain studies.

First attempts to assess psychophysiological concomitants of pain were undertaken in the 1950s (e.g., Malmo, Shagass, & Davis, 1950) but became more accepted in the 1960s when biofeedback methods came into wider use. Over the past 20 years much evidence for the interaction of psychological and physiological variables in pain has been accumulated (Wall & Melzack, 1989), and thus psychophysiological concepts of pain have gained importance (Keefe & Gil, 1986). The quality of the measurements has been enhanced due to significant progress made in electronics and computer technology. Despite these advances, much of the research related to the psychophysiology of pain still lacks adequate theoretical foundation and methodological rigor (Flor & Turk, 1989). Thus, few conclusive results have been obtained with respect to the psychophysiology of pain.

Psychophysiological data serve a number of useful functions in the assessment of chronic and acute pain states. They provide evidence on the role of psychological factors in maladaptive physiological functioning in specific patients. Moreover, results of psychophysiological recordings may be used for the differential indication of intervention methods. For example, we (Flor & Birbaumer, 1991) have used psychophysiological responses to personal and general stress in order to classify patients into biofeedback responders versus responders to operant or cognitive behavior therapy. Psychophysiological assessments, are, moreover, a necessary prerequisite for the use of biofeedback treatment. Psychophysiological measurements during treatment and posttreatment help to document the efficacy of the intervention as well as generalization and transfer. They may also serve as predictors of treatment outcome (Blanchard et al., 1983). Another important aspect of psychophysiological measurements is their motivational character. The patients may learn from the results that they are able to influence bodily processes by their own thoughts, emotions, and actions. Thus, feelings of helplessness may be reduced and the acceptance of psychological interventions may be increased not only in the patients but also in referring physicians to whom psychophysiological assessment data should be made available. In experimental pain research, psychophysiological data have been used to examine physiological concomitants of anxiety and general arousal associated with pain, and they have served as measures of central processes related to the pain experience (see section on EEG recordings).

PERIPHERAL MEASURES IN THE ASSESSMENT OF PAIN

Electromyography

Basic Issues

Elevated levels of muscle tension have been discussed as an etiological factor in a number of chronic pain syndromes (tension headache or temporomandibular pain and dysfunction). Furthermore, it has been assumed that in any type of pain syndrome, reflex muscle spasm may develop that further increases pain (Zimmermann, 1984). Thus, the surface electromyogram (EMG) is a frequently used psychophysiological parameter with chronic pain patients. In order to obtain EMG measures, muscle action potentials summed over a large area of the muscle are recorded as a voltage difference between adjacent sites. In contrast to a neuro-

logical EMG that mainly serves the purpose of testing the function of motor neurons, psychophysiological EMG assessments are designed to record muscle tension that may contribute to the pain experience. EMG evaluations are especially indicated for musculoskeletal pain syndromes such as chronic back pain, headache, or pain in the jaw region.

Several aspects of muscular function may be measured: elevated baseline levels, asymmetry of bilateral muscle tension, hyperreactivity to physical or psychological stress, time to return to baseline post stress, or irregularities during movement (Dolce & Razcynski, 1985; Flor & Turk, 1989; Nouwen & Bush, 1984). These characteristics may be present by themselves or they may appear in combination. It must be noted that a causal role of muscular dysfunctions has so far not been demonstrated for pain disorders. There is, however, conclusive evidence that pain may be maintained or exacerbated by increases in muscle tension (Borgeat, Hade, Elie, & Larouche, 1984; Christensen, 1986a, 1986b).

Whereas previously the m. frontalis has most often been the target of measurements—based on the assumption that generalized hyperarousal is present in chronic pain patients—today more emphasis is placed on localized increases in muscle tension levels. Therefore, measurements tend to be site-specific: the masseter and temporalis muscles are used with patients who suffer from chronic temporomandibular pain and dysfunction, the m. erector spinae in lower back pain patients, the m. trapezius in upper back pain patients, the m. splenius capitis, m. occipitalis, m. trapezius, or m. frontalis for muscle tension headache. There has also been a trend to assess several muscle groups at the same time because this procedure yields information on the prime location of increased tension and permits an assessment of the generality or specificity of the response.

Methodological Considerations

Most physiological signals are quite weak and thus need sufficient amplification. The amplification factor of the EMG is usually around 1 $\times 10^5$. A too low amplification leads to misinterpretations of the signal because relevant EMG changes may not be detected (Cobb, deVries, Urban, Leukens, & Bagg, 1975). Due to the high "noise" level that is present in unshielded clinical settings where most assessments are made, differential amplifiers with a high common mode rejection (80–100 dB) are required. Thus, signals are suppressed that act symmetrically on the electrodes and would lead to artifacts. It is necessary that the impedance between the surface of the skin and the electrode not exceed 10 kΩ. The use of nonpolarizing Ag/AgCl electrodes is recommended. Amplifiers with very high imput impedance allow for less strict skin preparation and permit the use of lower quality electrodes (see section on Muscle Scanning below). The amplifiers need to have an adequate filtering range. Many biofeedback machines have a range of 100–200 Hz only, which is not sufficient for EMG dysfunction assessment. As was shown by Cram and Garber (1986), such a limited signal range leads to an underestimation of true activity in the muscles tested and thus to incorrect treatment decisions.

The raw EMG signal must be processed in order to receive adequate information about the state of muscle tension. Usually a root mean square integrated EMG is calculated from the raw data. It is important not to use too long integration intervals because these will then disguise artifacts related to movements or other intrusions in the recording process. The raw EMG should always be displayed in order to detect artifacts. Another important aspect is the sampling rate of the signal. It must be at least two times higher than the highest frequency of the signal. If this requirement is not met, the signal will be distorted (''aliasing''). Cheaper biofeedback equipment usually does not have this high-speed sampling capability. Further details on recording sites, skin preparation and further technical considerations may be found in Basmajian (1986), Coles, Gratton, Kramer, and Miller (1986), Fridlund and Cacioppo (1986), and Venables and Martin (1967).

Resting Baseline Levels

In their critical review of 60 psychophysiological studies on chronic headache, back pain, and temporomandibular pain and dysfunction, Flor and Turk (1989) noted that elevated resting baseline levels have sometimes been found, but they are not necessarily characteristic of chronic pain patients. Overall, the evidence for permanently elevated baseline levels in patients suffering from chronic muscu-

loskeletal pain problems has been scarce. Although normative data for the EMG levels of various muscle groups have been established (e.g., Cram, 1988, 1990; Matheson, Toben, & de la Cruz, 1988), resting baseline levels must be interpreted with caution. Elevated levels may not always be considered as abnormal, nor may low values be interpreted as normal. Even though low baseline levels may be present, abnormal responses may be detected during movement or during psychological or physical stress. On the other hand, Wolf, Wolf, and Segal (1989) have shown that resting values may be inflated by slight changes in posture that are difficult to control. There are also doubts about the reliability of measurement in certain muscle groups (e.g., Arena, Blanchard, Andrasik, Cotch, & Myers, 1983), although the assessment of low back muscle tension in different postures has been demonstrated as reliable (Arena, Sherman, Bruno, & Young 1990).

Stress Reactivity

A possibly more important physiological parameter than the baseline value is the reactivity of the muscle during physical or psychological stress. The EMG is assessed while the person is exposed to a somatic (e.g., a certain body position, writing on the typewriter) or a psychological stressor (e.g., stressful imagery, discussion of an emotionally involving event). The stressor should have personal relevance for the person. The superiority of personally relevant stressors has been demonstrated in various experiments (e.g., Arntz, Merckelbach, Peters, & Schmidt, 1991; Dickson-Parnell & Zeichner, 1988; Flor, Turk, & Birbaumer, 1985; Thompson & Adams, 1984). Several studies have also shown that the EMG stress response is symptom-specific. In patients with chronic back pain the erector spinae muscles are most responsive to stress and in patients with temporomandibular pain and dysfunction the masseter muscle is most reactive, but not vice versa (Flor, Birbaumer, Schugens, & Lutzenberger, in press). In stress reactivity assessments the question of norms and criteria for a stress response is still open. The best procedure is to employ both neutral and general as well as stressful stimuli and to assess person-specific differences in the response to all three types of stimuli.

Overall, a number of empirical studies have

shown symptom-specific EMG hyperreactivity in chronic back pain (Arntz et al., 1991; Fischer & Chang, 1985; Flor et al., in press; Flor et al., 1985; Peters & Schmidt, 1991; Soderberg & Barr, 1983). Similar results have been obtained for temporomandibular pain and dysfunction (Dahlstrom, 1989; Dahlstrom, Carlsson, Gale, & Jansson, 1985; Flor, Birbaumer, Schulte, & Roos, 1991; Kapel, Glaros, & McGlynn, 1989; Mercuri, Olson, & Laskin, 1979; Thomas, Tiber, & Schireson, 1983; Yemm, 1969). There is also convincing evidence that symptom-specific responses are present in chronic headache patients. In 29 of 37 studies that were reviewed by Flor and Turk (1989), at least one significant difference was found with respect to the muscular reactivity of headache patients as compared to healthy controls. Significant differences were especially present if the EMG was recorded from several muscles and personal relevant stressors (e.g., socially involving situations) were used (e.g., Arena, Blanchard, Andrasik, Appelbaum, & Myers, 1985; Bischof, Traue, & Zenz, 1982; Cohen et al., 1983; Kröner, 1984; Thompson & Adams, 1984; Traue, Bischoff, & Zenz, 1985; Traue, Gottwald, Henderson, & Bakal, 1985). It must be noted that the reactivity is symptom specific and not general, as has been shown by the assessment of additional physiological parameters, such as heart rate, blood pressure, and skin conductance.

Return to Baseline

An additional parameter, the time to return to baseline after the induction and termination of a stressor, has so far not been sufficiently assessed. Traue, Gottwald et al. (1985) as well as Pritchard and Wood (1984) reported a slower return to baseline of the trapezius and frontalis EMG in patients with chronic tension headache; however, these results could not be replicated in other studies (cf. Feuerstein, Bush, & Corbisiero, 1982; Kröner, 1984). Flor and Turk (1989) presented a detailed analysis of the methodological problems as well as suggestions for improved recording methods.

Posture and Dynamic Movement

Wolf and Basmajian (1978) reported that patients with chronic back pain often show abnormal static posture. Similar results have been noted by Cram and Engstrom (1986). How-

ever, so far it is not known if the changes in posture maintain pain problems, elicit them, or if they are a mere consequence of the pain and an adaptation in posture. There seem to be differences in posture-related EMG based on diagnostic subgroups. Arena, Sherman, Bruno, and Young (1989, 1991) showed that although patients with low back pain display higher EMG levels in a standing position, patients with intervertebral disk disorder are significantly different from other back pain patients and healthy controls; therefore they display significantly higher tension levels. This points to the necessity of a differential diagnostic assessment in these patients, and on the other hand supports the assumption that these postural EMG abnormalities may be of a reactive nature.

Wolf, Nacht, and Kelly (1982) as well as Wolf et al. (1989) have reported the presence of abnormal patterns of movement in patients with chronic back pain. Based on these results, the authors suggested to correct these posture and movement abnormalities by a specific biofeedback training (Jones & Wolf, 1980; Wolf et al., 1982). However, there have not been any controlled studies related to the efficacy of this procedure.

Muscle Scanning

EMG scanning is a quick and easy method to detect abnormal levels of muscle activity in chronic pain patients (Cram & Engstrom, 1986; Cram & Steger, 1983). Using hand-held electrodes, 22 muscle sites may be scanned in about 15 minutes. Bilateral recordings in a sitting and standing posture with scan times of at least 2 seconds are suggested. The values obtained are then compared to normative integrated EMG values from healthy controls. Due to the use of high quality differential amplifiers the necessity of extensive skin abrasion is reduced. Test–retest reliability (Cram, Lloyd, & Cahn, 1989; Thompson, Erickson, Madson, & Offord, 1989) and validity (Thompson, Madson, & Erickson, 1991) of the measurements have been demonstrated. As noted above, the relationship of these elevated EMG levels to pain and psychological antecedents of pain has not been clarified, and thus the value of EMG scanning for the selection of psychological intervention methods still needs to be determined.

Relationship of EMG and Pain Intensity

It is important to note that pain intensity and EMG levels are usually not systematically correlated at any given point in time (Arena et al., 1991; Chapman et al., 1985). It has, however, been shown that an elevation of muscle tension over an extended period of time leads to pain induction or an enhancement of already existing pain in the facial, back, or head muscles (e.g., Borgeat et al., 1984; Christensen, 1986a, 1986b; Flor, in press). In order to understand the relationship of pain and EMG levels better, extended EMG assessments with concurrent assessment of pain levels are necessary, preferably by using ambulatory monitoring devices. First attempts in this direction have been made by Sherman, Arena, Sherman, and Ernst (1989) in patients with phantom limb pain, by Sherman, Arena, Searle, and Ginther (in press) in chronic back pain patients, and by Schlote (1989) with headache patients. Several studies have provided evidence that pain may be induced by experimentally produced increases of muscle tension (e.g., Bakke, Tfelt-Hansen, Olson, & Moller, 1982; Borgeat et al., 1984), and that there may be lag times of several days between the increase of muscle tension and the induction of pain (e.g., Feuerstein, Bortolussi, Houle, & Labbé, 1983).

Cardiovascular measures

Cardiovascular parameters seem to be of little relevance in pain syndromes of musculoskeletal nature. They may, however, play a major role in vascular pain problems such as migraine headache or Raynaud's disease, as well as in pain syndromes related to sympathetic dysfunction such as sympathetic reflex dystrophies. They have also been used in laboratory investigations with acute pain stimuli. Several methods are available to assess cardiovascular parameters: the electrocardiogram to measure heart rate, photoplethysmography, laser, or sonographic Doppler flowmetry to assess changes in blood flow; thermistor recordings or thermography to measure changes in skin temperature; and blood pressure recordings.

Measures of Blood Flow

Photoplethysmography involves the measurement of the volume of blood vessels by the use of a light source directed at the vessel and a photo-sensitive plate that records the reflected light. When blood flow increases, the saturation with red blood cells increases and less light is reflected. Tonic measurements involve the changes in blood flow over time (blood volume recordings); phasic measurements are related to beat-to-beat variations in the force of flow (pulse volume recordings). Both blood and pulse volume are reduced with certain emotional responses (e.g., Coles, Donchin, & Porges, 1986; Venables & Martin, 1967). Photoplethysmographic measures have, however, the disadvantage that they can only display relative changes in volume, not absolute values.

Changes in blood volume are of special interest in migraine headaches based on etiological theories that assume an important role of vasomotor processes in the development of pain. Comparable to the results of EMG recordings in patients with tension headache, most controlled studies did not find baseline differences in vascular parameters in migraine patients as compared to healthy controls (for a summary see Flor & Turk, 1989). It was interesting to note that few specific differences with respect to EMG baseline values and vascular parameters have been reported for the different types of headaches (e.g., Arena et al., 1985). In migraine patients, migraine attacks could even be elicited by inducing spasms in the head muscles (Bakke et al., 1982). The authors report a high correlation between the onset of pain and peaks in EMG readings. This finding suggests that in migraine pain a muscular component may be relevant as well.

Studies on the stress reactivity in migraine patients point toward a functional abnormality of the major head arteries, particularly the temporal artery, especially if personal relevant stressors were used (e.g., Arena et al., 1985; Bakal & Kaganov, 1977; Drummond, 1982; Rojahn & Gerhards, 1986). The empirical results with respect to a slower return to baseline after stressors are controversial (see Flor & Turk, 1989, for a summary). Photoplethysmography of the temporal artery in migraine patients was used in several studies as a biofeedback and assessment method. Patients were trained to reduce vascular contraction in order to block excessive dilation shortly before and during attacks (see Miltner et al., 1986, for a review).

Magerl, Geldner, and Handwerker (1990) have presented data that indicate that peripheral sympathetic reflexes related to noxious stimulation as measured by photoplethysmography may be valid indicators of painful experiences. This method is also useful in assessing the influence of the sympathetic nerve system on local blood flow in sympathetic reflex dystrophy (Blumberg, 1988; Wallin, 1989). Measurement of regional cerebral blood flow revealed that acute pain stimulation is associated with increased cerebral blood flow only when anxiety related to pain is increased at the same time (Ryding, Eriksson, Rosen, & Ingvar, 1985). Similarly, Talbot et al. (1991) demonstrated localized (primary and secondary somatosensory cortex, anterior gyrate cingulus) increases in cerebral blood flow by the use of positron emission tomography (PET) scans combined with magnetic resonance imaging (MRI).

Measurement of blood flow velocity with ultrasound Doppler sonography in migraine reveals abnormally increased flow velocity after presentation of stressful stimuli in migraine sufferers, but not in controls. Doppler sonography uses high-frequency sound waves (above 20 kHz, for large vessels 4–5 MHz) directed toward the vessel. The frequency of the reflection of the two slightly distant sound sources is proportional to the blood flow velocity (Anliker, Casty, Friedl, Kubli, & Keller, 1977). Recently, laser Doppler flowmetry has been introduced as an alternative method (e.g., Magerl, Szolcsanyi, Westerman, & Handwerker, 1987). First attempts to use the Doppler principle as a biofeedback device for assessment and treatment of migraine were reported by our group (Fuchs, Gerber, Birbaumer, & Miltner, 1985).

The interpretation of vascular parameters in clinical practice may be problematic because the signals are very much prone to artifact. Body temperature, the temperature of the environment, or the position of the body may all influence the recordings.

Skin Temperature

Skin temperature is largely dependent on peripheral circulation. Vasoconstriction is associated with lower and vasodilation with higher skin temperature. Usually, temperature-sensitive thermistors are used that measure temperature changes and convert them to changes in electrical resistance. However, recordings with thermistors are very prone to artifact, especially because they are easily disturbed by slight changes in temperature or air circulation in a room. Skin temperature does respond to stress. This is of special relevance in Raynaud's disease, which is associated with pain related to cold extremities. In a series of studies, Freedman and his coworkers (e.g., Freedman & Ianni, 1983; Freedman, Mayes, & Sabbarwal, 1989) were able to show that emotional as well as physical stressors lead to more local vasoconstriction in patients who suffer from Raynaud's disease than in healthy controls. Consequently, temperature biofeedback has proven to be a very efficient treatment method (Freedman, 1991).

Although temperature biofeedback has often been used with migraine patients the usefulness of temperature recordings has not yet been demonstrated for migraine headaches. The procedure is based on the observation that migraine attacks may improve with hand-warming biofeedback in attack-free periods. The studies that assessed the role of temperature and temperature reactivity in migraine headaches have not provided empirical evidence for a specific role in the therapeutic effect (for a summary, see Chapman, 1986; Flor & Turk, 1989).

In thermography, infrared photography of the body surface is used to measure vascular abnormalities related to pain. Abnormally high as well as low tempertures may be associated with pain. Thermography has been widely used as an assessment instrument as well as in the documentation of treatment-related changes (e.g., Fergason, 1964; Uematsu, Hendeler, & Hungerford, 1981). Thermography is especially used in the asssessment of pain caused by inflammatory processes such as in rheumatoid arthritis (Collins, Ring, Bacon, & Brookshaw 1976). Its usefulness as a psychophysiological research method has not yet been adequately assessed. Thermographic recordings tended to suffer from inadequate analyses and may have little specificity (Mills, Davies, Getty, & Coney, 1986), although computerized thermographic recordings have yielded more reliable results (Handwerker, Geldner, & Magerl, 1989).

From a psychophysiological perspective, thermographic recordings have been used in the analysis of facial temperature in migraine patients. For example, Drummond and Lance (1984) did not find resting baseline differences in facial temperature between migraine patients and healthy controls; they reported, however, lower temperature in the migraine patients following pressure on the temporal artery. Thus, reactivity measures might be a better indicator of dysfunction than resting levels and should be studied more carefully.

Heart Rate and Blood Pressure

The recording of heart rate is often used in psychophysiology because it is a very easy to measure parameter. Usually, the number of R-waves of the ECG is converted into beats per minute. Although frequently used in acute laboratory pain assessments, there is little research on the relationship of heart rate and chronic pain, and even less research on the relationship of blood pressure and chronic pain. Most of the research avaliable is inconclusive. For example, Collins, Cohen, Nahiboff, and Schandler (1982) as well as Flor et al. (1985) reported no differences in heart rate during resting baseline or during various stressors (brief cold pressor, mental math, discusion of personally relevant stress and pain episodes) between chronic back pain patients and healthy controls. On the other hand, Arntz et al. (1991) found lower heart rate reactivity to an extended cold pressor test, Flor et al. (in press) noted lower heart rate reactivity to personally relevant stress images in chronic back pain patients compared to healthy controls, and Kapel, Glaros, and McGlynn (1989) also reported less reactivity in patients with temperomandibular pain dysfunction compared to healthy controls. Both Arntz et al. (1991) and Flor et al. (in press) interpreted these findings as indicative of a lack of active coping in the patients as compared to the controls. This hypothesis is based on Obrist's (1976) findings of a coupling of somatic and cardiovascular responses during active and a decoupling during passive coping. This assumption is corroborated by the high negative correlation between heart rate reactivity and passive coping (catastrophizing) reported by Flor (in press).

Heart rate has also frequently been used as a physiological correlate of acute pain intensity (Sternbach, 1968). However, increases in tonic heart rate have been related more to subjective pain ratings than objective characteristics of the nociceptive stimulus (cf. Hampf, 1990; Moltner, Hölzl, & Strian, 1990).

In studies of postoperative pain cardiovascular measures have been used to document the effects of postoperative pain as well as the favorable effects of psychological interventions. Both blood pressure and heart rate reductions have been reported in patients who underwent psychological coping training as compared to patients not involved in these procedures (Flor & Birbaumer, 1990).

In experimental pain studies, a negative correlation of blood pressure and pain experience has been established for subjects with elevated tonic blood pressure, whereas this correlation is positive for normotensives (Birbaumer, Dworkin, Elbert, & Rockstroh, 1987; Larbig, Elbert, Rockstroh, Lutzenberger, & Birbaumer, 1985). The induction of elevated blood pressure levels by the use of baroreceptor stimulation leads to a reduction in pain sensitivity in borderline hypertensives and to an increase of pain sensitivity in normotensives (Elbert et al., 1988; Rockstroh et al., 1988).

Skin Conductance Measures

Skin conductance may be viewed as a measure of general arousal. It changes with the activation of the sweat glands, which are responsive to psychological stimuli (Fowles, 1986). Their activity is mediated by the sympathetic nervous system. An often used parameter of the sympathetic activity of the skin is the tonic skin conductance level or the phasic skin conductance response. Acute pain is associated with both increased heart rate and skin conductance levels (Dowling, 1982; Sternbach, 1968). In certain pain syndromes autonomic dysfunction seems to be of some importance, for example, in reflex sympathetic dystrophy or phantom limb pain. Here, measures of the activity of the sympathetic system such as skin conductance level seem indicated (Cronin & Kirshner, 1982; Howe, 1983). However, results on the significance in skin conductance measures for chronic pain have been controversial. Collins et al. (1982) and Peters and Schmidt (1991) reported increased skin conductance levels in response to stress in low back pain patients, but these results were not confirmed by Flor et al. (1985, in press). Both Jamner and Tursky (1987) and Salamy, Wolk, and Shukard (1983) reported that pain patients show increased electrodermal activity in response to words that are relevant to their pain syndrome. The authors' suggestion to use this measure in the detection of deception in medicolegal cases has not yet been realized.

Overall, responses to painful stimuli seem to be associated with characteristic peripheral physiological responses in the muscular, vascular, as well as the eccrine system (e.g., Myrtek & Spital, 1986). Further research is needed to determine the role of peripheral psychophysiological variables in both chronic and acute pain.

Recommendations

Based on the methodological suggestions made by Flor and Turk (1989), several guidelines for the assessment of psychophysiological variables in chronic pain syndromes may be established. First, the type of pain problem should be clearly described and a differential diagnosis should be made. Psychophysiological measurements should be tailored to the assumed etiology of the pain problem. Thus, EMG recordings seem to be of primary importance in chronic musculoskeletal pain problems, vascular measures in migraine headaches and Raynaud's disease, and vascular combined with skin conductance measures in nerve-related pain syndromes. As we do not yet know enough about the role of symptom-specific and general arousal in chronic pain patients, at least one specific and one general activation measure (skin conductance, heart rate) should be used.

Recordings from several muscles seem to be especially important because several muscles may be involved in the disorder. In addition, recordings from a distal site should be made because this allows conclusions about the site-specificity of the dysfunction and again has treatment implications. Recordings should not only be made in a resting state, but several psychological and physical stressors should be introduced. For chronic back pain patients this might, for example, involve recordings of the EMG during the discussion or imagery of stressful life events as well as the assumption of different postures that may contribute to the pain problem. The relevance of the stressor for the patient should be assessed by the use of stress ratings and or general activation measures.

Sufficient adaptation to the laboratory situation (about 15 minutes) and sufficiently long intertrial intervals (5–10 minutes) are required to allow for measures to return to baseline. Pretrial baselines should be recorded in order to take into account resting baseline changes due to different postures or lack of return to baseline on previous trials. Patients should refrain from taking analgesic and muscle-relaxing medication at least on the day of the assessment.

Following Dolce and Raczynski (1985), we recommend that EMG assessments should be accompanied by the recording of autonomic responses in order to identify patients who are generally overaroused and could profit from nonspecific stress management and relaxation. In patients with specific local dysfunctions such as heightened stress reactivity of the back muscles or heightened vascular reactivity of the extremities specific biofeedback is indicated (e.g., Flor & Birbaumer, 1991; Freedman, 1991). It has been shown that feedback that includes stress exposure has a more favorable outcome than feedback that is only aimed at resting levels (e.g., Freedman, Ianni, & Wenig, 1983). Laboratory measures should be supplemented by field recordings in the natural environment with portable equipment using radio telemetry (Schlote, 1989).

Case Study

The following case is presented in order to demonstrate the integration of verbal–subjective, somatic–motor, and physiological–organic data into a comprehensive assessment profile that allows for specific treatment prescriptions.

Mr. X, a 55-year-old married blue-collar worker with a high school diploma attended the pain ambulance with a complaint of facial pain. The pain had begun 5 years ago when he was involved in an accident at his work site. Since then his ability to work was greatly reduced (frequent days missed at work) and he was informed that he might lose his job, although the patient was quite willing to work. After a comprehensive pain interview the following assessment instruments were used: West Haven–Yale Multidimensional Pain Inventory (Kerns, Turk, & Rudy, 1985), Pain-Related Self-Statements and Pain-Related Convictions of Control Scales (Flor & Turk, 1988), Brief Stress Questionnaire (Flor, in press), and the Tubingen Pain Behavior Check List (Flor & Birbaumer, 1991).

The analysis of the questionnaires and the interview data indicated that the patient's pain and interference level were very high compared to other pain clinic patients. Both affective distress and depression scores were low. Life control as well as active coping with the pain were low; tendencies to catastrophize and to assume a helpless attitude toward the pain were high. Mr X's spouse was supportive but showed little tendency to reinforce pain behaviors that were overall unremarkable. The patient experienced a high level of stress in his everyday life. He also noticed that anger or stress—especially at the work site—increased his pain. Additional factors that influenced the pain were heat and cold, changes in light, changes in mood, and high levels of concentration on a task. Overall, the patient attemped to ignore the pain or to control it by rest and medication (narcotic and antidepressant). He reported sleep disturbances he attributed to the pain. The patient seemed to be eager to work despite of his incapacitating pain problem.

The psychophysiological assessment consisted of bilateral EMG measurements at the m. masseter, the m. frontalis, and the m. trapezius, and the recording of heart rate and skin conductance level. Following a 10-minute adaptation and a 2-minute baseline the patient imagined personally relevant pain and stress situations, and a neutral situation, participated in extended (10 minutes) mental arithmetic and a 10-minute movement task. Each phase had 1-minute pre- and postbaseline recordings.

The resting values of the m. masseter, the m. trapezius, and the m. frontalis were significantly elevated (EMG values > μV) with a marked asymmetry especially at the m. frontalis (related to damage during the accident). EMG levels at other sites as well as heart rate and skin conductance levels were not remarkable.

During *stress testing* a marked response to the stressors was noted with a very high reactivity for the pain episode. Overall, the assessment revealed that the patient showed elevated facial muscle tension levels both in the resting state and during exposure to relevant stressors as compared to healthy controls. These increases in muscle tension are most likely a reaction to the pain problem, which was additionally exacerbated and maintained by them. This elevated tension also extended to the upper back, but not to the m. erector spinae.

Based on these findings the primary goal of the treatment was viewed as the reduction of tension in the relevant muscles and the alteration of the patient's response to aversive stimulation. The patient received EMG-biofeedback training that focused on alternative ways of dealing with stressful situations. The patient imagined the aversive situations and simultaneously observed his EMG response in the m. masseter and a "control" muscle of the lower back. Real-life exposure such as aggressive verbalization of the therapist was also combined with the task of bringing the EMG response of the masseter back to the normal levels of the "control" muscle as quickly as possible. Homework included the recording of stress episodes, the patient's response to them, and the generation of alternate responses.

CENTRAL MEASURES OF THE PAIN EXPERIENCE

Since the mid-1960s, researchers and clinicians have become interested in the use of spontaneous brain electrical activities (spontaneous electroencephalogram, EEG) and event-related potentials (ERPs) as additional tools in the assessment of pain. The ideas of EEG and ERPs and their clinical use in the field of pain assessment will be presented.

Spontaneous EEG recordings

It is now widely accepted that the EEG reflects fluctuations of voltages caused by changes of the summed ionic currents of the many billions of pyramidal cells of the cerebral cortex (Birbaumer & Schmidt, 1990; Lutzenberger, Elbert, Rockstroh, & Birbaumer, 1985; Martin, 1985; Miltner, 1989). Their dendrites in the apical layers (layers I and II) of the cerebral cortex and their soma in the deeper brain structures (i.e., layers III–V) generate an electrical dipole when there is input from nonspecific thalamic structures or from the commissures or different parts of the association cortex. Thousands of pyramidal cells are simultaneously activated when the cortex is processing nonspecific thalamic input and the input from external or internal stimuli. These simulataneously active cells (modules) are structured strictly in a parallel order. Thus, the electrical field potentials of these modules sum up to large electrical field potentials that can be measured intracranially and also extracranially, that is, by the EEG. The amplitude of the EEG is attenuated by the skull and the scalp so that the normal EEG activity recorded from external electrodes ranges somewhere between 5 and 100 μV.

The EEG power spectrum provides a measure of the relative "power" of the EEG waves within a certain frequency band. Usually the bands delta (0.5–3.5 Hz: profound sleep and pathology), theta (3.5–7.5 Hz: deep sleep but also focused attention if localized in the frontal area), alpha (8–12 Hz: relaxed wakefulness with eyes closed), and beta (13–30 Hz: eyes open, attentive) are discriminated.

Studies investigating the ongoing EEG while subjects experience pain were aimed primarily at finding cortical correlates of different procedures of pain control. Within this context EEG recordings are used as cortical correlates of pharmacological or psychological pain treatments such as analgesic agents, general anesthetics, or hypnotically induced states of trance and relaxation. Interestingly, only a few studies were concerned with the investigation of the frequency characteristics of the spontaneous EEG in chronic pain patients or subjects exposed to experimental pain.

EEG and the Diagnosis of Pain

Using acute dental pain as a model, Chen, Dworkin, and Drangsholt (1983) evaluated the cortical power spectral density of the EEG. The EEG of patients with severe acute dental pain was recorded for 10 minutes before dental treatment and compared to a 10-minute epoch obtained 1 week later when patients were pain free. Subjective pain reports and other physiological measures before and after the EEG recording supplemented the data. Results of the fast Fourier transform function showed significant cortical power spectral density *reductions* in all frequency bands ranging from 0.5 to 50 Hz when pain states were compared to nonpain states. The assessment of the relation between the subjective pain reports and the magnitude of the freqency reduction revealed that pain and alpha blocking are closely associated. A further study of the ongoing EEG power spectral density used cold-pressor pain as a model. Chen, Dworkin, Haug, and Gehrig (1989) demonstrated significant differences in the cortical power spectral densities of painful and nonpainful stages with significantly *heightened delta* and beta power densities for painful stages. Subjects were divided into two groups; that is, into one group with pain-tolerant subjects and a group of pain-sensitive subjects, as defined by tolerance of cold-pressor exposure. While exposed to the cold-pressor stimulus, pain-sensitive subjects had significantly higher delta power than the pain-tolerant subjects, but showed no sign of increased beta. It was concluded that hightened delta activity may reflect the aversive component of this tonic pain experience, whereas beta is related to vigilance scanning.

EEG and Analgesic Treatments

Another series of experiments compared the EEG power spectral densities of subjects undergoing various analgesic treatments with that of drug-free baseline epochs. These studies suggest that analgesic pain control is associated with a significant reduction of power spectral density. In a placebo-controlled, double-blind repeated measures design that applied 1000 mg of acetylsalicylic acid (ASA) or placebo, Bromm, Rundshage, and Scharein (in press) demonstrated a significant reduction of pain-induced delta power compared to placebo. No changes were observed in other frequency bands. However, no effects were observed within the same subjects in the power spectral densities of the ongoing EEG following auditory stimuli while under ASA compared to placebo. Pain was induced by a brief electrical stimulus of 10 ms duration. This type of stimulation does not produce inflammatory effects on subdermal peripheral nociceptive structures. Therefore, Bromm et al. claimed a central action of ASA. Significant changes in the EEG spectral density function were seen for somatosensory painful electrical stimuli when subjects received ASA but not when they were stimulated auditorily. Thus, ASA clearly has a modality-specific action and acts not through a general impact on higher nervous system structures. In another study similar effects on the EEG power spectra densities were found for the nonnarcotic analgesic flupirtin and the opioid pentazocine (Bromm, Ganzel, Herrmann, Meier, & Scharein, 1987).

To summarize these studies, pain control by analgesics is associated with an decrease of delta and theta activity and a concurrent reduction of alpha activity. Furthermore, strong analgesics such as pentazocine and pethidine have a general arousal-reducing effect that is associated with relaxation and drowsiness in healthy subjects. Flupirtine and ASA differ from these strong analgesics in that they do not induce changes in the vigilance level but lead to a selective inhibition of pain correlates.

EEG and Psychological Pain Control

The literature on power spectral density changes due to psychological treatments of pain is mainly concerned with the effects of hypnotic trance. In a series of cross-cultural field observations and laboratory experiments,

Larbig (1982) studied changes in the power density of the spontaneous EEG of members of a Greek Orthodox community. These subjects were engaged in fire walking as part of their annual memorial to Saint Konstantin, who rescued holy icons out of a burning church barefoot and without sustaining injuries to his feet. Larbig further investigated Hindus in Sri Lanka while they were celebrating painful hook-hanging rituals in a hypnotic state as part of their annual religious group activities. Finally, EEG recordings were studied in a fakir while he was lancering his body with daggers, long needles, and spears (for an overview of these studies, see Larbig, 1982, 1988, 1989).

The ongoing EEG of the fire walkers was measured by a telemetric EEG recording device the subjects carried on their backs. The recordings were taken while the fire walkers were outside the fire approaching the glowing charcoals, when they left the fire, and for the entire period while they were dancing on the fire. The power spectral densities during fire walking showed significantly more theta activity compared to that outside the fire. These subjects did not sustain burns or other injuries to their feet. Recordings were also made from a male subject who did not belong to the group of fire walkers but participated spontaneously in the ritual. He developed no theta rhythm while approaching and dancing on the charcoal but showed severe burns after the unprepared fire walking.

In a series of additional studies the EEG recordings were replicated with student volunteers who did not prepare themselves for the fire walk dancing on a fire. Like the original Greek fire walkers, these subjects again showed no burns on their feet but similar changes of their power spectral density from faster to slower EEG rhythms; that is, to theta and delta activities.

In another series of observations Larbig (1982, 1989) telemetrically recorded the ongoing EEG of nine subjects before, during, and after a painful hook-hanging ritual. The skin and muscles of the subjects' backs were penetrated by six to eight hooks bound together by a string that was fixed to a wooden joist so that the subjects waved freely in the air for about 15 minutes. Like the Greek fire walkers, these subjects also showed an increase of theta activity at sensorimotor brain sites while preparing for, anticipating, and performing the hook hanging. In addition, five of the nine subjects remained in the theta stage for several hours after the hook-hanging ritual. According to their subjective pain reports none of the subjects experienced severe pain.

Finally, Larbig (1982, 1989) investigated the spontaneous EEG of a French fakir of Mongolian descent before, during, and after he penetrated several parts of his body—his tongue, frontal neck, and abdominal skin—with daggers. He reported that he did not feel pain but rather that he achieved complete pain control by a self-induced deep hypnotic trance. According to his report trance was induced by a shift of attention to pleasant ideas, thoughts, and positive images. His EEG replicated the earlier observations of a significant increase in theta before, during, and shortly after the painful procedure.

The significant increase of theta activity within these "visceral athletes" might be considered as a correlate of pain control induced by attentional manipulations. The EEG activity resembles EEG patterns that are observed during drowsiness and sleep and during stages of deep relaxation when pain sensation presumably is significantly reduced. Larbig et al. (1982) suggested that this sleeplike cortical activity indicates a stage of localized "microsleep" of brain structures involved in the processing of pain (i.e., the somatosensory primary and secondary cortex) while those brain areas that are not involved in the processing of pain, that is, areas engaged in the motor behavior of the fire walkers, are still functioning properly and may even show an increased level of activation.

These studies confirm that the investigation of the ongoing EEG represents a useful tool to supplement behavioral data and subjective reports of pain and pain reduction. It might especially be helpful in increasing our knowledge of the psychophysiological mechanisms of pain control.

Event-Related Potentials

Over the past years, ERPs have become a prime tool in the investigation of higher nervous system functions related to pain. The term "event-related potential" refers to brain electrical activities that can be recorded from different sites of the scalp or from inside the scalp, that is, from single neurons or assemblies of neurons, before, during, or after a subject is exposed to a physical or "mental" event. It is now widely accepted that ERPs model the temporary pattern of neural activities associated with cortical information processing of concrete stimuli (for an extensive overview of current ideas and methods see Birbaumer, Elbert, Canavan, & Rockstroh, 1990; Miltner, 1989; Picton, 1988; Rockstroh, Elbert, Canavan, Lutzenberger, & Birbaumer, 1989).

Measurement of ERPs

The measurement of ERPs is realized with the same technical equipment and the same conventions for electrode placements that are used for the recording of spontaneous EEG activity. However, the recording of ERPs from the scalp is more difficult because the brain electrical activity related to the processing of an event (the signal) is very small and normally masked by the larger changes of voltages caused by the spontaneous activities of the brain and by electrical oscillations of the recording system (noise). The ERP is therefore a linear combination of the event-related electrical brain activity and unspecific neuronal and electrotechnical background noise. It is further assumed that the relation between an event and its neural processing is constant and uniform, that is, that the processing of an event always takes place constantly in the identical neural structures. This does not imply that for each signal identical cells of a neural modul are active, but it is assumed that the electrical response of the neural structure involved is constant. However, Ruchkin (1988) criticized that this assumption does not necessarily hold when global changes in the central nervous activation are involved due to recovery, adaptation, habituation, or shifts in vigilance and of general attention. Such modulating influences are more relevant for endogeneous, late components of the ERP than for the early ones.

Furthermore, ERPs may become contaminated by artifacts due to eye movements, activity of other muscles in the face and neck, such as the masseter muscles, or by vegetative reflexes, such as changes in electrodermal activities that may transiently decrease the impedance of the EEG recording electrodes. The influence of such sources of artifacts can be essentially reduced by minimizing the electrical resistance between the electrode and the skin of the scalp. For these reasons, the skin at the site of the electrode has to be prepared carefully by cleansing the surface of the skin with alcohol.

Additionally, the use of Ag/AgCl electrodes and electrolyte significantly reduces this impedance. Most research groups prefer a preparation that reduces the impedance between skin and electrode below 3 kΩ.

Several methods were suggested that deal with eye movement artifacts and its correction from the ongoing EEG and ERP. The most widely used method is to record blinks and eye movements by the electrooculogram and to discard segments or trials of an experimental session that are contaminated with concurrent eye movements. More sophisticated methods include corrections by using cross-correlation functions, autoregressive models, time domain approaches, and frequency domain approaches (for an extensive review and comparison of different methods, see Brunia et al., 1989).

The separation of an ERP signal from the noise of the spontaneous background EEG is commonly based on averaging techniques. They are useful whenever the assumption of linearity between signal and noise is valid. The brain electrical activities (the ERP) are separately recorded at each electrode site and are averaged on- or off-line for each experimental condition (e.g., for each stimulus intensity). The averaging reduces the noise of the ERP and produces a nearly bias-free estimation of the true event-related signal.

For further improvements of the signal-to-noise ratio, digital filters are used that allow for attenuation of such frequencies of the signal that are not considered part of the brain electrical activity (for details see Lutzenberger et al., 1985; Ruchkin, 1988) or those activities not of experimental interest. When the assumption of the invariance of the signal is violated or when there are additional systematic influences on the signal (e.g., systematic variations of the latencies of components), then averaging techniques may lead to distortions of the signal with similar effects like that of a low-pass filter. Such effects are prevented by the application of a Woody-filter (Harris & Woody, 1969; Woody, 1967).

The ERP is described by its detectable positive and negative maxima of voltages within distinct time windows form the amplitudes or half-waves of the ERP. Commonly these maxima are labeled with the letters "N" or "P," indicating that the maximum is of negative (N) or positive (P) polarity. Additionally, the maxima are commonly defined by their latency related to the time of stimulus application. Thus, N100 or P300 describes single amplitudes that show their maximum at 100 ms or 300 ms, respectively.

The analysis of ERP wave forms is commonly based on single amplitudes such as P80, N100, P200, P300, and their corresponding latencies. In most studies the amplitudes are based on one of four reference baselines: (1) on technical zero, (2) an empirically determined baseline, (3) the preceding or subsequent maximum of an amplitude, or (4) a peak-to-peak instead of a base-to-peak measure. Additionally, a number of research groups use the average integral of the wave as a reference. Another method of analysis is based on factor analysis models (for detailed information, cf. Ruchkin, 1988; for a critique see Rösler & Manzey, 1981).

Event-Related Potentials and Pain

ERPs induced by brief noxious stimuli have become powerful tools for the quantification of phasic pain in humans (for reviews see Bromm, 1985, 1987; Chapman & Jacobson, 1984; Chudler & Dong, 1983; Miltner, 1989).

The application of ERPs is based on early studies by Spreng and Ichioka (1964) and by Chatrian and coworkers (Chatrian, Canfield, Knauss, & Lettich, 1974; Chatrian, Canfield, Lettich, & Black, 1975; Chatrian, Farrell, Canfield, & Lettich, 1975) demonstrating that the amplitudes of the late components of somatosensory ERPs evoked by *electrical stimulation of the tooth pulp* are highly correlated with subjective pain reports. All subjects reported brief and sharp sensations of moderate pain the intensity of which covaried with the size of the amplitudes of the vertex somatosensory evoked potential (SEP) recorded between 147 and 249 ms poststimulus. These findings were replicated by Chapman and his group (Chapman, Chen, Colpitts, & Martin, 1981; Chen, Chapman, & Harkins, 1979; Harkins & Chapman, 1978) and by Miltner, Johnson, Braun, and Larbig (1989).

In a further series of experiments Carmon and coworkers (Carmon, Friedman, Coger, & Kenton, 1980; Carmon, Mor, & Goldberg, 1976a, 1976b) and Bromm and his group (Bromm & Treede, 1984) achieved comparable results when short *heat stimuli* were applied by brief CO_2-laser pulses. Again the largest ERP was recorded from the vertex with a maximum negative amplitude between 130 and 190 ms and a maximum positive amplitude between 230 and 400 ms. Its peak-to-peak size was recorded between 5 and 40 μV. These findings were replicated by Bromm and coworkers (Bromm & Treede, 1987; Treede & Bromm, 1988; Treede, Kief, Hölzer, & Bromm, 1988). They also showed that the vertex response becomes largest when the different stimulus intensities are applied in a random order (Bromm, 1987).

Another pain model consists of brief *electrical skin stimuli* applied either *transcutaneously* (Stowell, 1977) or *intracutaneously* to the tip of the fingers (Bromm & Meier, 1984; Miltner, Larbig, & Braun, 1991; Miltner, Larbig, & Braun, 1988a, 1985b). Comparable to the studies mentioned above, a highly positive relationship between the amplitude size of the peak-to-peak measure and pain ratings was obtained. As another variation on the stimuls side, *olfactory painful stimuli* were investigated by Kobal and his group (Kobal & Hummel, 1988). They applied brief CO_2 pulses to the olfactory mucous membrane of the nose and reported similar relationships between the subjective pain reports and the size of the vertex responses.

However, ERP responses are not an "objective correlate of acute pain" as was stated enthusiastically by Carmon et al. (1976a, 1976b) at the first stage of this area of research. Both Chapman et al. (1981) and Miltner (1989) showed that the vertex ERP amplitude is not a simple measure of the physical aspects of different stimulus intensities but is influenced by psychological aspects. Thus, it is much rather a measure of the subjective evaluation of stimuli than their mere physical properties. The N150-P260 vertex amplitude showed the closest relationship to both the physical and subjective stimulus intensities. Other amplitudes of the ERP response, such as the N65-P120 or the P120-N175, and the late slow wave component were less highly correlated with the subjective pain report. However, when the variance due to the physical intensity of the stiumli was partialed out, a much closer relationship between the subjective repsonse and the ERP amplitude was also present for these components. Averaging the ERP according to the subjective intensity reports results in a more distinct ERP than the ERP averaged according to the physical aspects of the stimuli. The relationship between the subjective report and the size of the N150-P260 amplitude was high (i.e., $r = .71$) when the physical stimulus dimension was partialed out. By way of contrast, the correlation coefficient between the physical intensity and the ERP was only .11 when the subjective dimension was partialed out.

In addition to this well-established function of the N150-P260 vertex complex, Bromm and Treede (1984, 1987) and Treede and Bromm (1988) recently reported similar relationships between the subjective pain report and so called "ultra-late components" of laser-evoked somatosensory potentials. This ultra-late response (with a latency between 1050 and 1250 ms) that was subjectively described by the subjects as a burning second pain, was interpreted as the result of the processing of stimulus-related C-fibre inputs to the cerebral cortex. Bromm and his coworkers reported that this ultra-late response could only be observed when the faster A-delta inputs were blocked. They suggested that the ultra-late component occurs only when the brain is not preactivated by faster A-delta inputs that prevent the perception of second pain in untrained subjects.

Localization of ERPs to Painful Stimuli

Multichannel recordings of the ERP to pain stimuli that use special mathematical analyses to localize the source of the pain-related ERP at N150-P260 confirm its main origin at postcentral brain sites (cf. Miltner, 1989). These findings were recently replicated by Joseph et al. (1991) using magnetoencephalography to measure magnetic fields evoked by intracutaneous noxious stimuli. Finally, a recent study by Talbot et al. (1991) utilized MRI together with PET in humans who were stimulated with painful heat. This study showed that the somatosensory cortex was activated in response to painful heat stimuli. Additionally, clear evidence for limbic involvement (anterior cingulate gyrus) in the processing of painful events as compared to nonpainful heat stimulation was found. The cingulate gyrus seems to reflect the emotional component of the pain experience.

Taken together, these studies clearly support the assumption that the ERP vertex amplitude is a useful tool for the quantification of the subjective intensity aspects of phasic pain. The vertex response primarily reflects the subjective evaluation of the stimulus intensities applied. The relationship between subjective pain reports and the size of the amplitude of late ERP components encouraged several researchers to use ERPs elicited by painful experimental stimuli as an additional tool to subjective pain reports in the quantification of the effects of analgesic agents or psychological methods of pain control.

ERPs and Pain Control By Analgesics and Paramedical Procedures

Peripheral Analgesics. Chen and Chapman (1980) published a study quantifying the analgesic effects of acetylsalicylic acid (ASA). As was shown, both the vertex ERP response and the subjective pain reports, respectively, were significantly reduced under medication, whereas the auditory brain electrical responses did not change. There were no changes in earlier components of the ERP. These results were replicated by Buchsbaum and coworkers (Buchsbaum, 1984; Buchsbaum, Davies, Coppola, & Naber, 1981) and by Bromm, Rundshage, and Scharein (in press) in a placebo-controlled, double-blind repeated measures design.

Opioids. A number of studies investigated the effects of opioids (i.e., morphine, pethidine, fentanyl, alfentanyl, pentazocine, and tilidine) and other centrally acting agents, (e.g., nitrous oxide, imipramine, flupirtine (Bromm et al., 1987; Bromm, Ganzel, Hermann, Meier, & Scharein, 1986; Bromm, Meier, & Scharein 1986; Kobal & Hummel, 1988) by using ERPs and pain reports elicited by different pain stimulation paradigms. These studies all confirm the sensitivity of the ERP measures to the analgesic properties of the drug. However, morphine and other opioids lead to amplitude reductions and increased amplitude latencies for all components of the ERP from 100 ms on.

Chapman and coworker intensely studied the effects of fentanyl (Chapman, Colpitts, Benedetti, & Butler, 1982) and alfentanyl (Chapman, Hill, Seager, & Walter, 1988; Hill et al., 1986), demonstrating significant reductions in pain report and the P100, N120, and P200 of the ERP. Again the effects of fentanyl were antagonized by naloxone (Chapman et al., 1982). In the Hill et al. (1986) study a clear dose-dependent effect of the opioid on the late ERP components and the subjective pain intensities was reported. Similar results were obtained by Bromm et al. (1986, 1987) for pentazocine and by Bromm, Meier, and Scharein (1983) for tilidin. Finally, Bromm et al. (1986) reported a study testing imipramine, a tricyclic antidepressant.

Paramedical procedures. ERPs were also used to test the pain-reducing effects of electrical nerve stimulation (Raab, Kobal, Steude, Hamburger, & Hummel, 1987). Due to atypical pain in the face, four subjects received electrical stimulation of the trigeminal ganglion with chronically implanted electrodes coupled with an implanted stimulus generator that was activated by the subjects by magnetic induction whenever they felt pain. The analgesic effects of this stimulation was tested with tooth-pulp ERPs and subjective pain ratings while subjects stimulated their thalamic ganglion compared to a series of pain stimulation without electrical nerve stimulation. Both the late vertex-ERP response and the pain reports, respectively, were clearly reduced while subjects applied the electrical nerve stimulation up to 10 minutes after termination of the electrical self-stimulation. Similar results for transcutaneous electrical nerve stimulation (TENS) and acupuncture were published by Chapman, Colpitts, Benedetti, Kitaeff, and Gehring (1980), and Chapman, Schimek, Gehring, Gerlach, and Colpitts (1983).

ERPs and Pain Control by Psychological Procedures

Attention. In a series of three experiments Miltner and coworkers (Miltner, 1989; Miltner, Johnson, & Braun, 1990; Miltner, Johnson, Braun, & Larbig, 1989) investigated the effects of attention on experimentally induced pain by means of ERP and subjective pain reports. The results show significant amplitude reductions for ignored painful and nonpainful stimuli compared to attended stimuli that are most pronounced at Cz. An analysis of variance revealed significantly shorter latencies for N150, P260, and P300 of attended stimuli compared to ignored stimuli with no difference between painful and nonpainful stimuli.

Hypnosis. In a further study Miltner and coworkers (Miltner, 1989; Miltner, Braun, & Revenstorf, in press) investigated the effects of hypnosis on experimentally induced intracutaneous pain using 16 healthy subjects selected for their high suggestibility. The results revealed no systematic difference between the ERP amplitudes for the suggestion of desensitization and the suggestion of augmented pain. However, the subjective ratings were significantly different between sensitization and desensitization with greater intensities reported for suggestions of sensitization than for those of desensitization.

Hypnosis is obviously different from a shift in attention but seems to include a dissociation between perceptual processing of the stimulus and its subsequent cognitive (conscious) evaluation. This dissociation between perception and evaluation was suggested by Hilgard and Hilgard (1983). Hypnosis may not change the cortical arrival and processing of painful information but may be based on a change in the interpretation of the painful stimulus. According to Hilgard and Hilgard subjects feel the painful stimuli (hidden pain) but neglect what they feel.

Biofeedback. In another study by Miltner and his group (Miltner, Larbig, & Braun, 1988b), subjects were trained to self-control the size of the vertex response to painful stimuli by an operant conditioning approach. The purpose of the study was to determine whether a learned increase of the vertex response leads to higher subjective pain reports than a conditioned decrease of this amplitude. Based on biofeedback results with animals published by Rosenfeld and his coworkers (for a review, see Rosenfeld, 1990), 15 healthy subjects were trained to increase or decrease the N150-P260 peak-to-peak amplitude of painful intracutaneous stimuli by a visual biofeedback paradigm. The visual feedback stimuli for correct responses, e.g., for an increase of the N150-P260 amplitude consisted of a series of male figures displayed on a video screen immediately after the subjects' brain electrical response to the pain stimulus was recorded. The number of figures indicated the size of the response related to baseline. Correct responses for a decrease in amplitude were indicated with a corresponding series of female figures. Subjects quickly achieved control over the size of this amplitude within the first 50 trials of training, even when the sequence of trials for increased or decreased amplitudes changed in random order. Corresponding to the direction of change of the N150-P260 vertex response the subjective pain report was reduced for trials with reduced amplitudes and increased for trials with increased amplitudes. These results were recently replicated with a slightly different feedback paradigm (Miltner, 1989). The clinical usefulness of the self-control of pain-related ERPs in chronic pain patients remains to be demonstrated.

Slow Wave activity and pain

Based on the well-established fact that slow cortical activities reflect preparatory processes of the brain while subjects are attending an imperative stimulus, that is, a meaningful or aversive event (for a review of slow cortical potentials within these two-stimulus paradigms see Rockstroh et al., 1989), Larbig et al. (1982) recorded slow brain potentials of 12 male volunteers and of a fakir with an ability to control extreme pain. The results of this study show that subjects developed a larger negative slow wave activity over frontal and vertex sites in anticipation of the aversive and painful stimuli as compared to the neutral second stimuli, even if no motor response was required. There were no significant differences between the volunteers and the fakir. The results confirm the notion that slow cortical potentials are indicators of late behavioral processes related to the control of motivationally relevant stimuli (i.e., of aversiveness and painfulness within the present context) and may serve as an additional tool to quantify the motivational relevance or the emotional impact of an aversive or painful event.

Clinical populations

Evoked brain potentials are frequently used to quantify sensory loss, depth of anesthesia, and neurological disorders as well as disorders of the processing of nociceptive stimuli (cf. Bromm, Frieling, & Lankers, in press). Bromm, Frieling, and Lankers (in press) used CO_2 laser pulses for the stimulation of nociceptive cutaneous afferents in the superficial skin layers (i.e., C-fibers and A-delta fibers) in patients with dissociated loss of pain and temperature sensibility but intact functions of mechanosensibility. All 18 patients showed reduced or delayed somatosensory evoked potentials related to the area affected by the disease with significantly delayed latencies compared to the unaffected control site. Furthermore, these abnormalities were only seen when laser stimuli but not when electrical skin stimulation was

employed, which primarily affects mechanosensitive fast conducting fibers but not nociceptive structures. Patients with spinal lesions often suffer from sensory loss or hyperalgesia; the same is true for patients with encephalomyelitis, polyneuropathies, and other central and peripheral neuronal lesions. Delayed or reduced pain sensitivity is reliably correlated with delayed latency and reduced amplitude of the vertex response (N150-P260). However, with late components (100 ms and above) it is impossible to differentiate medical-organic from psychological origins of hyper- or hypoanalgesia because both conditions modify the ERP amplitudes. Whether ERPs will become a useful tool in the psychophysiological assessment of other chronic pain states such as migraine headaches, low back pain, and facial pain remains to be determined.

Conclusion

The studies cited above support the notion that ERPs elicited by brief noxious stimuli rated as painful serve as powerful and noninvasive tools for the quantification of phasic experimental pain in humans without the need of invasive procedures related to the neural pathways and structures involved in transmission of nociceptive information and pain perception (Bromm, 1987). As was shown in all studies, this function is primarily based on a close relationship between the late components of ERPs and the subjective pain report.

ERPs in a clinical setting with chronic pain patients are applied as phasic stimuli probing into the tonic background of chronic pain. The match or mismatch of the probe stimulus with the background tonic pain should evoke ERPs whose components and latencies might be specific for the nature of the respective chronic pain problem. The multichannel measurement of spontaneous EEG that allows for the localization of the sources of a respective EEG band provides additional information on possible local origins and disturbances of the neurophysiological basis of the clinical pain experience. MEG (magnetencephalogram) recordings will augment the precision of brain localization (e.g., Hari & Lounasmaa, 1989).

New methods of EEG analysis such as nonlinear fractional dimensional analysis (Lutzenberger, Elbert, Ray, & Birbaumer, in press) are another possibility of future applications of CNS recordings in the quantification of pain processing in the human brain. The use of nonlinear ("chaos") deterministic models allows the dimensional reduction of the EEG trace into a few basic factors (fractal dimensions) that determine the actual time series. With the reduction of the mental "complexity" in focused attentional tasks we (Lutzenberger et al., in press) have demonstrated a parallel reduction of fractal (chaotic) dimensions of the EEG. It may well be the case that chronic pain also leads to a "simplification" of cortical processes focusing the attentional resources mainly of the pain experience.

Although we still do not know exactly where these amplitudes are generated, these studies clearly indicate that the perception of pain is determined by the cerebral cortex and not by peripheral or subcortical neural structures. These peripheral structures serve as necessary conditions for the experience of pain but they are not sufficient for the determination of the pain experience. Spontanous EEG recordings and ERPs are therefore additional tools that supplement subjective pain reports and other techniques of pain measurement in the investigation of the neural basis of the highest representation of painful perception. The determination of these activities enables us to investigate the pain-related afferent system and the cortical representation of pain.

SUMMARY

The purpose of this chapter was to demonstrate the usefulness of psychophysiological recording methods in the assessment of both laboratory pain and clinical pain syndromes. Whereas peripheral measures—especially the EMG and vascular parameters—have been widely used in the assessment of chronic pain, the use of central measures such as the spontaneous EEG or ERPs has so far been almost exclusively limited to laboratory pain assessments. An integration of peripheral and central measures in both applications would be desirable. Furthermore, the relationship of physiological measures and psychological processes should be further investigated. Many clinicians and researchers limit their endeavors to the assessment of abnormalities in physiological functioning of pain patients without relating them to psychological processes. A truly multidimensional assessment of pain (cf. Turk & Rudy, 1987) must assess both physiological and psychological parameters of the pain experience and—most important—must elucidate their mutual interrelationship.

Acknowledgments. The completion of this chapter was facilitated by Grants Fl 156/1 and Fl 156/2 from the Deutsche Forschnungsgemeinschaft (DFG) to H.F., grant 0705103 from the Bundesministerium fur Forschung und Technologie and SFB 307/B1 from the DFG to N.B., and SFB 307/B2 from the DFG to W.M. The authors are solely responsible for the content of this publication.

REFERENCES

Anliker, M., Casry, N., Friedl, P., Kubli, R., & Keller, H. (1977). Noninvasive measurement in blood flow. In N. H. Hwang & N. A. Norman (Eds.), *Cardiovascular flow dynamics and measurement* (pp. 177–198). Baltimore: University Park Press.

Arena, J., Sherman, R. A., Bruno, M., & Young, T. R. (1990). Temporal stability of paraspinal electromyographic recordings in low back pain. *International Journal of Psychophysiology, 9*, 31–37.

Arena, J., Sherman, R. A., Bruno, M., & Young, T. R. (1991). Electromyographic recording of low back pain subjects and non-pain controls in six different position: Effect of pain levels. *Pain, 45*, 23–28.

Arena, J. G., Blanchard, E. B., Andrasik, F., Appelbaum, K., & Myers, P. E. (1985). Psychophysiological comparisons of three kinds of headache subjects during and between headache states: Analysis of post-stress adaptation periods. *Journal of Psychosomatic Research, 29*, 427–441.

Arena, J. G., Blanchard, E. B., Andrasik, F., Cotch, P. A., & Myers, P. E. (1983). Reliability of psychophysiological assessment. *Behaviour Research & Therapy, 21*, 447–460.

Arena, J. G., Sherman, R. A., Bruno, G. M., & Young, T. R. (1989). Electromyographic recordings of 5 types of low back pain subjects and non-pain controls in different positions. *Pain, 37*, 57–65.

Arntz, A., Merckelbach, H., Peters, M. C., & Schmidt, A. J. M. (1991). Chronic low back pain, response specificity and habituation to painful stimuli. *Journal of Psychophysiology, 5*, 177–188.

Bakal, D. A., & Kaganov, J. A. (1977). Muscle contraction and migraine headache: Psychophysiological comparison. *Headache, 17*, 208–214.

Bakke, M., Tfelt-Hansen, O., Olsen, J., & Moller, E. (1982). Action of some pericranial muscles during provoked attacks of common migraine. *Pain, 14*, 121–135.

Basmajian, J. V. (1986). The musculature. In M. G. H. Coles, E. Donchin, & S. W. Porges (Eds.), *Psychophysiology: Systems, processes, and applications* (pp. 97–106). New York: Guilford Press.

Birbaumer, N., Dworkin, B., Elbert, T., & Rockstroh, B. (1987). Stimulation der Barorezeptoren erhöht die Schmerzschwelle bei Bluthochdruck [Stimulation of the baroreceptors elevates pain thresholds in hypertension]. In F. Nutzinger (Ed.), *Herzphobie* [Heart phobia] (pp. 92–102). Stuttgart: Enke.

Birbaumer, N., Elbert, T., Canavan, A., & Rockstroh, B. (1990). Slow potentials of the cerebral cortex and behavior. *Physiological Reviews, 70*, 1–41.

Birbaumer, N., & Schmidt, R. F. (1990). *Biologische Psychologie* [Biological psychology]. Berlin, Heidelberg, New York: Springer.

Bischoff, C., Traue, H. C., & Zenz, H. (1982). Muskelspannung und Schmerzerleben von Personen mit und ohne Spannungskopfschmerz bei experimentell gesetzter aversiver Reizung [Muscle tension and pain sensations of persons with and without tension headache during experimentally induced aversive stimulation]. *Zeitschrift für experimentelle und angewandte Psychologie, 29*, 357–385.

Blanchard, E. B., Andrasik, F., Arena, J. G., Neff, D. F., Saunders, N. L., Jurish, S. E., Teders, S. J., & Rodichok, L. D. (1983). Psychophysiological responses and predictors of response to behavioral treatment of chronic headache. *Behavior Therapy, 14*, 357–374.

Blumberg, H. (1988). *Zur Klinik und Pathophysiologie der sympathischen Reflexdystrophie* [The clinical and pathophysiological aspects of sympathetic reflex dystrophies]. Unpublished Habilitation, Department of Neurology, University of Freiburg, FRG.

Borgeat, F., Hade, B., Elie, R., & Larouche, L. M. (1984). Effects of voluntary muscle tension increases in tension headache. *Headache, 24*, 199–202.

Bromm, B. (1985). Evoked cerebral potential and pain. In H. L. Fields, R. Dubner, & F. Cervero (Eds.), *Advances in pain research and therapy* (pp. 305–329). New York: Raven Press.

Bromm, B. (1987). Assessment of analgesia by evoked cerebral potential measurements in humans. *Postgraduate Medical Journal, 63* (3), 9–13.

Bromm, B., Frieling, A., & Lankers, J. (in press). Laser-evoked brain potentials in patients with dissociated loss of pain and temperature sensibility. *Electroencephalography and Clinical Neurophysiology.*

Bromm, B., Ganzel, R., Hermann, W. M., Meier, W., & Scharein, E. (1986). Pentazocine and flupirtine effects on spontaneous and evoked EEG activity. *Neuropsychobiology, 16, 152–156.*

Bromm, B., Ganzel, R., Herrmann, W., Meier, W., & Scharein, E. (1987). The analgesic efficacy of flupirtine in comparison to pentazocine and placebo assessed by EEG and subjective pain ratings. *Postgraduate Medical Journal, 63*, 109–12.

Bromm, B., & Meier, E. (1984). The intracutaneous stimulus: A new pain model for algesimetric studies. *Methods and Findings in Experimental and Clinical Pharmacology, 6*, 405–410.

Bromm, B., Meier, W. & Scharein, E. (1983). Antagonism between tilidine and naloxone on cerebral potentials and pain ratings in man. *European Journal of Pharmacology, 87*, 431–439.

Bromm, B., Meier, W., & Scharein, E. (1986). Imipramine reduces experimental pain. *Pain, 25*, 245–257.

Bromm, B., Rundshage, I., & Scharein, E. (in press). Central analgesic effects of acetylsalicylic acid in healthy men. *Drug Research.*

Bromm, B., & Treede, R. D. (1984). Nerve fibre discharges, cerebral potentials and sensations induced by CO_2 laser stimulation. *Human Neurobiology, 3*, 33–40.

Bromm, B., & Treede, R. D. (1987). Pain related cerebral potentials: Late and ultra-late components. *International Journal of Neuroscience, 33*, 15–23.

Brunia C. H. M., Mocks, J., van den Berg-Lenssen, M. M. C., Coelho, M., Coles, M. G. H., Elbert, T., Gasser, T., Gratton, G., Ifeachor, E. C., Jervis, J. W., Lutzenberger, W., Sroka, L., von Blokland-Vogelesang, A. W., von Driel, G., Woestenburg, J. C., Berg, P., McCallum, W. C., Tuan, P. D. T., Pocock, P. V., & Roth, T. W. (1989). Correcting ocular artifacts in the EEG. *Journal of Psychophysiology, 3*, 1–50.

Buchsbaum, M. F. (1984). Quantification of analgesic effects by evoked potentials. In B. Bromm (Ed.), *Pain measurement in man: Neurophysiological correlates of pain* (pp. 291–300). Amsterdam, New York, Oxford: Elsevier.

Buchsbaum, M. F., Davies, G. C., Coppola, R., & Naber, D. (1981). Opiate pharmacology and individual differences: II. Somatosensory evoked potentials. *Pain, 10*, 367–377.

Carmon, A., Freidman, Y., Coger, R., & Kenton, B. (1980). Single evoked potentials to noxious stimulation in man. *Pain, 8*, 21–31.

Carmon, A., Mor, J., & Goldberg, J. (1976a). Application of laser to psychophysiological study of pain in man. In J. J. Bonica & D. Albe-Fessard (Eds.), *Advances in pain research and therapy* (Vol. 1, pp. 375–380). New York: Raven Press.

Carmon, A., Mor, J., & Goldberg, J. (1976b). Evoked cerebral responses to noxious thermal stimuli in humans. *Experimental Brain Research, 25*, 103–107.

Chapman, C. R., Casey, K. L., Dubner, R., Foley, K. M., Gracely, R. H., & Reading, A. E. (1985). Pain measurement: An overview. *Pain, 22*, 1–31.

Chapman, C. R., Chen, A. C., Colpitts, Y. M., & Martin, R. W. (1981). Sensory decision theory describes evoked potentials in pain discrimination. *Psychophysiology, 18*, 114–120.

Chapman, C. R., Colpitts, Y. M., Benedetti, C., & Butler, S. (1982). Event-related potential correlates of analgesia: Comparison of fentanyl, acupuncture and nitrous oxide. *Pain, 14*, 327–337.

Chapman, C. R., Colpitts, Y. M., Benedetti, C., Kitaeff, R., & Gehring J. D. (1980). Evoked potential assessment of acupunctural analgesia: Attempted reversal with naloxone. *Pain, 9*, 183–197.

Chapman, C. R., Hill, H. F., Seager, L., & Walter M. H. (1988). Effects of controlled alfentanyl concentration on pain report and dental evoked potentials. In R. Dubner, G. F. Gebhardt, & M. R. Bond (Eds.), *Proceedings of the Vth World Congress on Pain* (pp. 403–406). Amsterdam, New York, Oxford: Elsevier.

Chapman, C. R., & Jacobson, R. C. (1984). Assessment of analgesic states: Can evoked potentials play a role? In B. Bromm (Ed.), *Pain measurement in man: Neurophysiological correlates of pain* (pp. 233–255). Amsterdam: Elsevier.

Chapman, C. R., Schimek, F., Gehring, J. D., Gerlach, R., & Colpitts, Y. H. (1983). Effects of nitrous oxide, transcutaneous electrical stimulation, and their combination on brain potentials elicited by painful stimulation. *Anesthesiology, 58*, 250–256.

Chapman, S. L. (1986). A review and clinical perspective on the use of EMG and thermal biofeedback for chronic headaches. *Pain, 27*, 1–43.

Chatrian, G., Canfield, R. C., Knauss, T. A., & Lettich, E.

(1975). Cerebral responses to electrical tooth pulp stimulation in man. *Neurology, 25,* 745–757.

Chatrian, G. E., Canfield, R. C., Lettich, E., & Black, R. G. (1974). Cerebral responses to electrical stimulation of tooth pulp in man. *Journal of Dental Research, 53,* 1299.

Chatrian, G. E., Farrell, D. F., Canfield, R. C., & Lettich, E. (1975). Congenital insensitivity to noxious stimuli. *Archives of Neurology, 32,* 141–145.

Chen, A. C., Dworkin, S. F., & Drangsholt, M. T. (1983). Cortical power spectral analysis of acute pathophysiological pain. *International Journal of Neuroscience, 18,* 269–78.

Chen, A. C., Dworkin, S. F., Haug, J., & Gehrig, J. (1989). Topographic brain measures of human pain and pain responsivity. *Pain, 37,* 129–41.

Chen, A. C. N., & Chapman, C. R. (1980). Aspirin analgesia evaluated by event-related potentials in man: Possible central action in brain. *Experimental Brain Research, 39,* 359–364.

Chen, A. C. N., Chapman, C. R., & Harkins, S. W. (1979). Brain evoked potentials are functional correlates of induced pain in man. *Pain, 6,* 365–378.

Christensen, L. V. (1986a). Physiology and pathophysiology of skeletal muscle contraction: Part 1. Dynamic activity. *Journal of Oral Rehabilitation, 13,* 451–461.

Christensen, L.V. (1986b). Physiology and pathophysiology of skeletal muscle contraction: Part 2. Static activity. *Journal of Oral Rehabilitation, 13,* 463–477.

Chudler, E. H., & Dong, W. K. (1983). The assessment of pain by cerebral evoked potentials. *Pain, 16,* 221–244.

Cobb, C. R., deVries, H. A., Urban, R. T., Leukens, C. A., & Bagg, R. J. (1975). Electrical activity in muscle pain. *American Journal of Physical Medicine, 54,* 80–87.

Cohen, R. A., Williamson, D. A., Monguillot, J. E., Hutchinson, P. D., Gottlieb, J., & Waters, W. F. (1983). Psychophysiological patterns in vascular and muscle-contraction headaches. *Journal of Behavioral Medicine, 6,* 93–107.

Coles, M.G.H., Donchin, E., & Porges, S.W. (Eds.) (1986). *Psychophysiology: Systems, processes, and applications.* New York: Guilford Press.

Coles, M. G. H., Gratton, G., Kramer, A., & Miller, G. A. (1986) Principles of signal acquisition and analysis. In M. G. H. Coles, E. Donchin, & S. W. Porges (Eds.), *Psychophysiology: Systems, processes, and applications (pp. 183–221).* New York: Guilford Press.

Collins, A. J., Ring, F., Bacon, P. A., & Brookshaw, J. D. (1976). Thermography and radiology complementary methods for the study of inflammatory diseases. *Clinical Radiology, 27,* 237–243.

Collins, G. A., Cohen, M. J., Naliboff, B. D., & Schandler, S. L. (1982). Comparative analysis of paraspinal and frontalis EMG, heart rate and skin conductance in chronic low back pain patients and normals to various postures and stress. *Scandinavian Journal of Rehabilitation Medicine, 14,* 39–46.

Cram, J. R. (1988). Surface EMG recordings and pain-related disorders: A diagnostic framework. *Biofeedback and Self-Regulation, 13,* 123–138.

Cram, J. R. (Ed.). (1990). *Clinical EMG surface recordings* (Vol. 2). Bothell, WA: Clinical Resources.

Cram, J. R., & Engstrom, D. (1986). Patterns of neuromuscular activity in pain and non-pain patients. *Clinical Biofeedback and Health, 9,* 106–116.

Cram, J. R., & Garber, A. (1986). The relationship between narrow and wide bandwidth filter settings during an EMG-scanning procedure. *Biofeedback and Self-Regulation, 11,* 105–114.

Cram, J. R., Lloyd, J., & Cahn, T. S. (1989). The reliability of EMG muscle scanning. Special issue: Between life and death: Aging. *International Journal of Psychosomatics, 37,* 68–72.

Cram, J. R., & Steger, J. S. (1983). EMG scanning and the diagnosis of chronic pain. Biofeedback and Self-Regulation, 8, 229–242.

Cronin, K. D., & Kirshner, R. L. F. (1982). Diagnosis of reflex sympathetic dysfunction: Use of the skin potential response. *Anaesthesia, 37,* 848–852.

Dahlström, L. (1989). Electromyographic studies of craniomandibular disorders: A review of the literature. *Journal of Oral Rehabilitation, 16,* 1–20.

Dahlström, L., Carlsson, S. G., Gale, E. N., & Jansson, T. B. (1985). Stress-induced muscular activity in mandibular dysfunction: Effects of biofeedback training. *Journal of Behavioral Medicine, 8,* 191–199.

Dickson-Parnell, B., & Zeichner, A. (1988). The premenstrual syndrome: Psychophysiologic concomitants of perceived stress and low back pain. *Pain, 34,* 161–170.

Dolce, J. J., & Raczynski, J. M. (1985). Neuromuscular activity and electromyography in painful backs: Psychological and biomechanical models in assessment and treatment. *Psychological Bulletin, 97,* 502–520.

Dowling, J. (1982). Autonomic measures and behavioral indices of pain sensitivity. *Pain, 16,* 193–200.

Drummond, P. (1982). Extracranial and cardiovascular reactivity in migrainous subjects. *Journal of Psychosomatic Research, 26,* 317–331.

Drummond, P. D., & Lance, J. W. (1984). Facial temperature in migraine, tension-vascular and tension headache. *Cephalalgia, 4,* 149–158.

Elbert, T., Rockstroh, B., Lutzenberger, W., Kessler, M., Pietrowski, K., & Birbaumer, N. (1988). Baroreceptor stimulation alters pain sensation depending on tonic blood pressure. *Psychophysiology, 25,* 25–29.

Fergason, J. L. (1964). Liquid crystals. *Scientific American, 211,* 76–82.

Feuerstein, M., Bortolussi, L., Houle, M., & Labbé, E. (1983). Stress, temporal artery activity, and pain in migraine headache: A prospective analysis. *Headache, 23,* 296–304.

Feuerstein, M., Bush, C., & Corbisiero, R. (1982). Stress and chronic headache: A psychophysiological analysis of mechanisms. *Journal of Psychosomatic Research, 26,* 167–182.

Fischer, A. A., & Chang, C. H. (1985). Electromyographic evidence of muscle spasm during sleep in patients with low back pain. *Clinical Journal of Pain, 1,* 147–154.

Flor, H. (1991). *Psychobiologie des Schmerzes* [Psychobiology of pain]. Bern: Huber.

Flor, H. (in press). *A biobehavioral perspective of chronic pain and its management.* New York: Plenum Press.

Flor, H., & Birbaumer, N. (1990). Psychologische Behand!ung bei akuten Schmerzen [Psychological control of acute pain]. In W. Lehmann (Ed.), *Der postoperative Schmerz* [Postoperative pain] (pp. 383–400). Heidelberg: Springer.

Flor, H. & Birbaumer, N. (1991). Comprehensive assessment and treatment of chronic back pain patients without physical disabilities. In M. Bond (Ed.), *Pro-*

ceedings of the VIth World Congress on Pain (pp. 229–234). Amsterdam: Elsevier.

Flor, H., Birbaumer, N., Schugens, M. M., & Lutzenberger, W. (in press). Symptom-specific psychophysiological responses in chronic pain patients. Psychophysiology.

Flor, H., Birbaumer, N., Schulte, W., & Roos, R. (1991). Stress-related EMG responses in chronic temporomandibular pain patients. Pain.

Flor, H., Birbaumer, N., & Turk, D. C. (1990). The psychobiology of chronic pain. Advances in Behaviour Research and Therapy, 12, 47–87.

Flor, H., & Turk, D. C. (1988). Chronic back pain and rheumatoid arthritis: Relationship of pain-related cognitions, pain severity, and pain behaviors. Journal of Behavioral Medicine, 11, 251–265.

Flor, H., & Turk, D. C. (1989). Psychophysiology of chronic pain: Do chronic pain patients exhibit symptom-specific psychophysiological responses? Psychological Bulletin, 105, 215–259.

Flor, H., Turk, D. C., & Birbaumer, N. (1985). Assessment of stress-related psychophysiological reactions in chronic back pain patients. Journal of Consulting and Clinical Psychology, 53, 354–364.

Fowles, D. (1986). The eccrine system and electrodermal activity. In M. G. H. Coles, E. Donchin, & S. W. Porges (Eds.), Psychophysiology: Systems, processes, and applications (pp. 51–96). New York: Guilford Press.

Freedman, R. R. (1991). Physiological mechanisms of temperature biofeedback. Biofeedback & Self-Regulation, 16, 95–115.

Freedman, R. R., & Ianni, P. (1983). Role of cold and emotional stress in Raynaud's disease and scleroderma. British Medical Journal, 287, 1499–1502.

Freedman, R. R. Ianni, P., & Wenig, P. (1983). Behavioral treatment of Raynaud's disease. Journal of Consulting and Clinical Psychology, 51, 539–549.

Freedman, R. R., Mayes, M. D., & Sabbarwal, S. C. (1989). Induction of vasospastic attacks despite digital nerve block in Raynaud's disease and phenomenon. Circulation, 80, 859–862.

Fridlund, A. J., & Cacioppo, J. T. (1986). Guidelines for human electromyographic research. Psychophysiology, 23, 567–589.

Fuchs, D., Gerber, W. D., Birbaumer, N., & Miltner, W. (1985). Anwendungsmoglichkeiten der Ultraschall-Dopplersonographie in der Biofeedbackbehandlung der Migrane [The use of laser doppler sonography in the biofeedback treatment of migraine patients]. In D. Vaitl & N. Birbaumer (Eds.), Klinische Psychologie. Bd. 1 [Clinical Psychology. Vol. 1] (pp. 56–83). Weinheim: Beltz.

Hampf, G. (1990). Influence of cold pain in the hand on skin impedance, heart rate, and skin temperature. Physiology and Behavior, 47, 217–218.

Handwerker, H. O., Geldner, G., & Magerl, W. (1989). Assessment of local skin reactions and of sympathetic vasoconstrictor reflexes with infrared thermography. European Journal of Neuroscience, S168.

Hari, R., & Lounasmaa, O. V. (1989). Recovery and interpretation of cerebral magnetic fields. Science, 244, 432–436.

Harkins, S. W., & Chapman, C. R. (1978). Cerebral evoked potentials to noxious dental stimulation: Relationship to subjective pain report. Psychophysiology, 15, 248–252.

Harris, E. K., & Woody, C. D. (1969). Use of an adaptive filter to characterize signal-noise relationships. Computers in Biomedical Research, 2, 242–273.

Hilgard, E. R. & Hilgard, J. R. (1983). Hypnosis in the relief of pain (2nd ed.). Los Altos, CA: Kaufmann.

Hill, H., Walter, M. H., Saeger, L., Sargur, M., Sizemore, W., & Chapman, C. R. (1986). Dose effects of alfentanyl in human analgesia. Clinical Pharmacology and Therapeutics, 40, 178–186.

Howe, F. (1983). Phantom limb pain—a reafferentiation syndrome. Pain, 15, 101–107.

Jamner, L. D., & Tursky, B. (1987). Discrimination between intensity and affective pain descriptors: A psychophysiological evaluation. Pain, 30, 271–283.

Jones, A., & Wolf, S. (1980). Treating chronic low back pain: EMG biofeedback-training during movement. Physical Therapy, 60, 58–63.

Joseph, J., Howland, E. W., Wakai, R., Backonja, M., Baffa, O., Potenti, F. M., & Cleeland, C. S. (1991). Late pain-related magnetic fields and electrical potentials evoked by intracutaneous electric finger stimulation. Electroencephalography and Clinical Neurophysiology, 80, 46–52.

Kapel, L., Glaros, A. G., & McGlynn, F. D. (1989). Psychophysiological dysfunction syndrome. Journal of Behavioral Medicine, 12, 397–406.

Keefe F. J., & Gil, K. M. (1986). Behavioral concepts in the analysis of chronic pain syndromes. Journal of Consulting and Clinical Psychology, 54, 776–783.

Kerns, R. D., Turk, D. C., & Rudy, T. E. (1985). The West Haven–Yale Multidimensional Pain Inventory (WHYMPI). Pain, 23, 345–356.

Kobal, G., & Hummel, Th. (1988). Effects of flupirtine on the pain-related evoked potential. Agents and Actions, 23, 117–119.

Kröner, B. (1984). Psychophysiologische Korrelate chronischer Kopfschmerzen.[Psychophysiological correlates of chronic headache]. Zeitschrift für experimentelle und angewandte Psychologie, 31, 610–639.

Larbig, W. (1982). Schmerz: Grundlagen—Forschung—Therapie [Pain: Foundations—research—treatment]. Stuttgart: Kohlhammer.

Larbig, W. (1988). Transkulturelle und larborexperimentelle Untersuchungen zur zentralnervosen Schmerzverarbeitung: Empirische Befunde und klinische Konsequenzen [Transcultural and experimental studies to the central processing of pain: Empirical results and clinical consequences.] In W. Miltner, W. Larbig, & J. C. Brengelmann (Eds.), Therapieforschung für die Praxis 8. Psychologische Schmerzbehandlung [Treatment outcome research for clinical practice 8. Psychological pain treatment] (pp. 1–18). München: Röttger Verlag.

Larbig, W. (1989). Kultur und Schmerz: Untersuchungen zur zentralnervosen Schmerzverarbeitung: Empirische Befunde und klinische Konsequenzen [Culture and pain: Studies on central processing of pain: Empirical results and clinical implications]. Psychomed, 1, 17–26.

Larbig, W., Elbert, T., Lutzenberger, W., Rockstroh, B., Schnerr, G., & Birbaumer, N. (1982). EEG and slow corticol potentials during anticipation and control of painful stimulation. Electroencephalography and Clinical Neurophysiology, 53, 298–309.

Larbig, W., Elbert, T., Rockstroh, B., Lutzenberger, W., & Birbaumer, N. (1985). Elevated blood pressure and reduction of pain sensitivity. In J. F. Orlebeke, G. Mulder, & L. J. P. van Doornen (Eds.), Psychophy-

siology of cardiovascular control (pp. 350–365). New York: Plenum Press.

Lutzenberger, W., Elbert, T., Ray, W. J., & Birbaumer, N. (in press). The scalp distribution of the fractal dimension of the EEG and its variation with mental tasks. *Psychophysiology.*

Lutzenberger, W., Elbert, T., Rockstroh, B., & Birbaumer, N. (1985). *Das EEG: Psychophysiologie und Methodik von Spontan-EEG und ereigniskorrelierten Potentialen* [The EEG: Psychophysiology und methods for spontaneous and event-related potentials]. Heidelberg, Berlin: Springer.

Magerl, W., Geldner, G., & Handwerker, H. O. (1990). Pain and vascular reflexes in man elicited by prolonged noxious mechano-stimulation. *Pain, 43,* 219–225.

Magerl, W., Szolcsanyi, J., Westerman, R. A., & Handwerker, H. O. (1987). Laser doppler flowetry measurements of skin vasodilatation elicited by percutaneous electrical stimulation of nociception in humans. *Neuroscience Letters, 82,* 349–354.

Malmo, R. B., Shagass, C., & Davis, F. H. (1950). Symptom specificity and bodily reactions during psychiatric interview. *Psychosomatic Medicine, 12,* 362–372.

Martin, J. H. (1985). Cortical Neurons, the EEG and the mechanisms of epilepsy. In E. R. Kandel & J. H. Schwartz (Eds.), *Principles of neural science* (2nd ed., pp. 636–647). New York, Amsterdam, Oxford: Elsevier.

Matheson, D. W., Toben, T. P., & de la Cruz, D. E. (1988). EMG scanning: Normative data. *Journal of Psychopathology and Behavioral Assessment, 10,* 9–20.

Mercuri, L. G., Olson, R. E., & Laskin, D. M. (1979). The specificity of response to experimental stress in patients with myofascial pain and dysfunction syndrome. *Journal of Dental Research, 58,* 1866–1871.

Mills, G. H., Davies, G. K., Getty, L. J. M., & Conay, J. (1986). The evaluation of liquid crystal thermography in the investigation of nerve root compression due to lumbosacral lateral spinal stenosis. *Spine, 11,* 420–432.

Miltner, W. (1989). *Ereigniskorrelierte Potentiale in der Schmerzmessung und Schmerzkontrolle* [Event-related potentials in pain assessment and pain Control.] Unpublished Habilitation, Department of Medical Psychology, University of Tubingen, FRG.

Miltner, W., Birbaumer, N., & Gerber, W.-D. (1986). *Verhaltensmedizin* [Behavioral medicine]. Berlin: Springer.

Miltner, W., Braun, C., & Revenstorf, D. (in press). Hypnosis does not change the late components of event-related potentials to painful stimuli. *Journal of Psychophysiology.*

Miltner, W., Johnson, R., Jr., & Braun, C. (1990). Effects of attention on the late components of somatosensory ERPs. In C. H. M. Brunia, A. W. K. Gaillard, & A. Kok (Eds.), *Psychophysiological brain research* (Vol. 1., pp. 212–216). Tilburg: Tilburg University Press.

Miltner, W., Johnson, R., Jr., Braun, C., & Larbig, W. (1989). Somatosensory event-related potentials to painful and non-painful stimuli: Effects of attention. *Pain, 38,* 303–312.

Miltner, W., Larbig, W., & Braun, C. (1988a). Attention and event related potentials elicited by intracutaneous electrical stimulation of the skin. *Journal of Psychophysiology, 2,* 269–276.

Miltner, W., Larbig, W., & Braun, C. (1988b). Biofeedback of somatosensory event-related potentials: Can individual pain sensations be modified by biofeedback-induced self-control of event-related potentials? *Pain, 35,* 205–214.

Miltner, W., Larbig, W., & Braun, C. (1991). Zahnpulpa- und intracutane elektrische Stimulation. Eigenschaften und Unterschiede [Tooth pulp and intracutaneous electrical stimulation. Major characteristics and differences]. Manuscript submitted for publication.

Moltner, A., Hölzl, R., & Srian, F. (1990). Heart rate changes as an autonomic change measure of the pain response. *Pain, 43,* 81–89.

Myrtek, M., & Spital, S. (1986). Psychophysiological response patterns to single, double, and triple stressors. *Psychophysiology, 23,* 663–671.

Nouwen, A., & Bush, C. (1984). The relationship between paraspinal EMG and chronic low back pain. *Pain, 17,* 353–360.

Obrist, P. A. (1976). The cardiovascular-behavioral interaction—as it appears today. *Psychophysiology, 13,* 95–107.

Peters, M. & Schmidt, A. J. (1991). Psychophysiological responses to repeated acute pain stimulation in chronic low back pain patients. *Journal of Psychosomatic Research, 35,* 59–74.

Picton, T. W. (Ed.). (1988). *Handbook of electroencephalography and clinical neurophysiology: Vol. 3. Human event-related potentials* (rev. series). Amsterdam, New York, Oxford: Elsevier.

Pritchard, D. W., & Wood, M. M. (1984). EMG levels in the occipito-frontalis muscles under an experimental stress condition. *Biofeedback and Self-Regulation, 8,* 165–175.

Raab, W. Kobal, G., Steude, M. Hamburger, C., & Hummel, C. (1987). Die elektrische Stimulation des Ganglion gasseri bei Patienten mit atypischem Gesichtsschmerz [Electrical stimulation of the ganglion gasseri in patients with atypical myofascial pain]. *Deutsche Zahnärztliche Zeitung, 42,* 793–797.

Rockstroh, B., Dworkin, B., Lutzenberger, W., Larbig, W., Ernst, M., Elbert, T., & Birbaumer, N. (1988). The influence of baroreceptor activity on pain perception. In T. Elbert, W. Langosch, A. Steptoe, & D. Vaitl (Eds.), *Behavioral medicine of cardiovascular disorders* (pp. 49–60). New York: Wiley.

Rockstroh, B., Elbert, T., Canavan, T., Lutzenberger, W., & Birbaumer, N. (1989). *Slow cortical potentials and behavior* (2nd ed., formerly entitled: *Slow brain potentials and behavior*). Baltimore, Munich, Vienna: Urban & Schwarzenberg.

Rösler, F., & Manzey, D. (1981). Principal components and varimax-rotated components in event-related potentials research: some remarks on their interpretation. *Biological Psychology, 13,* 3–26.

Rojahn, J., & Gerhards, F. (1986). Subjective stress sensitivity and physiological responses to an aversive auditory stimulus in migraine and control subjects. *Journal of Behavioral Medicine, 9,* 203–212.

Rosenfeld, J. P. (1990). Applied psychophysiology and biofeedback of event-related potentials (brain waves): Historical perspective, review, future directions. *Biofeedback and Self-Regulation, 15,* 99–119.

Ruchkin, D. S. (1988). Measurement of event-related potentials: signal extraction. In T. W. Picton (Ed.), *Handbook of electroencephalography and clinical neurophysiology: Vol. 3. Human event-related potentials* (rev. series, pp. 7–43). Amsterdam, New York, Oxford: Elsevier.

Ryding, E., Erikson, B. E., Rosen, I., & Ingvar, D. H. (1985). Regional blood flow (rCBF) in man during perception of radiant warmth and heat pain. *Pain, 22,* 353–362.

Salamy, J. G., Wolk, D. J., & Shucard, D. W. (1983). Psychophysiological assessment of statements about pain. *Psychophysiology, 20,* 579–584.

Schlote, B. (1989). *Langzeitregistrierung der Muskelspannung von Büroangestellten* [Long-term registration of muscle tension in office workers]. In C. Bischoff, H.C. Traue, & H. Zenz (Eds.), Klinische Perspektiven des chronischen Kopfschmerzes und chronischer Rückenschmerzen [Clinical perspectives of migraine and low back pain] (pp. 81–103). Göttingen: Hogrefe.

Sherman, R. A., Arena, J. G., Sherman, C. J., & Ernst, J. L. (1989). The mystery of phantom limb pain: Growing evidence for psychophysiological mechanisms. *Biofeedback and Self-Regulation, 14,* 267–280.

Sherman, R. A., Arena, J. G., Searle, J. D., & Ginther, J. R. (in press). Development of an ambulatory recorder for evaluation of muscle tension related low back pain and fatigue in soldiers normal environment. *Military Medicine.*

Spreng, M., & Ichioka, M. (1964). Langsame Rindenpotentiale bei Schmerzreizung am Menschen [Slow potentials by pain stimulation in pain]. *Pflügers Archive, 279,* 121–132.

Stowell, H. (1977). Cerebral slow waves related to the perception of pain in man. *Brain Research Bulletin, 2,* 23–30.

Soderberg, G. L., & Barr, J. O. (1983). Muscular function in chronic low-back dysfunction. *Spine, 8,* 79–85.

Sternbach, R. A. (1968). *Pain: A psychophysiological analysis.* New York: Academic Press.

Talbot, J. D., Marrett, S., Evans, A. C., Meyer, E., Bushnell, M. C., & Duncan, G. H. (1991). Multiple representations of pain in human cerebral cortex. *Science, 251,* 1355–1358.

Thomas, L. J., Tiber, P. D., & Schireson, S. (1983). The effects of anxiety and frustration on muscular tension related to the temporomandibular joint syndrome. *Oral Surgery, 5,* 763.

Thompson, J. K., & Adams, H. E. (1984). Psychophysiological characteristics of headache patients. *Pain, 18,* 41–52.

Thompson, J. M., Erickson, R. P., Madson, T. J., & Offord, K. P. (1989). Stability of hand-held surface electrodes. *Biofeedback and Self-Regulation, 14,* 55–62.

Thompson, J. M., Madson, T. J., & Erickson, R. P. (1991). EMG muscle scanning: Comparison to attached surface electrodes. *Biofeedback and Self-Regulation, 16,* 167–179.

Traue, H. C., Bischoff, C., & Zenz, H. (1985). Sozialer Streß, Muskelspannung und Spannungskopfschmerz [Social stress, muscle tension, and tension headache]. *Zeitschrift für Klinische Psychologie, 15,* 57–70.

Traue, H. C., Gottwald, A., Henderson, P. R., & Bakal, D. A. (1985). Nonverbal expressiveness and EMG activity in tension headache sufferers and controls. *Journal of Psychosomatic Research, 29,* 375–381.

Treede, R. D., & Bromm, B. (1988). Reliability and validity of ultra-late cerebral potentials in response to C-fibre activation in man. In R. Dubner, G. F. Gebhardt, & M. R. Bond (Eds.), *Proceedings of the Vth World Congress on Pain: Pain research and clinical management* (Vol. 3., pp. 429–441). Amsterdam, New York, Oxford: Elsevier.

Treede, R. D., Kief, S., Holzer, T., & Bromm, B. (1988). Late somatosensory evoked cerebral potentials in response to cutaneous heat stimuli. *Electroencephalography and Clinical Neurophysiology, 70,* 429–441.

Turk, D. C., & Rudy, T. E. (1987). Toward a comprehensive assessment of chronic pain patients. *Behaviour Research and Therapy, 25,* 237–249.

Turpin, G. (Ed.). (1989). *Handbook of clinical psychophysiology.* Chichester, UK: Wiley.

Uematsu, S., Hendeler, N., Hungerford, D. (1981). Thermography and electromyography in the differential diagnosis of chronic pain syndrome and reflex sympathetic dystrophy. *Electromyographic Clinical Neurophysiology, 21,* 165–182.

Venables, P. H., & Martin, I. (1967). *A manual of psychophysiological methods.* New York: Wiley.

Wall, P. D., & R. Melzack, R. (Eds.). (1989). *Textbook of pain* (2nd ed.). Edinburgh: Churchill Livingstone.

Wallin, G. B. (1989). Peripheral sympathetic neural activity in conscious humans. *Annual Review of Physiology, 50,* 565–576.

Wolf, S. L., & Basmajian, J. V. (1978). Assessment of paraspinal electromyographic activity in normal subjects and in chronic back pain patients using a muscle biofeedback device. In E. Asmussen & K. Jorgenson (Eds.), *Biomechanics. VI. Proceedings of the Sixth International Congress of Biomechanics* (pp. 160–178). Baltimore: University Park Press.

Wolf, S. L., Nacht, M., & Kelly, J. L. (1982). EMG feedback training during dynamic movement for low back pain patients. *Behavior Therapy, 13,* 395–496.

Wolf, S. L., Wolf, L. B., & Segal, R. L. (1989). The relationship of extraneous movements to lumbar paraspinal muscle activity: Implications for EMG biofeedback training applications to low back pain patients. *Biofeedback and Self-Regulation, 14,* 63–73.

Woody, C. D. (1967). Characterization of an adaptive filter for the analysis of variance latency in neuroelectric signals. *Medical and Biological Engineering, 5,* 539–553.

Yemm, R. (1969). Temporomandibular disorders and masseter muscle response to stress. *British Dental Journal, 127,* 508–510.

Zimmermann, M. (1984). Physiologie und Schmerz [Physiology and pain]. In M. Zimmermann & H. O. Handwerker (Eds.), *Schmerz: Konzepte und ärztliches Handeln* [Pain: Concepts and medical practice] (pp. 1–43). Berlin: Springer.

III

PSYCHOLOGICAL EVALUATION OF THE PATIENT WITH PAIN

Chapter 12

Assessment of Psychological Status Using Interviews and Self-Report Instruments

LAURENCE A. BRADLEY, PhD
JULIE McDONALD HAILE, BS
THERESA M. JAWORSKI, PhD

A thorough evaluation of individuals with chronic pain must include an assessment of the psychological and social factors associated with their subjective experiences and pain behaviors. Recent studies of persons with various pain syndromes (e.g., musculoskeletal and gastrointestinal pain) have shown that psychological distress and environmental stressors are associated with reports of pain and related symptoms (Bigos et al., 1991; Bradley et al., 1992; Haythornthwaite, Sieber, & Kerns, 1991; Linton, 1990), functional impairment (Haley, Turner, & Romano, 1985; Lorish, Abraham, Austin, Bradley, & Alarcón, 1991), health-care-seeking behavior (Drossman et al., 1988; Whitehead, Bosmajian, Zonderman, Costa, & Schuster, 1988), and resumption of work (Gallagher et al., 1989). Thus, the goals of psychological assessment are to identify (1) psychosocial factors that may affect pain perception and behavior as well as functional impairment, (2) specific treatment goals for each patient, and (3) intervention strategies that may produce maximum patient improvement (Romano, Turner, & Moore, 1989). This chapter focuses on the use of interviews and self-report measures of affective distress and suffering in psychological assessment. It first reviews several strategies for selecting patients for psychological evaluation. The chapter then describes both structured and semistructured interviews for assessing the psychosocial dimensions of chronic pain and for making reliable and valid psychiatric diagnoses. The final portion of the chapter examines a large number of self-report instruments that are used to evaluate patients' psychological status, environmental stressors, and pain-related disability. Other psychological evaluation procedures, such as the measurement of cognitive factors, pain perceptions, and pain behavior, may be found in chapters by DeGood and Shutty (Chapter 13), Jensen and Karoly (Chapter 9), Melzack and Katz (Chapter 10), Craig, Prkachin, and Grunau (Chapter 15), and Keefe and Williams (Chaptet 16).

SELECTING PATIENTS FOR PSYCHOLOGICAL EVALUATION

Patients with chronic pain are usually required to undergo psychological evaluation only when physical findings that may underlie their symp toms cannot be identified. However, psychological assessment is useful for any patient who (1) displays high levels of pain behavior or functional impairment despite receiving appropriate medical treatment, (2) exhibits substantial psychological distress, or (3) excessively uses health-care services, medications, or alcohol (Romano et al., 1989).

Other patient selection strategies may be used for patients seen in tertiary-care centers. For example, university-based, inpatient units for rheumatic disease patients are usually staffed by multidisciplinary treatment teams composed of rheumatologists, orthopedic surgeons, psychologists, nurses, physical and occupational therapists, and social workers. The treatment teams will often perform brief psychosocial assessments on all patients who are admitted to the unit and then identify individuals who require more intensive psychological evaluation. As a result, appropriate behavioral and pharmacologic interventions may be initiated during the early phases of hospitalization and then continued following discharge.

Another strategy, which we use in the Esophageal Manometry Unit in the Division of Gastroenterology at the University of Alabama at Birmingham, is to perform a complete psychological assessment on all patients who are referred for evaluation of chronic chest pain of unexplained origin or other esophageal symptoms. Patients are advised before their arrival at our center that the psychological evaluation will be performed as part of the medical diagnostic process. In order to reduce patients' concerns that their symptoms are not viewed as legitimate by the medical staff, they are informed that the psychological assessment is mandatory for all patients. In addition, the psychological assessments are performed on the second day of the 3-day evaluation, prior to completion of the medical diagnostic procedures. The physicians and psychologists then meet with the patients to provide feedback regarding the results of the entire evaluation and to discuss their treatment plans, which often involve both medical and psychological regimens. These professionals also convey the same information in a joint written report and by telephone to the referring physicians.

Regardless of the procedure that is used to identify patients for psychological evaluation, physicians and psychologists must educate and prepare patients before the evaluation occurs. Specifically, it is necessary to reassure patients that their pains are not considered to be imaginary or the result of mental illness. Rather, the psychological evaluation is required to identify interactions between pathophysiologic and psychological processes that affect patients' physical symptoms, disabilities, and social and familial activities. The evaluation also may suggest interventions that might help to reduce the patients' suffering. Finally, information should be given regarding the specific assessment procedures that will be administered, the professionals who will perform the assessment, the time required to complete the assessment, and the manner in which feedback will be given to the patients and their physicians (Romano et al., 1989).

PSYCHOLOGICAL ASSESSMENT PROCEDURES

The assessment of affective distress and suffering requires at least one interview and the administration of one or more self-report measures. Interviews may be used to evaluate behavioral factors that might influence patients' pain and suffering as well as to make specific psychiatric diagnoses based on the criteria of the *Diagnostic and Statistical Manual of Mental Disorders-III-R*, or DSM-III-R (American Psychiatric Association, 1987). The self-report measures are used to evaluate patients' affective responses and other psychological factors that may influence pain and suffering.

Behavioral Interviews

The behavioral interview should involve both the patient and spouse or some other family member. Because the interview usually is the first procedure performed in the psychological assessment, it is helpful to begin by explaining that its purpose is to determine how the pain has affected the patient's life and what factors may influence the pain. It also is helpful to encourage the spouse or family member to contribute information and his or her opinions during the interview, even if a question is not directed specifically to the family member. This allows the interviewer to compare the responses and assess the interactions of the patient and family member.

Structured Interviews

Few structured behavioral interviews have been developed for use with chronic pain patients.

However, the most well-known structured interview is the Psychosocial Pain Inventory (PSPI) (Getto, Heaton, & Lehman, 1983; Heaton et al., 1982). This measure may be used to gather information from the patient and family member about 25 psychosocial aspects of chronic pain such as stressful life events, social reinforcement of pain behavior, medication usage, health-care-seeking behavior, and familial models for chronic pain. Table 12.1 summarizes the 25 PSPI items, each of which is scored on a 4-point or 3-point scale using a standardized system. A high score on a PSPI item indicates a greater contribution of that item to the patient's pain problem. It should be noted that administration of the instrument requires 1.5 to 2 hours.

With regard to psychometric properties, an initial study involving 169 consecutive chronic pain patients attending a multidisciplinary pain clinic found evidence of high interrater reliability ($r = .98$) and a mean correlation between PSPI items and total PSPI score of .30

TABLE 12.1. Summary of Psychosocial Pain Inventory Items

1. Pain duration
2. Disability income and litigation
3. Major stressful life events prior to pain onset
4. Major stressful life events prior to pain worsening
5. Major stressful life events prior to pain assessment
6. Pain-related stressors avoided by patient
7. Number of pain-related surgeries
8. Duration (months) of pain-related hospitalizations
9. Number of primary physicians for pain
10. Amount of previous relief from pain
11. Current pain-related medications
12. Pain behavior at home
13. Social reinforcement of pain behavior
14. Pain-reducing behaviors
15. Daytime hours spent reclining due to pain
16. Decrease in home/family responsibilities
17. Employment history prior to pain
18. Change in work status after pain onset
19. Plans for activities if pain is decreased
20. Previous painful or disabling medical problems of at least 1-month duration
21. Physician visits prior to pain onset
22. Maximum number of medications (any kind) used daily for at least 6 months prior to pain onset
23. Exposure to models for chronic pain or illness in family
24. History of alcohol abuse
25. Pain behavior observed in interview

Note: Adapted from Getto et al. (1983). Copyright 1983 Raven Press. Adapted by permission.

(Heaton et al., 1982). No other reliability data have been reported. Heaton et al. (1982) also provided evidence regarding the convergent validity of the instrument. This was established by modest but significant correlations (r's = .26) between total PSPI scores and the Total and Sensory Pain Rating Indices of the McGill Pain Questionnaire (MPQ). With regard to divergent validity, it was found that total PSPI scores were significantly associated with only 1 of the 10 clinical scales of the Minnesota Multiphasic Personality Inventory (MMPI), Hypochondriasis ($r = .21$). Finally, Getto et al. (1983) provided evidence regarding the predictive validity of the PSPI. They reported a study of 32 patients with acute pain who were treated by neurosurgeons with either surgical or conservative interventions. It was reported that pretreatment PSPI scores accurately differentiated patients who were classified by the neurosurgeons as either treatment successes or failures. Using a cutoff score of 30, the PSPI identified 72% of the successes and 79% of the failures. Thus, it appears that high PSPI scores are associated with high subjective ratings of pain and with physicians' judgments of treatment response independently of patients' psychopathology levels.

The Interactive Microcomputer Patient Assessment Tool for Health (IMPATH) (Monsein, 1990; Nelson, 1986) represents another structured interview that is noteworthy for its computerized format. The instrument consists of 400 dichotomous, multiple choice, and visual analog questions that are presented to patients on a computer screen. The patient responds to each question by pressing the appropriate computer key. These responses are stored and analyzed and a printout is produced for the health-care provider. This printout provides (1) information about the patient's medical history; (2) a list of psychological, behavioral, cognitive, and social factors that may contribute to the patient's current pain problems; and (3) a series of scales regarding symptom severity and the degree to which pain has negatively affected the patient's daily activities. The printout also includes the patient's scores on four validity scales that are designed to detect positive and negative response biases, random answering, and low accuracy in the patient's IMPATH responses. These scales are similar to the validity scales constructed for the MMPI.

The IMPATH manual (Nelson, 1986)

presents reliability and validity data regarding the responses of 128 patients with head and neck pain of myofascial origin and 95 healthy volunteers. The internal reliability of each IM-PATH scale was reported to be at least .80 and the minimum test–retest reliability coefficients over a 2-week period for these scales was .87. Evidence regarding the construct validity of the instrument was provided by the finding that each IMPATH item differentiated the patient sample from the healthy controls. In addition, correlational analyses revealed that the IM-PATH scales measure relatively independent constructs. It should be stressed, however, that it has not yet been shown that the instrument represents a reliable and valid measure for patients with pain syndromes other than myo-fascial head and neck pain.

Neither the PSPI nor IMPATH has received a great deal of attention in the research literature. No investigators, other than the instrument developers, have published reports of the psychometric properties of these two measures. Thus, at present, we recommend usage of both instruments primarily for research purposes.

Semi-Structured Interviews

Given the limitations of the research on structured interviews, most practitioners have chosen to perform their behavioral interviews using a semistructured format. We have adopted a modified version of the interview that originally was appended to the MPQ (Melzack, 1975). Other useful interview formats may be found in Karoly and Jensen (1989) and Phillips (1988). Table 12.2 shows a summary of the items included in the Phillips interview.

Regardless of the specific format that is chosen, the behavioral interview has several objectives (Bradley, 1989; Romano et al., 1989). The first objective is to obtain a "pain history." This should include a description of the events that may have precipitated the onset of pain as well as the course of the patient's pain over time with regard to intensity, frequency, sensory and affective qualities, and location. Collection of this information may be aided by the use of the MPQ and the Pain Drawing (Ransford, Cairns, & Mooney, 1976). The history also should include questions regarding prior pain treatments and the patient's responses to these treatments. This information is critical so that the practitioner may avoid

TABLE 12.2. Summary of Items Included in the Semi-Structured Interview

Is there evidence of:
1. Depression: _____
2. Anxiety: _____
3. Avoidance/confrontation activity patterns: _____
   _____
4. Inactivity/unfit: _____
   _____
5. Lack of evolved pain coping strategies: _____
   _____
6. Drug dependency: _____
   _____
7. Poor/inadequate understanding of chronic pain/ physical mechanisms: _____
8. Work disruption: _____
   _____
9. Marital problems: _____
   _____
10. Other: _____
11. Motivation for treatment: _____
    _____
12. Sources of reinforcement for pain:
    (a) financial
    (b) sympathy, attention, support from significant others and health-care providers
    (c) provision of time to engage in pleasurable activities
    (d) avoidance of work, school, unpleasant activities (e.g., home or family related), social events
    (e) other

Note: Adapted from Phillips (1988), page 198. Copyright 1988 Springer Publishing. Adapted by permission.

duplication of "failed" interventions or determine if these unsuccessful treatments may be attributed to problems such as inadequate dosages of pharmacologic agents, use of "passive" (e.g., massage, heat) rather than "active" physical therapy (e.g., graduated exercise program), or patient nonadherence with the treatment regimen.

The second objective of the interview is to identify the events that reliably precede exacerbations in the patient's pain perceptions or pain behavior as well as the events that reliably follow these exacerbations. For example, a patient with irritable bowel syndrome (IBS) reports that she dislikes attending business-related dinners with her spouse and that she always experiences increases in her IBS symptoms a few hours prior to these dinners. The patient also states that she takes analgesic or antispasmodic medication in response to the increases in her pain; in addition, she recently has had to increase the medication dosage in order to control her pain. Based on this information, the interviewer may generate several hypotheses that can be evaluated with additional questions and review of other assessment measures. First, it may be speculated that, due to several chance pairings of increased pain during previous business dinners, the events associated with preparing for these dinners now serve as conditioned stimuli that automatically elicit severe pain and other IBS symptoms. It also may be speculated that the patient's medication usage is reinforced by the sedating side effects of the medication. Indeed, the increased dosages required by the patient suggest that she may be developing a physiologic tolerance for or dependence on the medication (cf. Fordyce, 1976).

During this portion of the interview, it also should be noted how persons in the patient's environment respond to the patient's use of medication and other pain behaviors. With regard to the patient with IBS, it should be determined whether family members bring medication to the patient or provide reinforcement to her after medication usage. One example of positive reinforcement (i.e., positive consequences) would be increased attention or nurturance from the patient's spouse or children when they see her use medication. Several investigators have found that patients' reports of pain and pain behaviors are greatest when patients perceive that their spouses provide supportive or solicitous responses to expressions of pain (Anderson & Rehm, 1984; Block, Kremer, & Gaylor, 1980; Flor, Kerns,& Turk, 1987; Gil, Keefe, Crisson, & Van Dalfsen, 1987; Kerns et al., 1991). This relationship may be especially strong when marital satisfaction is high (Kerns, Haythornthwaite, Southwick, & Giller, 1990). Negative reinforcement for pain behavior (i.e., avoidance of unpleasant events) might occur if the patient is encouraged by her spouse to remain at home rather than attend his business dinners. Another example of negative reinforcement might occur if the patient's family is characterized by interpersonal conflict. In this case, reduced interactions

with the spouse or children following medication intake might reward the IBS patient for frequent usage of her medication or for increasing the dosage.

The results of this portion of the interview might suggest that an appropriate treatment plan must attend to the reinforcement contingencies associated with this patient's medication usage and her avoidance of business-related dinners. For example, treatment might include training the patient's family to withdraw positive reinforcement for medication usage and to reward relatively healthy behavior such as discussing her concerns with her spouse about attending these dinners.

The third objective of the interview is to evaluate the patient's daily activities. It is necessary to determine (1) how the patient usually spends his or her time during the day and evening, (2) activities that have been performed more often or less often since the onset of pain, and (3) whether any activities have been modified or eliminated since pain onset (e.g., a salesperson with a back injury who has had to limit driving a car since the injury occurred). The information that is gathered during this portion of the interview may be supplemented by direct observations of the patient's behavior or responses to activity diaries (see Keefe & Williams, Chapter 16) and functional capacity evaluations (see Polatin & Mayer, Chapter 3).

Information regarding changes in the patient's daily activities may allow one to generate hypotheses regarding reinforcement contingencies related to the patient's pain behavior in addition to those described earlier in this section. For example, if the performance of physically demanding, pleasurable activities has not decreased greatly but the performance of similarly demanding, aversive responsibilities has been substantially reduced, one might hypothesize that the patient's behavior has been influenced by negative reinforcement (Romano et al., 1989). This discordance in behavior would be exemplified by a patient with chronic back pain who reports that he is unable to perform factory work that requires standing and repetitive movement of the upper extremities but is able to serve as an umpire for his daughter's softball games. Although the physical requirements of the two activities are not entirely equal, one would have to consider the possibility that the patient's work-related pain behavior has been reinforced by the avoidance of monotonous activity in an unpleasant environment. This hypothesis would gain credibility if one also learned that the patient had experienced interpersonal conflicts with his job supervisor or co-workers (Bigos et al., 1991). Indeed, this information would suggest that the outcome of any vocational rehabilitation services offered to the patient might be poor if the patient were placed in another work environment that he considered aversive.

Information concerning the patient's daily activities also may allow one to determine the extent to which the patient exacerbates his or her suffering. For example, the restriction or elimination of activities due to the expectation of increased pain may lead to excessive disability or pain behavior resulting from distorted gait or physical deconditioning (Bradley, 1989). Intensive physical reconditioning or anxiety management may be necessary for the patient to successfully perform the activities that have been avoided. Conversely, a patient may describe behavior that is characterized by constant activity that is not reduced until the intensity of pain becomes severe. This individual will require instruction in appropriately modulating his or her activity level so that pain does not become a signal that automatically elicits rest, medication intake, or reinforcement from others in the environment.

The fourth objective of the interview is to determine if the patient has any relatives or friends who suffer from chronic pain or disabilities similar to those of the patient. Careful questioning may reveal that the patient spends a considerable amount of time with individuals who also have chronic pain problems (Gamsa & Vikis-Freibergs, 1991; Keefe & Bradley, 1984). Similarly, the interview may show that the patient's childhood was characterized by parental reinforcement for or modeling of maladaptive illness behaviors (e.g., school or work absenteeism in response to minor symptoms). These childhood experiences may have important implications for the patient's current pain behavior or psychological adjustment (Spirito, DeLawyer, & Stark, 1991). Thus, experiences during childhood and as an adult may provide the patient with a great deal of opportunity to learn complex, maladaptive, chronic pain behaviors (e.g., inappropriate usage of medications or health-care services). This may occur particularly often among patients with chronic pain syndromes, such as IBS, that tend to be found among multiple family members (White-

head, Winget, Fedoravicius, Wooley, & Blackwell, 1982) and fibromyalgia (Pellegrino, Waylonis, & Sommer, 1989). Indeed, Mikail and von Baeyer (1990) as well as Gamsa and Vikis-Freibergs (1991) have reported that a history of chronic pain among one's relatives is a significant premorbid risk factor for suffering from a chronic pain syndrome.

Another family-related issue that has recently received a great deal of attention is whether or not the patient has suffered physical or sexual abuse. Haber and Roos (1985) were the first investigators to study histories of abuse among chronic pain patients. They reported that of 151 consecutive female patients who presented to a university-based chronic pain center, 53% reported histories of physical or sexual abuse during childhood or as adults. Of all women reporting abuse, 16% suffered sexual abuse, 43% experienced physical abuse, and 41% reported experiencing both types of abuse. Ninety percent of the women reported that abuse occurred during the adult years (over 18 years of age). The mean duration of abuse among the adults was 12 years; spouses were involved in 71% of these incidents. In addition, 17% of the victims reported that abuse had occurred during childhood or adolescence with 10% of those incidents involving incestuous relationships with a parent. Moreover, the abused patients, relative to those who had not been abused, were twice as likely to have suffered pain without a specific precipitating injury or identified cause and to have a significantly greater number of previous medical problems for which they had sought treatment.

Domino and Haber (1987) reported a similar prevalence of physical and sexual abuse among 30 female patients treated for chronic headaches at a university-based pain treatment center. Sixty-one percent of these patients reported histories of physical abuse, 11% reported sexual abuse, and 20% had suffered both physical and sexual abuse. The abused patients, relative to those who were not abused, were significantly more likely to report constant daily headaches. The abused patients also reported a significantly greater number of medical problems for which they had been hospitalized as well as previous surgical procedures.

Drossman et al. (1990) recently found that physical and sexual abuse also was common among female patients in a university-based specialty clinic. These investigators reported that of 206 consecutive females referred to a gastroenterology clinic, 30% reported histories of childhood sexual abuse and 4% reported frequent childhood physical abuse. The prevalence of sexual and physical abuse during adulthood was 40% and 4%, respectively. It should be noted that the greater prevalence of sexual relative to physical abuse among the gastroenterology patients is not consistent with the prevalence rates reported by Haber and Roos (1985) and Domino and Haber (1987). This difference was probably due to variations among the investigators regarding definitions of sexual and physical abuse. Nevertheless, consistent with the reports of previous investigators, Drossman et al. found that physical and sexual abuse was significantly more common among patients with functional disorders (e.g., IBS) relative to those with organic disorders (e.g., Crohn's disease). The abused patients, relative to the nonabused patients, also reported having a significantly greater number of previous surgical procedures as well as current symptoms, such as fatigue, shortness of breath, headache, and backache.

Relatively few data are available concerning male patients who have been physically or sexually abused. However, Wurtele, Kaplan, and Keairnes (1990) found that 7% of 45 consecutive male patients attending a chronic pain rehabilitation program reported a history of sexual abuse. Karol, Micka, and Kuskowski (1992) recently studied 100 consecutive male patients attending outpatient clinics for chronic back pain. Six percent reported a history of sexual abuse and 16% reported that they had been physically abused.

Given the evidence cited above, we suggest that assessments of all chronic pain patients should include a careful evaluation of possible sexual and physical abuse. Table 12.3 shows the interview questions that we use to assess abuse among patients who are referred to the Esophageal Manometry Unit. These questions were originally used in a Canadian national postal survey and were later used in two American research studies (Briere & Runtz, 1988; Drossman et al., 1990). With regard to the treatment of patients who report histories of abuse, merely giving the patient an opportunity to discuss these experiences with an empathic health professional often provides some emotional relief (Cahill, Llewelyn, & Pearson, 1991). Nevertheless, many patients must be referred to experienced therapists who may

TABLE 12.3. Interview Items Used to Assess Sexual and Physical Abuse[a]

Sexual Abuse[a]

During your childhood (< 14 years) or adulthood, has anyone ever:
A. exposed the sex organs of their body to you?
B. threatened to have sex with you?
C. touched the sex organs of your body?
D. made you touch the sex organs of their body?
E. tried forcefully or succeeded to have sex when you didn't want this?

Physical Abuse[b]

When you were a child (now that you are an adult), did an older person (does any other adult):
hit, kick, or beat you? (1 = never, 2 = seldom, 3 = occasionally, 4 = often)

Note: Adapted from Drossman et al. (1990), page 829. Copyright 1990 American College of Physicians. Adapted by permission.
[a] Patients are considered to be sexually abused if they answer "yes" to any sexual abuse question, except for category A during adulthood.
[b] Patients are considered to be physically abused if they answer "often" to the physical abuse question.

help them to resolve issues such as poor self-image, self-blame for the abuse, sexual dysfunction, and suppressed anger and rage.

The final objective of the behavioral interview is to evaluate the degree to which the patient is experiencing affective disturbance. Depression is commonly found among chronic pain patients (Romano & Turner, 1985). Although a few investigators have suggested that depression may initiate chronic pain (Blumer & Heilbronn, 1982), several recent studies have provided strong evidence that, among patients with chronic back pain, rheumatoid arthritis, or fibromyalgia, affective distress generally is a consequence of chronic pain (Ahles, Yunus, & Masi, 1987; Atkinson, Slater, Patterson, Grant, & Garfin, 1991; Brown, 1990; Gamsa, 1990). Thus, it should be determined whether the patient has experienced any change in mood or outlook on life since the onset of pain and whether the patient has experienced vegetative signs of depression such as sleep disturbance, change in food intake, or decreased desire for sexual intercourse. It also is important to evaluate patients' levels of satisfaction with their relationships with spouses or significant others. Several investigators have demonstrated that patient depression is inversely related to marital satisfaction (Kerns et al., 1990; Kerns & Turk, 1984; Saarijarvi, Rytokoski, &

Karppi, 1990). Kerns et al. (1990) also have shown that patient depression tends to be greatest when marital satisfaction is low and the patient perceives that his or her spouse responds punitively to expressions of pain. Finally, it is important to determine the degree to which patients may be experiencing difficulty in sexual functioning with their partners. Difficulty in sexual functioning may be associated with depression and decreased marital satisfaction as patients often report during the interview that they have experienced difficulty in achieving or maintaining erections, decreased vaginal lubrication, or dyspareunia. Decreased lubrication, dyspareunia, and restricted movement may be especially pronounced among persons with rheumatic diseases such as rheumatoid arthritis or systemic lupus erythematosus (Anderson, Bradley, Young, McDaniel, & Wise, 1985).

Psychiatric Interviews

Although questions regarding affective distress should be included in the behavioral interview, it recently has been suggested that structured psychiatric interviews also should be performed when evaluating patients with chronic pain syndromes (Clouse, 1991). For example, Beitman et al. (1991) have reported that between 34% and 59% of patients with chest pain (CP) of unexplained origin also meet the DSM-III-R criteria for panic disorder. Independent investigators have reported similar prevalence rates for panic disorder among these patients (Cormier et al., 1988; Katon et al., 1988). These prevalence rates are substantially higher than that found among patients with other chronic pain syndromes (16.2%; Katon, Egan, & Miller, 1985). Indeed, it has been suggested that panic disorder may cause CP in some patients because anxiety disorders may alter the thresholds of visceral afferent mechanisms and thereby cause individuals to perceive low-intensity esophageal stimuli as painful (Bradley, Scarinci, & Richter, 1991). Furthermore, psychiatric disorders, such as panic disorder, among CP patients have been shown to be associated with the use of negative coping strategies such as wishful thinking that may exacerbate pain (Vitaliano, Katon, Maiuro, & Russo, 1989). It should be noted that preliminary data indicate that pharmacologic and cognitive–behavioral interventions may be used to reduce panic disorder symptoms as well

as pain episodes among persons with CP (Beitman et al., 1989, 1991; Klimes, Mayou, Pearce, Coles, & Fagg, 1990). Thus, it appears that the use of a reliable and valid psychiatric interview might enable one to identify a specific target associated with episodes of CP that may respond well to appropriate treatment. The psychiatric interview also may allow one to identify patients who have mixed symptoms of anxiety and depression that do not meet diagnostic criteria for specific psychiatric disorders but that, nevertheless, place them at risk for more severe somatic complaints as well as mood and anxiety disorders when they are exposed to substantial life stresses (Katon & Roy-Byrne, 1991).

Two psychiatric interviews have been used extensively in studies of chronic pain patients. Both of these interviews have been developed to provide reliable and valid diagnoses based on the DSM-III-R criteria. The first is the Diagnostic Interview Schedule (DIS) (Helzer & Robins, 1988; Robins, Helzer, Croughan, & Ratcliff, 1981). The DIS is a highly structured interview that requires specialized training. However, training courses are offered twice each year at Washington University (DIS Training/Department of Psychiatry, 4940 Audobon Avenue, St. Louis, MO 63110). A computerized version of the DIS (C-DIS) also is available; nevertheless, we recommend that potential users of the C-DIS undergo training in the full interview in order to best understand the structure of the DIS and to learn to respond appropriately to patients' questions regarding interview items. Test–retest reliability studies of the DIS have reported median kappa coefficients for lifetime psychiatric diagnoses over 1-year intervals ranging from .37 to .59 (Helzer, Spitznagel, & McEvoy, 1987; Vandiver & Sher, 1991; Wells, Burnam, Leake, & Robins, 1988). The validity of the DIS was established by examining the lifetime diagnoses assigned to large samples of psychiatric patients and controls by groups of psychiatrists and lay interviewers, both of whom used the DIS interview. Kappa coefficients ranged between .47 and 1.00, indicating a high level of concordance between the diagnoses assigned by the psychiatrists and those assigned by the lay interviewers even after controlling for chance agreements (Robins et al., 1981).

The second psychiatric interview is the Structured Clinical Interview for DSM-III-R (SCID) (Spitzer, Williams, Gibbon, & First, 1990).

The SCID was designed for use by experienced clinicians who may supplement the structured interview with (1) additional questions to clarify differential diagnosis, (2) challenges to inconsistencies in subjects' self-reports, or (3) ancillary information drawn from hospital records, family members, or other clinical staff (Spitzer, Williams, Gibbon, & First, in press). A detailed training manual and training videotapes are available to persons who wish to administer the SCID (Spitzer et al., 1990). The reliability of the SCID was established by examining the consistency with which trained clinicians assigned lifetime diagnoses to a large sample of psychiatric patients and controls. It was found that the mean kappa coefficient for patient diagnoses was .68; the mean kappa for the controls, however, was .51 (Williams et al., in press). The lower reliability coefficients for the diagnoses assigned to the healthy controls were attributed primarily to the low base rates of psychiatric disorders within this subject sample.

In summary, it appears that the DIS and the SCID are approximately equal with regard to interrater reliability. However, few data concerning the other psychometric properties of the SCID have been published to date, whereas the reliability and validity of the DIS have been examined in several published studies. We agree with Spitzer et al. (in press) that the DIS decision tree procedure occasionally produces diagnoses that do not appear to be consistent with clinical impressions. At these times, the supplementary source material that one may use in making diagnoses with the SCID appears to be desirable. Given the difference between the two interview procedures with regard to training opportunities, we recommend that relatively inexperienced clinicians obtain training in and use the DIS as recommended by Helzer and his colleagues at Washington University. Relatively experienced clinicians may wish to obtain training in the use of both the DIS and the SCID; these individuals then may choose which instrument best meets the needs of their clinical settings or research efforts.

Self-Report Instruments

The preceding discussion demonstrated that questions regarding affective distress and the presence of psychiatric disorders may be addressed by the use of behavioral and psychiatric interviews. Nevertheless, most health care professionals also administer self-report measures of affective disturbance and related constructs to patients with chronic pain. These instruments are very important for clinical and research purposes because they provide standardized, reliable, and valid assessments of psychological variables that may influence pain perception and behavior. Moreover, the self-report instruments usually are more sensitive to treatment-related changes than are psychiatric diagnoses or other interview data. These instruments, then, may be used by clinicians and investigators to help guide or evaluate treatment interventions. The next portion of this chapter reviews the recent literature concerning the four primary measures of psychological status used with chronic pain patients. These are the MMPI, Symptom Checklist-90R, Millon Behavioral Health Inventory, and the Illness Behavior Questionnaire. This is followed by a discussion of the association between environmental stressors and chronic pain. The chapter then examines three measures designed to provide assessments of disability, suffering, and related dimensions of illness. These measures are the Sickness Impact Profile, Chronic Illness Problem Inventory, and the Multidimensional Pain Inventory.

Measures of Psychological Status: The MMPI

The MMPI is the instrument that is most commonly used to evaluate the psychological status of chronic pain patients. The original MMPI was a 566-item questionnaire that included ten scales designed to assess psychological disturbance and three additional validity scales. A revised version of this instrument, the MMPI-2 (Hathaway et al., 1989), recently was introduced and includes the same clinical and validity scales as those found in the original instrument. Both MMPI forms require patients' raw scores on each scale to be converted to standard T-scores so that they may be compared with the responses produced by a large normative sample.

The primary differences between the original and revised versions of the MMPI are that (1) the normative sample used for the MMPI-2 is more representative of the U.S. population with regard to ethnic group membership, religious preferences, and education; and (2) 90 of the MMPI items have been eliminated and 68 items have been modified for the MMPI-2 (Levitt, 1990). Only 12 items from the

MMPI's 13 scales have been eliminated from the MMPI-2, in an attempt to maximize consistency between profiles produced by patients on the two instruments. However, the method for transforming subjects' raw scores into T-scores on the MMPI-2 has been modified so that direct comparisons can be made of T-scores on the clinical and supplemental content scales (Ben-Porath & Graham, 1991). As a result, between 10% and 33% of the 2-point code types (e.g., elevations on the Hypochondriasis and Hysteria scales) produced by psychiatric patients on the original MMPI will not be replicated with the MMPI-2 (Ben-Porath & Graham, 1991).

Regardless of whether one chooses to use the MMPI or the MMPI-2, one should acknowledge that the standardization samples utilized for profile interpretation with both instruments are not appropriate for the assessment of chronic pain patients (Bradley, Prokop, Gentry, Van der Heide, & Prieto, 1981). For example, Pincus and his colleagues (Pincus, Callahan, Bradley, Vaughn, & Wolfe, 1986) identified five items from the MMPI Hypochondriasis, Depression, and Hysteria scales that reliably differentiated a sample of rheumatoid arthritis (RA) patients from healthy controls. It was found that RA patients' responses to these items reflected disease activity (as measured by grip strength and self-reports of disability) rather than psychological status (see Table 12.4). Similar findings have been reported by independent investigators (Moore, McFall, Kivlahan, & Capestany, 1988; Naliboff, Cohen, & Yellin, 1982; Prokop, 1986; Watson, 1982).

In response to the problem of MMPI interpretation, several groups of investigators have used hierarchical clustering methods to identify the MMPI profile patterns that are produced most frequently by chronic pain patients and the behaviors that are associated with each of these patterns. For example, Bradley and his colleagues (Bradley, Prokop, Margolis, & Gentry, 1978; Bradley & Van der Heide, 1984) identified and replicated three MMPI profile patterns across four samples of low back pain patients. It was found that MMPI profiles characterized by elevations on the Hypochondriasis, Depression, and Hysteria scales were associated with perceptions of severe pain, affective disturbance, and large disruptions in vocational, social, marital/sexual, and family endeavors. Profiles with elevations on the scales

TABLE 12.4. Responses of Rheumatoid Arthritis Patients to "Disease-Related" MMPI Items and Their Relation to Mean Health Assessment Questionnaire Scores and Grip Strength

MMPI	Mean HAQ scores		Mean grip strength values	
	True	False	True	False
9. I am about as able to work as I ever was	0.63	1.70[a]	126	95
51. I am in just as good physical health as most of my friends	0.73	1.62[b]	124	97
153. During the past few years I have been well	0.92	1.79[a]	124	87[c]
163. I do not tire quickly	0.79	1.47	153	98[c]
243. I have few or no pains	0.88	1.51	149	92[d]

Note: Adapted from Pincus et al. (1986), page 1463. Copyright 1986 American Rheumatism Association. Adapted by permission.
[a]$p \le .001$.
[b]$p = .006$.
[c]$p < .03$.
[d]$p = .002$.

noted above as well as on the Psychopathic Deviancy and Schizophrenia scales tended to be associated with difficulty in giving up positive reinforcements for pain behavior, high levels of psychopathology, and relatively moderate disruptions in vocational, social, marital/sexual, and family endeavors. Profiles without elevations on the clinical scales were associated with relatively few pain-related disabilities in daily functioning. Similar MMPI profile patterns and behavioral correlates have been identified among independent samples of back pain patients (McGill, Lawlis, Selby, Mooney, & McCoy, 1983) and patients with diverse chronic pain syndromes presenting to a university-based pain treatment center (Costello, Hulsey, Schoenfeld, & Ramamurthy, 1987; Costello, Schoenfeld, Ramamurthy, & Hobbs-Hardee, 1989). Costello, Hulsey, Shoenfeld, and Ramamurthy (1987) also have identified a profile pattern characterized by elevations only on the Hypochondriasis and Hysteria scales. However, no unique correlates for this profile pattern have been identified.

It originally was anticipated that the identification of distinct MMPI profile patterns would help clinicians tailor treatments for patient subgroups with similar MMPI profiles and pain-related behaviors (Bradley et al., 1978). Although this goal has not been achieved, several investigators have attempted to determine if specific MMPI profile patterns are associated with different responses to various treatment packages. Two studies have shown that MMPI profile patterns do not reliably predict outcome following interdisciplinary pain clinic treatment (Guck, Meilman, Skultety, & Poloni, 1988; Moore, Armentrout, Parker, & Kivlahan, 1986). However, McCreary (1985) has demonstrated that chronic back pain patients' responses to conservative orthopedic management were accurately predicted by their MMPI profile patterns. The proportions of accurate predictions ranged from 61% to 99% among the male patients and from 65% to 89% among the females. Moreover, a recent study of work-disabled patients' responses to the MMPI-2 (Moore, McCallum, Holman, & O'Brien, 1991) has produced two important findings. First, the profile patterns identified with the original MMPI were replicated with the MMPI-2. It also was reported that among the males, profiles characterized by elevations on the Hypochondriasis, Depression, Hysteria, Psychopathic Deviancy, and Schizophrenia scales were associated with a significantly poorer return-to-work rate (33%) than the remaining profile patterns (83% and 91%) at a 12-month follow-up assessment. This finding is consistent with the behavioral correlates identified for the same profile pattern derived from the MMPI (Bradley & Van der Heide, 1984). Profile patterns did not predict return to work among the female patients due to the high rates of work return associated with each pattern (78–88%).

We find it very encouraging that the profile patterns derived from chronic pain patients' MMPI responses have been replicated using the MMPI-2. We remain concerned, however, that MMPI profile patterns have not been shown consistently to predict treatment outcome. It has been demonstrated that the profile patterns are better predictors of responses to surgical and nonsurgical treatment when stringent criteria are used to evaluate profile pattern homogeneity (Henrichs, 1987). Therefore, we suggest that clinicians and investigators continue to study the profile patterns

associated with the MMPI-2 using conservative methods for defining these patterns (Sines, 1964). Moreover, given the evidence that statistical algorithms used to derive MMPI profile patterns in one setting may not generalize to other locales (Robinson, Swimmer, & Rallof, 1989), clinicians and investigators should continue to derive profile patterns and behavioral correlates based on the responses of patients at their respective institutions. This will allow for comparisons between local findings and the MMPI profile patterns and correlates already identified in the literature. Such cross-validation is necessary to ensure the validity of the interpretations and predictions that one makes regarding patients' MMPI and MMPI-2 profiles.

Given the problems associated with the MMPI, such as its length, the contamination of items with physical symptoms, and the uncertain predictive validity of chronic pain patients' profile patterns (Smythe, 1984), health care professionals have begun to use several alternative instruments to assess the psychological status of chronic pain patients. These instruments include the Symptom Checklist-90R or SCL-90R (Derogatis, 1983), Millon Behavioral Health Inventory or MBHI (Millon, Green, & Meagher, 1982), and the Illness Behavior Questionnaire or IBQ (Pilowsky & Spence, 1975).

Symptom Checklist-90R

The SCL-90R is a 90-item self-report measure of nine major psychological disturbances (Somatization, Obsessive–Compulsive, Interpersonal Sensitivity, Depression, Anxiety, Hostility, Phobic Anxiety, Paranoid Ideation, and Psychoticism). Three global measures of psychological distress also may be derived; the Global Severity Index is the measure that is most frequently reported in the literature. The SCL-90R requires patients to rate the extent to which each of 90 physical or psychiatric symptoms has bothered them during the past 7 days on a 6-point scale. The patients' raw scores on each scale are transformed to standard T-scores and are interpreted in a manner similar to that used with the MMPI.

The reliability and validity of the SCL-90R with psychiatric patients have been demonstrated in a large number of studies summarized by Derogatis (1983). The SCL-90R is much briefer than the MMPI; thus, it often produces less patient resistance to psychological assessment than does the MMPI. In addition, Parker et al. (1990) have reported that, among a sample of patients with RA, only the Depression and Hostility scales are associated with disease severity or activity as measured by rheumatologist judgments and anatomic stage comparisons.

Despite the advantages of the SCL-90R noted above, several studies have raised questions regarding its utility with chronic pain patients. For example, although Derogatis originally derived 10 factors from the responses of psychiatric patients, Shutty, DeGood, and Schwartz (1986) extracted only 5 factors from the SCL-90R responses of a sample of chronic pain patients. Similarly, Buckelew and her colleagues (Buckelew, DeGood, Schwartz, & Kerler, 1986) found different item response patterns among samples of psychiatric inpatients and chronic pain patients. Psychiatric patients tended to endorse equivalent levels of somatic and cognitive distress items on the SCL-90R, whereas the pain patients' reports of psychological distress generally were restricted to somatic signs of anxiety and depression. Therefore, it appears that different dimensions of distress underlie the SCL-90R responses of psychiatric and chronic pain patients. It is not valid, then, to interpret chronic pain patients' responses on the basis of norms produced by psychiatric patients.

Jamison, Rock, and Parris (1988) have adopted a strategy for interpreting SCL-90R scores similar to that used by Bradley with the MMPI (Bradley & Van der Heide, 1984). These investigators have empirically derived three subgroups of chronic pain patients based on their SCL-90R responses. It was found that patients with elevated scores on the majority of the scales, relative to those with scale scores within normal limits, reported the highest levels of (1) functional disability, (2) sleep disturbance, (3) usage of sleep medication, (4) family conflict, and (5) emotional distress. Butterworth and Deardorff (1987) have used the SCL-90R to identify three subgroups of craniomandibular pain patients identical to those derived by Jamison and his colleagues. However, no information has been produced regarding the predictive validity of the SCL-90R subgroups with regard to treatment outcome.

Millon Behavioral Health Inventory

The MBHI is a 150-item self-report measure that was designed to evaluate the psychological functioning of medical patients. It includes (1) eight scales that assess various dimensions of patients' styles of relating to health care providers (e.g., Cooperative, Forceful); (2) six scales that assess major psychosocial stressors (e.g., Future Despair, Social Alienation); and (3) six scales that assess probable responses to illness (e.g., Gastrointestinal Susceptibility) and treatment interventions (e.g., Pain Treatment Responsivity). Patients respond to each item using a "true" or "false" format and their raw scores on each scale are transformed into "base rate" scores. Thus, for example, an elevated base rate score on Gastrointestinal Susceptibility indicates that the score is significantly greater than that expected given the base rate of this variable within a normative sample of medical patients.

The MBHI has several advantages relative to the MMPI. First, it contains fewer items than the MMPI. Moreover, the items are not contaminated by symptoms of physical illness and the norms are based on the responses of patients with a variety of medical, rather than psychiatric, disorders. The reliability and construct validity of the MBHI scales have been established in a series of studies summarized by Millon and colleagues (Millon et al., 1983).

We have found the Somatic Anxiety and Gastrointestinal Susceptibility scales to be quite useful in our studies of patients with CP of unexplained origin. For example, we have shown that these scales reliably differentiated patients with chronic CP or IBS from patients with benign esophageal diseases and two groups of healthy control subjects (Richter et al., 1986). Among the CP patients, the prevalence rates of significant psychological disturbance identified by the MBHI and the DIS interview were nearly equivalent. In addition, we have found excellent agreement between the MBHI scales and the SCL-90R Somatization and Global Severity Index scales in the assessment of patients with CP and hypertensive lower esophageal sphincter pressures (Waterman et al., 1989). Finally, we have demonstrated that the frequently reported association between stress and gastroesophageal reflux symptoms (heartburn) may be attributed to a tendency of persons with high levels of chronic anxiety to report intense reflux symptoms during stress in the absence of changes in esophageal acid exposure (Bradley et al., in press).

The MBHI would be of exceptional value to clinicians and research investigators if it were confirmed that the instrument accurately predicted outcomes of treatment programs for patients with a variety of chronic pain syndromes. Unfortunately, two investigations have failed to show reliable relationships between the MBHI Pain Treatment Responsivity Scale and patients' changes on subjective and objective outcome measures following treatment in a multidisciplinary pain clinic (Gatchel, Mayer, Capra, Barnett, & Diamond, 1986; Sweet, Brewer, Hazlewood, Toye, & Paul, 1985). Negative results also have been reported for patients who participated in a behavioral program for chronic headaches (Gatchel, Deckel, Weinberg, & Smith, 1985).

Illness Behavior Questionnaire

The IBQ is a 62-item self-report measure that evaluates seven dimensions of abnormal illness behavior. Abnormal illness behavior is defined as "symptom complaints in the absence of somatic pathology, or the adoption by the patient of a sick role which the physician considers logically inconsistent with medical findings" (Hoon, Feuerstein, & Papciak, 1985, p. 385). The seven dimensions of abnormal illness behavior assessed by the IBQ are: (1) General Hypochondriasis, (2) Conviction of Disease, (3) Psychological Versus Somatic Focus of Disease, (4) Affective Inhibition, (5) Affective Disturbance, (6) Denial of Life Problems Unrelated to Pain, and (7) Irritability. Patients respond to each IBQ item using a "true" or "false" format. Although three relatively normal and three abnormal patterns of scores have been identified by Pilowsky and Spence (1976), there are no norms against which patients' IBQ scale scores can be compared. The instrument also has been criticized for the lack of information regarding its internal and test–retest reliability as well as the use of inappropriate factor procedures in the derivation of the IBQ scales (Bradley et al., 1981). It should be noted, however, that an interview form of the IBQ has been shown to be associated with adequate interrater reliability (mean percentage agreement of 88%; Pilowsky, Bassett, Barrett, Petrovic, & Minniti, 1983).

With respect to construct validity, several investigations have shown that patients with diverse chronic pain syndromes or pain symptoms without organic pathology produce higher IBQ scores than controls (Drossman et al., 1988; Pilowsky, Chapman, & Bonica, 1977; Speculand, Goss, Spence, & Pilowsky, 1981). It also has been shown that the IBQ is associated with observational measures of abnormal illness behavior (Waddell, Pilowsky, & Bond, 1989) and pain behavior (Keefe, Crisson, Maltbie, Bradley & Gil, 1986). Finally, the most recent factor analytic study of the IBQ (Zonderman, Heft, & Costa, 1985) produced six factors that closely resembled those originally derived by Pilowsky and Spence (1975). These were (1) Health Worry, (2) Illness Disruption, (3) Affective Inhibition, (4) Affective Disturbance, (5) Avowed Absence of Life Problems, and (6) Irritability. It also was found, however, that each of the factor scales was correlated significantly with Eysenck's Neuroticism Scale (Eysenck & Eysenck, 1968). Thus, it appears that the IBQ may primarily measure anxiety or other neurotic features rather than specific patterns of abnormal illness behavior. This probably accounts for the IBQ's low predictive validity with regard to outcome of low back surgery after controlling for psychological stress (Waddell et al., 1989). We believe that future investigators must provide evidence for the reliability of the IBQ and demonstrate that the IBQ scales are associated with relevant criterion variables (e.g., pain behavior, return to work following surgery) independently of neuroticism before they can be used with confidence to assess abnormal illness behavior.

To summarize, all of the psychological status measures described above have strengths and weaknesses. We recommend use of the MMPI and MBHI, however, given that these instruments appear to possess the greatest strengths and fewest weaknesses. The MMPI has been used in numerous studies of pain patient populations, and it recently has been revised using modified items and a new normative sample. The development of reliable MMPI profile patterns has helped to resolve some of the difficulties associated with the interpretation of profiles based on a psychiatric reference sample and with the instrument's predictive validity.

Nevertheless, the length of the MMPI continues to reduce cooperation with psychological assessment among some chronic pain patients.

The MBHI's greatest strengths are that it is relatively brief and its norms are based on the responses of medical patients. Several of the scales regarding psychosocial stressors (e.g., Gastrointestinal Susceptibility) have been shown to differentiate patients with chronic pain from those with other chronic illnesses and healthy controls. Greater attention, however, should be devoted to the utility of the remaining MBHI scales and to improving the predictive validity of the Pain Treatment Responsivity Scale.

Both the SCL-90R and IBQ are brief measures that may be easily administered to patients with chronic pain. However, the value of both of these instruments in chronic pain assessment has been reduced by important questions that have been raised regarding their factor structures and predictive validity.

Measures of Major Life Events and Daily Hassles

Several investigators recently have begun to examine the extent to which self-reports of environmental stressors are associated with psychological distress and pain behavior. This interest in environmental stressors stems from the associations that have been established within "healthy" populations among stress, psychological variables, and physical as well as psychiatric symptoms (e.g., Kohn, Lafreniere, & Gurevich, 1991). Investigators typically have chosen to examine major life stressors such as divorce, unemployment, and financial problems as well as "hassles" or everyday events that are perceived as annoying or irritating such as lack of sleep or rest, exposure to noise, and difficulty in relaxing. These investigators have most frequently assessed major life stressors using the Life Experiences Survey (Sarason, Johnson, & Siegel, 1978) and the Life Events and Difficulties Schedule (Brown & Harris, 1978). They have used the Daily Stress Inventory (Brantley, Waggoner, Jones, & Rappaport, 1987) as well as the Hassles Scale (Kanner, Coyne, Schafer, & Lazarus, 1981) to evaluate the influence of everyday stressors on pain and other symptoms. All of these methods have been shown to be reliable and valid measures of different dimensions of environmental stress.

With regard to major life stressors, it has been found that patients with back pain of unknown etiology are significantly more likely to report adverse life events prior to pain onset than are patients whose back pain is due to specific causes such as herniated disc (Crauford, Creed, & Jayson, 1990). Major life events also have been shown to differentiate patients with nonulcerative dyspepsia (upper abdominal pain that persists in the absence of an organic cause) from healthy control persons (Bennett, Beaurepaire, Langeluddecke, Kellow, & Tennant, 1991). However, patients with fibromyalgia and irritable bowel syndrome have tended to show equal or lower levels of major life stress than control groups composed of healthy persons or individuals with other chronic illnesses (Dailey, Bishop, Russell, & Fletcher, 1990; Drossman et al., 1988; Wolfe et al., 1984). It should be noted that several investigators have reported that the accuracy of patients' retrospective reports of major life events tends to sharply decrease as the time periods between those events and the assessments increase (e.g., Raphael, Cloitre, & Dohrenwend, 1991). There are methods for improving the accuracy of patients' recall of stressful events such as the use of interviewer-administered checklists and structured probes (Dohrenwend, Link, Kern, Shrout, & Markowitz, 1987). However, these methods have not yet been employed with chronic pain patients and may be too time-consuming for use in a busy clinic setting or in research studies in which patient response burden must be considered.

Relatively few studies have included measures of everyday stressors or hassles. Nevertheless, it has been found that daily hassles are positively associated with self-reports of psychological stress among patients with fibromyalgia (Dailey et al., 1990), negatively correlated with use of adaptive coping strategies among RA patients (Beckham, Keefe, Caldwell, & Roodman, 1991), and positively associated with reports of disease activity among patients with Crohn's disease (Garrett, Brantley, Jones, & McKnight, 1991).

Finally, Volinn and his colleagues (Volinn, Lai, McKinney, & Loeser, 1988) have demonstrated that socioeconomic factors that can produce both major life events and everyday stressors are associated with pain behavior displayed by large communities. These investigators examined differences in industrial insurance claim rates for back pain as a function of county in the state of Washington. It was found that after controlling for variables likely to predict back pain compensation claims, socioeconomic factors such as unemployment rate, per capita income, and percentage of individuals receiving food stamps accounted for approximately one-third of the variance in the rate of claims. Put another way, claims for disabling back pain increased in conjunction with greater economic hardship and job insecurity.

In summary, the literature regarding the association between environmental stressors and chronic pain is relatively small and is characterized by findings that differ as a function of type of pain syndrome and stressor. Given the associations that have been identified to date, we recommend that all patient assessments devote some attention to this issue using either interview questions or one of the self-report methods discussed above.

Measures of Disability and Suffering: The Sickness Impact Profile

The Sickness Impact Profile (SIP) (Bergner, Bobbitt, Carter, & Gilson, 1981) is a 136-item measure of functional disability that may be administered as an interview or as a self-report questionnaire. The SIP provides a profile of patient disability in 12 dimensions of functioning. These are ambulation, mobility, body care and movement, social interaction, communication, alertness, emotional behavior, sleep and rest, eating, work, home management, and recreation. These dimensions also may be combined to form Physical, Psychosocial, and Total Disability scales. Each SIP item describes a specific dysfunctional behavior and patients indicate whether or not each item applies to them. Scores are calculated for the Physical and Psychosocial dimensions of functioning as well as for the Total SIP by using predetermined weights that reflect the relative severity of each item. The test–retest reliabilities of these SIP scores over a 3-week interval have been shown to vary from .69 to .87 (Deyo, 1986). The validity of the SIP originally was established by comparing patients' SIP responses with direct home observations of the patients' behavior. However, it also has been shown that SIP scores are significantly associated with self-reports of pain, physical examination measures

such as spinal flexion and straight leg raising, as well as several other functional disability measures such as the Functional Status Index (Jette, 1980) and Index of Well-Being (Kaplan, Bush, & Berry, 1976; Liang, Larson, Cullen, & Schwartz, 1985).

Studies with arthritis patients have shown the efficiency and sensitivity of the SIP to be equal or superior to that of several other instruments with regard to changes in patient mobility, global functioning, and social functions (Liang et al., 1985). Follick and his colleagues (Follick, Smith, & Ahern, 1985) also have produced positive evidence regarding the concurrent validity and sensitivity to change of SIP scores produced by chronic back pain patients. As a result, numerous investigators have used the SIP as an outcome (Peters & Large, 1990; Turner & Clancy, 1988; Turner, Clancy, McQuade, & Cardenas, 1990) and criterion measure (Jensen, Turner, & Romano, 1991; Riley, Ahern, & Follick, 1988; Schwartz, Slater, Birchler, & Atkinson, 1991) in studies of chronic pain patients.

The major drawback of the SIP is its length. Patients who are highly disabled often have difficulty in responding to 136 items without assistance. Therefore, Roland and Morris (1983) developed a 24-item version of the SIP. Although Deyo (1986) has presented positive evidence regarding the reliability and validity of this short SIP form, it should be noted that its items focus almost exclusively on the physical dimension of disability. Thus, the correlations between the short form of the SIP and the Physical and Psychosocial dimensions of the full SIP are .89 and .59, respectively (Deyo, 1986).

The Chronic Illness Problem Inventory

Despite the strengths of the SIP, several investigators have devised alternative measures of disability (Bradley, 1989). One of the most promising of these alternatives is the Chronic Illness Problem Inventory (CIPI) (Kames, Naliboff, Heinrich, & Schag, 1984). The CIPI is a 65-item self-report measure that assesses behavioral problems associated with a variety of chronic illnesses. Similar to the SIP, each CIPI item describes a problem in functioning; patients rate the extent to which each item applies to them on a 5-point scale. The advantages of the CIPI relative to the SIP are that it is brief and that it evaluates several behavioral dimensions that are not included in the SIP. The 18 CIPI scales consist of activities of daily living, inactivity, social activity, family/friends contact, employment, sleep, eating, finances, medication, cognition, physical appearance, body deterioration, sex, assertion, medical interaction, marital overprotection, marital difficulty, and nonmarried relationships. The initial CIPI reliability studies revealed that the internal consistencies (alpha coefficients) for the 18 scales ranged from .78 to .98. The test–retest reliability coefficients over a 1-week interval ranged from .69 to .97. The validity of the CIPI was established by demonstrating an agreement rate of 80% between problems identified by patients on the instrument and those noted on their evaluations by a clinical psychologist (Kames et al., 1984). In addition, the CIPI was shown to reliably differentiate patients with chronic pain from those with chronic respiratory disease or obesity (Kames et al., 1984). A recent study (Romano, Turner, & Jensen, 1992) also has shown that the CIPI scores produced by chronic pain patients are significantly correlated with their SIP scores (r's = .72 before treatment and .62 following treatment). Both the CIPI and SIP are significantly correlated with patients' self-reports of pain, depression, and reclining time as well as with direct observations of patients' pain behaviors. However, analysis of changes in patients' CIPI and SIP scores revealed that a substantial amount of variance is not shared by the two instruments despite their strong association with each other (Romano, Turner, & Jensen, 1992). Thus, the CIPI and SIP appear to be complementary measures of dysfunction among chronic low back pain patients.

The Multidimensional Pain Inventory

Only one group of investigators has devoted effort to developing a comprehensive self-report instrument that evaluates the impact of diverse chronic pain syndromes on multiple dimensions of patients' lives. The Multidimensional Pain Inventory (MPI) (Kerns, Turk, & Rudy, 1985) is a 56-item measure that is comprised of three sections. The first section includes items regarding (1) interference of pain with daily activities, work, family relationships, and social activities; (2) support from spouse or significant other; (3) pain severity and suffering; (4) perceived life control; and (5) negative mood. The second section assesses patients' perceptions of the degree to which spouses or significant others display solicitous, distracting, or punishing responses to pain or suffering behavior. The final MPI section assesses the frequency with which patients engage in household chores, outdoor work, activities away from home, and social activities. Patients' responses to the MPI items are made on 6- or 7-point scales. These responses may be compared against normative data that are available from the MPI's developers (Turk, personal communication, 1991). Kerns et al. (1985) have demonstrated that the internal reliability coefficients of all MPI scales range from .70 to .90; the test–retest reliabilities of these scales over a 2-week interval range from .62 to .91.

The validity of the MPI originally was supported by the results of confirmatory and exploratory factor-analytic procedures. These procedures revealed that the MPI scales were significantly correlated with several criterion measures of anxiety, depression, marital satisfaction, pain severity, and health locus of control. Recent validity studies (Turk & Rudy, 1988, 1990) have shown that three MPI profile patterns may be reliably identified within samples of patients with chronic low back pain, temporomandibular disorders, and headaches. These patterns were labeled "dysfunctional," "interpersonally distressed," and "adaptive coper" profiles. "Dysfunctional" profile patterns were characterized by relatively high levels of pain severity, life interference, and affective distress, as well as relatively low levels of life control and activity. "Interpersonally distressed" profile patterns were characterized primarily by relatively low levels of support from significant others in the environment. The "adaptive coper" profile patterns were the converse of those of the "dysfunctional" patients. That is, they were characterized by relatively low levels of pain severity, activity interference, and affective distress, as well as by relatively high levels of life control.

The MPI originally was constructed to evaluate the psychosocial and behavioral-functional axes of a pain assessment model termed the Multiaxial Assessment of Pain (MAP) (Turk & Rudy, 1989). The third axis of the model consists of medical and physical findings; a system for quantifying these findings is currently in development (Rudy, Turk, Brena, Stieg, & Brody, 1990). Although the full MAP is not yet complete, several investigators have used the MPI as a criterion measure in studies of patients with rheumatic disorders, myofascial pain, and other chronic pain syndromes (Faucett & Levine, 1991; Jensen & Karoly, 1991; Romano, Turner, Friedman, et al., 1991; see also chapters by Kerns & Jacob, Chapter 14 and Turk & Rudy, Chapter 23).

In summary, there are three self-report measures that may be used to assess disability and suffering among patients with diverse chronic pain syndromes. One of these measures, the SIP, measures disability in both the physical and psychosocial domains of functioning. This instrument is the most extensively studied disability measure in the chronic pain literature and is especially useful in treatment outcome studies due to its high levels of sensitivity and measurement efficiency. However, investigators also may wish to use the CIPI as a complementary instrument given that it assesses several areas of suffering (e.g., finances, sex, medical interaction) that are not evaluated by the SIP. The MPI is a promising measure of disability and suffering that is noteworthy for its assessment of a large number of behavioral and psychosocial dimensions with only 56 items. Although additional research is necessary to validate the MAP classification system proposed by its developers (Turk & Rudy, 1990), the MPI represents a highly valuable assessment tool for clinicians or investigators who wish to measure multiple dimensions of pain and suffering without placing a large response burden on patients.

CONCLUSIONS

This chapter has reviewed a wide array of psychological assessment procedures that may be used with chronic pain patients. We have noted that the assessment of affective distress and suffering requires the administration of at least one interview with the patient and spouse (or other family member) and one or more patient self-report measures. A semistructured interview similar to that described in this chapter or those developed by Phillips (1988) and Karoly and Jensen (1989) is usually most appropriate. This interview should include questions regarding (1) the patient's pain history, (2) events that precede or follow exacerbations in the patient's pain perceptions or behavior, (3) patient's daily activities, (4) social models for pain and disability, (5) occurrence

of sexual or physical abuse, and (6) affective disturbance.

The information that is derived from the interview should be compared with the patient's responses to one or more self-report measures in order to help support evaluative inferences regarding the patient and to aid in treatment planning. These self-report measures should provide information regarding psychological status, environmental stressors, as well as disability and related aspects of suffering. If one is limited to using only one instrument, we suggest that the MPI would be the most appropriate and useful assessment measure. However, if multiple measures are used, investigators and clinicians may consider using either the MMPI or the MBHI to evaluate psychological status. These assessment devices also may be supplemented by a structured psychiatric interview such as the DIS or SCID. Environmental measures may be evaluated with measures such as the Life Experiences Survey, Life Events and Difficulties Schedule, Daily Stress Inventory, or the Hassles Scale. It should be recognized, however, that retrospective reports of major life events over long time periods often are inaccurate. Finally, the SIP and the CIPI may be used either singly or in combination to evaluate disability across a large number of domains of functioning.

REFERENCES

Ahles, T.M., Yunus, M.B., & Masi, A.T. (1987). Is chronic pain a variant of depressive disease? The case of primary fibromyalgia syndrome. *Pain, 29,* 105–111.

American Psychiatric Association. (1987). *Diagnostic and statistical manual of mental disorders* (3rd., rev.). Washington, DC: Author.

Anderson, K.O., Bradley, L.A., Young, L.D., McDaniel, L.K., & Wise, C.M. (1985). Rheumatoid arthritis: Review of psychological factors related to etiology, effects, and treatment. *Psychological Bulletin, 98,* 358–387.

Anderson, L.P., & Rehm, L.P. (1984). The relationship between strategies of coping and perceptions of pain in three chronic pain groups. *Journal of Clinical Psychology, 40,* 1170–1177.

Atkinson, J.H., Slater, M.A., Patterson, T.L., Grant, I., & Garfin, S.R. (1991). Prevalence, onset, and risk of psychiatric disorders in men with chronic low back pain: A controlled study. *Pain, 45,* 111–121.

Beckham, J.C., Keefe, F.J., Caldwell, D.S., & Roodman, A.A. (1991). Pain coping strategies in rheumatoid arthritis: Relationship to pain, disability, depression, and daily hassles. *Behavior Therapy, 22,* 113–124.

Beitman, B.D., Basha, I.M., Trombka, L.H., Jayaratna, M.A., Russell, B., Flaker, G., & Anderson, S. (1989).

Pharmacotherapeutic treatment of panic disorder in patients presenting with chest pain. *Journal of Family Practice, 28,* 177–180.

Beitman, B.D., Mukerji, V., Kushner, M., Thomas, A.M., Russell, J.L., & Logue, M.B. (1991). Validating studies for panic disorder in patients with angiographically normal coronary arteries. *Medical Clinics of North America, 75,* 1143–1155.

Bennett, E., Beaurepaire, J., Langeluddecke, P., Kellow, J., & Tennant, C. (1991). Life stress and non-ulcer dyspepsia: A case-control study. *Journal of Psychosomatic Research, 35,* 579–590.

Ben-Porath, Y.S., & Graham, J.R. (1991). Resolutions to interpretive dilemmas created by the Minnesota Multiphasic Personality Inventory 2 (MMPI-2): A reply to Strassberg. *Journal of Psychopathology and Behavioral Assessment, 13,* 173–179.

Bergner, M., Bobbitt, R.A., Carter, W.B., & Gibson, B.S. (1981). The Sickness Impact Profile: Development and final revision of a health status measure. *Medical Care, 19,* 787–805.

Bigos, S.J., Battie, M.C., Spengler, D.M., Fisher, L.D., Fordyce, W.E., Hansson, T.H., Nachemson, A.L., & Wortley, M.D. (1991). A prospective study of work perceptions and psychosocial factors affecting the report of back injury. *Spine, 16,* 1–6.

Block, A.R., Kremer, E.F., & Gaylor, M. (1980). Behavioral treatment of chronic pain: The spouse as a discriminative cue for pain behavior. *Pain, 9,* 243–252.

Blumer, D., & Heilbronn, M. (1982). Chronic pain as a variant of depressive disease: The pain-prone disorder. *Journal of Nervous and Mental Disease, 170,* 381–406.

Bradley, L.A. (1989). Psychological evaluation of the low back pain patient. In C.D. Tollison & M.L. Krieger (Eds.), *Interdisciplinary rehabilitation of low back pain* (pp. 33–50). Baltimore: Williams & Wilkins.

Bradley, L.A., Prokop, C.K., Gentry, W.D., Van der Heide, L.H., & Prieto, E.J. (1981). Assessment of chronic pain. In C.K. Prokop & L.A. Bradley (Eds.), *Medical psychology: Contributions to behavioral medicine* (pp. 91–117). New York: Academic Press.

Bradley, L.A., Prokop, C.K., Margolis, R., & Gentry, W.D. (1978). Multivariate analyses of the MMPI profiles of low back pain patients. *Journal of Behavioral Medicine, 1,* 253–272.

Bradley, L.A., Richter, J.E., Pulliam, T.J., Haile, J.M., Scarinci, I.C, Schan, C.A., Dalton, C.B., & Salley, A.N. (1992). *The relationship between stress and symptoms of gastroesophageal reflux: The influence of psychological factors.* Manuscript submitted for publication.

Bradley, L.A., Scarinci, I.C., & Richter, J.E. (1991). Pain threshold levels and coping strategies among patients who have chest pain and normal coronary arteries. *Medical Clinics of North America, 75,* 1189–1202.

Bradley, L.A., & Van der Heide, L.H. (1984). Pain-related correlates of MMPI profile subgroups among back pain patients. *Health Psychology, 3,* 157–174.

Brantley, P.J., Waggoner, C.D., Jones, G.N., & Rappaport, N.B. (1987). A daily stress inventory: Development, reliability, and validity. *Journal of Behavioral Medicine, 10,* 61–74.

Briere, J., & Runtz, M. (1988). Multivariate correlates of childhood psychological and physical maltreatment among university women. *Child Abuse and Neglect, 12,* 331–341.

Brown, G.K. (1990). A causal analysis of chronic pain and depression. *Journal of Abnormal Psychology, 99,* 127–137.

Brown, G.W., & Harris, T. (1978). *Social origins of depression: A study of psychiatric disorder in women.* New York: Free Press.

Buckelew, S.P., DeGood, D.E., Schwartz, D.P., & Kerler, R.M. (1986). Cognitive and somatic item response patterns of pain patients, psychiatric patients, and hospital employees. *Journal of Clinical Psychology, 42,* 852–860.

Butterworth, J.C., & Deardoff, W.W. (1987). Psychometric profiles of craniomandibular pain patients: Identifying specific subgroups. *Journal of Craniomandibular Practice, 5,* 225–232.

Cahill, C., Llewelyn, S.P., & Pearson, C. (1991). Treatment of sexual abuse which occurred in childhood: A review. *British Journal of Clinical Psychology, 30,* 1–12.

Clouse, R.E. (1991). Psychiatric disorders in patients with esophageal disease. *Medical Clinics of North America, 75,* 1081–1096.

Cormier, L.E., Katon, W., Russo, J., Hollifield, M., Hall, M.L., & Vitaliano, P.P. (1988). Chest pain with negative cardiac diagnostic studies: Relationship to psychiatric illness. *Journal of Nervous and Mental Disease, 176,* 351–358.

Costello, R.M., Hulsey, T.L., Schoenfeld, L.S., & Ramamurthy, S. (1987). P-A-I-N: A four-cluster MMPI typology for chronic pain. *Pain, 30,* 199–209.

Costello, R.M., Schoenfeld, L.S., Ramamurthy, S., & Hobbs-Hardee, B. (1989). Sociodemographic and clinical correlates of P-A-I-N. *Journal of Psychosomatic Research, 33,* 315–321.

Crauford, D.I.O., Creed, F., & Jayson, M.I.V. (1990). Life events and psychological disturbance in patients with low-back pain. *Spine, 15,* 490–494.

Dailey, P.A., Bishop, G.D., Russell, I.J., & Fletcher, E.M. (1990). Psychological stress and the fibrositis/fibromyalgia syndrome. *Journal of Rheumatology, 17,* 1380–1385.

Derogatis, L. (1983). The SCL-90R manual—II: Administration, scoring and procedures. Baltimore: Clinical Psychometric Research.

Deyo, R.A. (1986). Comparative validity of the Sickness Impact Profile and shorter scales for functional assessment in low-back pain. *Spine, 11,* 951–954.

Dohrenwend, B.P., Link, B.G., Kern, R., Shrout, P.E., & Markowitz, J. (1987). Measuring life events: The problems of variability within event categories. In B. Cooper (Ed.), *Psychiatric epidemiology: Progress and prospects* (pp. 103–119). London: Croom Helm.

Domino, J.V., & Haber, J.D. (1987). Prior physical and sexual abuse in women with chronic headache: Clinical correlates. *Headache, 27,* 310–314.

Drossman, D.A., Leserman, J., Nachman, G., Li, Z., Gluck, H., Toomey, T.C., & Mitchell, M. (1990). Sexual and physical abuse in women with functional or organic gastrointestinal disorders. *Annals of Internal Medicine, 113,* 828–833.

Drossman, D.A., McKee, D.C., Sandler, R.S., Mitchell, C.M., Cramer, E.M., Lowman, B.C., & Burger, A.L. (1988). Psychosocial factors in the irritable bowel syndrome: A multivariate study of patients and nonpatients with irritable bowel syndrome. *Gastroenterology, 95,* 701–708.

Eysenck, H.J., & Eysenck, S.B.G. (1968). *The manual of the Eysenck Personality Inventory.* San Diego: Educational and Industrial Testing Service.

Faucett, J.A., & Levine, J.D. (1991). The contributions of

interpersonal conflict to chronic pain in the presence or absence of organic pathology. *Pain, 44,* 35–43.

Flor, H., Kerns, R.D., & Turk, D.C. (1987). The role of the spouse in the maintenance of chronic pain. *Journal of Psychosomatic Research, 31,* 251–259.

Follick, M.J., Smith, T.W., & Ahern, D.K. (1985). The Sickness Impact Profile: A global measure of disability in chronic low back pain. *Pain, 21,* 67–76.

Fordyce, W.E. (1976). *Behavioral methods for chronic pain and illness.* St. Louis: Mosby.

Gallagher, R.M., Rauh, V., Haugh, L.D., Milhous, R., Callas, P.W., Langelier, R., McClallen, J.M.., & Frymoyer, J. (1989). Determinants of return-to-work among low back pain patients. *Pain, 39,* 55–67.

Gamsa, A. (1990). Is emotional disturbance a precipitator or a consequence of chronic pain? *Pain, 42,* 183–195.

Gamsa, A., & Vikis-Freibergs, V. (1991). Psychological events are both risk factors in, and consequences of chronic pain. *Pain, 44,* 271–277.

Garrett, V.D., Brantley, P.J., Jones, G.N., & McKnight, G.T. (1991). The relation between daily stress and Crohn's disease. *Journal of Behavioral Medicine, 14,* 87–96.

Gatchel, R.J., Deckel, A.W., Weinberg, N., & Smith, J.E. (1985). The utility of the Millon Behavioral Health Inventory in the study of chronic headaches. *Headache, 25,* 49–54.

Gatchel, R.J., Mayer, T.G., Capra, P., Barnett, J., & Diamond, P. (1986). Millon Behavioral Health Inventory: Its utility in predicting physical function in patients with low back pain. *Archives of Physical Medicine and Rehabilitation, 67,* 878–882.

Getto, C.J., Heaton, R.K., & Lehman, R.A. (1983). PSPI: A standardized approach to the evaluation of psychosocial factors in chronic pain. *Advances in Pain Research and Therapy, 5,* 885–889.

Gil, K.M., Keefe, F.J., Crisson, J.E., & Van Dalfsen, P.J. (1987). Social support and pain behavior. *Pain, 29,* 209–217.

Guck, T.P., Meilman, P.W., Skultety, M., & Poloni, L.D. (1988). Pain-patient Minnesota Multiphasic Personality Inventory (MMPI) subgroups: Evaluation of long-term treatment outcome. *Journal of Behavioral Medicine, 11,* 159–169.

Haber, J.D., & Roos, C. (1985). Effects of spouse abuse and/or sexual abuse in the development and maintenance of chronic pain in women. *Advances in Pain Research and Therapy, 9,* 889–895.

Haley, W.E., Turner, J.A., & Romano, J.M. (1985). Depression in chronic pain patients: Relation to pain, activity, and sex differences. *Pain, 23,* 337–343.

Hathaway, S.R., McKinley, J.C., Butcher, J.N., Dahlstrom, W.G., Graham, J.R., Tellegen, A., & Kaemmer, B. (1989). *Minnesota Multiphasic Personality Inventory-2: Manual for administration.* Minneapolis: University of Minnesota Press.

Haythornthwaite, J.A., Sieber, W.J., & Kerns, R.D. (1991). Depression and the chronic pain experience. *Pain, 46,* 177–184.

Heaton, R.K., Getto, C.J., Lehman, R.A.W., Fordyce, W.E., Brauer, E., & Groban, S.E. (1982). A standardized evaluation of psychosocial factors in chronic pain. *Pain, 12,* 165–174.

Helzer, J.E., & Robins, L.N. (1988). The Diagnostic Interview Schedule: Its development, evaluation, and use. *Social Psychiatry and Psychiatric Epidemiology, 23,* 6–16.

Helzer, J.E., Spitznagel, E.L., & McEvoy, L. (1987). The predictive validity of lay Diagnostic Interview Schedule diagnoses in the general population: A comparison with physician examiners. *Archives of General Psychiatry, 44,* 1069–1077.

Henrichs, T.F. (1987). MMPI profiles of chronic pain patients: Some methodological considerations that concern clusters and descriptors. *Journal of Clinical Psychology, 43,* 650–660.

Hoon, P.W., Feuerstein, M., & Papciak, A.S. (1985). Evaluation of the chronic low back pain patient: Conceptual and clinical considerations. *Clinical Psychology Review, 5,* 377–401.

Jamison, R.N., Rock, D.L., & Parris, W.C.V. (1988). Empirically derived Symptom Checklist 90 subgroups of chronic pain patients: A cluster analysis. *Journal of Behavioral Medicine, 11,* 147–158.

Jensen, M.P., & Karoly, P. (1991). Control beliefs, coping efforts, and adjustments to chronic pain. *Journal of Consulting and Clinical Psychology, 59,* 431–438.

Jensen, M.P., Turner, J.A., & Romano, J.M. (1991). Self-efficacy and outcome expectancies: Relationship to chronic pain coping strategies and adjustment. *Pain, 44,* 263–269.

Jette, A.M. (1980). Functional status instrument: Reliability of a chronic disease evaluation instrument. *Archives of Physical Medicine and Rehabilitation, 61,* 395–401.

Kames, L.D., Naliboff, B.D., Heinrich, R.L., & Schag, C.C. (1984). The Chronic Illness Problem Inventory: Problem-oriented psychosocial assessment of patients with chronic illness. *International Journal of Psychiatry in Medicine, 14,* 65–75.

Kanner, A.D., Coyne, J.C., Schaefer, C., & Lazarus, R.S. (1981). Comparison of two modes of stress measurement: Daily hassles and uplifts versus major life events. *Journal of Behavioral Medicine, 4,* 1–39.

Kaplan, R.M., Bush, J.W., & Berry, C.C. (1976). Health status: Types of validity for an index of well-being. *Health Services Research, 11,* 478–507.

Karol, R.L., Micka, R.G., & Kuskowski, M. (1992). *Physical, emotional, and sexual abuse among pain patients and health care practitioners.* Poster presented at the meeting of the Society of Behavioral Medicine, New York, NY, March 1992.

Karoly, P., & Jensen, M.P. (1989). *Multimethod assessment of chronic pain.* Elmsford, NY: Pergamon Press.

Katon, W., Egan, K., & Miller, D. (1985). Chronic pain: Lifetime psychiatric diagnoses and family history. *American Journal of Psychiatry, 142,* 1156–1160.

Katon, W., Hall, M.L., Russo, J., Cormier, L., Hollifield, M., Vitaliano, P.O., & Beitman, B.D. (1988). Chest pain: Relationship of psychiatric illness to coronary arteriographic results. *American Journal of Medicine, 84,* 1–9.

Katon, W., & Roy-Byrne, P.P. (1991). Mixed anxiety and depression. *Journal of Abnormal Psychology, 100,* 337–445.

Keefe, F.J., & Bradley, L.A. (1984). Behavioral and psychological approaches to the assessment and treatment of chronic pain. *General Hospital Psychiatry, 6,* 49–54.

Keefe, F.J., Crisson, J.E., Maltbie, A., Bradley, L., & Gil, K.M. (1986). Illness behavior as a predictor of pain and overt behavior patterns in chronic low back pain patients. *Journal of Psychosomatic Research, 30,* 543–551.

Kerns, R.D., Haythornthwaite, J., Southwick, S., & Giller, E.L. (1990). The role of marital interaction in chronic pain and depressive symptom severity. *Journal of Psychosomatic Research, 34,* 401–408.

Kerns, R.D., Southwick, S., Giller, E.L, Haythornth-waite, J.A., Jacob, M.C., & Rosenberg, R. (1991). The relationship between reports of pain-related social interactions and expressions of pain and affective distress. *Behavior Therapy, 22,* 101–111.

Kerns, R.D., & Turk, D.C. (1984). Depression and chronic pain: The mediating role of the spouse. *Journal of Marriage and the Family, 46,* 845–852.

Kerns, R.D., Turk, D.C., & Rudy, T.E. (1985). The West Haven–Yale Multidimensional Pain Inventory (WHYMPI). *Pain, 23,* 345–356.

Klimes, I., Mayou, R.A., Pearce, M.J., Coles, L., & Fagg, J.R. (1990). Psychological treatment for atypical non-cardiac chest pain: A controlled evaluation. *Psychological Medicine, 20,* 605–611.

Kohn, P.M., Lafreniere, K., & Gurevich, M. (1991). Hassles, health, and personality. *Journal of Personality and Social Psychology, 61,* 478–482.

Levitt, E.E. (1990). A structural analysis of the impact of MMPI-2 on MMPI-1. *Journal of Personality Assessment, 55,* 572–577.

Liang, M.H., Larson, M.G., Cullen, K.E., & Schwartz, J.A. (1985). Comparative measurement efficiency and sensitivity of five health status instruments for arthritis research. *Arthritis and Rheumatism, 28,* 542–547.

Linton, S.J. (1990). Risk factors for neck and back pain in a working population in Sweden. *Work and Stress, 4,* 41–49.

Lorish, C.D., Abraham, N., Austin, J., Bradley, L.A., & Alarcón, G.C. (1991). Disease and psychosocial factors related to physical functioning in rheumatoid arthritis. *Journal of Rheumatology, 8,* 1150–1157.

McCreary, C. (1985). Empirically derived MMPI profile clusters and characteristics of low back pain patients. *Journal of Consulting and Clinical Psychology, 53,* 558–560.

McGill, J., Lawlis, F., Selby, D., Mooney, V., & McCoy, C.E. (1983). The relationship of Minnesota Multiphasic Personality Inventory (MMPI) profile clusters to pain behaviors. *Journal of Behavioral Medicine, 6,* 677–692.

Melzack, R. (1975). The McGill Pain Questionnaire: Major properties and scoring methods. *Pain, 1,* 277–299.

Mikail, S.F., & von Baeyer, C.L. (1990). Pain, somatic focus, and emotional adjustment in children of chronic headache sufferers and controls. *Social Science and Medicine, 31,* 51–59.

Millon, T., Green, C., & Meagher, R. (1983). *Millon Behavioral Health Inventory manual* (3rd ed.). Minneapolis: National Computer Systems.

Monsein, M. (1990). Soft tissue pain and disability. *Advances in Pain Research and Therapy, 17,* 183–200.

Moore, J.E., Armentrout, D.P., Parker, J.C., & Kivlahan, D.R. (1986). Empirically-derived pain-patient MMPI subgroups: Prediction of treatment outcome. *Journal of Behavioral Medicine, 9,* 51–63.

Moore, J.E., McCallum, S., Holman, C., & O'Brien, S. (1991). *Prediction of return to work after pain clinic treatment by MMPI-2 clusters.* Paper presented at the meeting of the American Pain Society, New Orleans, LA.

Moore, J.E., McFall, M.E., Kivlahan, D.R., & Capestany, F. (1988). Risk of misinterpretation of MMPI Schizophrenia scale elevations in chronic pain patients. *Pain, 32,* 207–213.

Naliboff, B.D., Cohen, M.J., & Yellin, A.N. (1982). Does the MMPI differentiate chronic illness from chronic pain? *Pain, 13,* 333–341.

Nelson, A.F. (1986). *Impath TMJ: User reference manual.* Minneapolis: Chronic Illness Care, Inc.

Parker, J.C., Buckelew, S.P., Smarr, K.L., Buescher, K.L., Beck, N.C., Frank, R.G., Anderson, S.L, & Walker, S.E. (1990). Psychological screening in rheumatoid arthritis. *Journal of Rheumatology, 17,* 1016–1021.

Pellegrino, M.J., Waylonis, G.W., & Sommer, A. (1989). Familial occurrence of primary fibromyalgia. *Archives of Physical Medicine and Rehabilitation, 70,* 61–63.

Peters, J.L., & Large, R.G. (1990). A randomized controlled trial evaluating in- and outpatient pain management programmes. *Pain, 41,* 283–293.

Phillips, H.C. (1988). *The psychological management of chronic pain: A treatment manual.* New York: Springer Publishing.

Pilowsky, I., Bassett, D., Barrett, R., Petrovic, L., & Minniti, R. (1983). The Illness Behavior Assessment Schedule: Reliability and validity. *International Journal of Psychiatry in Medicine, 13,* 11–28.

Pilowsky, I., Chapman, C.R., & Bonica, J.J. (1977). Pain, depression, and illness behavior in a pain clinic population. *Pain, 4,* 183–192.

Pilowsky, I., & Spence, N.D. (1975). Patterns of illness behavior in patients with intractable pain. *Journal of Psychosomatic Research, 19,* 279–287.

Pilowsky, I., & Spence, N.D. (1976). Illness behavior syndromes associated with intractable pain. *Pain, 2,* 61–71.

Pincus, T., Callahan, L.F., Bradley, L.A., Vaughn, W.K., & Wolfe, F. (1986). Elevated MMPI scores for hypochondriasis, depression, and hysteria in patients with rheumatoid arthritis reflect disease rather than psychological status. *Arthritis and Rheumatism, 29,* 1456–1466.

Prokop, C.K. (1986). Hysteria scale elevations in low back pain patients: A risk factor for misdiagnosis? *Journal of Consulting and Clinical Psychology, 54,* 558–562.

Ransford, A.O., Cairns, D., & Mooney, V. (1976). The pain drawing as an aid to the psychologic evaluation of patients with low-back pain. *Spine, 1,* 127–134.

Raphael, K.G., Cloitre, M., & Dohrenwend, B.P. (1991). Problems of recall and misclassification with checklist methods of measuring stressful life events. *Health Psychology, 10,* 62–74.

Richter, J.E., Obrecht, W.F., Bradley, L.A., Young, L.D., Anderson, K.O., & Castell, D.O. (1986). Psychological profiles of patients with the nutcracker esophagus. *Digestive Diseases and Sciences, 31,* 131–138.

Riley, J.F., Ahern, D.K., & Follick, M.J. (1988). Chronic pain and functional impairment: Assessing beliefs about their relationship. *Archives of Physical Medicine and Rehabilitation, 69,* 579–582.

Robins, L.N., Helzer, J.E., Croughan, J., & Ratcliff, K.S. (1981). National Institute of Mental Health Diagnostic Interview Schedule. *Archives of General Psychiatry, 38,* 381–389.

Robinson, M.E., Swimmer, G.I., & Rallof, D. (1989). The P-A-I-N MMPI classification system: A critical review. *Pain, 37,* 211–214.

Roland, M., & Morris, R. (1983). A study of the natural history of back pain: Part I. Development of a reliable and sensitive measure of disability in low-back pain. *Spine, 8,* 141–144.

Romano, J.M., & Turner, J.A. (1985). Chronic pain and

depression: Does the evidence support a relationship? *Psychological Bulletin, 97,* 18–34.

Romano, J.M., Turner, J.A., Friedman, L.S., Bulcroft, R.A., Jensen, M.P., & Hops, H. (1991). Observational assessment of chronic pain patient–spouse behavioral interactions. *Behavior Therapy, 22,* 549–567.

Romano, J.M., Turner, J.A., & Jensen, M.P. (1992). The Chronic Illness Problem Inventory as a measure of dysfunction in chronic pain patients. *Pain, 49,* 71–75.

Romano, J.M., Turner, J.A., & Moore, J.E. (1989). Psychological evaluation. In C.D. Tollison (Ed.), *Handbook of chronic pain management* (pp. 38–51). Baltimore: Williams & Wilkins.

Rudy, T.E., Turk, D.C., Brena, S.F., Stieg, R.L., & Brody, M.C. (1990). Quantification of biomedical findings of chronic pain patients: Development of an index of pathology. *Pain, 42,* 167–182.

Saarijarvi, S., Rytokoski, V., & Karppi, S-L. (1990). Marital satisfaction and distress in chronic low-back pain patients and their spouses. *Clinical Journal of Pain, 6,* 148–152.

Sarason, I.G., Johnson, J.H., & Siegel, J.M. (1978). Assessing the impact of life changes: Development of the Life Experiences Survey. *Journal of Consulting and Clinical Psychology, 46,* 932–946.

Shutty, M.S., DeGood, D.E., & Schwartz, D.P. (1986). Psychological dimensions of distress in chronic pain patients: A factor analytic study of Symptom Checklist-90 responses. *Journal of Consulting and Clinical Psychology, 54,* 836–842.

Schwartz, L., Slater, M.A., Birchler, G.R., & Atkinson, J.H. (1991). Depression in spouses of chronic pain patients: The role of patient pain and anger, and marital satisfaction. *Pain, 44,* 61–67.

Sines, J.O. (1964). Actuarial methods as an appropriate strategy for the validation of diagnostic tests. *Psychological Review, 71,* 517–523.

Smythe, H.A. (1984). Problems with the MMPI (editorial). *Journal of Rheumatology, 11,* 417–418.

Speculand, B., Goss, A.N., Spence, N.D., & Pilowsky, I. (1981). Intractable facial pain and illness behavior. *Pain, 11,* 213–219.

Spirito, A., DeLawyer, D.D., & Stark, L.J. (1991). Peer relations and social adjustment of chronically ill children and adolescents. *Clinical Psychology Review, 11,* 539–564.

Spitzer, R.L., Williams, J.B.W., Gibbon, M., & First, M.B. (1990). *Structured Clinical Interview for DSM-III-R.* Washington, DC: American Psychiatric Association Press. (Available from Biometrics Research, New York State Psychiatric Institute, 722 West 168th Street, New York, NY 10032)

Spitzer, R.L., Williams, J.B.W., Gibbon, M., & First, M.B. (in press). The Structured Clinical Interview for DSM-III-R (SCID): I. History, rationale and description. *Archives of General Psychiatry.*

Sweet, J.J., Brewer, S.R., Hazlewood, L.A., Toye, R., & Paul, R.P. (1985). The Millon Behavioral Health Inventory: Concurrent and predictive validity in a pain treatment center. *Journal of Behavioral Medicine, 8,* 215–226.

Turk, D.C., & Rudy, T.E. (1988). Toward an empirically derived taxonomy of chronic pain patients: Integration of psychological assessment data. *Journal of Consulting and Clinical Psychology, 56,* 233–238.

Turk, D.C., & Rudy, T.E. (1989). A cognitive-behavioral perspective on chronic pain: Beyond the scalpel and syringe. In C.D. Tollison (Ed.)., *Handbook of chronic pain management* (pp. 222–236). Baltimore: Williams & Wilkins.

Turk, D.C., & Rudy, T.E. (1990). The robustness of an empirically derived taxonomy of chronic pain patients. *Pain, 43,* 27–35.

Turner, J.A., & Clancy, S. (1988). Comparison of operant behavioral and cognitive-behavioral group treatment for chronic low back pain. *Journal of Consulting and Clinical Psychology, 56,* 261–266.

Turner, J.A., Clancy, S., McQuade, K.J., & Cardenas, D.D. (1990). Effectiveness of behavioral therapy for chronic low back pain: A component analysis. *Journal of Consulting and Clinical Psychology, 58,* 573–579.

Vandiver, T., & Sher, K.J. (1991). Temporal stability of the Diagnostic Interview Schedule. *Psychological Assessment, 3,* 277–281.

Vitaliano, P.O., Katon, W., Maiuro, R.D., & Russo, J. (1989). Coping in chest pain patients with and without psychiatric disorders. *Journal of Consulting and Clinical Psychology, 57,* 338–343.

Volinn, E., Lai, D., McKinney, S., & Loeser, J.D. (1988). When back pain becomes disabling: A regional analysis. *Pain, 33,* 33–40.

Waddell, G., Pilowsky, I., & Bond, M.R. (1989). Clinical assessment and interpretation of abnormal illness behavior in low back pain. *Pain, 39,* 41–53.

Waterman, D.C., Dalton, C.B., Ott, D.J., Castell, J.A., Bradley, L.A., Castell, D.O., & Richter, J.E. (1989). Hypertensive lower esophageal sphincter: What does it mean? *Journal of Clinical Gastroenterology, 11,* 139–146.

Watson, D. (1982). Neurotic tendencies among chronic pain patients: An MMPI item analysis. *Pain, 14,* 365–385.

Wells, K.B., Burnam, M.A., Leake, B., & Robins, L.N. (1988). Agreement between face-to-face and telephone administered versions of the depression section of the NIMH Diagnostic Interview Schedule. *Journal of Psychiatric Research, 22,* 207–220.

Whitehead, W.E., Bosmajian, L., Zonderman, A.B., Costa, P.T., & Schuster, M.M. (1988). Symptoms of psychologic distress associated with irritable bowel syndrome: Comparison of community and medical clinic samples. *Gastroenterology, 95,* 709–714.

Whitehead, W.E., Winget, C., Fedoravicious, A.S., Wooley, S., & Blackwell, B. (1982). Learned illness behavior in patients with irritable bowel syndrome and peptic ulcer. *Digestive Diseases and Sciences, 27,* 202–208.

Williams, J.B.W., Gibbon, M., First, M.B., Spitzer, R.L., Davies, M., Borus, J., Howes, M.J., Kane, J., Pope, H.G., Rounsaville, B., & Wittchen, H-V. (in press). The Structured Clinical Interview for DSM-III-R (SCID): II. Multi-site test–retest reliability. *Archives of General Psychiatry.*

Wolfe, F., Cathey, M.A., Kleinheksel, S.M., Amos, S.P., Hoffman, R.G., Young, D.Y., & Hawley, D.J. (1984). Psychological status in primary fibrositis and fibrositis associated with rheumatoid arthritis. *Journal of Rheumatology, 11,* 500–506.

Wurtele, S.K., Kaplan, G.M., & Keairnes, M. (1990). Childhood sexual abuse among chronic pain patients. *Clinical Journal of Pain, 6,* 110–113.

Zonderman, A.B., Heft, M.W., & Costa, P.T. (1985). Does the Illness Behavior Questionnaire measure abnormal illness behavior? *Health Psychology, 4,* 425–436.

Chapter 13

Assessment of Pain Beliefs, Coping, and Self-Efficacy

DOUGLAS E. DeGOOD, PhD
MICHAEL S. SHUTTY, JR., PhD

Our interest in the beliefs and attitudes of chronic pain patients began in the clinic rather than in the laboratory or library. As anticipated from a reading of the medical and psychological literature, when we began to work with patients with chronic pain, we frequently observed mood disturbances, narcotic drug dependency, activity restriction, work avoidance, and marital/family upset. Somewhat to our surprise, however, the most striking feature presented by these patients was the persistence of certain maladaptive beliefs about the diagnosis and treatment of pain. Despite reporting multiple prior radiologic studies, invasive treatments, and lengthy periods of inactivity, it was not uncommon for a patient to expect, and sometimes plaintively demand, more of the same failed effort.

Our clinic's approach, which is to review and ensure completeness of past workups, rather than to order more tests, as well as to recommend conservative treatments and deemphasize surgery and medication, was not infrequently met with skepticism and disappointment, if not anger. Obviously, conservative recommendations, including exercise, relaxation, and less medication, was not the treatment that many patients expected from a major university med-

ical clinic. Even when politely expressing agreement with the rationale and the probable therapeutic value, it was not uncommon to hear, "Yes, but in my case I'm sure there just must be something that needs to be fixed first," or more dramatically, "You don't seem to really understood how much I hurt." Additionally, these patients often intoned that no one had ever explained anything understandable to them about the cause or management of their pain problem. Thus, the patient felt compelled to continue in a desperate search for a doctor who "will just tell me what is wrong."

DeGood (1979, 1983) elaborated on a number of specific patient beliefs about self-management therapies which can contribute to misunderstanding, low motivation, and treatment noncompliance. For example, many patients find it inconceivable that some disorders can be improved through self-regulation, as this might imply that their disease is nonphysical and therefore less respectable. Such patients often approach the psychologist "feeling compelled to prove their sanity rather than to consider new treatment options" (1983, p. 572). Furthermore, such patients may exaggerate their symptoms or pursue dangerous, invasive treatments in order to legitimize their pain complaints. These observations underscore a need for assessment of patient beliefs about their pain and its treatment. Indeed, as Turk, Meichenbaum, and Genest (1983) emphasized, "a dubious attitude about one element of a treatment program may lessen the credibility of the entire program and increase the likelihood of resistance or nonadherence" (p. 261).

One can speculate that the beliefs underlying such persistent ritualized behavior lie in the prior learning that pain is a warning that something is wrong with the body and one should seek medical experts to identify and treat the underlying problem—an appropriate response to acute trauma or illness. However, when expectations for relief are not met, fear soon emerges and often turns to anger and depression as the patient begins to feel a loss of control over the course of his or her life.

Problematic beliefs about pain and its management, we feel, should not be viewed as mere artifacts of the chronic pain experience that will disappear once a correct diagnosis and treatment is found. Rather, such cognitions can lie at the heart of the chronic pain problem. Whether true or false, adaptive or maladaptive, such beliefs can become the internal reality controlling the patient's behavior. Active compliance with treatment, and ultimately treatment success, begins with the establishment of beliefs compatible with the treatment program.

The purpose of this chapter is to describe and critically evaluate the assessment methods available for researchers and clinicians to evaluate such beliefs in the patient with chronic pain. Special attention will be given to beliefs about the nature of pain and its treatment, self-efficacy expectancies, and coping skills.

THEORETICAL BACKGROUND AND DEFINITIONS

Cognitive-Behavioral Model of Pain

Clinical attention to pain patient beliefs is not new. Nearly two decades ago Sternbach (1974) described a taxonomy of pain games which characterized the transactional styles of patients who adopt a lifestyle and set of beliefs fostering invalidism. In an influential book detailing therapeutic strategies for chronic pain patients Turk et al. (1983) make extensive reference to the importance of beliefs on the cognitions

(thoughts and images) a patient may have about pain.

A cognitive-behavioral perspective provides a useful theoretical framework for understanding patient reactions to pain as it emphasizes the reciprocal interaction between cognitive, affective, and behavioral components with sensory input in determining patient beliefs. Consequently, from this integrated perspective, coping with pain is viewed as a dynamic process wherein patient beliefs, attitudes, and thinking style mediate emotional and behavioral responses (Lazarus, 1991; Turk et al., 1983). Consistent with our emphasis on pain beliefs, Turk and Rudy (1986) argue that the cognitive-behavioral theory has focused greater attention on the "attitudes and beliefs of patients regarding their understanding of their plights, of the health care system, of appropriate behavioral responses to disease, of their own capabilities and of their responses to stress" (p. 762).

Definitions and Relationships Among Terms

Within the cognitive-behavioral model the primary terms of interest, although related to the layman's use, have taken on specific operational definitions. "Beliefs" have been defined as personally formed or culturally shared cognitive configurations (Wrubel, Benner, & Lazarus, 1981). They are preexisting notions about the nature of reality which mold our perception of ourselves and our environment and shape its meaning (Lazarus & Folkman, 1984). Beliefs may be so generalized or wide ranging as to serve as a stable personality disposition, or be highly specific to a particular context (Lazarus & Folkman, 1984). Beliefs, as just defined, can be elaborated in a number of different ways. Some additional belief-related constructs of special interest in our review include *expectancy,* and *cognitive coping.*

"Expectancy" is a term often considered nearly synonymous with beliefs, but in the research literature it normally refers to beliefs about the future, and more particularly, relationships between one set of events and future consequences. Most relevant to pain management are the so-called "self-efficacy expectancies." These have to do with beliefs about one's capacity to execute the behavior required to produce a certain outcome (Bandura, 1977). Self-efficacy beliefs are contrasted to outcome expectancy beliefs which have to do with the belief that a particular behavior can lead to a particular outcome regardless of whether or not a patient has the ability to execute the behavior. Thus, a self-efficacy expectancy represents a self-appraisal of how much control, or coping, potential one has in a particular situation.

In contrast "cognitive coping" is the actual process of executing a cognitive response to threat. A coping response may either be adaptive or maladaptive, depending upon a number of variables including demands of the stressor and resources available (Lazarus & Folkman, 1984). Because the use of behavioral coping strategies (e.g., resting, exercise) has been assessed along side cognitive coping strategies (e.g., diverting attention) in the pain literature, both topics will be reviewed.

A concrete example may help to illustrate the operational meaning of the above terms and show how patient beliefs interact with actual behavior. Imagine that a patient with musculoskeletal back pain is informed by a clinician that a particular set of stretching exercises has been found to be helpful for managing such pain. The patient may or may not believe this information to be accurate (outcome expectancy belief). Additionally, even if it is believed to be true, the patient may doubt his or her own ability to perform such exercises (self-efficacy belief). Therefore, if this stretching routine, after it has been demonstrated, is to translate into an actual pain coping skill, the individual must (1) believe that the prescribed exercise might be helpful, (2) believe he or she is capable of doing it, (3) actually perform the exercise, and (4) then experience a perception of pain control as an outcome.

Dimensions of Beliefs

Beliefs that are relevant to the pain domain range from the very general to the highly specific and include (1) basic philosophical assumptions about the nature of the self and the world; (2) beliefs sufficiently generalized and stable to take on the quality of a personality trait; and (3) beliefs directly related to the context of pain and its treatment.

The first category has to do with loosely organized but deep-seated philosophical and ethical assumptions about values such as justice, fairness, suffering, and responsibility. These represent preexisting value judgments about the nature of reality—how things should, or should not, be. If one believes that life should be pain free that particular value can intensify the feelings of suffering associated with pain. Likewise, if pain is viewed as an injustice that inevitably lies in the maliciousness, ignorance, or lack of concern of someone (including divine forces), tolerance of pain can be affected. Category-1 beliefs are difficult to assess because they can be highly personalized, inconsistent, and contradictory.

Beliefs of the second category tend to be more organized and rooted in everyday life. These beliefs are more generalizable across situations and generally more stable over time. Often conceptualized as personality traits, such belief patterns have generated considerable attention in the research literature. Lazarus (1991) suggests that "people carry around with them private and recurrent personal meanings that lead them to react inappropriately to an encounter with a sense of betrayal, victimization, refection, abandonment, inadequacy, or whatever." (p. 363). Fortunately, others may have personality predispositions which translate into positive coping skills. Popular psychological constructs such as "hardiness" (Kobasa, 1979; Pollock & Duffy, 1990), "locus of control" (Rotter, 1966; Wallston, Wallston, & DeVellis, 1978; "attributional style" (Abramson, Seligman, & Teasdale, 1978); "cognitive errors" (Ellis, 1962; Gil, Williams, Keefe, & Beckham, 1990), and "self-efficacy" (Bandura, 1977) are examples of dispositions that may be constant for the individual across a range of stressful situations, including pain and illness.

The third, and final, category of pain beliefs has to do with the specific "nuts and bolts" regarding what the patient believes he or she and others should do to control pain. A category-2 belief such as self-efficacy becomes a category-3 belief when the emphasis moves from a generalized attitude to specific beliefs about one's capacity to perform a target behavior related to pain control. Finally, as reflected in the introduction to this chapter, category-3 beliefs, such as the insistence that further diagnostic workup is needed, are intimately associated with patient responses to treatment recommendations. Some of the category-3 beliefs about the etiology of pain and the corresponding expectations about diagnosis and treatment, which have particular relevance for subsequent adherence and outcome, are listed in Table 13.1.

Place of Belief Assessment in the Evaluation Process

For the clinician concerned with where beliefs assessment fits into the overall biopsychosocial evaluation of the chronic pain patient, Table 13.2 may be helpful.

As portrayed in the table, we consider pain sensation and behavior to be the result of a complex interaction of somatic ("bio"), individual personality ("psycho"), and environmental ("social") factors, magnified by time. These are the primary, or independent, variables in the pain determination process. These primary variables, however, exert their influence on a thinking and feeling organism resulting in a set of personal cognitions and emotions that in time become directly tied to the current pain experience. The intervening cognitive variables may be a more direct entry point to working with a patient than are the more primary psychosocial variables. At initial contact, pain patients will more readily discuss their pain-related experiences and expectations than psychosocial factors that may be viewed as

TABLE 13.1. Contrasting Dimensions of Patient Beliefs about Chronic Pain Regularly Encountered in Treatment Settings

Etiology of pain
  Somatic only vs. interaction of multiple factors
  External vs. internal, e.g., accident vs. aging
  Someone is to blame vs. unfortunate chance
  Pain as symptom vs. benign

Diagnostic expectations regarding
  History taking
  Clinical exams
  Laboratory tests, esp. radiological
  Psychosocial evaluation

Treatment expectations
  Patient passive vs. active, e.g., surgery or medications
    vs. exercise or pain counseling
  Invasive vs. noninvasive
  Fix/repair vs. rehabilitation
  Somatic/medical vs. psychological/behavioral

Outcome goals
  Cure vs. relief
  Rapid vs. gradual change
  Complete vs. partial freedom from pain
  Sensory change only vs. quality of life

TABLE 13.2. Etiologic Model Suggesting Variables to Be Evaluated in Assessment of Patients with Chronic Pain

Variables		
Independent	Intervening	Dependent
$(S \times P \times E)T \longrightarrow$	C and A $\longrightarrow$	cP

Independent variables causing pain
  S = somatic events: physiopathology
  P = personality template: premorbid coping skills
  E = environment: socio/economic consequences
  T = time since pain began
Intervening variables generated by independent variables
  C = cognitions
      beliefs
      attitudes
      expectations
  A = affects
      depression
      frustration/anger
      anxiety
Dependent variables
  cP = chronic pain
      pain sensation
      pain behavior

irrelevant to pain. This entry point is crucial because if the patient does not understand, or accept as personally relevant, the philosophy, methods, and goals of the pain-management program, the intervention plan itself must begin with an effort to enhance understanding and modify expectations.

In the sections to follow we describe recent advances in assessment of beliefs, self-efficacy, and coping and attempt to identify those procedures which seem to be most promising. Emphasis is placed on the clinical utility of the procedure under consideration. Because beliefs can be considered the supraordinate construct, we will begin with this topic.

ASSESSMENT OF THE BELIEFS OF PAIN PATIENTS

Not surprisingly, when mental health clinicians first become involved in the evaluation of pain patients, emphasis was given to psychometric testing for conventional symptoms of psychopathology (see Bradley, Haile, & Jaworski, Chapter 12). Unfortunately, procedures developed and standardized to measure psychiatric symptoms cannot be used to directly assess pain beliefs. Certainly elevated Hypochondrias or Hysteria scores on the MMPI are suggestive of a misinterpretation of physical symptoms; however, any further discrimination of beliefs content is not possible. Although other tests designed and standardized on nonpsychiatric medical patients—the Cornell Medical Index (Abramson, 1966), the Millon Behavioral Health Inventory (Millon, Green, & Meagher, 1979), the Illness Behavioral Questionnaire (Pilowsky, Spence, Cobb, & Katsikitis, 1984), or the Psychosocial Adjustment to Illness Scale (Derogatis, 1986)—have subscales tailored to measure patient adjustment to illness and disability, they still may require considerable inference to justify conclusions about pain-specific beliefs.

In the past decade there has emerged a number of psychometric instruments designed to measure patient beliefs specific to the context of pain and its treatment. Extending early research (e.g., Davis, 1968; Leventhal, Zimmerman, & Gutmann, 1984) which emphasizes the impact of patient beliefs about medical treatment can have on compliance, this recent literature has largely focused on identifying beliefs and attitudes about pain which may potentially compromise compliance with conservative pain management.

A recent study of patient dissatisfaction, following an initial clinic visit for low back pain, underscores the potential impact of patient beliefs about their pain problems upon treatment response. In their series of 140 outpatients, Deyo and Diehl (1986) found that the most frequently reported source of patient dissatisfaction was failure to receive an adequate explanation of their pain problems. Additionally, 15% of the patients did not believe that the doctors and nurses understood their pain problems. Consequently, when compared to patients who reported receiving an adequate explanation of their problems, those who did not believe that the explanation given was adequate requested more diagnostic tests and reported being less likely to want to see the same doctor again. Not surprisingly, dissatisfied patients tended to be less compliant with prescribed medication use and reported less overall improvement at a 3-week follow-up visit.

In light of such findings underscoring the importance of specific patient beliefs about pain and its treatment, a growing number of assessment methods have been recently developed. Listed in Table 13.3 and described below are several procedures which we consider most promising in order of appearance in the pain literature.

Cognitive Error Questionnaire

Lefebvre (1981) developed the Cognitive Error Questionnaire (CEQ) to measure four cognitive errors typically made by pain patients when describing their pain situation: catastrophizing,

TABLE 13.3. Summary of Instruments Designed to Measure Pain Beliefs

Titles and reference	Item total	Subscales or dimensions
Cognitive Error Questionnaire (CEQ) (Lefebvre, 1981)	24	Catastrophizing Overgeneralization Personalization Selective abstraction
Pain Beliefs Questionnaire (PBQ) (Gottlieb, 1984)	43	Disability expectations Self-efficacy Depression Pain as threat
Pain Information and Beliefs Questionnaire (PIBQ) (Schwartz, DeGood, Shutty, 1985; revised Shutty & DeGood, 1990)	32	Factual knowledge about chronic pain Extent of agreement with conservative treatment strategies
Survey of Pain Attitudes (SOPA) (Jensen, Karoly, & Huger, 1987; revised Jensen & Karoly, 1989)	35	Pain control Solicitude Medical cure Disability Medication Emotion
Pain and Impairment Relationship Scales (PAIRS) (Riley, Ahern, & Follick, 1988)	15	Ability to function despite pain
Pain Beliefs and Perception Inventory (PBAPI) (Williams & Thorn, 1989)	16	Judgment about stability of pain Self-blame Perception of pain as mysterious
Pain Cognitions Questionnaire (PCQ) (Boston, Pearce, & Richardson, 1990)	30	Acting coping strategies Hopelessness Helplessness Passive optimism

overgeneralization, personalization, and selective abstraction. The CEQ is composed of 24 short vignettes followed by a description of a dysphoric cognition about the vignette that reflects one of the four cognitive errors. The patient is asked to rate how similar the cognition is to the thought they would have had in a similar situation. Two forms of the CEQ were developed: one describing general life experiences and the other describing limitations of, or problems experienced by, chronic low back pain (LBP) patients.

Research using the CEQ (Lefebvre, 1981) has indicated that depressed subjects, with or without LBP, endorsed cognitive errors more strongly than did nondepressed subjects with or without LBP. Depressed LBP subjects endorsed errors pertaining to pain experiences significantly more strongly than depressed no-pain patients, whereas both groups responded similarly to the general CEQ. These findings while supporting Beck's (1976) contention that cognitive distortion is a central feature of depression, suggest that pain and depression interact to determine the extent of cognitive distortion which occurs in pain-relevant situations. The absence of a similar difference in the nondepressed LBP group suggests this effect was not the result of LBP patients responding more strongly to the pain vignettes.

Lefebvre has pointed out that the kinds of cognitive errors endorsed more strongly by depressed LBP patients tend to distort the impact of low back pain on the subject's life. Unfortunately, the tendency for LBP patients to make greater cognitive distortions on the CEQ is not robust (Diaz-Clark, Pure, Willis, & Hines, 1985), although positive within-group associations between cognitive distortions and ratings of disability/psychological distress have been reported (Smith, Aberger, Follick, & Ahern, 1986; Smith, Follick, Ahern, & Adams, 1986). More recently, the CEQ has been infrequently used probably due in part to the unwieldiness of the instrument and length of administration. Consequently, it appears more suitable for research, rather than clinical applications.

Pain Beliefs Questionnaire

The Pain Beliefs Questionnaire (PBQ) (Gottlieb, 1984, 1986) is a 43-item questionnaire which assesses four factorially derived dimensions: (1) disability expectations, (2) self-efficacy, (3) depression, and (4) pain as threat. The PBQ is brief, easily administered, and has high internal consistency reliability. In addition, the PBQ is face-valid and likely to minimize patient reluctance to complete a psychologically oriented test.

Preliminary research with 116 outpatients undergoing an 8-week behaviorally oriented rehabilitation program found the PBQ to be associated with treatment outcome. Patients who endorsed "dysfunctional cognitions" at the beginning of treatment tended to make significantly less progress during the course of treatment than those who showed few negative thoughts at the outset. In addition, patients judged as treatment successes evidenced a reliable decrease in dysfunctional cognition scores throughout the course of treatment. While these findings suggest that the PBQ may be useful in predicting treatment response, it appears that the measure blends several distinct constructs such as self-efficacy expectancies, cognitive coping strategies, and specific beliefs about treatment, making the PBI difficult to interpret. Nevertheless, the PBQ has demonstrated potential as a clinical tool in at least two studies and warrants further attention to better establish its clinical utility.

Pain Information and Beliefs Questionnaire

The Pain Information and Beliefs Questionnaire (PIBQ) (Schwartz, DeGood, & Shutty, 1985; Shutty & DeGood, 1990) is a two-part questionnaire designed to measure factual knowledge about conservative pain management and extent of agreement with this treatment philosophy. The first section provides a factual information score based on 18 items in which patients are instructed to identify facts about chronic pain. The second section provides a factorially derived patient agreement score based on 13 items in which the patient indicates extent of agreement with each statement reflecting a belief about the applicability of conservative treatment methods to the patient's own pain problem (see Appendix 13.A). Psychometric analyses reveal the agreement scale to possess high internal consistency reliability and taps a single factor, namely, agreement with conservative strategies (Shutty & DeGood, 1990).

One unique feature of the PIBQ is that the authors recommend that it be administered following patient viewing of an educational videotape describing conservative treatment strategies for pain management. The authors argue that this procedure allows for direct measurement of the discrepancy between patient and clinic expectations regarding pain treatment.

Interestingly, the authors note that responses to the agreement scale are independent of patient performance on the factual portion of the questionnaire, underscoring the distinction between patients' generic knowledge about chronic pain problems, and what they actually believe about their own particular pain problem. Analyses of 100 patients (Shutty, DeGood, & Tuttle, 1990) undergoing outpatient treatment found that those who did not initially agree that the information presented on the videotape applied to their unique case reported more pain and disability and were less satisfied with their treatment, at a 1-month follow-up, as compared to those who did agree with the videotape presentation. Although the PIBQ can be used without the videotape, preliminary studies have not evaluated such use. Consequently, the PIBQ is not as easily adaptable to other clinical settings, nor are the findings generalizable to a wide range of treatment programs.

The PIBQ assessment procedure using the videotape is promising and deserves further study, as it has the advantage of tailoring assessment of patient beliefs about their pain and its treatment to a specific referent (i.e., the videotape content). Further research is needed to evaluate the videotape assessment procedure on other clinics.

Survey of Pain Attitudes

The Survey of Pain Attitudes (SOPA) is a 35-item self-report scale (Jensen, Karoly, & Huger, 1989; Jensen & Karoly, 1989) partitioned to the following six subscales measuring the following dimensions of pain beliefs (1) pain control, (2) solicitude, (3) medical cure, (4) disability, (5) medication, and (6) emotion (see Appendix 13.B). Factor analysis and inter-item correlations were evaluated to select items from a larger pool of 74. Initial psychometric analyses revealed the SOPA to have high internal consistency within subscales and to be stable over time. Subsequent analyses revealed the SOPA to be associated with patient report of pain behavior and coping responses as well as

sensitive to attitudinal changes following conservative pain treatment.

More recently, Jenson and Karoly (1991) found that several patient beliefs measured by the SOPA were associated with patient judgments of psychological, social, and medical adjustment 1 to 7 years following completion of inpatient pain treatment. For example, the belief that one is disabled was associated with lower ratings of activity level, higher use of medical facilities for pain, and lower levels of well-being.

The SOPA has undergone two major revisions since its inception and appears to possess strong psychometric qualities. The instrument has demonstrated good clinical utility in characterizing patient responses to conservative pain management.

Pain Beliefs and Perceptions Inventory

The Pain Beliefs and Perceptions Inventory (PBAPI) (Williams & Thorn, 1989) is a 16-item questionnaire measuring the following three factorially derived dimensions of patient beliefs: (1) judgments about the stability of pain, (2) self-blame, and (3) perceptions of pain as mysterious (see Appendix 13.C). The instrument is briefly administered, face valid, and possesses high internal consistency reliability for each of the three dimensions. In a preliminary study, the PBAPI factor of "pain stability" (i.e., that pain is chronic and likely to persist at the same level despite treatment effort) evidenced positive associations with pain intensity ratings and decreased treatment compliance with conservative therapy. In addition, the belief that "pain is mysterious" (i.e., that pain has no explanation) was inversely associated with posttreatment ratings of psychological distress and somatization. Finally, both "pain stability" and "pain as mysterious" beliefs were associated with negative self-perceptions and decreased control over pain.

More recently, Williams and Keefe (1991) examined the relationship between patient beliefs as measured by the PBAPI and coping strategies. A cluster analysis of PBAPI responses to the Stability of Pain and Pain as Mysterious subscales revealed three patient subgroups that differed in patterns of coping strategies used. For example, patients who believed that their pain was enduring and without explanation reported a greater tendency to catastrophize about their pain and employed fewer cognitive coping strategies as compared to patients who believed their pain was of short duration and understandable. These findings have implications for identifying patients who may view training in coping skills to enable better self-control over pain as not appropriate.

Although further research is needed to test the clinical utility of the PBAPI, preliminary findings are promising, particularly given the associations found with short-term treatment outcome.

Pain and Impairment Relationship Scales

The Pain and Impairment Relationship Scales (PAIRS) (Riley, Ahern, & Follick, 1988) is composed of 15 attitudinal statements pertaining to one's ability to function despite pain to which the patient rates level of agreement. The instrument is briefly administered, face valid, and possesses adequate internal consistency. Initial validity research found the PAIRS to be significantly associated with functional impairment in a heterogeneous patient group. More recently, Slater, Itall, Atkinson, and Garfin (1991) have extended the validation and reliability of the PAIRS by demonstrating that patient beliefs associated with impairment were more prominent in LBP patients than controls, were stable over time, and readily distinguishable from measures of emotional distress or response style. In addition, PAIRS scores were associated with patient ratings of disease severity but not associated with physician judgments of severity.

The PAIRS appears to successfully operationalize and directly assess specific patient beliefs about pain and its treatment. Unfortunately, the PAIRS has not been tested as a predictor of treatment compliance or outcome; nevertheless, preliminary findings are encouraging.

Pain Cognitions Questionnaire

The Pain Cognition Questionnaire (PCQ) (Boston, Pearce, and Richardson, 1990) is a 30-item questionnaire composed of patient-elicited pain cognitions which preliminary factor analyses have revealed the following four factors: (1) active positive coping strategies, (2) hopelessness, (3) helplessness, and (4) passive optimism. The PCQ is briefly administered, face valid, and shows adequate internal consistency reliability for the factor scores. Prelimi-

nary analyses reveal that scores on the negative factors (hopelessness and helplessness) were positively associated with measures of pain intensity, distress, and behavioral disruption. Conversely, the positive factors do not appear to be associated with various indices of patient functioning, lending support to previous observations (Chaves & Brown, 1978; Rosenstiel & Keefe, 1983) that successful coping is the consequence of avoiding negative, and, in particular, extremely negative "catastrophizing cognitions." Because the PCQ is the most recently developed measure of pain beliefs found in our review, further research is needed to establish its clinic and research utility. Nevertheless, it appears that the PCQ suffers from similar problems of overlapping constructs of coping strategies and specific pain beliefs as noted above for the PBQ.

ASSESSMENT OF SELF-EFFICACY EXPECTATIONS IN PAIN PATIENTS

A set of specific beliefs about pain and its treatment involves Bandura's (1977) global construct of self-efficacy—that is, the belief that one is capable of producing the necessary behavior to obtain a certain outcome. Bandura (1984) has reviewed laboratory evidence which suggests that individuals who regard themselves as efficacious tend to be more perseverant despite repeated failures, work harder at difficult tasks, and show fewer signs of anxiety than inefficacious individuals. Conversely, individuals who perceive themselves as inefficacious tend to show the opposite pattern of behavior (Schmidt, 1985). These concepts suggest that pain patients who perceive themselves as lacking the capacity to acquire self-management skills might be less persistent, more prone to frustration, and more apt to be noncompliant with treatment recommendations. Hence, some patients might demonstrate adequate understanding of particular treatment rationale, yet be noncompliant due to their perceived inability to produce the behavior necessary to follow treatment recommendations.

Given the potential impact of self-efficacy beliefs on treatment response, assessment of this domain of beliefs appears to be clinically important. Unfortunately, development of specific instruments to assess self-efficacy in pain patients has been severely lacking. Most of the existing research has involved category-3 behavior-specific beliefs, generally asking patients to rate their ability to perform a specific behavior along a graded dimension of difficulty (e.g., Jensen, Turner, & Romano, 1991; Kores, Murphy, Rosenthal, Elias, & North, 1990). For example, three studies have evaluated self-efficacy beliefs regarding ability to exercise using this approach (Council, Ahern, Follick, & Kline, 1988; Dolce, Crocker, & Doleys, 1986; Dolce, Crocker, Moletteire, & Doleys, 1986). More specifically, Dolce, Crocker, Moletteire, & Doleys (1986) assessed self-efficacy expectancies using the single question: "How many repetitions of this exercise do you feel you are capable of doing right now"? They studied 14 chronic pain patients participating in a 4-week rehabilitation program utilizing exercise quota systems and found that self-efficacy ratings consistently improved across the 4-week period, accompanied by a concomitant decrease in ratings of worry and concern about pain and reinjury.

Jensen et al. (1991) used a similar method to assess self-efficacy beliefs to examine the association between patient beliefs about coping ability and reported patterns of coping strategy use. To measure self-efficacy, patients were asked how frequently they could perform eight specific pain-coping behaviors such as aerobic exercise and active relaxation. Their results revealed consistent associations between patient judgments of their ability to use a particular coping strategy and their actual use of that strategy, thus suggesting that patient coping behavior is dependent upon judgments about their ability to perform that behavior. This pattern of results emphasizes the importance of tailoring self-efficacy assessment to a specific behavioral domain which has been defined differently across studies. Consequently, few standardized measures of self-efficacy exist, due to the very specific and narrow range of behavior assessed. One example of a standardized questionnaire measure of self-efficacy tailored for use with arthritis patients in a rehabilitative setting is the Arthritis Self-efficacy Scale (Lorig, Chastain, Ung, Shoor, & Holman, 1989).

Arthritis Self-Efficacy Scale

The Arthritis Self-Efficacy Scale (ASE) is a 20-item self-report questionnaire developed from a pool of 43 items derived in part from rheumatologists and arthritis patients themselves to ensure high face-validity (see Appendix 13.D). The item pool was reduced via exploratory factor analysis of responses from 97 arthritis patients followed by confirmatory factor analysis using a second sample of 144 patients. This rigorous analysis produced three factors (1) self-efficacy for physical function, (2) self-efficacy for controlling other arthritis symptoms, and (3) self-efficacy for pain. Preliminary analysis of the ASE indicated good internal consistency, stability over time, and predicted associations between self-report of self-efficacy with independent ratings of activity level. In addition, the ASE has been shown to be associated with present health status and is sensitive to change during the course of rehabilitative treatment. For example, perceived self-efficacy for pain and other symptoms of arthritis rose significantly from baseline levels for a group of patients undergoing treatment without showing a concomitant change for a no-treatment control group.

The ASE is promising and deserves further study as it has both the advantage of tailoring assessment of self-efficacy expectancies to a specific set of target behaviors while possessing good psychometric properties. The ASE could potentially be modified for use in a variety of treatment settings in addition to arthritis.

ASSESSMENT OF COPING STRATEGIES IN PAIN PATIENTS

Cognitive coping is what people do with their thoughts to try to control or tolerate stressful events, including pain. There is a growing literature which examines the relationship between the way people cope with life stresses and their psychological, physical, and social well-being (see Cohen & Lazarus, 1979; Folkman & Lazarus, 1980; and Lazarus & Folkman, 1984). In this regard, use of varying coping strategies have been found to differentially effect psychological adjustment in patients with chronic illness independent of actual patient controllability of the illness (Felton & Revenson, 1984). For example, Felton, Revenson, and Hinrichsen (1984) measured six qualitatively distinct coping strategies derived through factor analysis in patients suffering from chronic illness; the scales were labeled as follows: cognitive restructuring, emotional expression, wish-fulfilling fantasy, self-blame, information seeking, and threat minimization. Results indicated that a modest but unique part of the variation in adjustment was explained by considering the nature of individual coping responses. In sum, assessment of coping strategies used by chronically ill patients has demonstrated that there are distinct and identifiable dimensions of coping strategies that patients spontaneously use in an effort to function with their illness.

Coping strategy use has been found to be differentially related to general psychological adjustment in many studies. For example, Rybstein-Blinchik (1979) compared posttreatment verbal descriptors of pain using the McGill Pain Questionnaire (see Melzack & Katz, Chapter 10) in patients instructed in different cognitive coping strategies. Chronic pain patients were taught to replace their labeling of "pain" with either (1) an acknowledgment of a specific sensation, such as "burning," (2) a pleasant event that is unrelated to the pain experience, such as a memory, or (3) a reinterpretation of the pain sensation, such as "numbness." The results indicated that although there were no differences across groups before treatment, group C (as compared to groups A, B, and a control) used significantly fewer and milder sensory, affective, and evaluative adjectives to describe their pain experiences. In summary, this literature suggests that coping strategies used by chronic pain patients merit further research and represent an important area of assessment which may affect treatment response.

The effectiveness of training cognitive coping strategies for dealing with experimental pain has received considerable research attention. Training in the use of coping strategies such as imaginative inattention (e.g., ignoring pain by engaging in imagery incompatible with pain) or attention diversion (e.g., focusing attention on the environment) has been shown to decrease pain report and increase pain tolerance and threshold (Tan, 1982). More recently, Fernandez and Turk (1986) utilized meta-analysis of 42 studies to examine the effects of cognitive strategies on reducing experimentally induced pain, providing an empirically derived taxonomy of cognitive coping strategies for pain. Their taxonomy consisted of six dimensions: (1) external focus of attention, (2) neutral imagery, (3) dramatized coping, (4) rhythmic cognitive activity, (5) pain acknowledging, and (6) pleasant imagery. Their analysis revealed

that cognitive strategies are generally effective in reducing experimental pain when compared to no-pain control groups and that there is some suggestion that "pleasant imagery" is the most efficacious while "pain acknowledging" is the least efficacious. The authors suggest that it may be the attention–distraction component of certain cognitive strategies that influence pain perception. On balance, they conclude that the greater the attentional demand of a cognitive strategy, the greater the reduction in perceived pain.

Despite the seeming level of interest and enthusiasm regarding assessment of coping strategies in chronic pain patients, there has been relatively few instruments developed; rather, the clinical literature on coping strategies in pain patients has been largely dominated by a couple of instruments, namely, the Ways of Coping Questionnaire (Folkman & Lazarus, 1980) and the Coping Strategies Questionnaire (Rosenstiel & Keefe, 1983). However, recent additions to the assessment literature (Brown

TABLE 13.4. Summary of Instruments Designed to Measure Coping Strategies

Title and reference	Item total	Subscales or dimensions
Ways of Coping Questionnaire (WOC) (Folkman & Lazarus, 1980)	55	Cognitive restructuring Information seeking Self-blame Wish-fulfilling fantasy Emotional expression Threat minimization
Coping Strategies Questionnaire (CSQ) (Rosenstiel & Keefe, 1983)	50	Diverting attention Reinterpreting pain sensation Coping self-statements Ignoring pain sensation Praying and hoping Catastrophizing Increasing activity level Increasing pain behavior
Vanderbilt Pain Management Inventory (VPMI) (Brown & Nicassio, 1987)	19	Passing coping strategies Active coping strategies

& Nicassio, 1987) underscore continued growth in the area of coping assessment.

Ways of Coping Questionnaire

The Ways of Coping questionnaire (WOC), developed by Folkman and Lazarus (1980) and revised by both Felton et al. (1984) and Vitaliano, Russo, Carr, Maiuro, and Becker (1985), is a three-part 55-item scale composed of six subscales, including (1) cognitive restructuring, (2) information seeking, (3) self-blame, (4) wish-fulfilling fantasy, (5) emotional expression, and (6) threat minimization. Parts I and III of the WOC measures the kinds of stressors experienced and ratings of ability to cope with these stressors respectively. The scale takes about 30 minutes to complete and possesses adequate internal consistency reliability.

Turner, Clancy, and Vitaliano (1987) added items to Part I of the WOC to represent stressors specific to chronic pain. Because the WOC was developed for wide use with a variety of medical populations, its use with chronic pain patients has been somewhat limited. Turner et al. (1987) found associations between coping strategies and patient beliefs about their pain; for example, patients who reported using problem-solving coping strategies were more likely to believe that they must accept pain and not let their pain hold them back from what they wanted to do. Another study (Buckelew et al., 1990) found that WOC coping strategy scores were associated with locus of control orientation for women. For example, women patients with high internal scores only were more likely to utilize information-seeking, self-blame, and threat minimization coping strategies than patients with high scores on both the internal and powerful other locus of control orientations.

Research with the WOC has focused primarily upon relationships between coping strategies and patient beliefs; consequently, the WOC has not typically been used as a clinical tool but rather has been employed primarily for research purposes. Further research is needed to establish its clinical utility.

The Coping Strategies Questionnaire

The Coping Strategies Questionnaire (CSQ) is a 50-item rationally derived self-report instrument (Rosenstiel & Keefe, 1983) designed to assess six cognitive and two behavioral coping strategies including (1) diverting attention, (2) reinterpreting pain sensation, (3) coping self-statements, (4) ignoring pain sensations, (5) praying or hoping, (6) catastrophizing, (7) increasing activity level, and (8) increasing pain behaviors (see Appendix 13.E). The CSQ also includes two items which require the patient to report perceived control over pain and ability to decrease pain. The CSQ has received considerable research attention aimed at improving interpretability via factor-analytic studies of dimensions of coping, clinical studies comparing patient subgroups, and evaluating treatment outcomes.

Factor-analytic studies examining the relationships between the subscales (Keefe et al., 1987; Rosenstiel & Keefe, 1983; Turner & Clancy, 1986) have failed to find a reliable factor structure underscoring the difficulties in conceptualizing important dimensions of coping. The most rigorous of these studies (Lawson, Reesor, Keefe, & Turner, 1990) used confirmatory factor analysis to identify three replicable factors across five heterogeneous samples of pain patients collected from five independent sites. This analysis revealed two global factors with some consistency: (1) reported attempts to use ignoring and self-statements, and (2) self-efficacy appraisals of ability to control or decrease pain. A third factor consisting of diverting attention and praying and hoping was identified but with less consistency. Only one study (Tuttle, Shutty, & DeGood, 1991) evaluated the factor structure of the scales themselves and found factorial support for the catastrophizing, praying and hoping, reinterpreting pain sensation, and diverting attention subscales. In addition, coping self-statements and ignoring pain sensation were found to be indistinguishable, supporting the findings of Lawson et al. (1990). These findings underscore the difficulties and empirically identify distinct dimensions of coping and suggest a need for further research examining the "active ingredients" of patient self-reported coping responses.

Clinical studies using the CSQ to compare reported use of coping strategies to indices of patient functioning and treatment outcome have been more promising. In a recent review of these findings, Turner (1991) concluded that two major relationships between CSQ factors and adjustment to chronic pain have consistently emerged. First, several studies have found that patients who report catastrophizing thinking styles and who perceive themselves as ineffectual at controlling their pain appear to be more disabled and depressed at initial assessment (Rosenstiel & Keefe, 1983; Turner & Clancy, 1986; Keefe, et al., 1987) and at follow-up (Keefe, Brown, Wallston, & Caldwell, 1989). The second major finding has been that for low back pain patients, higher endorsement of ignoring pain, reinterpreting pain sensations, attention diversion, and praying and hoping coping strategies are associated with greater pain and disability levels, suggesting that these coping strategies are not effective methods of coping with chronic pain.

In summary, the clinical utility of the CSQ is well established despite weakness in the interpretation of reliable dimensions of coping strategies themselves. This latter difficulty probably more reflects theoretical shortcomings regarding the taxonomy of coping strategies used, rather than specific weaknessess of the CSQ. In this regard, an adaptation of the CSQ deserves further mention. Buckelew et al. (1990) recently developed a situation version of the CSQ which was used to assess spontaneous coping strategies used during painful EMG testing. The instrument used was based upon the CSQ except that each coping strategy was reworded to reflect present coping. Preliminary findings revealed that most patients used a wide variety of coping strategies that generally appeared to be ineffective. Only use of reinterpreting pain sensations in a minority of patients was negatively associated with reported pain intensity; whereas catastrophizing, diverting attention, and use of self-statements were associated with increased pain. This approach to measuring coping strategies offers the advantage of a clear referent (i.e., EMG testing) and deserves further research attention

Vanderbilt Pain Management Inventory

The Vanderbilt Pain Management Inventory (VPMI) (Brown & Nicassio, 1987) is a 19-item self-report scale which measures the frequency patients report engaging in various thoughts or behaviors to cope with their pain. The items are partitioned into passive coping and active coping subscales, thus differentiating coping strategies by the amount of effort the patient puts forth to function, despite his or her pain, as compared to a patient's tendency to depend upon others. Item selection was based upon factor analysis of 259 rheumatoid arthritis pa-

tients which was replicated using a confirmatory factor analysis on a second sample of 101 RA patients. This rigorous analysis resulted in a brief face-valid measure with stable subscale structure which has been shown to be both internally consistent and invariant over a 6-month period.

Preliminary analysis revealed good construct validity as use active coping strategies was associated with lower pain intensity, fewer depressive symptoms, and less functional impairment as compared to patients who reported using primarily passive coping strategies. In addition, active coping was positively associated with global measures of self-efficacy.

A subsequent study (Brown, Nicassio, & Wallston, 1989) using the VPMI found passive coping to be associated with increased depressive symtomatology in the face of high pain conditions for 287 RA patients. A longitudinal analysis over a 6-month period further strengthened these results, suggesting that continued use of passive coping strategies in the face of high pain contributed to the most severe levels of depression. These findings are consistent with those of Keefe et al. (1987), suggesting that coping strategies contribute significantly to pain adjustment over time. Given the rigorous psychometric development of the VPMI coupled with meaningful associations with pain adjustment, the VPMI appears to represent a promising conceptualization of pain-coping strategies based upon the active/passive dichotomy.

CONCLUSIONS

The current pain assessment literature, we believe, demonstrates a movement away from efforts to extend a preexisting psychiatric nosology to pain patients. Along with identification of primary biopsychosocial variables there is a trend toward assessment of ongoing psychological/behavioral variables, such as beliefs, self-efficacy, and coping skills that are primary components of chronic pain behavior. To date, much of the measurement is theoretically driven and highly individualized to particular research settings. Much more work needs to be done in refining and making available to clinicians convenient, reliable, and valid measures. Until such measures are well established, and are readily available, most clinicians will continue to assess such variables via interview and behavioral observation.

The literature reviewed here demonstrates the unequivocal importance of patient beliefs in coping with pain and ultimately in the adherence and response to treatment. Nevertheless, the question remains as to whether the available procedures are ready for use in individual case assessment by the clinician.

Most of the measures that have been described are very brief and convenient to administer, and several show good psychometric properties. But all of them lack a broad base of testing for clinical utility. Selection alone can be confusing; as seen in Table 13.3, despite similarity in titles, different tests may measure quite different cognitive constructs.

Jensen, Turner, Romano, and Karoly (1991) have recently provided an excellent critique of strengths and weaknesses characterizing the pain beliefs and coping literature. They point to several serious methodological problems in the assessment procedures themselves and in the experimental designs which limit the conclusions that can be drawn from the relevant studies. Among the most serious of these problems is the confounding of conceptually distinct constructs, such as cognitive styles, appraisals, and coping strategies, within a given measure. Confusing the picture further is the frequent use of a composite score, combining several conceptually distinct scales into a single score. Even when validity studies demonstrate that a composite score is predictive of response to treatment, the clinician can be left quite perplexed regarding what is actually being measured. This is not a trivial concern to the clinician, who must try to translate assessment information into individual treatment strategies. It is not sufficient to know that a patient has some vague composite of faulty beliefs and inadequate coping skills, when one must attempt to address specific problematic beliefs or skills.

Along with the above caveat for caution it must be acknowledged that we are dealing with a young, vigorous area of research which represents an exciting opportunity to apply behavioral science theory to the very real world problem of chronic pain. We should not be disappointed with the current absence of a definitive assessment instrument able to generate computerized clinical reports. It is premature to argue that it is time to seek greater uniformity in measurement by discouraging

the development of further new procedures. With greater uniformity can also come a closing off of creative new ideas.

As far as the future of beliefs research is concerned, we believe that the category-1 abstract value-laden beliefs will remain critical to the psychotherapist, but are probably not readily amenable to standardized measurement. Category-2 beliefs, sufficiently pervasive across situations to be considered personality traits, are well grounded in traditional social/ personality psychology theory and measurement and will continue to be important to the theory-driven pain researcher. However, we believe it is measurement of the highly specific category-3 beliefs about pain and its treatment that will continue to attract the most interest and has the greatest potential for clinical application. For example, in our clinic we are currently pilot testing a self-report instrument designed to test the specific expectations about etiology, diagnosis, treatment, and outcome listed in Table 13.1.

RECOMMENDED PROCEDURES

Of the research instruments described, we believe several show particular promise by virtue of their rigorous psychometric development and demonstrated associations with indices of patient functioning and treatment outcome. For example, among the belief measures the PBAPI and SOPA were both developed using rigorous methods such as factor analysis and have demonstrated associations with treatment response. In addition, the PIBQ was developed using factor analysis and has been shown to predict short-term treatment response, although the PIBQ requires use of an educational videotape as part of the assessment process. All of the above instruments possess high face validity, adequate internal consistency, and in the case of the SOPA, stability over time. In addition, the above instruments all assess category-3 beliefs (i.e., beliefs highly specific to pain and its treatment). With regard to assessing self-efficacy, the ASE provides a rigorous model for test development, shares many of the psychometric qualities listed above, and appears to have several advantages over past assessments of self-efficacy.

Finally, in the area of coping, the CSQ continues to enjoy research popularity despite weaknesses in the interpretation of the coping strategies measured. Nevertheless, the CSQ possesses a broad research base for comparing findings across settings. In contrast, the VPMI represents a promising conceptualization of pain-coping strategies based upon an active/passive dichotomy. In addition, the VPMI was developed using factor analysis and has demonstrated adequate internal consistency and stability over time. Finally, VPMI scores have shown predicted associations with indices of patient functioning as well as treatment response.

APPENDIX 13.A
Pain Information and Beliefs Questionnaire*

The videotape you have just seen was developed to teach some important factors about chronic pain and ways we approach its treatment at the Pain Management Center. We would appreciate your help in finding out whether it is effective in teaching these facts.

The first part of the questionnaire deals with facts which were presented in the tape. We do not expect anyone to get them all right. Just do the best you can. Circle *all* the choices that are correct.

1. According to the videotape which of the following are characteristics of chronic pain?

    (a) body-tissue damage which has not healed
    (b) muscle weakness
    (c) Social isolation from family and friends
    (d) a problem which has not been properly diagnosed
    (e) feelings of depression or irritability
    (f) pain that lasts for a long time

2. According to the videotape which of the following are reasonable treatment goals for chronic pain?

    (a) complete pain relief
    (b) increased ability to be active despite some pain
    (c) increased use of pain-killing medications
    (d) gradual return to work and social activities
    (e) increased use of hospital services
    (f) reduction in use of pain medications

3. According to the videotape which of the following are treatments which may help patients learn to live with their pain?

    (a) increased bedrest whenever the pain gets worse
    (b) surgical correction of tissue damage
    (c) use of tranquilizers (Valium, Ativan, Xanax)
    (d) stretching and exercise
    (e) use of narcotic pain-killing medications (Percodan, Codeine)
    (f) relaxation training and pain counseling

The next part of the questionnaire applies to your reactions to the videotape. Please, circle the number that best expresses your level of *agreement* with how much each statement applies to *your* pain problem.

	Not at all					A great deal
1. The tape was easy to understand	1	2	3	4	5	6
2. I believe that the information about chronic pain was accurate	1	2	3	4	5	6
†3. The tape left out important information about my pain	1	2	3	4	5	6
4. Exercise can help me manage my pain	1	2	3	4	5	6

I Agree

(*continued*)

APPENDIX 13.A *(Continued)*

	I Agree					
	Not at all					A great deal
[†]5. It seems to me that I have never really been thoroughly examined for my pain	1	2	3	4	5	6
6. Many of the facts in the videotape also apply to my pain	1	2	3	4	5	6
[†]7. My pain could be completely cured if some doctor found my real problem	1	2	3	4	5	6
8. The approach to chronic pain the video talks about can help me learn to manage my pain	1	2	3	4	5	6
[†]9. A doctor should be able to prescribe a medicine that can control my pain	1	2	3	4	5	6
10. After watching the video, I feel that the doctors understand pain problems like mine	1	2	3	4	5	6
11. It is my responsibility to gradually increase my activity level	1	2	3	4	5	6
12. I believe learning relaxation and stress management skills would help me with my pain	1	2	3	4	5	6
13. My attitude and the way I think are important in learning to manage my pain	1	2	3	4	5	6
[†]14. I believe that improvement of my pain condition will require an operation	1	2	3	4	5	6

*Copyright 1992 Douglas E. DeGood and Michael S. Shutty, Jr.
[†]Reverse-scored items.

APPENDIX 13.B
Survey of Pain Attitudes*

Instructions: Please indicate how much you agree with each of the following statements about your pain problem by using the following scale:

0 = This is very untrue for me.
1 = This is somewhat untrue for me.
2 = This is neither true nor untrue for me (or it does not apply to me).
3 = This is somewhat true for me.
4 = This is very true for me.

1. There are many times when I can influence the amount of pain I feel	0	1	2	3	4
2. The pain I usually experience is a signal that damage is being done	0	1	2	3	4
3. I do not consider my pain to be a disability	0	1	2	3	4
4. Nothing but my pain really bothers me	0	1	2	3	4
5. Pain is a signal that I have not been exercising enough	0	1	2	3	4
6. My family does not understand how much pain I am in	0	1	2	3	4
7. I count more on my doctors to decrease my pain than I do on myself	0	1	2	3	4
8. I will probably always have to take pain medications	0	1	2	3	4
9. When I hurt, I want my family to treat me better	0	1	2	3	4
10. If my pain continues at its present level, I will be unable to work	0	1	2	3	4
11. The amount of pain I feel is completely out of my control	0	1	2	3	4

(continued)

APPENDIX 13.B *(Continued)*

0 = This is very untrue for me.
1 = This is somewhat untrue for me.
2 = This is neither true nor untrue for me (or it does not apply to me).
3 = This is somewhat true for me.
4 = This is very true for me.

12. I do not expect a medical cure for my pain   0 1 2 3 4
13. Pain does not necessarily mean that my body is being harmed   0 1 2 3 4
14. I have had the most relief from the pain with the use of medications   0 1 2 3 4
15. Anxiety increases the pain I feel   0 1 2 3 4
16. There is little that I or anyone can do to ease the pain I feel   0 1 2 3 4
17. When I am hurting, people should treat me with care and concern   0 1 2 3 4
18. I pay doctors so they will cure me of my pain   0 1 2 3 4
19. My pain problem does not need to interfere with my activity level   0 1 2 3 4
20. My pain is not emotional, it is purely physical   0 1 2 3 4
21. I have given up my search for the complete elimination of my pain through the work of the medical profession   0 1 2 3 4
22. It is the responsibility of my loved ones to help me when I feel pain   0 1 2 3 4
23. Stress in my life increases my pain   0 1 2 3 4
24. Exercise and movement are good for my pain problem   0 1 2 3 4
25. Just by concentrating or relaxing, I can "take the edge" off my pain   0 1 2 3 4
26. I will get a job to earn money regardless of how much pain I feel   0 1 2 3 4
27. Medicine is one of the best treatments for chronic pain   0 1 2 3 4
28. I am unable to control a significant amount of pain   0 1 2 3 4
29. A doctor's job is to find effective pain treatments   0 1 2 3 4
30. My family needs to learn how to take better care of me when I am in pain   0 1 2 3 4
31. Depression increases the pain I feel   0 1 2 3 4
32. If I exercise, I could make my pain problem much worse   0 1 2 3 4
33. I believe that I can control how much pain I feel by changing my thoughts   0 1 2 3 4
34. Often I need more tender loving care than I am now getting when I am in pain   0 1 2 3 4
35. I consider myself to be disabled   0 1 2 3 4
36. I wish my doctor would stop prescribing pain medications for me   0 1 2 3 4
37. My pain is mostly emotional, and not so much a physical problem   0 1 2 3 4
38. Something is wrong with my body which prevents much movement or exercise   0 1 2 3 4
39. I have learned to control my pain   0 1 2 3 4
40. I trust that the medical profession can cure my pain   0 1 2 3 4
41. I know for sure I can learn to manage my pain   0 1 2 3 4
42. My pain does not stop me from leading a physically active life   0 1 2 3 4
43. My physical pain will never be cured   0 1 2 3 4
44. There is a strong connection between my emotions and my pain level   0 1 2 3 4
45. I can do nearly everything as well as I could before I had a pain problem   0 1 2 3 4
46. If I do not exercise regularly, my pain problem will continue to get worse   0 1 2 3 4
47. I am not in control of my pain   0 1 2 3 4
48. No matter how I feel emotionally, my pain stays the same   0 1 2 3 4
49. Pain will never stop me from doing what I really want to do   0 1 2 3 4
50. When I find the right doctor, he or she will know how to reduce my pain   0 1 2 3 4
51. If my doctor prescribed pain medications for me, I would throw them away   0 1 2 3 4
52. Whether or not a person is disabled by pain depends more on your attitude than the pain itself   0 1 2 3 4

(continued)

APPENDIX 13.B *(Continued)*

0 = This is very untrue for me.
1 = This is somewhat untrue for me.
2 = This is neither true nor untrue for me (or it does not apply to me).
3 = This is somewhat true for me.
4 = This is very true for me.

53. I have noticed that if I can change my emotions, I can influence my pain	0	1	2	3	4
54. I will never take pain medications again	0	1	2	3	4
55. Exercise can decrease the amount of pain I experience	0	1	2	3	4
56. I'm convinced that there is no medical procedure that will help my pain	0	1	2	3	4
57. My pain would stop anyone from leading an active life	0	1	2	3	4

SOPA Scoring Key

Control: 1, 11†, 16†, 25, 28†, 33, 39, 41, 47†, 53

Disability: 3†, 10, 19†, 26†, 35, 42†, 45†, 49†, 52†, 57

Harm: 2, 5†, 13†, 24†, 32, 38, 46†, 55†

Emotion: 4†, 15, 20†, 23, 31, 37, 44, 48†

Medication: 8, 14, 27, 36†, 51†, 54†

Solicitude: 6, 9, 17, 22, 30, 34

Medical Cure: 7, 12†, 18, 21†, 29, 40, 43†, 50, 56†

APPENDIX 13.C
Pain Beliefs and Perceptions Inventory*

The following is a listing of the PBAPI items reorganized by their factored scales. Each item is associated with a 4-point Likert scale (e.g., −2 = strongly disagree, to 2 = strongly agree). There is no 0 point. Items were are starred are scored with inverted values so as to be consistent with the scale construct.

Pain stability (TIME)

*   3. There are times when I am pain-free.
  6. I am continuously in pain.
 10. It seems like I wake up with pain and I go to sleep with pain.
 16. My pain varies in intensity but is always with me.
  2. I used to think my pain was curable but now I'm not so sure.
  5. My pain is here to stay.
*   9. My pain is a temporary problem in my life.
* 12. There is a cure for my pain.
* 15. Someday I'll be 100% pain free again.

Pain as a mystery (MYST)

  1. No one's been able to tell me exactly why I'm in pain.
  4. My pain is confusing to me.
  8. I don't know enough about my pain.
14. I can't figure out why I'm in pain.

Self-blame (S-B)

  7. If I am in pain it is my own fault.
11. I am the cause of my pain.
13. I blame myself if I am in pain.

APPENDIX 13.D
Arthritis Self-Efficacy Scale*

Self-efficacy pain subscale

In the following questions, we'd like to know how your arthritis pain affects you. For each of the following questions, please circle the number which corresponds to your certainty that you can *now* perform the following tasks.

1. How certain are you that you can decrease your pain *quite a bit?*
2. How certain are you that you can continue most of your daily activities?
3. How certain are you that you can keep arthritis pain from interfering with your sleep?
4. How certain are you that you can make a *small-to-moderate* reduction in your arthritis pain by using methods other than taking extra medication?
5. How certain are you that you can make a *large* reduction in your arthritis pain by using methods other than taking extra medication?

Self-efficacy function subscale

We would like to know how confident you are in performing certain daily activities. For each of the following questions, please circle the number which corresponds to your certainty that you can perform the tasks as of *now, without* assistive devices or help from another person. Please consider what you *routinely* can do, not what would require a single extraordinary effort.

AS OF NOW, HOW CERTAIN ARE YOU THAT YOU CAN:

1. Walk 100 feet on flat ground in 20 seconds?
2. Walk 10 steps downstairs in 7 seconds?
3. Get out of an armless chair quickly, without using your hands for support?
4. Button and unbutton 3 medium-size buttons in a row in 12 seconds?
5. Cut 2 bite-size pieces of meat with a knife and fork in 8 seconds?
6. Turn an outdoor faucet all the way on and all the way off?
7. Scratch your upper back with both your right and left hands?
8. Get in and out of the passenger side of a car without assistance from another person and without physical aids?
9. Put on a long-sleeve front-opening shirt or blouse (without buttoning) in 8 seconds?

Self-efficacy other symptoms subscale

In the following questions, we'd like to know how you feel about your ability to control your arthritis. For each of the following questions, please circle the number which corresponds to the certainty that you can *now* perform the following activities or tasks.

1. *How certain* are you that you can control your fatigue?
2. *How certain* are you that you can regulate your activity so as to be active without aggravating your arthritis?
3. *How certain* are you that you can do something to help yourself feel better if you are feeling blue?
4. As compared with other people with arthritis like yours, *how certain* are you that you can manage arthritis pain during your daily activities?
5. *How certain* are you that you can manage your arthritis symptoms so that you can do the things you enjoy doing?
6. *How certain* are you that you can deal with the frustration of arthritis?

Note. Each question is followed by the scale:

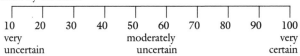

Each subscale is scored separately, by taking the mean of the subscale items. If one-fourth or less of the data are missing, the score is a mean of the completed data. If more than one-fourth of the data are missing, no score is calculated. (The authors invite others to use the scale and would appreciate being informed of study results.)

*From Lorig et al. (1989), page 40. Copyright 1989 J.B. Lippincott Co. Reprinted by permission.

APPENDIX 13.E
Coping Strategies Questionnaire*

Cognitive coping strategies

1. *Diverting attention:* thinking of things that serve to distract one away from the pain.
   Sample item: I count numbers in my head or run a song through my mind.
2. *Reinterpreting pain sensations:* imagining something, which if real, would be inconsistent with the experience of pain.
   Sample item: I just think of it as some other sensation, such as numbness.
3. *Coping self-statements:* telling oneself that one can cope with the pain, no matter how bad it gets.
   Sample item: I tell myself to be brave and carry on despite the pain.
4. *Ignoring pain sensations:* denying that the pain hurts or affects one in any way.
   Sample item: I tell myself it doesn't hurt.
5. *Praying or hoping:* telling oneself to hope and pray that the pain will get better someday.
   Sample item: I pray to God it won't last long.
6. *Catastrophizing:* negative self-statements, catastrophizing thoughts and ideation.
   Sample item: I worry all the time about whether it will end.

Behavioral coping strategies

1. *Increasing activity level:* engaging in active behaviors which divert one's attention away from the pain.
   Sample item: I do something active, like household chores or projects.
2. *Increasing pain behavior:* overt pain behaviors that reduce pain sensations.
   Sample item: I take my medication.

Effectiveness ratings

1. Control over pain.
2. Ability to decrease pain.

*From Rosenstiel and Keefe (1983), page 35. Copyright 1983 Elsevier Science Publishers, B.V. Reprinted by permission.

REFERENCES

Abramson, J.H. (1966). The Cornell Medical Index as an epidemiological tool. *American Journal of Public Health, 56,* 287–298.

Abramson, L.Y., Seligman, M.E.P., & Teasdale, J.D. (1978). Learned helplessness in humans: Critique and reformulation. *Journal of Abnormal Psychology, 87,* 49–74.

Bandura, A. (1977). Self-efficacy: Toward a unifying theory of behavioral change. *Psychological Review, 84,* 191–215.

Bandura, A. (1984). Recycling misconceptions of perceived self-efficacy. *Cognitive Therapy and Research, 8,* 231–255.

Beck, A. (1976). *Cognitive therapy and the emotional disorders.* New York: International University Press.

Boston, K., Pearce, S.A., & Richardson, P.H. (1990). The Pain Cognition Questionnaire. *Journal of Psychosomatic Research, 34,* 103–109.

Brown, G.K., & Nicassio, P.M. (1987). The development of a questionnaire for the assessment of active and passive coping strategies in chronic pain patients. *Pain, 31,* 53–65.

Brown, G.K., Nicassio, P.M., & Wallston, K.A. (1989). Pain coping strategies, and depression in rheumatoid arthritis. *Journal of Consulting and Clinical Psychology, 57,* 652–657.

Buckelew, S.P., Shutty, M.S., Hewett, J., Landon, T., Morrow, K., & Frank, R.G. (1990). Health locus of control, gender differences and adjustment to persistent pain. *Pain, 42,* 287–294.

Chaves, F.F., & Brown, J. (August, 1978). *Self-generated strategies for control of pain and stress.* Paper presented at meeting of the American Psychological Association, Toronto, Ontario.

Cohen, F., & Lazarus, R.S. (1979). Coping with the stresses of illness. In G.C. Stone, F. Cohen, & N.E. Adler (Eds.), *Health psychology: A handbook* (pp. 217–254). San Francisco: Jossey-Bass.

Council, J.R., Ahern, D.K., Follick, M.J., & Kline, C.L. (1988). Expectancies and functional impairment in chronic low back pain. *Pain, 33,* 323–331.

Davis, M.S. (1968). Variation in patients' compliance with doctors' advice: An empirical analysis of patterns of communication. *American Journal of Public Health, 58,* 274–288.

DeGood, D.E. (1979). A behavioral pain management program: Expanding the psychologist's role in a medical setting. *Professional Psychology, 2,* 491–502.

DeGood, D.E. (1983). Reducing medical patients' reluctance to participate in psychological therapies: The initial session. *Professional Psychology, 14,* 570–579.

Derogatis, L.R. (1986). The psychosocial adjustment to illness scale (PAIS). *Journal of Psychosomatic Research, 30,* 77–91.

Deyo, R.A., & Diehl, A.K. (1986). Patient satisfaction with medical care for low-back pain. *Spine, 11,* 28–30.

Diaz-Clark, A., Pure, D., Willis, G., & Hines, V.A. (1985, October). *The assessment of cognitive distortion in a V.A. pain population.* Paper presented at American Pain Society, Dallas, TX.

Dolce, J.J., Crocker, M.F., & Doleys, D.M. (1986). Prediction of outcome among chronic pain patients. *Behaviour Research and Therapy, 14,* 313–319.

Dolce, J.J., Crocker M.F., Moletteire, C., & Doleys, D.M. (1986). Exercise quotas, anticipatory concern and self-efficacy expectancies in chronic pain: A preliminary report. *Pain, 24,* 365–372.

Ellis, A. (1962). *Reason and emotion in psychotherapy.* New York: Lyle Stuart.

Felton, B.J., & Revenson, T.A. (1984). Coping with chronic illness: A study of illness controllability and the influence of coping strategies on psychological adjustment. *Journal of Consulting and Clinical Psychology, 52,* 343–353.

Felton, B.J., Revenson, T.A., & Hinrichsen, G.A. (1984). Stress and coping in the explanation of psychological adjustment among chronically ill adults. *Social Sciences in Medicine, 18,* 889–898.

Fernandez, E., & Turk, D.C. (1989). The utility of cognitive coping strategies for altering pain perception: A meta-analysis. *Pain, 38,* 123–135.

Folkman, S., & Lazarus, R.S. (1980). An analysis of coping in a middle-aged community sample. *Journal of Health and Social Behavior, 21,* 219–239.

Gil, K.M., Williams, D.A., Keefe, F.J., & Beckham, J.C. (1990). The relationship of negative thoughts to pain and psychological distress. *Behavior Therapy, 21,* 349–352.

Gottlieb, B.S. (1984, November). *Development of the Pain Beliefs Questionnaire: A preliminary report.* Paper presented at Association for the Advancement of Behavior Therapy, Philadelphia, PA.

Gottlieb, B.S. (1986, August). *Predicting outcome in pain programs: A matter of cognition.* Paper presented at the American Psychological Association, Washington, DC.

Jensen, M.P., & Karoly, P. (1991). Control beliefs, coping efforts, and adjustment to chronic pain. *Journal of Consulting and Clinical Psychology, 59,* 431–438.

Jensen, M.P., & Karoly, P. (1989, March). *Revision and cross-validation of the Survey of Pain Attitudes (SOPA).* Poster presented at the 10th Annual Meeting of the Society of Behavioral Medicine, San Francisco, California.

Jensen, M.P., Karoly, P., & Huger, P. (1987). The development and preliminary validation of an instrument to assess patients' attitudes toward pain. *Journal of Psychosomatic Research, 31,* 393–400.

Jensen, M.P., Turner, J.A., & Romano, J.M. (1991). Self-efficacy and outcome expectancies: Relationship to chronic pain coping strategies and adjustment. *Pain, 44,* 263–269.

Jensen, M.P., Turner, J.A., Romano, J.M. & Karoly, P. (1991). Coping with chronic pain: A critical review of the literature. *Pain, 47,* 249–283.

Keefe, F.J., Brown, G.K., Wallston, K.A., & Caldwell, D.S. (1989). Coping with rheumatoid arthritis pain: Catastrophizing as a maladaptive strategy. *Pain, 37,* 51–56.

Keefe, F.J., Caldwell, D.S., Queen, K.T., Gil, K.M.,

Martinez, S., Crisson, J.E., Ogden, W., & Nunley, J. (1987). Pain coping strategies in osteoarthritis patients. *Journal of Consulting and Clinical Psychology, 55,* 208–212.

Kobasa, S.C. (1979). Stressful life events, personality, and health: An inquiry into hardiness. *Journal of Personality and Social Psychology, 37,* 1–11.

Kores, R.C., Murphy, W.D., Rosenthal, T.L., Elias, D.B., & North, W.C. (1990). Predicting outcome of chronic pain teatment via a modified self-efficacy scale. *Behaviour Research and Therapy, 28,* 165–169.

Lawson, K., Reesor, K.A., Keefe, F.J., & Turner, J.A. (1990). Dimensions of pain-related cognitive coping: Cross validation of the factor structure of the Coping Strategy Questionnaire. *Pain, 43,* 195–204.

Lazarus, R.A. (1991). Cognition and motivation in emotion. *American Psychologist, 46,* 353–367.

Lazarus, R.A., & Folkman, S. (1984). *Stress, appraisal, and coping.* New York: Springer.

Lefebvre, M.F. (1981). Cognitive distortion in depressed psychiatric and low back back pain patients. *Journal of Consulting and Clinical Psychology, 49,* 517–525.

Leventhal, H., Zimmerman, R., & Gutmann, M. (1984). Compliance: A self-regulatory perspective. In W.D. Gentry (Ed.), *Handbook of behavioral medicine* (pp. 369–436). New York: Guilford Press.

Lorig, K., Chastain, R.L., Ung, E., Shoor, S., & Holman, H.R. (1989). Development and evaluation of a scale to measure perceived self-efficacy in people with arthritis. *Arthritis and Rheumatism, 32,* 37–44.

Millon, T., Green, C.J., & Meagher, R.B. (1979). The MBHI: A new inventory for the psychodiagnostician in medical settings. *Professional Psychology, 10,* 529–539.

Pilowsky, I., Spence, N., Cobb, J., & Katsikitis, M. (1984). The Illness Behavior Questionnaire as an aid to clinical assessment. *General Hospital Psychiatry, 6,* 123–130.

Pollock, S.E., & Duffy, M.E. (1990). The Health-Related Hardiness Scale: Development and psychometric analysis. *Nursing Research, 39,* 218–222.

Riley, J.F, Ahern, D.K, & Follick, M.J. (1988). Chronic pain and functional impairment: Assessing beliefs about their relationship. *Archives of Physical Medicine and Rehabilitation, 59,* 579–582.

Rosenstiel, A.K., & Keefe, F.J. (1983). The use of coping strategies in low-back pain patients: Relationship to patient characteristics and current adjustment. *Pain, 17,* 33–40.

Rotter, J.B. (1966). Generalized expectancies for internal versus external control of reinforcement. *Psychological Monographs: General and Applied, 80*(Whole No. 609).

Rybstein-Blinchik, E. (1979). Effects of different cognitive strategies on chronic pain experience. *Journal of Behavioral Medicine, 2,* 93–101.

Schmidt, A.J.M. (1985). Cognitive factors in the performance level of chronic low back pain patients. *Journal of Psychosomatic Research, 29,* 183–189.

Schwartz, D.P., DeGood, D.E., & Shutty, M.S. (1985). Direct assessment of beliefs and attitudes of chronic pain patients. *Archives of Physical Medicine and Rehabilitation, 66,* 806–809.

Shutty, M.S., & DeGood, D.E. (1990). Patient knowledge and beliefs about pain and its treatment. *Rehabilitation Psychology, 35,* 43–54.

Shutty, M.S., DeGood, D.E., & Tuttle, D.H. (1990).

Chronic pain patients' beliefs about their pain and treatment outcomes. *Archives of Physical Medicine and Rehabilitation, 71,* 128–132.

Slater, M.A., Itall, H.F., Atkinson, J.H., & Garfin, S.R. (1991). Pain and impairment beliefs in chronic low back pain: Validation of the Pain and Impairment Relationship Scale (PAIRS), *Pain, 44,* 51–56.

Smith, T.W., Aberger, E.W., Follick, M.J., & Ahern, D.K. (1986). Cognitive distortion in chronic low back pain patients. *Journal of Consulting and Clinical Psychology, 54,* 573–575.

Smith, T.W., Follick, M.J., Ahern, D.K., & Adams, A. (1986). Cognitive distortion and disability in chronic low back pain. *Cognitive Therapy and Research, 10,* 201–210.

Sternbach, R.A. (1974). *Pain patients: Traits and treatment.* New York: Academic Press.

Tan, S.Y. (1982). Cognitive and cognitive behavioral methods for pain control: A selective review. *Pain, 12,* 201–228.

Turk, D.C., Meichenbaum, D., & Genest, M. (1983). *Pain and behavioral medicine: A cognitive-behavioral perspective.* New York: Guilford Press.

Turk, D.C., & Rudy, T.E. (1986). Assessment of cognitive factors in chronic pain: A worthwhile enterprise? *Journal of Consulting and Clinical Psychology, 54,* 766–768.

Turner, J. A. (1991). Coping and chronic pain. In M.R. Bond, J.E. Charlton, & C.J. Woolf (Eds.), *Proceedings of the VIth World Congress on Pain* (pp. 219–227). New York: Elsevier.

Turner, J.A., & Clancy, S. (1986). Strategies for coping with chronic low back pain: Relationship to pain and disability. *Pain, 24,* 355–364.

Turner, J.A., Clancy, S., & Vitaliano, P.P. (1987). Relationships of stress, appraisal and coping, to chronic low back pain. *Behaviour Research and Therapy, 25,* 281–288.

Tuttle, D.H., Shutty, M.S., & DeGood, D.E. (1991). Empirical dimensions of coping in chronic pain patients: A factorial analysis. *Rehabilitation Psychology, 36,* 179–188.

Vitaliano, P., Russo, J., Carr, J., Maiuro, R., & Becker, J. (1985). The Ways of Coping Checklist: Revision and psychometric properties. *Multivariate Behavioral Research, 20,* 3–26.

Wallston, K.A, Wallston, B.S., & DeVellis, R. (1978). Development of the Multidimensional Health Locus of Control (MHLC) scales. *Health Education Monographs, 6,* 160–170.

Williams, D.A., & Keefe, F.J. (1991). Pain beliefs and the use of cognitive-behavioral coping strategies. *Pain, 46,* 185–190.

Williams, D.A., & Thorn, B.E. (1989). An empirical assessent of pain beliefs. *Pain, 36,* 351–358.

Wrubel, J., Benner, P., & Lazarus, R.S. (1981). Social competence from the perspective of stress and coping. In J. Wine & M. Smye (Eds.), *Social competence* (pp. 61–99). New York: Guilford Press.

Chapter 14

Assessment of the Psychosocial Context of the Experience of Chronic Pain

ROBERT D. KERNS, PhD
MARY CASEY JACOB, PhD

HISTORICAL AND THEORETICAL PERSPECTIVE

Attention to the role of psychological and social factors in the thorough assessment of pain states has long been emphasized in both the clinical and experimental literature. The influence of mood and cognition on the experience of pain and, conversely, the effects of pain on one's psychological state and behavior are universally accepted. In fact, predominant historical perspectives on pain consider the phenomenon to be defined by its psychosocial context. As a function of the rapid pace of clinical research in the past decade, the domain of psychosocial factors relevant to the assessment of the pain experience is rapidly expanding.

Emphasis on the broad domain of psychosocial factors is no more apparent than in the chronic pain area. This state of affairs is largely a function of the development of clinical constructs such as the "chronic pain syndrome" (Black, 1975), "psychogenic pain disorder" (Engel, 1959), and "pain behavior" (Fordyce, 1974), terms that by their definition encourage a focus on psychosocial factors as cardinal features of the pain experience. Recent elabora-

tions of traditional psychodynamic models (Blumer & Heilbronn, 1982) and the articulation of operant conditioning (Fordyce, 1976) and cognitive-behavioral (Turk, Meichenbaum, & Genest, 1983) conceptualizations of chronic pain have encouraged consideration of psychological and interpersonal factors in the development and maintenance of the pain problem. The cognitive-behavioral perspective, in particular, has emphasized the importance of a broad domain of potentially relevant variables in defining the often deleterious impact of the chronic pain experience and in identifying possible psychosocial contributors to the problems of the individual with chronic pain.

Clinical investigators and scholars in the area of chronic pain emphasize thorough assessment of the broad domain of psychosocial factors in order to fully understand the idiosyncracies of the experience for any given individual, and to identify multiple targets for intervention in a comprehensive pain treatment and rehabilitation program. Indeed, multidimensional and multimodal clinical programs based, in part, on a consideration of psychosocial, in addition to biomedical, factors are rapidly replacing discipline-specific and unidimensional treatment centers as the state of the art in chronic pain management. Research designed to examine interactions of psychological and interpersonal variables with biomechanical and physiological parameters is a burgeoning area of investigation that will likely continue to influence clinical assessment and the development of treatment and rehabilitation alternatives.

The primary historical emphasis and bulk of empirical work in the area of chronic pain has been on describing the often deleterious impact or influence of pain on psychological and social functioning. Psychological distress, particularly clinical depression and anxiety disorders, has been cited as a frequent concomitant of chronic pain (Romano & Turner, 1985; Sternbach, 1974; see also Bradley, Haile, & Jaworski, Chapter 12). Additional clinical and social problems commonly noted to occur include unemployment or underemployment, marital and family dysfunction, alcohol and substance abuse, and general declines in social and recreational functioning. With ongoing investigation, the list of documented problems or changes in the psychosocial functioning of patients with chronic pain continues to grow.

Conversely, the development and refinement of contemporary models that incorporate or emphasize psychological processes in the experience of pain has led to a search for specific psychological and social variables that contribute to the development, maintenance, or expression of pain and its impact. Most noteworthy is the Gate Control Theory of pain that emphasizes cognitive-evaluative and motivational-affective processes in addition to sensory-discriminative processes, in the experience of pain (Melzack & Wall, 1965). The viability of this model has been instrumental in opening the door to others who have proposed specific psychological models to explain the development and maintenance of chronic pain (e.g., Fordyce, 1976; Turk et al., 1983).

It is unfortunate, however, that research and clinical wisdom generally continue to view the relationship between the experience of pain and psychosocial variables in unidirectional terms; that is, that chronic pain may be *either* caused by psychosocial factors or provokes psychosocial sequelae. This apparent divergence in theoretical perspectives and the resultant split of scientific and clinical focus of attention compromises a view of these associations as reciprocal and dynamic. It seems much more reasonable to appreciate that the psychosocial context in which chronic pain develops

and continues to exist is inextricably linked with the phenomenon of pain itself. Consistent with this perspective, Karoly (1985) has encouraged a view that the "context" of the pain experience should be viewed as the primary unit of inquiry or investigation in pain assessment. The psychosocial context, then, should be considered as relevant to the understanding of the development as well as the impact of the experience of chronic pain. A cross-sectional approach to assessment of psychosocial factors is to be avoided, or at least interpretation of psychosocial data should consider the reciprocal and dynamic relationships among variables, including the individual's report of pain.

Thus far we have emphasized the broad domain of psychosocial variables that may be relevant to the assessment of chronic pain, the reciprocal and dynamic relationship among these variables, and the importance of thorough assessment of these variables in order to develop a reasonable understanding of the individual's pain and associated problems and to develop realistic and comprehensive plans for intervention. Several additional factors should be considered when developing an assessment plan and deciding upon specific measures. These choices can clearly influence the quality of the data collected as well as their interpretation and ultimate utility.

OVERVIEW OF THE ASSESSMENT PROCESS

Regardless of theoretical perspective, clinicians involved in the assessment of the psychosocial context of the chronic pain experience are generally encouraged to adopt a hypothesis-testing approach to evaluation. A broadly based consideration of the full scope of psychological and social functioning typically begins the assessment process. Most commonly this review is conducted in an interview format that is relatively standardized across individuals regardless of the specifics of their pain complaints. Two examples are offered later in this chapter, the Pain Assessment Report (Holzman, Kerns, & Turk, 1981) and the Psychosocial Pain Inventory (Getto & Heaton, 1985a). Questionnaires are frequently used as an adjunct to the interview. Examples of the most commonly used psychosocial questionnaires and critical discussions of their psychometric properties and clinical uses are provided below.

The content domain includes educational accomplishments and vocational functioning, family and marital status and functioning, and social and recreational functioning. Psychological well-being should be specifically addressed, paying particular attention to levels of affective distress, and to alcohol and drug use (illicit and prescription). Consideration should be given to both historical information and present functioning. Emphasis should be placed on changes in functioning over time, especially those that are temporally associated with alterations in the individual's pain complaint or medical condition or psychosocial concerns.

Based upon this broad screening or review process, specific psychosocial problem areas should be identified, and hypotheses developed to explain the link between them and the pain problem. These problem areas then serve as targets for further assessment and investigation. Efforts should be made to specify psychosocial problems in quantifiable terms, to identify important mediators of their development and maintenance, and to identify potential mediators for change. A range of standardized assessment procedures (e.g., the psychosocial questionnaires described below, and standardized depression inventories) as well as strategies specifically developed by the clinician for this purpose (e.g., a diary developed by the clinician to assess social/recreational activity level and its relationship to pain intensity) are likely to be used.

Whenever possible, clinicians and researchers should avoid relying on a single measure to assess specific content domains (e.g., marital functioning). Optimally, data are collected via multiple methods (e.g., interviews, questionnaires, and diaries) to avoid the biases or sources of error inherent in any single method or specific instrument. Information from sources other than the patient is also valuable, and in certain situations critical, in making accurate judgments about psychosocial functioning. The inclusion of spouses or other family members or close friends is a routine part of many pain programs' assessment protocols.

Clinicians will do best to consider the assessment process as an ongoing component of intervention for most patients. Initial interactions with the patient and others set the stage for the future viability of more structured interventions. With this in mind, concerns that many pain patients have about contact with mental health professionals or the specific focus on psychosocial functioning should be addressed in a straightforward and preemptive fashion. Emphasis during the assessment process should be on engaging the patient and others in a collaborative effort that will maximize treatment participation and outcomes. Goals of the assessment process should be specified and the importance of assuming a broad view of chronic pain and its impact should be emphasized. Assessment should continue beyond the specification of problems and the development of treatment or rehabilitation goals. Ongoing reevaluation of these goals and outcomes throughout the application of intervention strategies is desirable in order to permit identification of new problems or concerns, adjustment of intervention goals, and refinement in intervention strategies.

Thus far our discussion has offered a broad framework in which to consider the assessment of the psychosocial context in chronic pain. In the following pages, we describe a number of methods and instruments that are either commonly used or little known but deserving of attention and evaluation. All are creative efforts to add a psychosocial component to the evaluation of chronic pain.

ASSESSMENT INSTRUMENTS

Interviews

The most commonly used method for the collection of psychosocial information is the clinical interview. The interview is typically the initial contact between the patient and clinician, and often between significant others in the patient's life and the clinician. Because it is the initial contact, the interview has a significant influence on the expectancies of the patient and on the outcome of subsequent assessment and intervention. The interview serves multiple purposes including the identification of potential problem areas and targets for further assessment, the development of possible intervention strategies, and importantly, as a means of motivating patients for further contact with the clinician. Interviews vary with regard to degree of structure, whether or not significant others are included, the scope of the interview, and the breadth versus depth of information gathered. These variables are likely influenced by the theoretical perspective of the clinician. Readers interested in further information about interview strategies, in general, are referred to Gordon (1975) and Haynes (1978). Discussions of the clinical pain interview specifically are also readily available (cf. Karoly & Jensen, 1987; Turk et al., 1983).

Pain Assessment Report

A specific example of a semistructured pain assessment interview is the Pain Assessment Report (Holzman et al., 1981). The interview was developed as a preintervention interview format for the collection of a broad range of specific and quantifiable information relevant to the psychosocial assessment of chronic pain. Purposes of the interview include those common among clinical interview formats, but because of its structure and emphasis on quantification, it also has the advantage of being useful for research.

Clinicians using the Pain Assessment Report follow a specific format for collection of information, referring to a manual that describes methods for coding patient responses in measurable terms. Content domains include a review of the history, site, and presumed diagnosis of the pain complaint; variables perceived by the patient as influencing the pain experience; history and present use of prescribed and over-the-counter pain medications, illicit substances, and alcohol; history of past medical, surgical, physical therapy, and other interventions related to the pain problem; perceived cognitive and behavioral/physical means of coping with pain; educational, vocational, and avocational history and current status with an emphasis on changes related to the pain problem; current status, satisfaction, and pain-related changes in family and marital relations and domestic activities; social functioning; and psychological functioning with an emphasis on mood, sleep, and mental status assessment and current or past psychological treatment. Although the structured nature of the interview and the availability of a detailed coding manual should increase the reliability of the information collected, reliability and validity of the measure have not been reported.

Psychosocial Pain Inventory

A slightly different approach to interviewing has been taken by Heaton and his colleagues in their development of the Psychosocial Pain Inventory (PSPI) (Getto & Heaton, 1985a;

Getto, Heaton, & Lehman, 1983; Heaton et al., 1981, 1982). The PSPI was developed to allow reliable quantification of psychosocial variables hypothesized to influence the experience and the expression of pain. This, in turn, would allow testing of hypotheses such as Fordyce (1976) and Sternbach (1974) have put forth.

The PSPI is a 25-question structured interview developed and tested initially on 169 consecutive pain patients at the Pain Clinic at the University of Colorado Health Sciences Center. The authors report choosing a structured format because in their experience they get more information this way, and it communicates to the patient that many of his or her experiences are normal for a pain patient. In addition, it can reassure a patient who might react to a more traditional psychiatric interview with suspicion and concern about what the interviewer is trying to uncover. The patient is encouraged to add anything of significance, and the interviewer is free to pursue other topics as advisable. The PSPI is meant to generate a minimum patient database, and to guide further assessment. Topics addressed include pain-contingent financial gain, rest, solicitous responding by others, medication use, and illness behaviors. Uniquely, the PSPI also includes items inquiring about past learning history related to the sick role.

The original item pool contained 31 questions. In development, the interview was conducted jointly with 169 pain patients and significant others (Getto & Heaton, 1985b), taking 1 to 2 hours for each interview. Originally, each item was scored on a 4-point scale (0–3), with equal weighting (pending further testing), and specific descriptors anchored each point. Seven items, however, turned out to be clearly bimodal, and so now are scored as 0 = normal or nonsignificant, and 2 = a significant nonorganic contribution is noted. Also, 6 items were deleted because of low variability. Possible scores range from 0 to 68; in the test sample the range was 9–54, with a mean of 30 and a standard deviation of 7.9. Interrater reliability on a sample of 24 patients was .98 for total inventory scores.

During development, PSPI scores were compared to MMPI scores, McGill Pain Questionnaire (MPQ) (Melzack, 1975) responses, physician impressions of exaggerated reports of pain, and objective physical findings. PSPI scores were largely unrelated to MMPI scores except that patients with low PSPI scores appear slightly more defensive and less somatically concerned than patients scoring higher on the PSPI. Patients with higher PSPI scores tended to use more MPQ adjectives and adjectives of greater severity, particularly sensory adjectives.

Almost 27% of the sample had been seen as exaggerating their symptoms by the examining physician. These patients also tended to have higher PSPI scores and elevated MMPI depression scales. In terms of objective physical findings, patients with objective findings were more likely to score higher on the PSPI. Heaton et al. (1982) point out the critical issue here is that psychosocial influences operate strongly for all pain patients, regardless of physical findings.

A small study of 32 neurosurgery consults tested the hypothesis that patients who score high on the PSPI are unlikely to respond to purely medical intervention or advice. Of the 32 referrals who completed the PSPI, 19 received surgery and the others received rest, traction, medication, and/or physical therapy. At 6-month follow-up, the 18 patients considered significantly improved were those who had scored lower on the PSPI.

The PSPI is likely to be of use to many clinicians, and provides for uniform assessment by teams with many members and by clinicians of varied backgrounds. The authors point out that it does not obviate the need for standard psychiatric assessment, such as screening with the MMPI or diagnostic interviewing. It is likely that the PSPI will be sensitive to treatment gains, but the evidence remains to be gathered.

Self-Report Measures

West Haven–Yale Multidimensional Pain Inventory

In assessing the dynamic relationship between psychosocial variables and pain, interviews are generally supplemented by self-report measures. The West Haven–Yale Multidimensional Pain Inventory (WHYMPI) (Kerns, Turk, & Rudy, 1985) is a multifactor instrument designed to assess the broad domain of psychosocial variables relevant to the chronic pain experience. The instrument is theoretically linked to a cognitive-behavioral perspective on chronic pain (Turk et al., 1983) and health assessment (Turk & Kerns, 1985). As such, it places an emphasis on patients' idiosyncratic beliefs or appraisals of their pain problems, its impact in their lives, and the responses of others. The instrument is designed to provide a brief, psychometrically sound, and comprehensive assessment of important components of the pain experience. The authors encourage its use in the context of a multimodal and multidimensional assessment regimen.

The WHYMPI is a 52-item, 12-scale inventory divided into three parts, each containing several scales. Part I consists of five scales designed to evaluate important dimensions of the chronic pain experience: perceived Interference of pain in vocational, social/recreational, and family/marital functioning; Support and concern from significant others; Pain Severity; Life-Control with regard to activities of daily living and daily problems, and Affective Distress. Part II assesses patients' perceptions of the responses of others to their demonstrations and complaints of pain. Three scales assess the perceived frequencies of Negative, Solicitous, and Distracting responses. Part III assesses patients' reports of their participation in four categories of common daily activities: Household Chores, Outdoor Work, Activities Away from Home, and Social Activities. In addition to the individual scale scores, derivation of a General Activity score that is the combination of the four activity scale scores has been recommended for some purposes (Turk & Rudy, 1990). For the 12 WHYMPI scales, the number of items loading on each scale range from two in the case of the Life-Control scale to nine for the Interference scale. The composition of the WHYMPI is offered in Appendix 14.A as an example of a comprehensive self-report instrument for the assessment of chronic pain.

Original development of the WHYMPI was conducted on a sample of 120 chronic pain patients who were heterogeneous with regard to site and etiology of their pain complaints. The sample was drawn from two VA Medical Centers and therefore was largely male. Otherwise, the sample can generally be viewed as typical of many hospital-based pain treatment centers and included patients who had a long duration of pain (mean > 10 years) and a substantial history of failed treatment efforts.

Twenty-two items for Part I of the instrument were developed to assess six a priori domains relevant to the comprehensive assessment of pain severity and the impact of pain on patients' lives. The domains were identical to the final scales named above except that the Interference scale was originally conceptualized as two separate domains measuring pain-related interference and dissatisfaction with present levels of functioning. Confirmatory factor analysis was used to verify the reliability of the six scales. However, a high correlation between the interference and dissatisfaction scales led to combining these scales into a single Interference scale. Two items were dropped because they failed to meet established criteria for convergent and discriminant validity. The resulting five scales were subsequently found to have adequate degrees of internal consistency (alphas ranging from .72 to .90) and stability over a 2-week test–retest period (r ranging from .69 to .86).

Part II was developed to evaluate patients' perceptions of the range and frequency of responses by significant others (most often a spouse or close family member) to displays of pain and suffering. Items consisted of 21 responses derived from interviews with significant others. Exploratory factor analysis was conducted on the responses from a subsample of 95 patients who reported living with a spouse or family member. A 3-factor solution was selected based on established criteria, and three scales comprised of 14 of the original 21 items were identified and named. These scales were each found to have reasonable levels of internal consistency (alphas ranged from .74 to .84) and stability (r ranging from .62 to .89).

Thirty items for Part III of the WHYMPI were derived from published activity lists and lists of activity goals for patients already seen at a pain program at one of the VA Medical Centers. Four reliable factors were identified on the basis of factor analysis. Eighteen of the original pool of items were retained. Each resulting scale demonstrated good levels of reliability (alphas ranging from .70 to .86) and stability (r ranging from .83 to .91).

Validity of the scales of the WHYMPI was examined in two ways. Interscale correlations were all lower than each scale's index of internal consistency, suggesting that each scale contains a unique reliable variance or discriminant distinctiveness from the other scales. Factorial validity was also examined by submitting the 12 scales from the WHYMPI along with several other standardized measures of pain-relevant constructs to exploratory factor analy-

sis. The WHYMPI scales loaded significantly and meaningfully on factors also comprised of conceptually related standardized measures. For example, the Negative Mood and Life-Control scales from the WHYMPI loaded significantly on the first factor along with standardized measures of depression and anxiety.

Since its publication in 1985, the WHYMPI has been used in several research projects that support its heuristic value and clinical utility. Studies have documented its sensitivity to improvements in pain and functioning (Kerns & Haythornthwaite, 1988; Kerns, Turk, Holzman, & Rudy, 1986); the ability of several of its scales to discriminate level of depression symptom severity (Kerns & Haythornthwaite, 1988); the viability of the Pain Severity and Activity scales as brief and reliable measures of pain intensity and adaptive functioning, respectively (Holmes & Stevenson, 1990); and the predictive utility of the Part II response scales in analyses of the role of social interactions in the maintenance of pain and disability (Faucett & Levine, 1991; Flor, Kerns, & Turk, 1987; Flor, Turk, & Rudy, 1989; Kerns, Haythornthwaite, Southwick, & Giller, 1990; Kerns et al., 1991). Rudy (1989) proposed a revision of the WHYMPI that contains two additional items in both the Life Control and Interference scales. Computer scoring of this version is also available (Rudy, 1989).

Turk and Rudy and their colleagues (Rudy, Turk, Zaki, & Curtin, 1989; Turk & Rudy, 1988, 1990; Turk, Rudy, & Stieg, 1988) have proposed an empirically derived taxonomy of chronic pain patients called the Multiaxial Assessment of Pain (MAP) based on analyses of the WHYMPI scale scores. In a series of studies these investigators have identified three reliable profiles or categories of chronic pain patients: Dysfunctional, Interpersonally Distressed, and Adaptive Copers. These profiles have been confirmed as similar in groups of patients suffering from chronic low back pain, headache, and temporomandibular joint pain (Turk & Rudy, 1990; see also Turk & Rudy, Chapter 23). Together, these findings support the discriminant validity of the WHYMPI and its utility as a clinical assessment procedure. Kerns et al. (1985) continue to encourage that the WHYMPI be used in the context of a comprehensive evaluation protocol that also assesses medical/physical parameters.

In summary, the WHYMPI holds substantial promise as a measure of psychosocial functioning for clinical as well as research purposes. The strengths of the WHYMPI are its brevity, the ease with which it is scored (by hand or computer), its demonstrated reliability and validity, and its demonstrated utility in multiple clinical research investigations.

A spouse version of the WHYMPI has also been developed that follows a format similar to the patient version. Part I includes items designed to assess the spouses' perceptions of the patients' pain complaints as well as the spouses' reports of their own level of affective distress, perceptions of the impact of pain on their lives, and their global perceptions of support for the patients. Part II assesses the spouses' reports of their characteristic means of responding to the patients' pain complaints. Part III asks the spouses to report on the patients' level of activity. As such, the spouse version of the WHYMPI may be useful as a check on the validity of the patients' reports, as well as providing information about the perceived impact of pain on significant others. Although components of the measure have been used in published reports and limited reliability and validity data have been presented (e.g., Flor et al., 1987), the psychometric properties of the spouse version of the WHYMPI have yet to be examined systematically. In the absence of these data, the spouse version should be used with considerable caution.

Chronic Illness Problem Inventory

The Chronic Illness Problem Inventory (CIPI) (Kames, Naliboff, Heinrich, & Schag, 1984) is a 65-item instrument intended to assess patient functioning in the areas of physical limitations, psychosocial functioning, health-care behaviors, and marital adjustment. Its form has been influenced by the emphasis Turk and his colleagues (Turk, Sobel, Follick, & Youkilis, 1980) have placed on measures of competency as a way of focusing on patient-environment relationships.

In developing the CIPI, mental health clinicians working in areas of chronic illness generated 74 items in 24 "problem areas" thought to be of concern to the chronically ill and amenable to treatment. These items were initially administered to 115 pain patients. Initial analyses included (1) tests of internal consistency using Cronbach's alpha, (2) factor analyses, and (3) frequency distributions (items

with extremely low frequencies were discarded unless they were thought to represent significant concerns of the chronically ill but not of pain patients). These analyses resulted in a 65-item inventory with 18 scales. Coefficient alphas ranged from .78 to .98 (mean = .85). A 1-week test–retest sample of 30 patients resulted in coefficients ranging from .69 to .97 (mean = .87).

The validity of the 65-item inventory was evaluated by comparing scores on individual scales to the results of a psychological evaluation by a clinical psychologist on the pain team. There was an 80% chance that problems noted by the psychologist were indicated on the CIPI, and a 72% chance that the psychologist and the CIPI agreed on the absence of a specific problem.

A second approach to validity testing involved administering the CIPI to pain patients (back, head and neck, and multiple pain sites), people in treatment for obesity, and people with respiratory problems, mostly chronic obstructive pulmonary disease. Sample size for these analyses are unknown. Results indicated that pain patients report more problems and problems of greater severity than other groups. Further, the specific problem areas endorsed by particular patient groups were as expected, such as pain patients reporting the greatest difficulty with activity. Additionally, some problem areas like sex and marital concerns were endorsed by all groups, suggesting the existence of problem areas common to chronic illness generally.

In a recent study by Romano and her colleagues (Romano, Turner, & Jensen, 1992), the CIPI was found to share a substantial amount of variance with the Sickness Impact Profile (SIP) (described later in this chapter). However, these authors also acknowledge that there is a significant amount of unshared variance between these measures, suggesting they may be addressing somewhat different aspects of dysfunction.

The CIPI is intended to be used as a screening device that can assist in focusing an assessment, and as an outcome measure that can assist in evaluating progress in treatment (Kames, Rapkin, Naliboff, Afifi, & Ferrer-Brechner, 1990). Romano et al. (1992) suggest that its ease of administration and scoring, as well as its preliminary psychometric properties, makes it very attractive, but that its 18 scales make it somewhat unwieldy. For the time being the CIPI should be used with caution and with additional indices of dysfunction.

Illness Behavior Inventory

A measure with potential usefulness for screening and measuring treatment gains is the Illness Behavior Inventory (IBI) (Turkat & Pettegrew, 1983). Developed from a behavioral perspective, the IBI is a 20-item self-report measure of illness behaviors defined as "an overt behavior performed by an individual which indicates that he or she is physically ill or in physical discomfort" (p. 36). The authors state that the original domain of 46 items was generated clinically after an exhaustive review of the literature proved relatively unhelpful given that much of the literature addressing "illness behavior" relies on intrapsychic concepts (see the discussion of the Illness Behavior Questionnaire, below).

The 46 items were administered to 40 graduate nursing students, a population selected for relative healthiness but sensitivity to health and illness. Because of the large number of items relative to the sample size, the data were explored with Elementary Linkage Analysis. Two factors were found, and they have been named Work Related Illness Behavior (9 items) and Social Illness Behavior (11 items). Other items were discarded. Cronbach's alphas were .89 and .88, respectively. Test–retest reliability on a sample of 32 undergraduate linguistic students at 2-week intervals was .97 for Work Related Illness Behavior and .93 for Social Illness Behavior; individual item coefficients ranged from .82 to 1.0. A confirmatory structural analysis of the original nursing data set compared to data from an unreported number of back pain patients indicated good stability of IBI items across subject populations.

In a test of discriminant validity, 22 diabetic neuropathy patients were classified as high or low illness behavior patients by medical staff. Scores for the total IBI as well as the two subscales were significantly different, in the expected direction, for the two groups.

The authors also report the IBI has good concurrent validity based on data from three studies (Turkat & Pettegrew, 1983). In the first the diabetic neuropathy patients mentioned above also completed a diabetes symptom questionnaire, a health interview survey with questions on disability and medical utilization, and the McGill Pain Questionnaire. In the

second study, 50 lower back pain patients provided information about their medical utilization and cost, hospitalization, and days lost from work. In the third study, 152 healthy college students completed the IBI; scores were positively and significantly related to medical utilization, Mechanic and Volkart's (1961) Sick Role Tendency Scale and Pilowsky's (1967) hypochondriasis scale.

Finally, predictive validity was assessed by administering the IBI and other measures to 63 female undergraduates. Regression analyses predicted outpatient medical utilization, bed disability days, and responses on a scale measuring the tendency to seek and receive medications from physicians (Wolinsky & Wolinsky, 1981).

These early tests of the IBI are promising. It is simple to use, appears psychometrically sound, and seems to have both clinical and research uses. Although individual items are written about "illness," the IBI has been used with low back pain patients without difficulty, and it would be easy to substitute "pain" for "illness" in individual items. The IBI's emphasis on self-observed behaviors can help to educate patients about the importance of behavioral expressions of pain in the development of a chronic pain mindset and in the maintenance of the pain itself.

Illness Behavior Questionnaire

The concept of illness behaviors is also the focus of the Illness Behavior Questionnaire (IBQ) (Pilowsky & Spence, 1983). It is based on the sociology of illness as Parsons (1951) and Mechanic (e.g., Mechanic & Volkart, 1960) have written about it. Pilowsky (1967, 1970) has worked to integrate these sociological concepts into a clinical understanding of hypochondriasis and abnormal illness behavior.

Scale development took place on 100 unselected pain patients (Pilowsky & Spence, 1975). The original questionnaire contained 52 items asking about patients' attitudes toward their illnesses, perceived reactions of others to the illness, and psychosocial variables. These 52 items were factor-analyzed in several steps, with seven factors ultimately interpreted and they are currently called General Hypochondriasis, Disease Conviction, Psychological-versus Somatic Focusing, Affective Disturbance, Affective Inhibition, Denial, and Irritability. In its most recent form, the IBQ has 62 items. Two second-order factors have also been identified: Affective State (a composite of General Hypochondriasis, Affective Disturbance, and Irritability) and Disease Affirmation (a composite of Disease Conviction and Psychological versus Somatic Focusing).

Pilowsky and his colleagues (e.g., Pilowsky & Spence, 1975; Waddell, Pilowsky, & Bond, 1989) have used the IBQ in several studies with patients with chronic pain. In these studies it was found that pain patients characteristically endorse items contributing to the Disease Affirmation Scale. These patients are somatically preoccupied, have a firm belief that their pain is "real," and reject suggestions or implications that psychological factors play a role in their pain. These findings are consistent with clinical practice, where many patients are initially resistant to a rehabilitation approach to pain management, fearing that it implies the pain is "in their heads."

Other studies have used the IBQ to examine the personality and patterns of illness behavior of subgroups of chronic pain patients (e.g., Keefe, Crisson, Maltbie, Bradley, & Gil, 1986; Schnurr, Brooke, & Rollman, 1990) and other clinical populations (Byrne, 1982; Joyce, Bushnell, Walshe, & Morton, 1986). The IBQ has also been demonstrated to be sensitive to treatment effects including surgery for pain (Waddell et al., 1989) and recently in a study comparing psychotherapy and antidepressants in the treatment of chronic pain (Pilowsky & Barrow, 1990).

The IBQ has moderate reliability and good validity (Williams, 1988), but its clinical usefulness in a comprehensive pain assessment may be limited. True, it could be used as a screening instrument to identify patients who use illness behaviors to cope, but the form in which the information is packaged does not assist the clinician in planning or monitoring interventions. Other instruments, such as the IBI or the CIPI, may be more helpful. Nevertheless, it is clear that the measure is a valuable research instrument given its important theoretical foundations.

Sickness Impact Profile

Of all the instruments we review in this chapter, the Sickness Impact Profile (SIP) (Bergner, Bobbitt, Carter, & Gilson, 1981) is the most comprehensively tested and revised. Boldly stated, the SIP was designed to be a measure of

perceived health status so sensitive that it would detect changes within groups and over time, regardless of the medical, demographic, or cultural variables involved. Because many developed countries are beginning to shift attention from cure and rehabilitation to prevention, traditional variables like morbidity and mortality were considered inadequate outcome measures. Bergner et al. hypothesized that a broad measure of daily activities would be sensitive to changes in health status, and this is the focus of the SIP.

The SIP was developed during multiple field trials over a 6-year period (Bergner et al., 1981; Bergner, Bobbitt, Kressel, et al., 1976; Bergner, Bobbitt, Pollard, Martin, & Gilson, 1976; Gilson et al., 1975; Pollard, Bobbitt, Bergner, Martin, & Gilson, 1976). Samples included a mixed group of 246 inpatients, outpatients, home-care patients, walk-in clinic patients and nonpatients; rehabilitation medicine patients; speech pathology patients; outpatients with chronic problems; prepaid health plan enrollees; a random sample of 696 prepaid health plan patients, and 199 patients from a family medicine clinic who considered themselves sick.

The process of developing the SIP was much too extensive to be reviewed in detail here. The numerous analyses, reported in their final form in Bergner et al. (1981), resulted in an instrument with 136 items and 12 categories or scales: Sleep and Rest, Eating, Work, Home Management, Recreation and Pastimes, Ambulation, Mobility, Body Care and Movement, Social Interaction, Alertness Behavior, Emotional Behavior, and Communication. The first five scales are considered "independent" categories, the second three are considered "physical" categories, and the last four are called "psychosocial" categories. It can be self-administered or administered by an interviewer in 20–30 minutes. The overall alpha was .94, and the test–retest on a sample of 53 was .92. Convergent and discriminant validity were evaluated with the multitrait, multimethod technique and were found to be good. Turner (1982; Turner & Clancy, 1988) has found it to be a sensitive measure of change as a function of psychological treatments for chronic pain.

Although lengthy and cumbersome to score, the SIP is a psychometrically sound instrument that provides a wealth of information, some of it psychosocial. According to Williams (1988), several investigators have found it to be clinically useful in working with patients with chronic pain (e.g., Deyo, 1984; Follick, Smith, & Ahern, 1985). A 1978 manual (*The Sickness Impact Profile,* 1978) notes that an investigator can administer only those scales of interest without compromising their reliability or construct validity, but warns against picking and choosing among individual items. It is not clear from the 1981 (Bergner et al., 1981) summary of the development of the SIP if this is still seen as reasonable.

The Pain Disability Index

The Pain Disability Index (PDI) (Pollard, 1984) was developed as a brief self-report measure of pain-related disability. The inventory consists of seven questions designed to measure the degree to which patients believe that their pain interferes with functioning in the areas of family/home responsibilities, recreation, social activities, occupation, sexual behavior, self-care, and life-support activity. Patients respond to each item on 0- to 10-point scales anchored with the descriptors "no disability" to "total disability."

In an extensive examination of the measure's psychometric properties, Tait and his colleagues (Tait, Chibnall, & Krause, 1990) examined a sample of 444 chronic pain patients who completed the PDI and several other pain-relevant measures as part of a comprehensive evaluation prior to participation in a rehabilitation program. Factor analysis of the PDI revealed a single factor that accounted for 56% of the variance in the data. Internal consistency for this single factor as measured by Cronbach's alpha was .86. Because previous research had discovered a 2-factor solution, these same data were forced into a 2-factor solution. Two reliable factors were again discovered, one described as assessing voluntary activities and the second was thought to assess disability in obligatory activities (self-care and life-support). Patients were then grouped into high versus low levels of disability on the PDI and compared on the other standardized measures. Results generally supported the concurrent validity of the BDI.

A subset of the original sample also completed the PDI a second time prior to their participation in treatment. Test–retest reliability was statistically significant, but lower than would be expected or desired ($r = .44$). Using this subsample, the investigators found signifi-

cant differences in observed pain behaviors among high versus low scorers on the PDI, findings that further support the validity of the measure. Studies have also demonstrated that the PDI discriminates patients immediately postsurgery (high disability) and those several months removed from surgery (low disability) (Pollard, 1984), outpatients (low disability) and inpatients (high disability) with pain (Tait, Pollard, Margolis, Duckro, & Krause, 1987), and employed versus unemployed pain patients and patients involved in litigation from those who are not (Tait, Chibnall, & Richardson, 1990).

The measure has strengths related to its brevity and theoretical and practical importance. Evaluations of its psychometric properties encourage its reliability and utility, but questions about its face-apparent nature (i.e., patients are clearly aware of its intended use) and possible systematic biases in reporting (e.g., desire of some patients to distort their reports toward an appearance of increased disability) should be examined before it is accepted as a valid measure of disability.

Combined Measures

McGill Comprehensive Pain Questionnaire

We noted in our earlier discussion that a comprehensive evaluation generally makes use of both interviews and self-report measures. An instrument that combines a questionnaire packet with a semistructured interview is the McGill Comprehensive Pain Questionnaire (MCPQ) offered by Monks and Taenzer (1983). The MCPQ is a self-report inventory complemented by an interview. The inventory is meant to inquire into the pain, its history and treatments, other physical symptoms, psychosocial concomitants, and personal variables, for the purposes of treatment planning, program evaluation, and research. The interview is used to clarify responses on the inventory and investigate personal and subjective variables, such as the patient's expectations and changes in sexual activity due to pain. The interviewer guide also contains the McGill Pain Questionnaire (MPQ) (Melzack, 1975; see also Melzack & Katz, Chapter 10), an inventory easily completed by patients alone. Monks and Taenzer report that the MCPQ was derived from clinical experience and from previously published instruments.

The MCPQ appears to be easy to use, and the authors report success in having patients complete the inventory part prior to their first appointments. It is probably most helpful in eliciting the patient's report of the pain history and its effect on work, finances, leisure, sleep, and weight. It is less clear how the sections on parents and family are to be used, particularly by non-mental-health workers. The interview itself explores a number of pertinent areas but offers no guidance in recording data that would allow pre–post comparisons or tests of research hypotheses, if properly quantified. Davis (1989) does report a study in which she used the MCPQ with patients with rheumatic disease and patients with acute surgical pain. She reports that it was time-consuming to use and difficult to score, but that it was helpful in understanding the experience of the individual.

Also of concern is the emphasis in both the inventory and the interview on the *effects* of pain on other variables, rather than vice versa or both. In summary, the MCPQ is a combined inventory/follow-up interview meant to be comprehensive in nature. It is rather long and difficult to score reliably or at all (depending on the question). It would be very useful to the neophyte pain management clinician trying to get a feel for the population, but less useful in a busy clinic where routine evaluation should point fairly reliably at appropriate and measurable targets for intervention.

Diaries

In the psychosocial assessment of the experience of pain, interviews and inventories provide an overview, historical perspective, and composite measures of critical variables. The interview also provides an opportunity to interact extensively with a patient, and to gather impressions concerning his or her psychological readiness for rehabilitation. Additional valuable information can be acquired with the use of mood and activity diaries because they allow an investigation into the actual temporal relationship between psychosocial variables and pain, rather than self-perceived reports of such. Affleck, Tennen, Urrows, and Higgins (1991), for example, report on the use of a daily events diary to examine relationships between negative events and pain in patients with rheumatoid arthritis.

Support for the reliability and validity of diary methodology is available from a number of investigators (e.g., Follick, Ahern, & Laser-Wolston, 1984; Haythornthwaite, Hegel, & Kerns, 1991). Follick and his colleagues investigated the psychometric properties of an activity diary for low back pain patients by comparing diary reports with those of spouses ($N = 20$) and with data from an automated, electromechanical "uptime/downtime" device ($N = 8$). The diary asked for ratings to be made three times a day for each preceding half-hour, in the following categories: position (lying, sitting, standing, walking, asleep); time spent alone, with family, with others; time at home; medication use; use of pain relief activities of devices; and average daily ratings of pain, tension, and mood. Pearson product moment correlations were used to determine the relationship between patient ratings and spouse and mechanical data. The correlations were all positive and statistically significant. The strongest correlations were those that were most clearly behaviorally defined, like medication use; the weakest were those most subjective, like mood and pain intensity ratings. The authors note that one way in which these findings are useful is to validate diary reports as pretreatment and outcome measures of functional impairment.

Haythornthwaite et al. (1991) have reported on the use of daily diaries to monitor sleep of pain patients. In that study, 46 patients participating in inpatient treatment for chronic pain kept diaries every morning after waking. Items were derived from clinical experience such as the number of times one awoke, as well as subjective reports, for example, of sleep quality. Patients also reported on sleep in the last week; completed measures of pain severity, depression, and anxiety; and reported average level of activity as well as wore a pedometer during the admission. Haythornthwaite et al. report that for pain patients poor sleep is only partly a function of pain but is more reliably related to mood. They also report results which suggest acceptable levels of reliability and stability, and present some helpful comments on the special issue of assessing stability in diary studies.

CONCLUSIONS

Consideration of psychosocial factors has become a routine component of the assessment of chronic pain conditions. Most would agree that to ignore the possible deleterious effects of chronic pain on the individual's life, or to fail to take into account possible psychological, interpersonal, and sociological contributors to the development and maintenance of the pain complaint, leaves the clinician vulnerable to erroneous assumptions about the extent of the problem, its etiology, and possible solutions. Similarly, systematic investigation of psychosocial factors will continue to have an enormous impact on our understanding of chronic pain conditions and their possible treatment.

This chapter provided a brief introduction into the broad domain of relevant psychosocial factors, an overview of the psychosocial assessment process, and descriptions of some of the most widely used or promising clinical and research measures of psychosocial functioning available. The review of the measures was intended to provide the interested reader with enough information to make preliminary decisions about the choice of measures. More critical discussion of the measures was beyond the scope of this chapter.

Selection of individual measures should be based on the specific needs of the clinician or clinical setting or the goals of the investigator, but should balance the desire to be thorough with the interests of patients. Use of measures that have been validated on the specific population being served is always an important consideration. In the end analysis, clinicians and researchers alike will do well to avoid relying on information from only one source regardless of the presumed reliability or validity of the measure. Clinicians are reminded to incorporate selected psychosocial measures into a more comprehensive, and optimally, interdisciplinary evaluation. Investigators should consider a multivariate approach that incorporates multiple measures of single constructs in order to minimize measurement error and bias. This is particularly important given the self-report nature of these measures. Continued examination of the psychometric properties and utility of the measures offered in this chapter, as well as the development of alternative methods and measures is strongly encouraged.

APPENDIX 14.A
The West Haven–Yale Multidimensional Pain Inventory*

SECTION 1

In the following 20 questions, you will be asked to describe your pain and how it affects your life. Under each question is a scale to record your answer. Read each question carefully and then *circle* a number on the scale under that question to indicate how that specific question applies to you.

1. Rate the level of your pain at the present moment.

0	1	2	3	4	5	6
No pain						Very intense pain

2. In general, how much does your pain problem interfere with your day to day activities?

0	1	2	3	4	5	6
No interference						Extreme interference

3. Since the time you developed a pain problem, how much has your pain changed your ability to work?

0	1	2	3	4	5	6
No change						Extreme change

    _____ Check here, if you have retired for reasons other than your pain problem.

4. How much has your pain changed the amount of satisfaction or enjoyment you get from participating in social and recreational activities?

0	1	2	3	4	5	6
No change						Extreme change

(continued)

APPENDIX 14.A *(Continued)*

5. How supportive or helpful is your spouse (significant other) to you in relation to your pain?

| 0 | 1 | 2 | 3 | 4 | 5 | 6 |

Not at all supportive ... Extremely supportive

6. Rate your overall mood during the *past week*.

| 0 | 1 | 2 | 3 | 4 | 5 | 6 |

Extremely low mood ... Extremely high mood

7. On the average, how severe has your pain been during the *last week?*

| 0 | 1 | 2 | 3 | 4 | 5 | 6 |

Not at all severe ... Extremely severe

8. How much has your pain changed your ability to participate in recreational and other social activities?

| 0 | 1 | 2 | 3 | 4 | 5 | 6 |

No change ... Extreme change

9. How much has your pain changed the amount of satisfaction you get from family-related activities?

| 0 | 1 | 2 | 3 | 4 | 5 | 6 |

No change ... Extreme change

10. How worried is your spouse (significant other) about you in relation to your pain problems?

| 0 | 1 | 2 | 3 | 4 | 5 | 6 |

Not at all worried ... Extremely worried

11. During the *past week* how much control do you feel that you have had over your life?

| 0 | 1 | 2 | 3 | 4 | 5 | 6 |

Not at all in control ... Extremely in control

12. How much *suffering* do you experience because of your pain?

| 0 | 1 | 2 | 3 | 4 | 5 | 6 |

No suffering ... Extreme suffering

13. How much has your pain changed your marriage and other family relationships?

| 0 | 1 | 2 | 3 | 4 | 5 | 6 |

No change ... Extreme change

14. How much has your pain changed the amount of satisfaction or enjoyment you get from work?

| 0 | 1 | 2 | 3 | 4 | 5 | 6 |

No change ... Extreme change

_____ Check here, if you are not presently working.

15. How attentive is your spouse (significant other) to your pain problem?

| 0 | 1 | 2 | 3 | 4 | 5 | 6 |

Not at all attentive ... Extremely attentive

(continued)

APPENDIX 14.A *(Continued)*

16. During the *past week* how much do you feel that you've been able to deal with your problems?

0	1	2	3	4	5	6
Not at all						Extremely well

17. How much has your pain changed your ability to do household chores?

0	1	2	3	4	5	6
No change						Extreme change

18. During the past week how irritable have you been?

0	1	2	3	4	5	6
Not at all irritable						Extremely irritable

19. How much has your pain changed your friendships with people other than your family?

0	1	2	3	4	5	6
No change						Extreme change

20. During the past week how tense or anxious have you been?

0	1	2	3	4	5	6
Not at all tense or anxious						Extremely tense or anxious

SECTION 2

In this section, we are interested in knowing how your spouse (or significant other) responds to you when he or she knows that you are in pain. On the scale listed below each question, *circle* a number to indicate *how often* your spouse (or significant other) generally responds to you in that particular way *when you are in pain*. Please answer *all* of the 14 questions.

    ***Please identify the relationship between you and the person you are thinking of. _____

1. Ignores me.

0	1	2	3	4	5	6
Never						Very often

2. Asks me what he/she can do to help.

0	1	2	3	4	5	6
Never						Very often

3. Reads to me.

0	1	2	3	4	5	6
Never						Very often

4. Expresses irritation at me.

0	1	2	3	4	5	6
Never						Very often

5. Takes over my jobs or duties.

0	1	2	3	4	5	6
Never						Very often

(continued)

APPENDIX 14.A *(Continued)*

6. Talks to me about something else to take my mind off the pain.

    0   1   2   3   4   5   6
    Never   Very often

7. Expresses frustration at me.

    0   1   2   3   4   5   6
    Never   Very often

8. Tries to get me to rest.

    0   1   2   3   4   5   6
    Never   Very often

9. Tries to involve me in some activity.

    0   1   2   3   4   5   6
    Never   Very often

10. Expresses anger at me.

    0   1   2   3   4   5   6
    Never   Very often

11. Gets me some pain medications.

    0   1   2   3   4   5   6
    Never   Very often

12. Encourages me to work on a hobby.

    0   1   2   3   4   5   6
    Never   Very often

13. Gets me something to eat or drink.

    0   1   2   3   4   5   6
    Never   Very often

14. Turns on the T.V. to take my mind off my pain.

    0   1   2   3   4   5   6
    Never   Very often

SECTION 3

Listed below are 18 common daily activities. Please indicate *how often* you do each of these activities by *circling* a number on the scale listed below each activity. Please complete *all* 18 questions.

1. Wash dishes.

    0   1   2   3   4   5   6
    Never   Very often

2. Mow the law.

    0   1   2   3   4   5   6
    Never   Very often

3. Go out to eat.

    0   1   2   3   4   5   6
    Never   Very often

(continued)

APPENDIX 14.A (*Continued*)

4. Play cards or other games.

    0   1   2   3   4   5   6
Never   Very often

5. Go grocery shopping.

    0   1   2   3   4   5   6
Never   Very often

6. Work in the garden.

    0   1   2   3   4   5   6
Never   Very often

7. Go to a movie.

    0   1   2   3   4   5   6
Never   Very often

8. Visit friends.

    0   1   2   3   4   5   6
Never   Very often

9. Help with the house cleaning.

    0   1   2   3   4   5   6
Never   Very often

10. Work on the car.

    0   1   2   3   4   5   6
Never   Very often

11. Take a ride in a car.

    0   1   2   3   4   5   6
Never   Very often

12. Visit relatives.

    0   1   2   3   4   5   6
Never   Very often

13. Prepare a meal.

    0   1   2   3   4   5   6
Never   Very often

14. Wash the car.

    0   1   2   3   4   5   6
Never   Very often

15. Take a trip.

    0   1   2   3   4   5   6
Never   Very often

16. Go to a park or beach.

    0   1   2   3   4   5   6
Never   Very often

(*continued*)

APPENDIX 14.A *(Continued)*

17. Do a load of laundry.

0	1	2	3	4	5	6
Never						Very often

18. Work on a needed house repair.

0	1	2	3	4	5	6
Never						Very often

WHYMPI Scoring

Section 1:

Interference:	(Question 2 + 3 + 4 + 8 + 9 + 13 + 14 + 17 + 19)/9
Support:	(Question 5 + 10 + 15)/3
Pain Severity:	(Question 1 + 7 + 12)/3
Life-Control:	(Question 11 + 16)/2
Affective Distress:	((6 − Question 6) + 18 + 20)/3

Section 2:

Negative Responses:	(Question 1 + 4 + 7 + 10)/4
Solicitous Responses:	(Question 2 + 5 + 8 + 11 + 13 + 14)/6
Distracting Responses:	(Question 3 + 6 + 9 + 12)/4

Section 3:

Household Chores:	(Question 1 + 5 + 9 + 13 + 17)/5
Outdoor Work:	(Question 2 + 6 + 10 + 14 + 18)/5
Activities Away From Home:	(Question 3 + 7 + 11 + 15)/4
Social Activities:	(Question 4 + 8 + 12 + 16)/4
General Activity:	(Sum of all questions in Section 3)/18

*Copyright 1985 Robert D. Kerns, Dennis C. Turk, and Thomas E. Rudy. Reprinted by permission.

REFERENCES

Affleck, G., Tennen, H., Urrows, S., & Higgins, P. (1991). The distribution and patterning of daily pain from rheumatoid arthritis. *Twelfth Annual Proceedings of the Society of Behavioral Medicine.* Rockville, MD: Society of Behavioral Medicine. (abstract)

Bergner, M., Bobbitt, R. A., with Carter, W. B., & Gilson, B. S. (1981). The Sickness Impact Profile: Development and final revision of a health status measure. *Medical Care, 19,* 787–805.

Bergner, M., Bobbitt, R. A., Kressel, S., Pollard, W. E., Gilson, B. S., & Morris, J. R. (1976). The Sickness Impact Profile: Conceptual formulation and methodology for the development of a health status measure. *International Journal of Health Services, 6,* 393–415.

Bergner, M., Bobbitt, R. A., Pollard, W. E., Martin, D. P., & Gilson, B. S. (1976). The Sickness Impact Profile: Validation of a health status measure. *Medical Care, 14,* 57–67.

Black, R. G. (1975). The chronic pain syndrome. *Surgical Clinics of North America, 55,* 999–1011.

Blumer, D., & Heilbronn, M. (1982). Chronic pain and a variant of depressive disease: The pain-prone disorder. *Journal of Nervous and Mental Diseases, 170,* 381–394.

Byrne, D. (1982). Illness behaviour and psychosocial outcome after a heart attack. *British Journal of Clinical Psychology, 21,* 145–146.

Davis, G. C. (1989). The clinical assessment of chronic pain in rheumatic disease: Evaluating the use of two instruments. *Journal of Advanced Nursing, 14,* 397–402.

Deyo, R. A. (1984). Measuring functional outcomes in therapeutic trials for chronic disease. *Controlled Clinical Trials, 5,* 223–240.

Engel, G. (1959). "Psychogenic" pain and the pain-prone patient. *American Journal of Medicine, 26,* 899–918.

Faucett, J. A., & Levine, J. D. (1991). The contributions of interpersonal conflict to chronic pain in the presence or absence of organic pathology. *Pain, 44,* 35–43.

Flor, H., Kerns, R. D., & Turk, D. C. (1987). The role of spouse reinforcement, perceived pain, and activity levels of chronic pain patients. *Journal of Psychosomatic Research, 31,* 251–259.

Flor, H., Turk, D. C., & Rudy, T. E. (1989). Relationship of pain impact and significant other reinforcement of pain behaviors: The mediating role of gender, marital status and marital satisfaction. *Pain, 38,* 45–50.

Follick, M. J., Ahern, D. K., & Laser-Wolston, N. (1984).

Evaluation of a daily activity diary for chronic pain patients. *Pain, 19,* 373–382.

Follick, M. J., Smith, T. W., & Ahern, D. K. (1985). The Sickness Impact Profile: A global measure of disability in chronic low back pain. *Pain, 21,* 67–76.

Fordyce, W. E. (1974). Pain viewed as a learned behavior. In J. J. Bonica (Ed.), *Advances in neurology* (Vol. 4, pp. 415–422). New York: Raven Press.

Fordyce, W. E. (1976). *Behavioral methods for chronic pain and illness.* St. Louis: Mosby.

Getto, C. J., & Heaton, R. K. (1985a). *A manual for the psychosocial pain inventory.* Odessa, FL: Psychological Assessment Resources Inc.

Getto, C. J., & Heaton, R. K. (1985b). Assessment of patients with chronic pain. In D. P. Swiercinsky (Ed.), *Testing adults: A reference guide for special psychodiagnostic assessments* (pp. 113–122). Kansas City: Test Corporation of America.

Getto, C. J., Heaton, R. K., & Lehman, W. E. (1983). PSPI: A standardized approach to the evaluation of psychological factors in chronic pain. In J. J. Bonica (Ed.), *Advances in pain research and therapy* (pp. 885–890). New York: Raven Press.

Gilson, B. S., Gilson, J. S., Bergner, M., Bobbitt, R. A., Kressel, S., Pollard, W. E., & Vesselago, M. (1975). Sickness impact profile: Development of an outcome measure of health care. *American Journal of Public Health, 65,* 1304–1310.

Gordon, R. L. (1975). *Interviewing: Strategy, techniques, and tactics.* Homewood, IL: Dorsey Press.

Haynes, S. N. (1978). *Principles of behavioral assessment.* New York: Gardner Press.

Haythornthwaite, J. A., Hegel, M. T., & Kerns, R. D. (1991). Development of a sleep diary for chronic pain patients. *Journal of Pain and Symptom Management, 6,* 65–72.

Heaton, R. K., Getto, C. J., Lehman, R. A. W., Fordyce, W. E., Brauer, E., & Groban, S. E. (1981). A standardized evaluation of psychosocial factors in chronic pain. *Pain* [suppl], *1,* 154, (abstract).

Heaton, R. K., Getto, C. J., Lehman, R. A. W., Fordyce, W. E., Brauer, E., & Groban, S. E. (1982). A standardized evaluation of psychosocial factors in chronic pain. *Pain, 12,* 165–174.

Holmes, J. A., & Stevenson, C. A. Z. (1990). Differential effects of avoidant and attentional coping strategies on adaptation to chronic and recent-onset pain. *Health Psychology, 9,* 577–584.

Holzman, A., Kerns, R. D., & Turk, D. C. (1981). *Pain assessment report.* Unpublished manuscript.

Joyce, P. R., Bushnell, J. A., Walshe, J. W. B., & Morton, J. B. (1986). Abnormal illness behaviour and anxiety in acute non-organic pain. *British Journal of Psychiatry, 149,* 57–62.

Kames, L. D., Naliboff, B. D., Heinrich, R. L., & Schag, C. C. (1984). The chronic illness problem inventory: Problem-oriented psychosocial assessment of patients with chronic illness. *International Journal of Psychiatry in Medicine, 14,* 65–75.

Kames, L. D., Rapkin, A. J., Naliboff, B. D., Afifi, S., & Ferrer-Brechner, T. (1990). Effectiveness of an interdisciplinary pain management program for the treatment of chronic pelvic pain. *Pain, 41,* 41–46.

Karoly, P. (1985). The assessment of pain: Concepts and procedures. In P. Karoly (Ed.), *Measurement strategies in health psychology* (pp. 461–515). New York: Wiley.

Karoly, P., & Jensen, M. P. (1987). *Multimethod assessment of chronic pain.* New York: Pergamon Press.

Keefe, F. J., Crisson, J. E., Maltbie, A., Bradley, L., & Gil, K. M. (1986). Illness behaviour as a predictor of pain and overt behaviour patterns in chronic low back pain patients. *Journal of Psychosomatic Research, 30,* 543–552.

Kerns, R. D., & Haythornthwaite, J. (1988). Depression among chronic pain patients: Cognitive-behavioral analysis and rehabilitation outcome. *Journal of Consulting and Clinical Psychology, 56,* 870–876.

Kerns, R. D., Haythornthwaite, J., Southwick, S., & Giller, E. L., Jr. (1990). The role of marital interaction in chronic pain and depressive symptom severity. *Journal of Psychosomatic Research, 34,* 401–408.

Kerns, R. D., Southwick, S., Giller, E. L., Jr., Haythornthwaite, J., Jacob, M. C., & Rosenberg, R. (1991). The relationship between reports of pain-relevant social interactions and expressions of pain and affective distress. *Behavior Therapy, 22,* 101–111.

Kerns, R. D., Turk, D. C., Holzman, A. D., & Rudy, T. E. (1986). Comparison of cognitive-behavioral and behavioral approaches to the outpatient treatment of chronic pain. *Clinical Journal of Pain, 1,* 195–203.

Kerns, R. D., Turk, D. C., & Rudy, T. E. (1985). The West Haven–Yale Multidimensional Pain Inventory (WHYMPI). *Pain, 23,* 345–356.

Mechanic, D., & Volkart, E. H. (1960). Illness behavior and medical diagnosis. *Journal of Health and Human Behavior, 1,* 86–96.

Mechanic, D., & Volkart, E. H. (1961). Stress, illness behavior and the sick role. *American Sociological Review, 26,* 51–58.

Melzack, R. (1975). The McGill Pain Questionnaire: Major properties and scoring methods. *Pain, 1,* 277–299.

Melzack, R., & Wall, P. (1965). Pain mechanisms: A new theory. *Science, 50,* 971–979.

Monks, R., & Taenzer, P. (1983). A comprehensive pain questionnaire. In R. Melzack (Ed.), *Pain measurement and assessment* (pp. 233–237, 1A–14A). New York: Raven Press.

Parsons, T. (1951). *The social system.* New York: Free Press.

Pilowsky, I. (1967). Dimensions of hypochondriasis. *British Journal of Psychiatry, 113,* 89–93.

Pilowsky, I. (1970). Primary and secondary hypochondriasis. *Acta Psychiatrica Scandinavica, 46,* 273–285.

Pilowsky, I., & Barrow, C. G. (1990). A controlled study of psychotherapy and amitriptyline used individually and in combination in the treatment of chronic intractable, 'psychogenic' pain. *Pain, 40,* 3–19.

Pilowsky, I., & Spence, N. D. (1975). Patterns of illness behaviour in patients with intractable pain. *Journal of Psychosomatic Research, 19,* 279–287.

Pilowsky, I., & Spence, N. D. (1983). *Manual for the Illness Behavior Questionnaire (IBQ)* (2nd ed.). Adelaide, Australia: University of Adelaide, Department of Psychiatry.

Pollard, C. A. (1984). Preliminary validity study of the Pain Disability Index. *Perceptual and Motor Skills, 59,* 974.

Pollard, W. E., Bobbitt, R. A., Bergner, M., Martin, D. P., & Gilson, B. S. (1976). The Sickness Impact Profile: Reliability of a health status measure. *Medical Care, 14,* 146–155.

Romano, J. M., & Turner, J. A. (1985). Chronic pain and depression: Does the evidence support a relationship? *Psychological Bulletin, 97,* 18–34.

Romano, J. M., Turner, J. A., & Jensen, M. P. (1992).

The Chronic Illness Problem Inventory as a measure of dysfunction in chronic pain patients. *Pain, 49,* 71–75.

Rudy, T. E. (1989). *Multiaxial assessment of pain: Multidimensional Pain Inventory. Computer program users manual. Version 2.1.* Technical report. Pittsburgh: Pain Evaluation and Treatment Institute.

Rudy, T. E., Turk, D. C., Zaki, H. S., & Curtin, H. D. (1989). An empirical taxonometric alternative to traditional classification of temporomandibular disorders. *Pain, 36,* 311–320.

Schnurr, R. F., Brooke, R. I., & Rollman, G. B. (1990). Psychosocial correlates of temporomandibular joint pain and dysfunction. *Pain, 42,* 153–165.

Sternbach, R. A. (1974). *Pain patients: Traits and treatment.* New York: Academic Press.

Tait, R. C., Chibnall, J. T., & Krause, S. (1990). The Pain Disability Index: Psychometric properties. *Pain, 40,* 171–182.

Tait, R. C., Chibnall, J. T., & Richardson, W. D. (1990). Litigation and employment status: Effects on patients with chronic pain. *Pain, 43,* 37–46.

Tait, R. C., Pollard, C. A., Margolis, R. B., Duckro, P. N., & Krause, S. J. (1987). The Pain Disability Index: Psychometric properties and validity data. *Archives of Physical Medicine and Rehabilitation, 68,* 438–441.

The Sickness Impact Profile: A brief summary of its purpose, uses, and administration. (1978). Unpublished manual, University of Washington, Department of Health Services, Seattle.

Turk, D. C., & Kerns, R. D. (1985). Assessment in health psychology: A cognitive-behavioral perspective. In P. Karoly (Ed.), *Measurement strategies in health psychology* (pp. 335–372). New York: Wiley.

Turk, D. C., Meichenbaum, D., & Genest, M. (1983). *Pain and behavioral medicine: A cognitive-behavioral perspective.* New York: Guilford Press.

Turk, D. C., & Rudy, T. E. (1988). Toward an empirically derived taxonomy of chronic pain patients: Integration of psychological assessment data. *Journal of Consulting and Clinical Psychology, 56,* 233–238.

Turk, D. C., & Rudy, T. E. (1990). The robustness of an empirically derived taxonomy of chronic pain patients. *Pain, 43,* 27–36.

Turk, D. C., Rudy, T. E., & Stieg, R. L. (1988). The disability determination dilemma: Toward a multiaxial solution. *Pain, 34,* 217–231.

Turk, D. C., Sobel, H. J., Follick, M. J., & Youkilis, H. D. (1980). A sequential criterion analysis for assessing coping with chronic illness. *Journal of Human Stress, 6,* 35–40.

Turkat, I. D., & Pettegrew, L. S. (1983). Development and validation of the Illness Behavior Inventory. *Journal of Behavioral Assessment, 5,* 35–47.

Turner, J. A. (1982). Comparison of group progressive-relaxation training and cognitive-behavioral group therapy for chronic low back pain. *Journal of Consulting and Clinical Psychology, 50,* 757–765.

Turner, J. A., & Clancy, S. (1988). Comparison of operant behavioral and cognitive-behavioral group treatment for chronic low back pain. *Journal of Consulting and Clinical Psychology, 56,* 261–266.

Waddell, G., Pilowsky, I., & Bond, M. R. (1989). Clinical assessment and interpretation of abnormal illness behavior in low back pain. *Pain, 39,* 41–53.

Williams, R. C. (1988). Toward a set of reliable and valid measures for chronic pain assessment and outcome research. *Pain, 35,* 239–251.

Wolinsky, F. D., & Wolinsky, S. R. (1981). Expecting sick-role legitimation and getting it. *Journal of Health and Social Behavior, 22,* 229–242.

IV

ASSESSMENT OF THE BEHAVIORAL EXPRESSION OF PAIN

Chapter 15

The Facial Expression of Pain

KENNETH D. CRAIG, PhD
KENNETH M. PRKACHIN, PhD
RUTH V.E. GRUNAU, PhD

Pain is a private experience with complex sensory, affective and evaluative qualities that must be measured if people in distress are to be helped. The sensations, thoughts, and feelings are salient for the sufferer, but incomprehensible to an observer unless there are observable manifestations. Nevertheless, observers often have complex verbal and nonverbal information available to infer others' private states as pain is very difficult to maintain as an exclusively private experience. Although it is the subjective experience of pain that dominates the observer's interest, it is the meaning attached to the complex pattern of behavioral responses, verbal and nonverbal, that constrains all efforts to care for the suffering person.

NONVERBAL ACTIVITY IN UNDERSTANDING OTHERS' PAIN

People in pain communicate their experience through a remarkable variety of actions, ranging from self-report, in its numerous forms, to nonverbal actions that have a similar range of variations. The latter include nonverbal or paralinguistic vocalizations in the form of crying, screaming, or moaning, physiological activity such as pallor, sweating, or muscle tension; bodily activity, including reflexive withdrawal of the limbs or torso or purposeful action designed to ward off injury or palliate pain; and facial expressions (see Keefe & Williams, Chapter 16). Facial grimaces and wincing can be as immediate as many of these other forms of pain behavior but do not have the same direct, instrumental ability to control physical threat. Instead, facial activity serves primarily as a source of communication to others who may provide help (Prkachin, 1986).

It is very difficult to suppress the tendency to look at others in distress, probably because the other person's distress could signal imminent personal threat (Craig, 1986). In clinical medicine, the importance of nonverbal expression is also well established, as the successful physical examination often depends upon sensitivity to nonverbal response. This apparent salience and utility of nonverbal components of pain and illness behavior is curious when contrasted with the clinical and research literature on pain that relies almost totally on self-report (Craig & Prkachin, 1983; Keefe, 1989; LeResche & Dworkin, 1984). The striking inconsistency between what clinicians and nonprofessional bystanders attend to when others are in pain and that which represents the focus of attention in textbooks and scientific articles needs to be redressed, not only to enhance understanding of ecologically important processes, but also because there is now ample reason to believe that nonverbal expression has uniquely important properties that may be unavailable in other pain behaviors.

Preoccupation with verbal report in the pain literature appears to reflect a variety of factors. The use of language in thinking suggests that self-report would be necessary to capture its essence. However, dual-process models of cognitive activity (Paivio, 1986) make it clear that imagery also assumes an important role in the stream of consciousness. As well, capturing the essence of affective states with language is as difficult a challenge as defining and measuring pain (Nisbett & Wilson, 1977; Zajonc, 1980). Methodological convenience and the conventions of everyday social discourse also play a role in the emphasis on verbal report. It is commonplace and extraordinarily easy for people to ask others about subjective states, but substantially more challenging to transduce nonverbal expression into quantitative indices. Certain humane biases also appear to operate. To discourage withholding care when the credibility of patient complaints is questioned, it has become axiomatic among clinicians that pain exists when the patient says it does. For example, Meinhart and McCaffery (1983) observe, "The patient's verbal report is the only way to determine the presence, intensity, and quality of pain" (p. 323). Strict adherence to this principle may result in ignoring nonverbal expression and the fundamental information it contains.

Despite the enthusiasm for self-report, it is well-established that it is not always a reliable or satisfactory source of information about states of subjective distress. Self-report is likely to represent only a subset of what the individual is feeling, thinking, or prepared to admit at a particular time. The language we use to characterize the experience also is figurative and often vague. For example, Procacci and Maresca (1991) noted that today nobody genuinely can know the real significance of the term "excruciating pain," as the practice of crucifixion has long been abandoned. People also bring reporting biases, modulate reports purposefully and unwittingly to maximize personal benefits, are reactive to situational demands, and vary in their memory and verbal ability (Gracely, 1989; Kremer, Block, & Atkinson, 1983; Teske, Daut, & Cleeland, 1983). Asking for self-report of pain attracts attention to its importance and functional significance, likely making respondents all the more reactive to situational demands. In contrast, nonverbal measures have the potential to permit continuous, nonintrusive measurement of pain in natural settings.

In some situations, nonverbal indices of pain may be the only information available. Very young children and people with intellectual deficits, verbal disorders, and linguistic problems represent people who are never capable of verbally reporting pain. Patients recovering from anesthetics or those who refuse to report pain provide illustrations of a more situationally determined need to rely on nonverbal expressions of pain.

Given that people do not monitor nonverbal actions as attentively as they do their speech (Craig & Prkachin, 1980), nonverbal expressions may be less subject to purposeful distortion than verbalizations. Von Baeyer, Johnson, and McMillan (1984) reviewed research indicating that "nonverbal behaviors may be a more accurate source of information than verbal reports because they are less subject to 'motivated dissimulation' " (p. 1319). People judging the emotional significance of another's actions appear to assume that nonverbal behavior is less amenable to dissimulation than self-report (Ekman & Friesen, 1969), and consider it more important when self-report and nonverbal behavior are discordant (DePaulo, Rosenthal, Eisenstat, Rogers, & Finkelstein, 1978; Jacox, 1980). Jacox (1980) reports that nurses found nonverbal behaviors and physiological signs to be more salient and easier to use in pain assessment than patient verbalizations about pain. Kraut (1978) observed that the accuracy of detection of others' attempts to deceive is enhanced when observers are allowed to observe nonverbal as well as verbal behavior during the deception.

The different manifestations of pain should not be conceptualized as redundant. It is possible for pain vocalizations to be consistent or inconsistent with facial expressions and other nonverbal activity. Nonverbal activity is often more immediate and reflexive than self-report. Self-report in turn often assumes importance because it alone provides for retrospective recall of events, even though there is evidence that recall of painful events often does not correspond to the experience itself (Eich, Reeves, Jaeger, & Graff-Radford, 1985).

The Role of Facial Activity

The prominence of the face among the various channels of nonverbal information is well established (Collier, 1985). Facial activity can be remarkably plastic and informative. Ekman and Friesen (1969) characterize channels of communication in terms of their sending capacity, referring to transmission time, number of discriminable patterns, and visibility. The sending capacity of the face is substantial, as its plasticity permits rapid variation in a considerable variety of expressions, and it commands the attention of observers. It is capable of conveying information about subjective states ranging through the domains of affect, thoughts, cognitive states, motivational states, and behavioral intentions. People who fail to monitor and correctly interpret the ongoing dynamic pattern of others' facial activity suffer serious social deficits.

The origins of individual differences in facial displays are difficult to determine, as both phylogenetic and socialization influences are evident. There are profound innate roots, as the newborn facial response to tissue damage is similar to that of older children and adults (Craig & Grunau, 1991; Grunau, Johnston, & Craig, 1990). Nevertheless, children become acculturated to display different patterns of pain and illness behavior in conformity with family and cultural expectations (Craig & Wyckoff, 1987). The relatively global reflexive reactions of very young infants to tissue damage become shaped and transform during the course of development into differentiated and socially responsive patterns of behavior (Craig, McMahon, Morison, & Zaskow, 1984).

Theories of the differentiation of facial expressions of emotion have generally reflected Darwin's (1872/1965) argument that in the course of evolution there were adaptive consequences to having a means to signal subjective states and behavioral intentions to conspecifics. Zajonc (e.g., Adelmann & Zajonc, 1989; Zajonc, 1985), in contrast, has argued that the communicative functions are secondary to internal homeostatic processes. It seems reasonable to believe that facial expressions reflect internal adaptive mechanisms as well as functional external consequences. Hypotheses

about the adaptive functions of the expression are not difficult to generate. The physical threat signaled by pain should provoke protective actions. The most prominent feature of pain, the lowered brow and narrowing of the eye orbit, could reflect immediate concern for the safety of the eyes. To close them fully could risk missing vital information needed to engage in other protective activity.

There is also reason to believe that facial activity contributes to the totality of the experience of pain. Facial feedback models of emotion argue that physiological feedback from the face permits subjective differentiation of different emotions (Adelmann & Zajonc, 1989). The position has been extended to the study of pain. Attenuated facial expression of pain has been associated with diminished autonomic activity, reduced subjective distress, and increased pain tolerance (Colby, Lanzetta, & Kleck, 1977; Kopel & Arkowitz, 1974; Lanzetta, Cartwright-Smith, & Kleck, 1976). Perhaps this is intuitively acknowledged when clinicians tell patients to "keep a stiff upper lip" or "grin and bear it."

SPECIFIC FACIAL ACTIONS ASSOCIATED WITH PAIN

Clinicians and laypeople alike have little difficulty talking globally about grimaces of pain, but the complexity and speed of facial actions make objective description difficult. Attempts to characterize facial expressions of pain without the benefit of objective, comprehensive coding systems have led to errors in both historical and contemporary descriptions of facial pain expressions. Darwin (1872/1965), for example, suggested that in pain "the mouth may be closely compressed, or more commonly the lips are retracted, with the teeth clenched or ground together" and "the eyes stare wildly as in horrified astonishment" (pp. 69–70). Recent systematic studies do not confirm these observations. Rather, open lips or a dropped jaw are likely to be seen and the eyes are likely to be narrowed, or closed.

Decoding facial expressions requires a comprehensive measurement system that objectively identifies all possible basic actions and their temporal relationships. At present, the most satisfactory approach is the Facial Action Coding System (FACS) (Ekman & Friesen, 1978). This microanalytic, anatomically based system identifies 44 discrete facial actions. Each action unit represents the movement of a single facial muscle, or, more rarely, a muscle strand or a group of facial muscles that move as a unit. Definition of the behavior units in terms of observable movement avoids a priori inferences about the presumed meaning or function of the observed behavior. The typical application has used videotaped, slow motion, or stop-frame feedback. Coders are trained to apply specific operational criteria to determine which actions have taken place and to identify their onset, offset, and in some instances intensity over brief intervals of time. Table 15.1 illustrates the rules for identifying one action that has consistently been associated with pain in systematic studies. Facial "expressions" (as opposed to specific movements) generally can be defined by specific facial actions that have a common onset or clear overlap in time.

Intercoder reliability in identifying pain-related action units is consistently high in published investigations (e.g., Craig, Hyde, & Patrick, 1991). When a second trained coder has recoded a randomly selected set of the videotaped reactions to pain, reliabilities, calculated as the proportion of agreements relative to the total number of action units identified by either of the two coders, consistently have exceeded .75 (LeResche & Dworkin, 1988; Prkachin & Mercer, 1989).

Studies published to date indicate that there is a relatively distinct subset of facial actions, recognizable as a facial expression, that is associated with acute, phasic pain. Although these actions occur consistently with pain, there are also substantial individual differences. The expression has been observed in studies using

experimental pain, exacerbation of persistent clinical pain, and pain instigated by invasive medical procedures. To date, most studies have examined short, sharp pain (e.g., Craig, Hyde, & Patrick, 1991; LeResche & Dworkin, 1988; Prkachin & Mercer, 1989); however, Prkachin (1991, unpublished manuscript) has recently found that a similar configuration occurs with more tonic pressure and ischemic pain. The tonic pain suffered by chronic pain patients still awaits investigation. This probably reflects the clinical observation that persistent pain is associated with a less vigorous expression of distress. The chronic pain patient is more likely to appear to be experiencing depression, except for those occasions in which there is exacerbation of clinical pain.

As Craig, Hyde, and Patrick (1991) note, all studies of adults describing the facial response during pain identify brow lowering and narrowing of the eye orbit as a result of tightening the eye lids as key to the expression. The majority (four to six of the seven available studies)* found raising the cheek (again narrowing the eye), eyes closed or blinking, raising the upper lip, and parting of lips or dropping the jaw to be pain related actions. The following actions were identified as pain-related in only one or two of the seven studies reported to date: horizontally stretching the lips, oblique pulling at the corner of the lips, vertically stretching the mouth open, wrinkling the nose, deepening the nasolabial fold, and drooping eyelids. Figure 15.1 illustrates the key facial muscles controlling each of the FACS action units that have been associated with pain.

Figure 15.2 provides an artist's drawing of a low back pain patient's reaction to a painful straight leg raising, range of motion exercise. This patient's reaction was selected because it represented a composite of many of the facial actions commonly observed. One can observe the brows slightly lowered, the nose wrinkled, the infraorbital triangle (the cheek area) raised, the lower eyelid raised and tightened, a slightly elevated upper lip, eyes closed with a marked tightening, and the lips slightly parted. More often patients display subsets of these facial actions.

TABLE 15.1. Minimum Requirements for Coding the Occurrence of Action Unit 7—Lid Tightening

---

1. *Slight* narrowing of the eye opening (due primarily to lower lid raise); or
2. The lower lid is raised and the skin below the eye is drawn up and/or medially towards the inner corner of the eye *slightly;* or
3. *Slight* bulge or pouch of the lower eyelid skin as it is pushed up.

If you did not see the lower lid *move* up, then requirement 1 must be *marked not slight* and requirement 3 must be met.

Note: From Ekman and Friesen (1978). Copyright 1978 Consulting Psychologist's Press. Reprinted by permission.

*Craig & Patrick, 1985; Craig, Hyde, & Patrick, 1991; LeResche, 1982; LeResche & Dworkin, 1988; Patrick, Craig, & Prkachin, 1986; Prkachin & Mercer, 1989; Swalm & Craig, 1990.

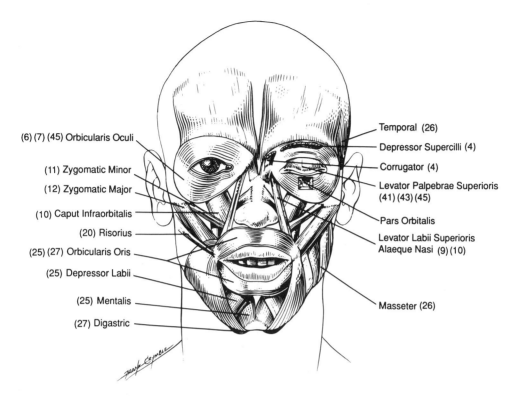

FIGURE 15.1. Facial muscles controlling the various facial actions associated with pain. The key action units are identified numerically and have been labelled according to the Facial Action Coding System (Ekman & Friesen, 1978) as follows: (4) brow lower, (6) cheek riase, (7) lids tight, (9) nose wrinkle, (11) nasolabial deepen, (10) upper lip raise, (12) lip corner pull, (20) lip stretch, (25) lips part, (26) jaw drop, (41) lids droop, (43) eyes closed, (45) blink.

Whereas the specific units of facial action identified here are central to the expression of pain, judges respond to the configuration of observed actions, including their temporal relationships, rather than to discrete cues. The importance of the configuration of facial actions, the facial expression itself, was demonstrated by Lee and Craig (1991), who reported that temporal overlap in pain-related facial movements was necessary for judgments of more severe pain. LeResche and Dworkin (1988) also identified overlapping facial actions associated with painful events. Although the integrated configuration of facial movements is important, in research studies it is not uncommon for facial patterns to be incomplete. Similarly, during natural interactions, one may have to observe "microexpressions" to decode the experiences of another.

Further refinement in the coding of facial activity can be anticipated given the capabilities of computer scanning and analytic systems (e.g., Pilowsky, Thornton, & Stokes, 1986) and the potential for using electromyographic

(Schwartz, Brown, & Ahern, 1980; Tassinary, Cacioppo, & Geen, 1990) and kinematic measures (Roy, in press).

Several strategies designed to validate the use of facial expressions as indices of pain have been adopted. As described above, empirical validity has been demonstrated in studies indicating that facial activity changes systematically when physical insults known to be painful are introduced. Content validity has been demonstrated in studies indicating that observers have little difficulty identifying people as experiencing pain, and their rating of pain varies systematically with the severity of noxious insult delivered (e.g., Patrick, Craig, & Prkachin, 1986).

Concurrent validity has been demonstrated in studies examining relationships between facial activity and the corresponding report of subjective states. A moderate relationship between the intensity of subjective distress and the magnitude of facial involvement has been observed (Craig, Hyde, & Patrick, 1991; Prkachin & Mercer, 1989), as described below. Relationships between facial expressions of pain

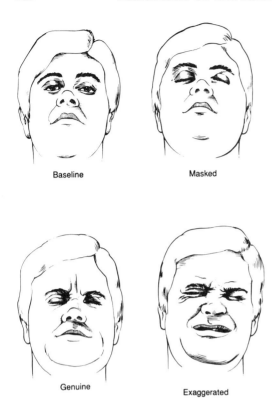

Baseline   Masked

Genuine   Exaggerated

FIGURE 15.2. Facial expressions of a chronic low back pain patient during: (A) A neutral baseline period prior to onset of motor exercises, (B) straight leg raising provoking sharp exacerbation of clinical pain, (C) repetition of the straight leg raising accompanied by instructions to mask the facial display, and (D) repetition of this exercise along with instructions to exaggerate the response. The video camera was placed above the patient's feet.

and other self-report characteristics of the experience also have been examined. LeResche and Dworkin (1988) found moderate positive correlations between various self-report measures of pain and various characteristics of the facial expression of pain. For example, the correlation between a McGill Pain Questionnaire (MPQ) measure of affective distress and the duration of the pain expression was $r = 0.69$.

Finally, one can discriminate facial activity during pain from the facial response when other known subjective states are being experienced. Judges are capable of discriminating expressions of pain from facial displays of various emotional states (Boucher, 1969). LeResche (1982) compared objective descriptions of facial activity observed in candid photographs of adults experiencing acute pain with

descriptions of various emotional states. Although the pain display shared some common elements with fear, anger, and sadness, the overlap was minimal. LeResche and Dworkin (1988) found no relationship between their measures of the facial expression of pain and a variety of measures of emotional states their patients were suffering. They concluded that the pain facial expression taps relatively specific qualities of the pain experience rather than other elements of psychological distress. In general, the significance of facial expression as a "window" on the many facets of pain has demonstrated that the approach has both sensitivity and specificity.

JUDGMENT STUDIES

The detailed and sophisticated information that is available from fine-grained observational systems, FACS in particular, makes this the method of choice for investigators whose concerns are equally as specific. FACS analysis is demanding of time and human resources. Some investigators may not have the resources available, however, and others may not be as interested in fine detail, but rather may wish to have a general "reading" of global characteristics of the pain display, such as its intensity. In other circumstances, for example, when the investigator is interested in how people decode pain information in others, FACS analysis may be inappropriate.

It is possible to acquire meaningful information about pain expression by performing a "judgment study." Examples of facial behavior are shown to observers who are asked to make decisions about the evidence that confronts them; for example, "How much pain does this person seem to experience?" The observer (often called the "receiver") may then rate the response of the subject ("sender") on a Likert-type scale ranging from "No pain" to "Strong pain."

Rosenthal (1982) provides a useful discussion of reliability statistics and other methodological issues involved in the conduct of such studies. It is sufficient for the present purposes to note that the reliabilities of judgments made in studies of pain expression are generally high. For example, in our studies (e.g., Prkachin & Craig, 1985; Prkachin, Currie, & Craig, 1983) effective reliabilities with relatively few receivers have tended to fall in the range .81–.97.

Judgment studies can be quite sensitive, valid, and discriminating. For example, Prkachin and Craig (1985) reported a judgment study in which receivers rated the amount of pain displayed by senders exposed to experimental pain in the presence of a tolerant model or in a control condition. Receivers viewed videotaped excerpts of senders' facial responses to no stimulation, mild pain, and strong pain and rated the amount of pain apparent in their reactions. The data were analyzed with signal detection methods. The results confirmed both the validity and sensitivity of the receivers' judgments. Receivers' ratings indicated that they could detect the difference between different levels of pain administered to observers. Ratings reflected both the actual intensity of the stimuli administered to senders and their subjective rating of the pain. Finally, the receivers' ratings distinguished between the tolerant modeling and control conditions, indicating that the method was sensitive to variables that may modulate the pain response.

INDIVIDUAL DIFFERENCES

Although a distinctive pattern of facial activity has been associated with pain, substantial variation has been observed. For this reason, describing a prototypical expression of pain seems inappropriate. Some of the variation appears to have a biological basis in the severity of tissue trauma, as well as in specific disease states, whereas other differences appear to relate to psychosocial factors, including culture-specific social conventions and situational influences. Personal dispositions and sex differences are ambiguous as to whether they have genetic or social learning origins.

Severity of Distress

We have observed consistently the overall magnitude of facial involvement and discrete movements to encode in a graded manner the severity of pain being experienced. Patrick et al. (1986) reported moderate correlations between facial activity and the severity of pain provoked by electric shock (mean multiple $r = .43$). In a study of facial activity during tonic pain, the cold pressor test, Craig and Patrick (1985) found that facial activity was greatest immediately following exposure to the painful event. Thereafter, facial activity diminished, whereas

pain ratings increased. This may not be unusual, suggesting that the initial insult has elements of startle, and that facial activity can serve primarily to indicate the onset of a painful event, dampening thereafter. In contrast to these findings, Feuerstein, Barr, Francoeur, Houle, and Rafman (1982) reported observing an increased incidence over time of facial grimaces in children aged 9 to 14 years old during the cold pressor experience.

Prkachin and Mercer (1989) found that subjective ratings of the sensory intensity and affective discomfort provoked by painful shoulder movement were related to facial actions, but the facial actions were not all equally sensitive. Cheek raising had the strongest relationship to subjective pain. Brow lowering, nose wrinkling, lip pulling, increasing degrees of mouth opening, and eye closing also correlated with pain in various circumstances, but not consistently. Correlations ranged between .44 and .71. Information concerning onset and offset of acute pain also is available in the facial display. With some forms of pain, onset produces the most distorted facial display, with the display dampened as the experience persists. The moderate correlation suggests that facial and self-report measures reflect different aspects of a complex reaction pattern, but also confirm that there can be desynchrony between self-report and nonverbal measures of pain.

Specific Disease States

Prkachin and Mercer (1989) have suggested that virtually all forms of pain, including the least severe, will trigger certain facial movements that have a "primary" status. They suggest brow lowering and eye closing were fundamental, but eye narrowing could serve in this capacity as well. Leventhal and Sharp (1965) made a complementary observation while observing women during childbirth. Heavy knitting and furrowing of the brow appeared to be elicited only when distress exceeded a minimum level or threshold. Prkachin and Mercer (1989) propose that other actions would be recruited thereafter, depending upon the specific source of the pain and the individual's experience with the condition. Increasing severity and duration of distress would also provoke greater facial involvement. Brow lowering and eye closing would be followed in sequence by the mid-face actions of upper lip raise, then nose wrinkling. The final phase would include mouth opening, followed, in the extreme, by horizontal stretching of the lips.

LeResche and Dworkin (1988) described the most prominent patterns of facial expression occurring in temporomandibular disorder (TMD) patients undergoing painful palpation of the muscles of mastication. The pattern that occurred most frequently during pain consisted of tightening of the skin around the eye, lowering the brow, and/or closing the eyes (including blinking). These actions were proposed to be the defining characteristics of pain. A range of lower face movements also accompanied these actions in the area of the eyes, including raising the upper lip, wrinkling the nose, stretching the lips horizontally, or opening the mouth, but these latter actions were observed to occur no more than 5% of the time. A variety of facial actions that define specific emotional states (e.g., lip corner pull representing a smile or an expression of happiness) were designated as exclusionary criteria for expressions of pain. Given the complexities of emotional states interacting with pain, one could question the assumption that the presence of specific emotional states would preclude the experience of pain.

Culture-Specific Differences

It is not unusual for clinicians to attribute highly reactive or impassive reponses to injury to an individual's ethnic or racial background. However, no studies examining cross-cultural variations in displays of pain have been undertaken despite their potential importance (LeResche & Dworkin, 1984). Evidence for cross-cultural consistency in facial expressions of emotion (Ekman et al., 1987; Russell & Fehr, 1987) suggest that the facial expression of pain should be relatively invariant, although some systematic differences can be expected. Certain "display rules" (Ekman & Friesen, 1969) govern the manner in which emotion will be expressed. For example, people often conform to a social convention that dictates that relatively few emotions should be displayed (Ekman & Friesen, 1969). Socialization within specific familial and cultural contexts is responsible for some cross-cultural variation in the display of emotion (Darwin, 1872/1965; Ekman, Sorensen, & Friesen, 1969), as well as in the display of pain and illness behavior (Craig,

1986; Craig & Patrick, 1985; Craig & Wyckoff, 1987; Sargent, 1984; Weisenberg, 1982).

Situational Influences

Systematic situational variation (Bayer, Baer, & Early, 1991) in pain behavior is well established, as numerous interventions, including hypnosis, cognitive coping strategies, relaxation, and social modeling have substantial effects on self-report of pain. Limited investigation has been undertaken of the impact of these procedures on nonverbal expression, although tolerance levels or willingness to accept noxious stimulation tend to covary with self-report. Exposure to social models who display intolerant or tolerant patterns of response to noxious stimulation has been shown to have a potent effect on most measures of pain experience and behavior (cf. Craig, 1986). Prkachin et al. (1983) and Prkachin and Craig (1985) demonstrated that exposure to tolerant pain models diminished nonverbal displays of pain. Patrick et al. (1986) found the impact of social models to be substantially greater on self-report in contrast to facial activity. This desynchrony in the impact of a form of situational influence on self-report and facial expression of pain suggests that social influences would be relatively slow in changing stylistic patterns of pain expression.

Personal Dispositions

Some of the variation in the facial display of pain can be attributed to traitlike dispositions to react differently. Some people maintain a very impassive, nonreactive expression, whereas others show numerous, intense facial contortions. The relationship of age to nonverbal behavior also is an important variable that has received little study, other than with very young children, as discussed later in this paper. Prkachin and Mercer (1989) found that intensities and durations of pain-related facial movements were related to the psychological and physical impact of patients' pain problems. Those patients who were more greatly affected by the problem displayed the greater facial activity.

Sex Differences

A variety of differences between men and women have been found in pain and illness behavior. Feine, Bushnell, Miron, and Duncan (1991) reviewed studies indicating a greater incidence of acute and persistent pain and demand for health services among women, a general tendency to report lower pain threshold and tolerance levels among women, and ratings of pain to comparable noxious events to be more severe among women (although there are equivocal findings). As yet, minimal description of the actual pattern of pain response has been provided (Lander, Fowler-Kerry, & Hill, 1990). Grunau and Craig (1987) reported that latencies of facial pain activity were shorter in newborn male infants. Craig, Hyde, & Patrick (1991) observed no differences using the FACS measure between male and female chronic lowback pain patients reacting to a movement exacerbating persistent pain, but independent judges viewing the videotapes rated the women as more expressive than the men. It was uncertain whether the judges were applying common cultural stereotypes arguing that women are more sensitive to pain than men or whether the FACS measures were insensitive to differences between men and women that were identified using the judgment method.

CONCURRENT AFFECTIVE/COGNITIVE STATES DURING PAIN

Although the focus in research examining facial activity during painful experiences has largely been on the presence and intensity of pain, one can also tap other components of the painful experience. People react to pain-provoking events in complex social and physical contexts, and one would expect other concurrent facial actions. One cannot fail to be impressed in clinical settings by patients whose faces disclose great forebearance, resolve, dismay, panic, anger, or resignation. Candid photographs in magazines are impressive when they show women experiencing pleasure during a painful birth, or firewalkers clearly trained in distraction strategies.

Mixed or blended facial expressions would be expected in which the facial expression of pain coincided with other subjective states. Subtle features of facial expression may disclose the significance or meaning of a painful experience for the person, and untangle the intricate confound between emotion and pain. For ex-

ample, Prkachin and Mercer (1989) suggest that increased blinking rates at the onset of pain may reflect startle. Deciphering the range of concurrent states is made easier by the presence of universal facial expressions for emotions including happiness, sadness, surprise, fear, anger, disgust, and contempt (Ekman & Friesen, 1986; Ekman et al., 1969).

Unfortunately, few systematic studies are available. LeResche and Dworkin (1988) applied a priori criteria for facial expressions of various emotional states based on the FACS action units (Friesen, 1987). The patients' reactions were quite variable but were observed to include disgust, contempt, fear, anger, and sadness, with most subjects displaying only one of these states concurrent to pain. It was noteworthy that pain report and pain facial expressions were higher for persons showing a greater number of different negative affective states. Thus, greater involvement of affective distress during pain is likely to intensify both verbal and nonverbal expression of pain.

THE FACIAL EXPRESSION OF PAIN IN YOUNG CHILDREN

Pain in young children provides a special case for intensive study of facial activity. The younger the child, the greater is the dependency of adults on nonverbal assessment (see McGrath & Brigham, Chapter 17). The infant's vulnerability and the substantial risks of physiological shock introduces urgency to the challenge of deciphering pain. Clinicians have available to them during invasive and other noxious events a broad range of cues for pain, including crying, facial expressions, body movements, and autonomic activity; but clinicians find them ambiguous, as many of the cues are not specific to pain, and they often underestimate the significance of pain in infants and children (Craig & Grunau, 1991; Craig & Grunau, in press; Dale, 1986; McGrath, 1987; Pigeon, McGrath, Lawrence, & MacMurray, 1989).

The most specific behavioral evidence for pain in the infant appears to be in the facial response (Craig & Grunau, in press). Johnston and Strada (1986) reported that the facial response to injection pain was more consistent across infants than were cry patterns, heart rate, or body movement. The Neonatal Facial Coding System (NFCS) provides an objective, reliable, and detailed approach for studying the infant's facial reaction to potentially painful situations (Grunau & Craig, 1990). Using this measure, a relatively stereotyped pattern of facial display has emerged (Grunau & Craig, 1987; Grunau et al., 1990) (see Figure 15.3). This is comprised of lowered brow, squeezed shut eyes, deepened nasolabial furrow (a line that begins adjacent to the nostrils and extends down and out beyond the lip corners), an opened mouth, and a taut, cupped tongue. As well, a protruding tongue appears to indicate states other than pain (Grunau et al., 1990). There appears to be greater consistency in this expression than in the adult's facial response. Figure 15.3 illustrates two infants' reactions to heel lancing, and the finding of Grunau and Craig (1987) that the severity of the infant's reaction is related to behavioral state of the infant at the time of the lance.

There are striking similarities between the newborn and adult facial response to events that are painful to adults. This provides substantial support for the position that newborns have a capacity to experience and communicate pain when subjected to invasive procedures. However, it would be inappropriate to conclude that the experience of pain in the infant is fully comparable to that of the adult. Infants do not have the capacity for cognizing the significance of the experience as do adults, and their experience of pain must be dominated by sensations and emotions. Minor facial differences between infants and adults suggest features of infants' experiences that probably are unique to them. Most significant would be that most often infants squeeze their eyes shut, while adults keep their eyes open, but narrowed, only closing them to particularly severe pain. Adults need to receive information if adaptive reactions are to be employed. In contrast, infants cannot attach meaning to the situation, and the greater protection afforded by closed eyes would appear to be the more adaptive reaction.

Several studies have demonstrated the usefulness of the NFCS measure. Comparisons have been made of the facial expression of pain observed in full-term and preterm infants (Craig, Whitfield, Grunau, Linton, & Had-

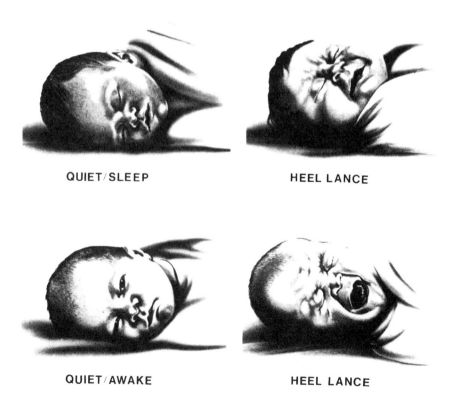

QUIET/SLEEP   HEEL LANCE

QUIET/AWAKE   HEEL LANCE

FIGURE 15.3. Infant facial responses to the heel lance procedure vary with their behavioral state at the time of the lance. From Grunau and Craig (1987), page 404. Copyright 1987 Elsevier Science Publishers, B.V. Reprinted by permission.

jistavropoulos, 1991). Assessment of infants who are born too early or too small is of particular interest because they often must be subjected to painful medical procedures, yet they are fragile, vulnerable to physiological shock, and particularly dependent upon adults. Shapiro (1991) found that nurses judged premature neonates to be suffering less than full-term newborns even though both groups had undergone the same noxious procedure: "Lack of recognition of pain in premature neonates may result in unnecessary suffering, increased morbidity and mortality for this vulnerable group" (p. 148).

The Craig, Whitfield, et al. (1991) findings indicated that the general pattern of facial activity observed in the preterm neonate was consistent with that of the full-term neonate; however, the magnitude and strength of activity varied with gestational age at birth. Greater activity was observed in infants of longer gestational age. Although preterm infants generally do not respond as vigorously, there is reason to believe they are hypersensitive. Fitzgerald and her colleagues (Fitzgerald, 1991) have examined cutaneous flexor reflexive movements in response to painful stimuli. The reflexive withdrawal of the foot is clearly present in preterm newborns and has a lower threshold than in full-term infants and adults. Studies of this reflex (Fitzgerald, Millard, & MacIntosh, 1989) led to the conclusion that "the preterm infant is if anything, supersensitive to painful stimuli when compared with the full term infant" (p. 442) (Fitzgerald & McIntosh, 1989).

The finding (Craig, Whitfield, et al., 1991) that neonates with lower gestational ages react less vigorously provokes the question "Does less activity mean less painful discomfort?" This seems improbable. Although the younger infants were less responsive, their attenuated reactions more likely reflected limited energy resources available for vigorous and sustained response. Metabolic resources in these infants are primarily devoted to ensuring survival. Little energy is left to cope after the handling and swab procedures. It would appear best to adhere to the principle that judgments of pain in the neonate should be made relative to gestational age cohorts, and, if these are not available, the judgments should reflect changes in apparent state as judged by an observer particularly familiar with the child. Facial expression would appear to be the most salient source of information available to the observer. Stevens and Johnston (1991) examined facial activity and physiological measures during the heel stick procedures with newborns. They found the physiological outcomes varied across infants and phases of the heel stick procedure, and these appeared to be less prevalent indicators of pain than facial activity.

A recent study (Grunau, Craig, & Drummond, 1989) reported the impact of various perinatal influences on newborn facial activity during heel lance. Obstetric medication and mode of delivery were related to the newborn's reaction. Facial movement was more extreme in infants who had experienced more stressful deliveries. This suggested that the more demanding birth led to greater irritability and to a reduced capacity to modulate the response to noxious stimulation.

McCrory (1990) has demonstrated the usefulness of NFCS in assessing effects of nondrug interventions for pain in the newborn. Using facial activity as a criterion measure, a combined auditory/proprioceptive-tactile stimulation procedure was effective in reducing pain during the heel lance procedure.

The NFCS has been useful in elucidating certain characteristics of infant colic. Barr et al. (1991) used the NFCS measure to assess the facial activity of infants identified by their parents as suffering from problematic crying. The infants who displayed a greater incidence of the facial actions associated with pain before feeding also were the infants who satisfied criteria for particularly severe and prolonged bouts of crying and fussing. Thus, there is evidence that pain represents a problem for a subset of infants with problematic crying.

Pomietto and Marvin (1991) recently examined facial responses of infants ranging between newborn and 12 months who were subjected to any of a variety of painful, invasive procedures (finger stick, heel stick, or venipuncture). Although sample sizes were small, there were a number of interesting correlations between facial activity and characteristics of both the children and the procedures used. The older infants were less reactive, children who were held on their parent's lap were less reactive, finger sticks yielded less activity than the other procedures, and there were differences attributable to the various persons conducting the procedure, apparently because variable skills in distracting the children were used. Thus, a systematic measure of facial activity appears capable of isolating a variety of subtle variations in factors influencing infant procedural pain.

Although Mills (1989) did not use a systematic coding system, she provided interesting observations on the facial response of older infants and toddlers. She generated qualitative, narrative descriptions of behavioral activity, including facial movement, in children ranging in age from birth to 36 months following surgery, fractures, and burns. The descriptive accounts of the children less than 3 months included frowns, grimaces, and a clenched jaw. Movements that might have exacerbated postoperative and other types of persistent pain yielded changes in expression, and flinching was apparent in children older than 9 months. Fear, sadness, anger, vigilance, and pouting were also evident in the older children.

A recent study (Hadjistavropoulos, Grunau, & Craig, 1991) compared the NFCS with the FACS (Ekman & Friesen, 1978), as adapted for infants by Oster and Rosenstein (1982), in the study of preterm infants' facial responses to the heel stick blood sampling procedure. Descriptions of the facial expressions obtained from the two measures were remarkably comparable. An advantage of the NFCS would be its ease in scoring and its potential promise as an assessment instrument in clinical settings.

Important observations concerning the emotional context of pain in infants and toddlers have been made using Izard's maximally discriminative facial movement coding system (MAX) (Izard, 1979). In this approach, preconceived categories of emotion, including anger, fear, surprise, and joy, as well as pain, are sought through scanning three regions of the face (brow, eyes, and mouth), with particular combinations of activity representing discrete emotional expressions. Johnston (1989) characterizes the pain configuration as having "the brows lowered and drawn together, bulged and/or vertical furrows between brows, nasal root broadened and bulged; eye fissure tightly closed, and angular, squarish mouth" (p. 18). Izard (Izard, Hembree, Dougherty, & Spizzirri, 1983; Izard, Huebner, Risser, McGinnes, & Dougherty, 1980) reported that during infancy the early pattern of facial response to immunization injections predominantly suggests pain, but around 6–8 months the pattern becomes one of anticipatory fear prior to the injection, pain following the needle stick, and anger thereafter. The pain response decreases with age whereas the anger response increases,

such that the latter is the dominant pattern by 19 months. The anger response was differentiated from the pain response primarily because the child's eyes were open and staring in anger. Individual differences were also observed, with the infants who were slow to be soothed showing significantly more anger, while those who were soothed more quickly showing less physical distress (Izard, Hembree, & Huebner, 1987).

HOW DO CLINICIANS AND OTHERS USE FACIAL EXPRESSION?

An important distinction can be made between what the face objectively does and how the face is perceived and interpreted by the observer (Poole & Craig, 1991). Objective identification of distinctive features of the facial expression of pain is a necessary precondition to establishing the extent to which these specific features are salient to observers and serve as determinants of others' judgments of pain and other subjective states.

Health professionals make judgments in real-time and integrate facial information with numerous other sources. Influential factors include self-report, other behavioral observations, knowledge of prior health status, the individual's sociocultural background, and an appreciation of the social context in which pain is displayed. The observer must assemble and integrate these numerous sources of information to arrive at a judgment concerning what is being experienced.

It is clear that decisions about pain reflect more than the specific facial display identified above. Hadjistavropoulos, Ross, and von Baeyer (1990) observed that the physical attractiveness of the person in pain heavily influenced physicians' judgments of facial expressions of pain and decisions concerning how the person should be treated. Von Baeyer et al. (1984) similarly found that variations in nonverbal expressiveness, including facial expression, influenced judgments of psychological distress during pain, with the ratings influenced by personality dispositions toward nurturance of the judges.

The specific facial cues used by judges to identify pain have been identified in several studies of adults and children. Patrick et al. (1986) concluded that brow lowering, eye blinking, cheek raise, and upper lip raise predicted on average 55% of the variance in ratings of pain (mean multiple $r = .74$). Studies with children also have found considerable consistency in the cues that are salient to adults. Parents display considerable agreement when judging pain in infants (not their own) using facial displays. Craig, Grunau, Johnston, and Hadjistavropoulos (1991) found mean interrater reliabilities to be $r = .62$. Using the NFCS, Craig, Grunau, and Aquan-Assee (1988) reported prominent predictor variables of adult ratings of infant pain to be taut tongue, open lips, latency to facial activity, vertical stretched mouth, and deepened nasolabial furrow. As well, the more facial involvement the adults observed, the greater were the ratings of pain experienced by the infants. Fully 43% of the variance in the adults' ratings of affective discomfort were determined by the variables identified above.

Comparisons have been made between the information value of facial activity and cry as sources of information about infant pain. Cry can be seen as a "biological siren" or a "distant early warning system" (Craig & Grunau, 1991; Levine & Gordon, 1982). It serves to alert adults to the onset of a child's distress as well as its continuing presence. A recent paper (Craig, Grunau, Johnston, & Hadjistavropoulos, 1991) compared the relative contributions of cry and facial activity to judgments of pain in infants and concluded that facial activity permitted substantially better discrimination of states of pain than the cry information. Thus, the social significance of facial activity during pain appears quite prominent during infancy. To the extent that parents and other adults must have accurate information concerning the state of well being of an infant, the facial expression of pain clearly is of great importance.

VOLUNTARY CONTROL AND DECEPTION

The linkage of facial expressions to noxious events appears to change during the transition from infancy to adulthood. By the time adulthood is achieved, expressive repertoires consist of several different categories of display, including expressions of genuine emotion, as well as false, inhibited, exaggerated and blended expressions (Ekman & Friesen, 1975; Ekman,

Friesen, & Ellsworth, 1972; Oster & Ekman, 1978). Most people are aware that their nonverbal behavior is used by others to infer emotional and cognitive states and can intentionally manipulate actions to control how others understand them (Yarczower & Daruns, 1982). When one person deliberately makes the choice to mislead another person, that behavior is reasonably described as deception or lying (Ekman, 1988). This is to be distinguished from spontaneous, nonintentional individual differences that have been shaped by social factors over time.

One interesting property of facial expression is its ability to shed light on underlying regulatory systems. Certain features of facial expression are less amenable to voluntary control than others. When people are startled, they display a characteristic configuration of nonverbal actions, including eye closure, lip stretching, and neck movements. When they explicitly try to inhibit the reaction, they find it difficult, if not impossible; whereas when they attempt to simulate the reaction, they make characteristic errors of omission and commission (Ekman, Friesen, & Simons, 1985; Hager & Ekman, 1985). Similarly, smiles when a person is genuinely happy differ in form from smiles when a person is experiencing negative affect (Ekman, Friesen, & O'Sullivan, 1988).

Distinctions between voluntary and involuntary expression reflect the neurological mechanisms that regulate facial behavior. It has long been known that deliberate and spontaneous facial expressions are under the control of partially independent neurological systems (Monrad-Krohn, 1924; Rinn, 1984). Both cortical and subcortical systems and pathways are arranged in at least two motor systems responsible for deliberate movements on the one hand and spontaneous movements on the other. Observers appreciate that certain features of facial expression are more trustworthy than others. When reporting which regions of the face are most important when making judgments of another's emotional state, observers attach primary importance to the upper face and eyes (Lee & Craig, 1991).

Clinicians are often concerned that patients may be exaggerating the display of pain (Cleeland, 1989; Fordyce, 1976; Kremer et al., 1983; Leavitt & Sweet, 1986). Instruments that discriminated genuine from posed pain would be of great interest in a variety of settings including judicial hearings concerning personal injury suits, compensation board settlements, and the progress of treatment for chronic pain (see Vasudevan, Chapter 7).

Of less obvious concern in clinical settings, but of great human interest, would be whether people can fully suppress the response to pain and conceal pain from others. Cancer patients appear to do so because of a fear of addiction from narcotics. Manual workers and athletes may hide pain because to be perceived as in pain could lead to the loss of work (Kotarba, 1983). Lander (1990) notes that reasons for patients minimizing pain include fears of injections and aversions to side effects of analgesics.

People are quite capable of either misrepresenting themselves as in pain or as not suffering painful distress when it indeed is present. Craig, Hyde, & Patrick (1991) examined facial activity when chronic low back pain sufferers posed expressions of pain, were genuinely experiencing pain, or suppressed their reactions when actually in pain. People who were faking pain displayed facial activity that did not differ from the genuine expression in the types of discrete facial action units that were displayed, but the display of distress was more severe or intense. It would seem that discrimination of faked from genuine patterns of response could not be based upon the specific action units available for observation. Those who were attempting to suppress visual evidence of distress also succeeded in dampening facial activity, leaving little to be observed, although there was residual facial activity, primarily tension around the eyes.

Figure 15.2 provides an artist's drawings of the facial behavior of a patient suppressing a pain reaction and exaggerating a pain reaction. In the masked expression the eyes are closed, and although there is some tension in the lids, there is no marked squeezing or tightening. In the exaggerated expression, the inner and central portion of the brow is lowered, pushing down and reducing visibility of the medial portion of the eyelid; there are marked wrinkles and muscle bulges between the eyebrows; the central portion of the brow and the skin above the brow are pulled together; there are marked crow's feet; the infraorbital triangle (cheek area) is raised, producing bags and wrinkles under the eyes; the nose is wrinkled; the eyes are squeezed shut; there is elongation of the mouth, along with a slight flattening of skin beyond the lip corners; and the lips are parted.

Prkachin (in press) compared reactions of healthy volunteers exposed to varying levels of pain induced by shock with their efforts to produce facial expressions of the different levels of pain deliberately. Judgment study methods confirmed that deliberate expressions tended to be exaggerated relative to spontaneous ones. Observers were able to discriminate spontaneous from deliberate expressions of pain with modest degrees of sensitivity. Moreover, when spontaneous and deliberate expressions were similar in intensity, observers were still able to discriminate them, suggesting the existence of topographic or temporal differences between the two types of display.

Other evidence indicates that judges can be readily convinced that the person is suffering to a greater or lesser extent than is genuinely the case (Poole & Craig, 1991). When asked to rate the amount of pain experienced by patients whose facial reactions were videotaped as they engaged in variably painful actions, judges did not effectively discriminate between genuine, posed, and suppressed facial activity or recognize the dissimulated states. Consistent with the earlier observation (Craig, Hyde, & Patrick, 1991) that faked facial displays of pain consisted of exaggerated caricatures of the genuine facial display, the subjects attributed greater pain to the posed faces than to the genuine display. As well, suppression of facial behavior during genuine pain also effectively deceived the judges as they substantially underestimated the amount of pain being experienced by these patients. However, the patients were not fully successful, as the judges continued to attribute some pain to the patients. Coding of facial activity when patients attempt to suppress displays of pain suggests that tension is most likely to "leak" through in the region of the eyes, with patients raising their cheeks, narrowing their eyes, deepening clefts in the skin folds in the eye orbit area, and blinking less when attempting to withhold evidence of pain. This would be consistent with early investigations of cutaneous heat-induced pain indicating that a contraction of the eye muscles at the outer canthus was the first sign of withdrawal from the heat stimulus (Craig & Prkachin, 1983). It seems to be very difficult to maintain suffering entirely as a personal, private experience.

Poole and Craig (1991) also supported earlier studies indicating that people generally attach greater credibility to nonverbal behavior than verbal report when making social judgments, particularly when they are inconsistent with one another (DePaulo et al., 1978). Self-report was discounted relative to nonverbal expression when the two were discrepant (i.e., the facial grimace signaled pain, but verbal reports denied it, or pain was reported, but there were no facial signs confirming the report).

There is little surprise in the evidence that displays of pain are readily exaggerated or suppressed, given that actors, of varying degrees of skill, have long practiced the art of portraying suffering. Numerous behavioral models depicting how one would or should behave when in pain are available through personal experience and observation of others (Craig, 1986).

Although it appears very difficult to discriminate genuine, posed, or suppressed expressions of pain, other prospects for identifying deception need to be examined. It is noteworthy that the full complex of cues associated with pain identified above rarely is observed when people are genuinely in pain. Only selected features of the expression are likely to be observed. In contrast, the prototypal expression is more likely to be observed when pain is being faked. Ekman (1985) noted this to be the case for attempts to deceive in general. Temporal relations among specific action units may provide cues to deception (Lee & Craig, 1991; Prkachin, 1990). Latencies, duration, and contiguities among facial actions may be difficult to dissimulate when deception is attempted. LeResche, Ehrlich, and Dworkin (1990) noted that smiles apparently designed to mask the facial expression of pain could be distinguished from genuine pain by an absence of orbicularis oculi activity. It also may be that if there were strong motivation to deceive and greater consequences for being found guilty of lying, more cues signifying the presence of a lie would have been observed (Ekman, 1988). Under these circumstances anxiety or shame may be apparent.

It was also of interest to know if expectations of deception improve the ability to discriminate genuine from either posed or suppressed expressions of pain. Poole and Craig (1991) reported that foreknowledge of deceptive facial expressions of pain did not lead to greater clinical sensitivity to deception, or more accurate judgments of the actual severity of pain being experienced. Rather, when primed to be suspicous judges generally became less willing

to attribute pain to the patients, irrespective of whether the patients were genuinely experiencing pain, faking the expression, or suppressing the facial display.

MEASURES OF FACIAL ACTIVITY AS A DIAGNOSTIC TOOL

The challenge is to improve upon the quality of information derived from facial activity that clinicians presently extract during their interactions with patients. There are powerful natural propensities to use nonverbal expressions, the information is readily accessible without special equipment, and there appears to be good reason to use it given that the information does encode important features of the experience of pain. More systematic use of this information should maximize its usefulness. The situation is akin to the importance of developing orderly self-report scales (see Jensen & Karoly, Chapter 9). Systematic self-report measures provide substantially better information than the informal questions concerning the severity of pain traditionaly used by clinicians.

Behavioral observation assessment strategies are needed for both adults and children who cannot articulate pain. Clinical assessment is most difficult with seriously ill people. The least healthy tend to be the least expressive. Until systematic measures are available, clinical intuition based on idiosyncratic experience will prevail. Several behavioral observation methods presently are available for both research and clinical assessment of pain for both adults and children (see Keefe & Williams, Chapter 16, and McGrath & Brigham, Chapter 17). Some include assessment of facial expression, and others do not explicitly mention it. It would seem appropriate to include a facial expression of pain measure, and one that corresponds to that which has been objectively described. Existing behavioral scales that include attention to facial activity sometimes misrepresent what should be observed. For example, the clinically important Keefe and Block (1982) behavioral measure of pain calls for ratings of facial grimaces, but the operational definition used by coders refers to "corners of the mouth pulled back and clenched teeth." These are rarely observed among people in pain.

It would be useful if clinicians had reference standards against which they could judge the severity of pain being experienced. Although the delivery of analgesics often is on an "as-needed" basis, the explicit criteria for satisfying the patient's needs are rarely specified. Establishing the specific cues that lead nurses to decide an analgesic is appropriate would be of considerable interest (e.g., Riemondy, Rang, Hershey, & Ballantine, 1991). Developing descriptive or pictorial standards characterizing pain reactions of varying degrees should be easier with young children, as the individual differences among adults are more substantial. The measures should be specific to the developmental age of the individual. As well, the relationships among verbal and nonverbal expressions of pain need further clarification. McGrath, Mathews, and Pigeon (1991) describe circumstances in which discordance between self-report of pain and nonverbal activity may be observed.

Nurse clinicians in the neonatal intensive care nursery setting have reported they consider facial "grimaces" to be diagnostic of pain in preterm infants (Craig, Grunau, Whitfield, & Linton, 1988). Although measures of physiological stress are also useful, they are not specific to pain. All pain is stressful, but all stress is not painful. Behavioral measures have the potential to disclose the source of distress, as well as how the trauma is integrated as subjective experience. Effective nursing intervention during invasive procedures and following surgery requires recognition and identification of behavioral signs of pain (Sparshott, 1989, 1990). The NFCS features that are associated with pain offer potential clinical application in identifying pain in the preterm as well as in the term infant.

There are many palliative interventions for children that need assessment, including analgesics and nonpharmaceutical strategies. In intensive medical care of premature infants it is now recommended that pain-relieving medication be considered as a fundamental component because if left untreated, pain can cause physiological and psychological stress (Anand & Hickey, 1987). The availability of behavioral measures of neonatal pain such as the NFCS will contribute to this endeavor by providing a behavioral referent for evaluation of the broad range of drug and nondrug interventions.

There are substantial differences between the tasks of clinicians assessing patients in pain and research technicians examining videotapes, using slow-motion or single-frame advance video feedback. We now have described a restricted set of well-defined facial actions that could provide the basis for an observational coding instrument that would indicate the presence, duration, and severity of pain, but it is uncertain whether real-time or videotaped measurement is necessary. The level of methodological precision needed to achieve reliable and valid measures remains uncertain.

WHERE DO WE GO FROM HERE?

Interest in the systematic use of information from the face to draw inferences about pain has a long history (Sears, 1932), but it is only within the past decade that our understanding of the nature and properties of pain expressions has advanced noticeably. Fine-grained analyses of facial actions have identified a subset of movements that capture information about pain that is carried by the face. These findings may make it possible to develop abbreviated coding systems that take advantage of the sensitivity of anatomically based notation, while avoiding the labor intensive aspects of comprehensive analysis. Ekman and Friesen (Friesen, 1987) have developed a simplified version of FACS in which observers are only required to attend to actions that play a role in the communication of fundamental emotions (EMFACS). A comparable simplified coding system could be developed for assessment of pain.

Clinical applications of the NFCS with infants, full-term and preterm, appear to have particular potential and importance. The immediate impact of pain in the form of physiological stress has recently been described (e.g., Anand & Carr, 1989; Anand & Hickey, 1987) and the long-term implications are beginning to be discovered. Until now it has been assumed that although extremely premature infants undergo multiple medical interventions and prolonged hospitalization, they do not remember these events, and that life-threatening medical needs are substantially more important than the experiential components of pain and distress. Recent findings indicate that the repeated painful procedures associated with intensive care of the very smallest and most premature infants may have long-term implications. Toddlers at age 18 months (adjusted for prematurity) whose birth weight had been below 1,000 grams were rated by their parents as less sensitive to the commonplace pain of childhood, compared with heavier preterm and full birth weight toddlers (Grunau, Whitfield, Petrie, & Fryer, 1991a).

At age 4½ years, preschool children who had been extremely premature showed a high incidence of somatic complaints of no known cause compared with children who had been born at term (Grunau, Whitfield, Petrie, & Fryer, 1991b). The infant suffers from not only pain during early nursery care but there are multiple external sources of distress (e.g., light, noise, intubation, physiological monitoring, mechanical respiration, multiple caregivers) (Field, 1990). Important intrinsic factors such as emotional variation, temperament, and coping style also are important (Lewis & Worobey, 1989). These may have a unique impact as well as an interaction with pain. Facial measures have not been satisfactorily explored in this context.

Despite the advances that have been made, a thorny issue that remains to be resolved concerns the optimal way of combining information obtained from facial measurement to provide a single metric of pain. The problem can be illustrated simply. Some half-dozen movements can be considered as candidate pain-related facial actions. They often combine (i.e., occur together) in a single pain "expression," but occasionally only elements appear. Singly, or in combination, most of the actions can vary in their intensity, and all can vary in duration. Research is needed to establish how to combine these observations into convenient indices. Examining the natural structure of these actions with multivariate methods is one obvious approach to this problem. Combining this with studies of how observers naturally process facial information would also be advantageous.

Acknowledgments. Support for the authors' research reported here was provided by the Canadian Social Sciences and Humanities Research Council, Natural Sciences and Humanities Research Council, and Medical Research Council.

REFERENCES

Adelmann, P.K., & Zajonc, R.B. (1989). Facial efference and the experience of emotion. *Annual Review of Psychology, 40,* 249–280.

Anand, K.J.S., & Carr, D.B. (1989). The neuroanatomy, neurophysiology, and neurochemistry of pain, stress, and analgesia in newborns and children. *Pediatric Clinics of North America, 36,* 795–822.

Anand, K.J.S., & Hickey, P.R. (1987). Pain and its effects in the human neonate and fetus. *The New England Journal of Medicine, 317,* 1321–1329.

Barr, R.G., Rotman, A., Yaremko, J., Leduc, D., & Francoeur, T.E. (in press). The crying of infants with colic: A controlled empirical description. *Pediatrics.*

Bayer, T.L., Baer, P.E., & Early, C. (1991). Situational and psychophysiological factors in psychologically induced pain. *Pain, 44,* 435–50.

Boucher, J.D. (1969). Facial displays of fear, sadness and pain. *Perceptual and Motor Skills, 28,* 239–242.

Cleeland, C.S., (1989). Measurement of pain by subjective report. In C.R. Chapman & J.D. Loeser (Eds.), *Advances in pain research and therapy: Issues in pain measurement* (pp. 391–404). New York: Raven Press.

Colby, C., Lanzetta, J., & Kleck, R. (1977). Effects of the expression of pain on autonomic and pain tolerance responses to subject-controlled pain. *Psychophysiology, 14,* 537–540.

Collier, G. (1985). *Emotional expression.* Hillsdale, NJ: Erlbaum.

Craig, K.D. (1986). Pain in context: Social modeling influences. In R.A. Sternbach (Ed.), *The psychology of pain* (pp. 67–96). New York: Raven Press.

Craig, K.D., & Grunau, R.V.E. (1991). Developmental issues: Infants and toddlers. In J.P. Bush & S.W. Harkins (Eds.), *Pain in children: Clinical and research issues from a developmental perspective* (pp. 171–193). New York: Springer-Verlag.

Craig, K.D., & Grunau, R.V.E. (in press). Neonatal pain perception and behavioural measurement. In K.J.S. Anand & P.J. McGrath (Eds.), *Neonatal pain and distress.* Amsterdam: Elsevier Science.

Craig, K.D., Grunau, R.V.E., & Aquan-Assee, J. (1988). Judgement of pain in newborns: Facial action and cry as determinants. *Canadian Journal of Behavioural Science, 20,* 442–451.

Craig, K.D., Grunau, R.V.E., Johnston, C.C., & Hadjistavropoulos, H. (1991). Facial and cry determinants of adult judgments of pain in newborns. Submitted for publication.

Craig, K.D., Grunau, R.V.E., Whitfield, M.F., & Linton, J. (1988). *Neonatal intensive care nurses' evaluations of pain.* Paper presented at the First European Conference on Pain in Children, Maastricht, The Netherlands.

Craig, K.D., Hyde, S., & Patrick, C.J. (1991). Genuine, suppressed, and faked facial behavior during exacerbation of chronic low back pain. *Pain, 46,* 161–172.

Craig, K.D., McMahon, R.S., Morison, J.D., & Zaskow, C. (1984). Developmental changes in infant pain expression during immunization injections. *Social Science and Medicine, 19,* 1331–1337.

Craig, K.D., & Patrick, C.J. (1985). Facial expression during induced pain. *Journal of Personality and Social Psychology, 48,* 1080–1091.

Craig, K.D., & Prkachin, K.M. (1980). Social influences on public and private components of pain. In I.G. Sarason & C.D. Spielberger (Eds.). *Stress and anxiety* (Vol. 7, pp. 57–72). New York: Hemisphere.

Craig, K.D., & Prkachin, K.M. (1983). Nonverbal measures of pain. In R. Melzack (Ed.), *Pain measurement and assessment* (pp. 173–179). New York: Raven Press.

Craig, K.D., Whitfield, M.S., Grunau, R.V.E., Linton, J., & Hadjistavropoulos, H.D. (1991). Pain in the preterm neonate: Behavioural and physiological indices. In preparation.

Craig K.D., & Wyckoff, M. (1987). Cultural factors in chronic pain management. In G.D. Burrows, D. Elton, & G. Stanley (Eds.), *Handbook of chronic pain management* (pp. 99–108). Amsterdam: Elsevier Science.

Dale, J.C. (1986). A multidimensional study of infants' responses to painful stimuli. *Pediatric Nursing, 12,* 27–31.

Darwin, C.R. (1965). *The expression of emotions in man and animals.* Chicago: University of Chicago Press. (Original work published in 1872)

DePaulo, B.M., Rosenthal, R., Eisenstat, R.A., Rogers, P.L., & Finkelstein, S. (1978). Decoding discrepant nonverbal cues. *Journal of Personality and Social Psychology, 36,* 313–323.

Eich, E., Reeves, J.L., Jaeger, B., & Graff-Radford, S.B. (1985). Memory for pain: Relation between past and present pain intensity. Pain, 23, 375–380.

Ekman, P. (1985). *Telling lies: Clues to deceit in the marketplace, politics, and marriage.* New York: Norton.

Ekman, P. (1988). Lying and nonverbal behavior: Theoretical issues and new findings. *Journal of Nonverbal Behavior, 12,* 163–176.

Ekman, P., & Friesen, P. (1969). The repertoire of nonverbal behavior: Categories, origins, usage and coding. *Semiotica, 1,* 49–98.

Ekman, P., & Friesen, W. (1975). *Unmasking the face.* Englewood Cliffs, N.J.: Prentice-Hall.

Ekman, P., & Friesen, W.V. (1978). *Facial Action Coding System: A technique for the measurement of facial movement.* Palo Alto, CA: Consulting Psychologists Press.

Ekman, P., & Friesen, W.V. (1986). A new pan-cultural facial expression of emotion. *Motivation & Emotion, 10,* 159–168.

Ekman, P., Friesen, W. V., & Ellsworth, P. (1972). *Emotion in the human face.* Elmsford, NY: Pergamon Press.

Ekman, P., Friesen, W.V., & O'Sullivan, M. (1988). Smiles when lying. *Journal of Personality and Social Psychology, 54,* 414–420.

Ekman, P., Friesen, W.V., O'Sullivan, M., Chan, A., Diacoyanni-Tarlatzis, I., Heider, K., Krause, R., LeCompte, W.A., Pitcairn, R., Ricci-Bitti, P.E., Scherer, K., Tornita, M., & Tzavaras, A. (1987). Universals and cultural differences in the judgments of facial expressions of emotion. *Journal of Personality and Social Psychology, 53,* 712–717.

Ekman, P., Friesen, W., & Simons, R. (1985). Is the startle reaction an emotion? *Journal of Personality and Social Psychology, 49,* 1416–1426.

Ekman, P., Sorenson, E.R., & Friesen, W.V. (1969). Pan cultural elements in facial displays of emotion. *Science, 164,* 86–88.

Feine, J.S., Bushnell, M.C., Miron, D., & Duncan, G.H. (1991). Sex differences in the perception of noxious heat stimuli. *Pain, 44,* 255–262.

Feuerstein, M., Barr, R.G., Francoeur, T.E., Houle, M., & Rafman, S. (1982). Potential biobhavioral mechanisms of recurrent abdominal pain in children. *Pain, 13,* 287–298.

Field, T. (1990). Alleviating stress in newborn infants in the intensive care unit. In B.M. Lester & E. Tronick (Ed.), *Stimulation and the preterm infant: The limits of plasticity: Clinics in perinatology* (Vol. 17, pp. 1–9). Philadelphia: Saunders.

Fitzgerald, M. (1991). The developmental neurobiology of pain. In M.R. Bond, J.E. Charlton, & C.J. Woolf, (Eds.), *Pain research and clinical management: Vol. 4. Proceedings of the VIth World Congress on Pain* (pp. 253–261). Amsterdam: Elsevier.

Fitzgerald, M., & McIntosh, N. (1989). Pain and analgesia in the newborn. *Archives of Disease in Childhood, 64,* 441–443.

Fitzgerald, M. Millard, C., & McIntosh, N. (1989). Cutaneous hypersensitivity following peripheral tissue damage in newborn infants and its reversal with topical anaesthesia. *Pain, 39,* 31–36.

Fordyce, W. (1976). *Behavioral methods for chronic pain and illness.* St. Louis: Mosby.

Friesen, W. (1987). *EMFACS.* Unpublished manuscript, Human Interaction Laboratory, University of California, San Francisco.

Gracely, R.H. (1989). Pain psychophysics. In C.R. Chapman & J.D. Loeser (Eds.), *Issues in pain measurement* (pp. 211–230). New York: Raven Press.

Grunau, R.V.E., & Craig, K.D. (1987). Pain expression in neonates: Facial action and cry. *Pain, 28,* 395–410.

Grunau, R.V.E., & Craig, K.D. (1990). Facial activity as a measure of neonatal pain expression. In D.C. Tyler & E.J. Krane (Eds.), *Advances in pain research and therapy* (Vol. 15, pp. 147–155). New York: Raven Press.

Grunau, R.V.E., Craig, K.D., & Drummond, J.E. (1989). Neonatal pain behavior and perinatal events: Implications for research observations. *Canadian Journal of Nursing Research, 21,* 7–17.

Grunau, R.V.E., Johnston, C., & Craig, K.D. (1990). Neonatal facial and cry responses to invasive and non-invasive procedures. *Pain, 42,* 295–305.

Grunau, R.V.E., Whitfield, M.F., Petrie, J.H., & Fryer, L. (1991a). Pain sensitivity in toddlers of birthweight < 1000 grams compared with heavier preterm and full birthweight toddlers. *Pediatric Research, 29,* 256A (Abst.).

Grunau, R.V.E., Whitfield, M.F., Petrie, J.H., & Fryer, L. (1991b). Neonatal pain, child temperament, and family characteristics as precursors of somatization in preterm and fulterm children. Submitted for publication.

Hadjistavropoulos, H.D., Grunau, R.V.E., & Craig, K.D. (1991). Facial activity during invasive events in the preterm neonate. *Canadian Psychology, 32,* 253 (Abst.).

Hadjistavropoulos, H.D., Ross, M.A., & von Baeyer, C. (1990). Are physicians' ratings of pain affected by patients' physical attractiveness? *Social Science and Medicine, 31,* 69–72.

Hager, J., & Ekman, P. (1985). The asymmetry of facial actions is inconsistent with models of hemispheric specialization. *Psychophysiology, 22,* 307–318.

Izard, C.E. (1979). *The maximally discriminative facial movement coding system (MAX).* Newark: University of Delaware Instructional Resources Center.

Izard, C.E., Hembree, E.A., Dougherty, L.M., & Spizzirri, C.C. (1983). Changes in facial expressions of 2 to 19-month-old infants following acute pain. *Developmental Psychology, 19,* 418–426.

Izard, C.E., Hembree, F.A., & Huebner, R.R. (1987). Infants' emotion expressions to acute pain: Develop-

mental changes and stability of individual differences. Developmental Psychology, 23, 105–113.

Izard, C.E., Huebner, R.R., Risser, D., McGinness, G.C., & Dougherty, L.M. (1980). The young infant's ability to produce discrete emotion expressions. *Developmental Psychology, 16,* 132–140.

Jacox, A.K. (1980). The assessment of pain. In W.L. Smith, H. Merskey, & S.C. Gross (Eds.), *Pain: Meaning and management* (pp. 75–88). New York: SP Medical & Scientific Books.

Johnston, C.C. (1989). Pain assessment and management in infants. *Pediatrician, 16,* 16–23.

Johnston, C.C., & Strada, M.E. (1986). Acute pain response in infants: A multidimensional description. *Pain, 24,* 373–382.

Keefe, F.J. (1989). Behavioral measurement of pain. In C.R. Chapman & J.D. Loeser (Eds.), *Advances in pain research and therapy: Issues in pain measurement* (Vol. 12., pp. 405–424). New York: Raven Press.

Keefe, F.J., & Block, A.R. (1982). Development of an observation method for assessing pain behavior in chronic low back pain patients. *Behavior Therapy, 13,* 363–375.

Kopel, S., & Arkowitz, H. (1974). Role playing as a source of self-observation and behavior change. *Journal of Personality and Social Psychology, 29,* 677–686.

Kotarba, J.A. (1983). *Chronic pain: Its social dimensions.* Beverly Hills, CA: Sage.

Kraut, R.E. (1978). Verbal and nonverbal cues in the perception of lying. *Journal of Personality and Social Psychology, 36,* 380–391.

Kremer, E.F., Block, A., & Atkinson, J.H. (1983). Assessment of pain behavior: Factors that distort self-report. In R. Melzack (Ed.), *Pain measurement and assessment* (pp. 165–172). New York: Raven Press.

Lander, J. (1990). Clinical judgments in pain management. *Pain, 42,* 15–22.

Lander, J., Fowler-Kerry, S., & Hill, A. (1990). Comparison of pain perceptions among males and females. *Canadian Journal of Nursing Research, 22,* 39–49.

Lanzetta, J.T., Cartwright-Smith, J., & Kleck, R.E. (1976). Effects of nonverbal dissimulation on emotional experience and autonomic arousal. *Journal of Personality and Social Psychology, 33,* 354–370.

Leavitt, F., & Sweet, J.J. (1986). Characteristics and frequency of malingering among patients with low back pain. *Pain, 25,* 357–364.

Lee, D.E., & Craig, K.D. (1991). Facial action determinants of observer judgment of subjective states: Complexity and configuration. Submitted for publication.

LeResche, L. (1982). Facial expression in pain: A study of candid photographs. *Journal of Nonverbal Behavior, 7,* 46–56.

LeResche, L., & Dworkin, S.F. (1984). Facial expression accompanying pain. *Social Science and Medicine, 19,* 1325–1330.

LeResche, L., & Dworkin, S.F. (1988). Facial expressions of pain and emotions in chronic TMD patients. *Pain, 35,* 71–78.

LeResche, L., Ehrlich, K.J., & Dworkin, S.F. (1990). Facial expressions of pain and masking smiles: Is "Grin and bear it" a pain behavior? *Pain, Supplement 5,* S286 (Abst.).

Leventhal, H., & Sharp, E. (1965). Facial expressions as indicators of distress. In S.S. Tomkins & C.E. Izard (Eds.), *Affect, cognition and personality* (pp. 296–318). New York: Springer.

Levine, J.D., & Gordon, N.C. (1982). Pain in prelingual children and its evaluation by pain-induced vocalization. *Pain, 14,* 85–93.

Lewis, M., & Worobey, J. (1989). *Infant stress and coping.* Oxford: Jossey-Bass.

McCrory, L. (1990). *The use of continuous sensory stimulation: Proprioceptive-tactile and auditory stimulation to reduce newborn's response to pain.* Master's thesis, University of Florida.

McGrath, P.A. (1987). An assessment of children's pain: A review of behavioral, physiological, and direct scaling techniques. *Pain, 31,* 147–176.

McGrath, P.J., Mathews, J.R., & Pigeon, H. (1991). Assessment of pain in chldren: A systematic psychosocial model. In M.R. Bond, J.E. Charlton, & C.J. Woolf (Eds.), *Pain research and clinical management* (Vol. 4, pp. 509–526). Amsterdam: Elsevier.

Meinhart, N.T., & McCaffery, M (1983). *Pain: A nursing approach to assessment and analysis.* Norwalk, CT: Appleton-Century-Crofts.

Mills, N. (1989). Pain behaviors in infants and toddlers. *Journal of Pain and Symptom Management, 4,* 184–190.

Monrad-Krohn, G.H. (1924). On the dissociation of voluntary and emotional innervation in facial paralysis of central origin. *Brain, 47,* 22–35.

Nisbett, R.N., & Wilson, T.D. (1977). Telling more than we can know: Verbal reports on mental processes. *Psychological Review, 84,* 231–259.

Oster, H., & Ekman, P. (1978). Facial behavior in child development. In W.A. Collins (Ed.), *Minnesota symposium on child psychology, 11,* 231–276.

Oster, H., & Rosenstein, D. (1982). *Analyzing facial movement in infants.* Unpublished manuscript.

Paivio, A. (1986). *Mental representations: A dual coding approach.* New York: Oxford University Press.

Patrick, C.J., Craig, K.D., & Prkachin, K.M. (1986). Observer judgments of acute pain: Facial action determinants. *Journal of Personality and Social Psychology, 50,* 1291–1298.

Pigeon, H.M., McGrath, P.J., Lawrence, J., & MacMurray, S.B. (1989). Nurses perceptions of pain in the neonatal intensive care unit. *Journal of Pain and Symptom Management, 4,* 179–183.

Pilowsky, I., Thornton, M., & Stokes, B.B. (1986). Towards the quantification of facial expressions with the use of a mathematical model of the face. In H.D. Ellis, M.A. Jeeves, F. Newcombe, & A. Young (Eds.), *Aspects of face processing* (pp. 340–348). Dordrecht: Martinus Nijhoff.

Pomietto, M. & Marvin, J.A. (1991). Pain expression in infants: A multi-dimensional study. *Journal of Pain and Symptom Management, 6,* 206 (Abst.).

Poole, G.D., & Craig, K.D. (1991). Judgments of genuine, masked, and posed facial expressions. Submitted for publication.

Prkachin, K.M. (1986). Pain behavior is not unitary. *Behavioral and Brain Sciences, 9,* 754–755.

Prkachin, K.M. (in press). Dissociating spontaneous and deliberate facial expressions of pain. *Pain.*

Prkachin, K.M. (1991). *A cross-modal comparison of pain indices: The consistency of facial expressions.* Unpublished manuscript.

Prkachin K.M., & Craig, K.D. (1985). Influencing nonverbal expressions of pain: Signal detection analyses. *Pain, 21,* 399–409.

Prkachin, K.M., Currie, A.N., & Craig, K.D. (1983).

Judging nonverbal expression of pain. Canadian Journal of Behavioural Science, 15, 408–420.

Prkachin, K.M., & Mercer, S.R. (1989). Pain expression in patients with shoulder pathology: Validity, properties and relationship to sickness impact. *Pain, 39,* 257–265.

Procacci, P., & Maresca, M. (1991). Central pruritus. *Pain, 45,* 307–308.

Riemondy, S., Rung, G.W., Hershey, J., & Ballantine, T.V.N. (1991). Nurse controlled analgesia: A new method of pediatric pain control. *Journal of Pain and Symptom Management, 6,* 160 (Abst).

Rinn, W.E. (1984). The neuropsychology of facial expression: A review of the neurological and psychological mechanisms for producing facial expression. *Psychological Bulletin, 95,* 52–77.

Rosenthal, R. (1982). Conducting judgement studies. In K. Scherer & P. Ekman (Eds.), *Handbook of methods in nonverbal behavior research* (pp. 287–361). New York: Cambridge University Press.

Roy, E.A. (in press). Movement variability in limb gesturing: Implications for understanding apraxia. In K. Newell & D. Corcos (Eds.), *Variability in motor control.* Champaign, IL: Human Kinetics.

Russell, J.A., & Fehr, B. (1987). Relativity in the perception of emotion in facial expressions. *Journal of Experimental Psychology: General, 116,* 233–237.

Sargent, C. (1984). Between death and shame: Dimensions of pain in Bariba culture. *Social Science and Medicine, 19,* 1299–1304.

Schwartz, G.E., Brown, S., & Ahern, G.L. (1980). Facial muscle patterning and subjective experience during affective imagery: Sex differences. *Psychophysiology, 17,* 75–82.

Sears, R.R. (1932). An experimental study of hypnotic anesthesia. *Journal of Experimental Psychology, 15,* 1–22.

Shapiro, C.R. (1991). Nurses judgments of pain intensity in term and preterm newborns. *Journal of Pain and Symptom Management, 6,* 148 (Abst.).

Sparshott, M. (1989). Minimising discomfort of sick newborns. *Nursing Times, 85,* 39–42.

Sparshott, M. (1990). The human touch. *Paediatric Nursing, 16,* 8–10.

Stevens, B., & Johnston, C.C. (1991). Premature infants' responses to heelstick. *Journal of Pain and Symptom Management, 6,* 206 (Abst.).

Swalm, D., & Craig, K. D. (1990). *Differential impact of placebo on verbal and noverbal measures of pain in men and women.* Unpublished manuscript.

Tassinary, L.G., Cacioppo, J.T., & Geen, T.R. (1990). A psychometric study of surface electrode placements for facial electromyographic recording: I. The brow and cheek muscle regions. *Psychophysiology, 26,* 1–16.

Teske, K., Daut, R.L., & Cleeland, C.S. (1983). Relationships between nurses' observations and patients' self-reports of pain. *Pain, 16,* 289–296.

Von Baeyer, C.L., Johnson, M.E., & McMillan, M.J. (1984). Consequences of nonverbal expression of pain: Patient distress and observer concern. *Social Science and Medicine, 19,* 1319–1324.

Weisenberg, M. (1982). Cultural and ethnic factors in reaction to pain. In I. Al-Issa (Ed.), *Culture and psychopathology* (pp. 187–198). Baltimore: University Park Press.

Yarczower, M., & Daruns, L. (1982). Social inhibition of spontaneous facial expressions. *Journal of Personality and Social Psychology, 43,* 831–837.

Zajonc, R.B. (1980). Feeling and thinking: Preferences need no inferences. *American Psychologist, 35,* 151–175.

Zajonc, R.B. (1985). Emotion and facial efference: A theory reclaimed. *Science, 228,* 15–21.

Zuckerman, M., Driver, R., & Koestner, R. (1982). Discrepancy as a cue to actual and perceived deception. *Journal of Nonverbal Behavior, 7,* 95–108.

Chapter 16

Assessment of Pain Behaviors

FRANCIS J. KEEFE, PhD
DAVID A. WILLIAMS, PhD

Although pain is a very personal and subjective experience, the fact that someone is experiencing pain is often apparent to others. People who have pain may vocalize their distress by moaning, crying, or complaining or may exhibit pain-related body postures or facial expressions. These verbal and nonverbal behaviors have been called pain behaviors because they serve to communicate the fact that pain is being experienced (Fordyce, 1976). The construct of pain behavior has emerged as a key component of behavioral formulations of chronic pain (Keefe & Gil, 1986). These formulations emphasize the role that social learning influences can play in the development and maintenance of pain behaviors (Fordyce, 1976; Keefe & Gil, 1986; Turk, Meichenbaum, & Genest, 1983). A patient who has had a low back injury, for example, may exhibit pain behavior long after the normal healing time if his or her spouse responds to pain behavior in an overly solicitous fashion.

The concept of pain behavior is particularly salient in the evaluation of chronic pain patients who are seen in pain clinics and pain management programs (Keefe, 1989). Many of these patients exhibit a maladaptive pattern of pain behavior that is characterized by an overly sedentary and restricted lifestyle and excessive dependence on pain medications or family members. Behavioral interventions designed to modify this pain behavior pattern (e.g., activation programs, social reinforcement for engaging in adaptive, well behaviors, and time-contingent delivery of pain medications) have been shown to reduce disability and improve psychological functioning of chronic pain patients (Keefe & Gil, 1986; Turk et al., 1983).

Over the past 10 to 15 years, behavioral and cognitive-behavioral therapists have developed a number of strategies for assessing pain behavior. Early work in this area relied on patient diaries for recording activity level or clinician recordings of the duration or frequency of behavior (Fordyce, 1976). More recently, behavioral researchers have developed and refined sophisticated observation systems that enable one to simultaneously record multiple categories of pain behavior. These observation systems have been evaluated in a number of research studies and appear to offer a promising means for analyzing pain behavior in chronic pain patients.

One of the major gaps in the emerging literature on pain behavior observation is the lack of practical information on how one develops and carries out such behavioral assessments. Published research reports usually provide a brief description of observation methods, but fail to provide detailed information on the basic features of these methods or procedures for recording or scoring. Although many research laboratories provide periodic observer training sessions, many who wish to obtain such training are unable to do so because of the costs involved. We have recently written about practical issues of pain behavior observation, but focused primarily on a methodology applicable to chronic low back pain patients (Keefe, Crisson, & Trainor, 1987).

The purpose of this chapter is to provide clinicians and researchers with detailed information on pain behavior observation methods. The chapter guides the reader through the steps involved in developing an observation method and evaluating its reliability and validity. Although examples drawn from our own research on low back pain and arthritic pain will be provided throughout, our intent is to provide guidelines for pain behavior assessment that are applicable to many chronic pain conditions.

The chapter is divided into three sections. The first section discusses basic elements of pain behavior observation such as methods of sampling pain behavior, coding category definitions, and observer training. The second section uses an observation method we developed for osteoarthritis patients to illustrate practical aspects of each of the basic elements of observation. In the third section, we consider important issues related to the application of pain behavior observation in clinical settings.

BASIC ELEMENTS OF PAIN BEHAVIOR OBSERVATION SYSTEMS

Although a variety of observational strategies can be used to record pain behavior, these strategies share certain basic elements. Five elements common to most observation methods are: (1) a rationale for observation, (2) a method for sampling pain behavior, (3) definitions of behavior codes, (4) a method for observer training, and (5) reliability and validity assessments.

Rationale for Observing Pain Behavior

Mr. Smith was having great difficulty tolerating the physical examination. Despite the fact that he had few physical findings, Mr. Smith complained bitterly of chronic back pain. He flinched visibly when the examiner palpated his back. His movements were slow, and he limped in an exaggerated fashion when asked to walk. He gave very detailed descriptions of his back pain and stated that he was not sure that he could cope with the pain much longer.

Most clinicians working in the pain management area have met patients like Mr. Smith. In a medical setting, the behavior of such a chronic pain patient may influence decisions about the need for further assessment or treatment (Cailliet, 1968). Patients who show exaggerated or inconsistent pain behavior are often considered to be poor candidates for invasive diagnostic testing (e.g., electroymyography) or for medical or surgical interventions (Waddell, McCulloch, Kimmel, & Venner, 1980). For a behavioral clinician, the behavior of a patient like Mr. Smith is interesting and important in and of itself.

One of the most common reasons for conducting observations of pain behavior is to provide a detailed description of the patient's behavior. Descriptive data, for example, could be used to document the amount of time that a patient spends up and out of the reclining position (uptime), to provide a record of medication intake, or to describe the verbal or nonverbal behaviors a patient displays during a physical examination. In behavioral assessment, such descriptive data are used for several purposes. First descriptive data can be used to pinpoint problem behaviors that may serve as targets for treatment efforts. Careful observations may reveal problem behaviors that patients are reluctant to report. A cancer patient, for example, may initially deny that pain is a problem but when asked to swallow or cough may exhibit pain-related facial expressions suggesting that considerable pain is being experienced (Keefe, Brantley, Manual, & Crisson, 1985). Second, descriptive data can be used to establish an initial baseline measure against which the effects of treatment can be compared. By carrying out observations before treatment, after treatment, and at follow-up intervals, one can evaluate the degree to which behavioral interventions can modify pain behavior. Finally, descriptive data on pain behavior may be used to predict patient's response to treatment. Connolly and Sanders (1991), for example, found that overt pain behavior recorded prior to a lumbar sympathetic block predicted the amount of pain relief patients reported following initial and subsequent blocks.

The second reason for conducting observations of pain behavior is to analyze the variables controlling that behavior. This application of behavioral observation has been called *functional analysis* (Ferster, 1965) to contrast it with more descriptive static analysis procedures. Functional analysis is designed to identify specific variables that serve to control pain behavior. Social and environmental variables often play an important role in eliciting pain behavior. A patient having an overly solicitous spouse, for example, may report a much higher level of pain when in the presence of that spouse than when in the presence of a neutral observer such as ward clerk (Block, Kremer, & Gaylor, 1980). Pain behavior may also be affected by its consequences. White and Sanders (1986), for example, found that when they had an experimenter attend to chronic pain patients' discussions about pain, the patients' ratings of pain routinely increased.

The rationale for observing pain behavior is important in determining the specific methods to be used. If the goal is to provide descriptive data, the focus of observation is on specific behaviors exhibited by the patient. Most of the current observation systems for recording pain behavior provide data on patient behavior only. They are thus suitable for a static analysis of behavior. If the goal is to perform a functional analysis, however, the scope of observation must be expanded to include not only patient behavior but also social or environmental variables (e.g., spouse behavior) that may be controlling that behavior. Although observation systems for performing functional analysis have been used in behavior therapy research for the past 15 to 20 years, these methods have only recently been extended to the chronic pain area (Romano et al., 1991).

Sampling and Recording Pain Behavior

One of the major decisions facing anyone who develops an observation system is how the behavior is to be sampled and recorded. There are a number of options. The first is to utilize *continuous observation*. In continuous observation one samples behavior, continuously noting any behaviors that occurred. One example of a continuous observation would be a detailed diary kept by an anthropologist who might live with and observe a primitive aboriginal tribe.

Continuous observations provide rich detail on behavior and often yield important clues as to environmental variables controlling a particular behavior. Consider the following case example.

A behavior therapist made a home visit to assist in the behavioral assessment of a chronic pain patient. The therapist arrived in the late afternoon and observed the patient continuously over a 3-hour time span. The patient was observed in a variety of situations: while grocery shopping, during physical therapy exercises, and as he carried out a variety of household chores. The patient was energetic, active, and showed few pain behaviors until his wife came home from work. As soon as the wife entered the house, the patient began complaining of back pain, went to his recliner, and asked her to bring him medication. A similar pattern was observed during a second home visit.

In this case, continuous observation suggested that downtime (i.e., reclining) and verbal pain behaviors (i.e., complaining of pain, requests for medications) were strongly influenced by the presence of the patient's spouse. Based on these findings, the behavioral treatment program focused not only on modifying the patient's behavior but on modifying the spouse's response to that behavior.

Behavior has been likened to a stream that is constantly moving. A major advantage of continuous observation is that it attempts to capture the complexity of the stream of behavior. A second advantage of this type of observation is that it can be carried out by observers who have minimal training. Continuous observation has two major limitations. First, the time and expense involved is often prohibitive. Continuous observation requires spending an extensive amount of time carefully watching a patient and recording the variety of behaviors he or she exhibits. Few practicing clinicians have the resources to devote to carrying out continuous observations in the patient's home, work, or treatment settings. Second, is the problem of data analysis. In continuous observation the observer provides a written record of everything the patient does. This yields an enormous amount of information, some of which is important and some of which is not. Synthesizing the data gathered from continuous observation is often a very difficult and demanding task. Because of these problems, continuous observation is used sparingly in behavioral assessment. If used, this type of observation is carried out early in the course of assessment when one is developing ideas about key target behaviors and controlling variables. Most often, continuous observation is carried out in the context of a visit to the patient's home or workplace.

A second option for sampling and recording pain behavior is to take a *duration* measure. This involves simply recording the length of time that the patient takes to perform a specific behavior. For example, when working with a patient who has become dependent on a back brace, one might record how much time the patient wears the brace each day. Alternatively, one could focus on measuring the duration of well behaviors (e.g., time spent walking or standing) that are incompatible with certain pain behaviors (e.g., time spent reclining) (Fordyce, 1976).

Duration measures provide a simple and practical means for directly observing pain behavior in naturalistic settings. These measures require minimal training for observers and have been widely used in the chronic pain literature (Fordyce, Fowler, Lehmann, & DeLateur, 1968). Chronic pain patients, for example, are routinely asked to complete diary records of their daily activities so that the duration of time they spend sitting, standing, or walking (uptime) can be recorded. Staff members working in pain management programs often keep duration measures of the amount of time a patient takes to complete a physically demanding task such as walking a series of laps around a track or climbing a set of stairs. The major disadvantage of duration measures is that one must be physically present throughout the entire observation period to record behavior in a reliable and valid fashion. Although this is not a problem for behaviors that have a short duration (e.g., time taken to complete a set of 20 sit-ups), it is a serious disadvantage when recording behaviors that can have a long duration (e.g., time spent reclining each day). Although the patient can be asked to observe and record his or her own behavior, the records provided may not be as reliable as those provided by independent observers.

Another option for observing pain behavior is to make *frequency counts*. In a frequency count one simply observes and records the number of instances of each of the target behaviors. One might keep a frequency count of important pain behaviors such as the number of times a patient requested medications or the number of times he or she complained of pain. Alternatively, one can record specific treatment-related behaviors that may serve as an index of pain behavior such as the number of repetitions that a patient completed a physical therapy exercise. Frequency counts are often gathered in treatment settings and can be used to measure behaviors that both patient and staff view as meaningful and salient. The major limitation of frequency counts is similar to that described for duration measures: the observer may need to carry out observations over long time periods to gather reliable and valid data.

A third option for sampling and recording pain behavior is *time sampling*. In time sampling, a trained observer samples the patient's behavior for a brief period (e.g., 30 sec–5 min) at specified times over a day (e.g., every 45 min). The observer's task is to carefully watch the patient and to note the occurrence of any behaviors included in the coding system. We have utilized a time sampling format for recording the behavior of inpatients hospitalized on a pain management unit (Keefe, Crisson, & Trainor, 1987). Nurses on this unit checked patients for 20 seconds approximately every half hour of the day noting the location of the patient (e.g., in room, off unit), social interaction (e.g., patient alone vs. interacting with other patients or staff), body position (e.g., reclining, sitting upright, walking), and pain behaviors (e.g., guarding, verbal pain statements, or using an assistive device such as cane or walker). The data were summarized each evening on entries made on graphs placed in the patient's medical chart. The graphs displayed (1) the percentage of time that the patient was observed out of bed (i.e., uptime) and (2) the percentage of time the patient displayed pain behavior. These data were reviewed in meetings of each patient's treatment team and provided the basis for decisions about the patient's response to particular treatment interventions (e.g., medications, activation program, or relaxation training).

Time sampling is an excellent method for carrying out direct behavioral observations of behavior in inpatient clinic settings. In these settings the patient can be readily observed throughout the day, enabling one to get a good estimate of the level and variability of important target behaviors. Time sampling is inexpensive (1) if it is carried out during regular contacts that a clinician already has with the patient, and (2) if the period of observation is brief. We have found that with relatively little training (e.g., 3 hr) nursing staff can master a recording system and coding category definitions. The reliability of time sampling can be checked by having a highly trained master observer and newly trained observer independently and simultaneously record the patient's behavior.

The major problem with time sampling is determining the duration and frequency of the observation periods. If one samples behavior for very brief periods of time (e.g., 30 sec) and carries out only a few observations over the day, few behaviors may be coded. On the other hand, if one samples for long periods of time (e.g., 15 min) and carries out observations each hour, the demands on the observer's time can be overwhelming.

The frequency of the target behaviors is a major factor determining the utility of time sampling. Time sampling works best for behaviors that occur at a high frequency. It is not as useful for low-frequency behaviors. For example, we found that our time sampling method was quite useful in documenting changes in uptime, namely, time spent up and out of bed (Keefe, Crisson, & Trainor, 1987). Uptime was typically observed during 30% or more of the observation intervals per day. Our time sampling strategy, however, was not as effective for tracking changes in other pain behaviors such as guarding, grimacing, or rubbing of the painful area. These behaviors were infrequent, occurring during 30% or less of the observation intervals each day. One way to enhance the effectiveness of time sampling in measuring low-frequency behaviors is to increase the length of time each patient was observed each day. As the amount of observation time goes up, however, the practical utility of time sampling goes down.

Interval recording represents yet another option for carrying out behavioral observations. In interval recording the observation period (e.g., 10 min or several hours) is broken down into equal intervals (e.g., 30 sec or 1-min long). The observer's task is to watch the patient throughout the interval and to simply note at the end of the interval whether specific behaviors were or were not observed. Interval recording is often used in coding videotaped samples of behavior gathered during standardized or simulated tasks. For example, we have used interval recording methods to observe pain behaviors that occur in chronic low back pain patients when they are asked to sit, stand, walk, and recline (Keefe & Block, 1982). More recently, Romano et al. (1991) have used interval recording methods to measure pain behaviors that occurred during a videotaped observation session in which chronic pain patients and their spouses were asked to discuss a conflict situation and carry out some daily tasks.

Using videotaped behavior samples for observation has many advantages. First, videotape provides a permanent record of the patient's behavior, enabling one to carry out repeated observations, check reliability, and refine or develop new coding systems. Second, one can structure a videotaped behavior sample to elicit pain behaviors. Patients can be observed as they engage in simple daily tasks that they tend to avoid doing, for example, walking, transferring from a reclining to a standing position. Third, by applying interval recording methods to videotaped behavior samples one can obtain data that are easily quantified.

There are several disadvantages of combining videotaped behavior sampling with interval recording methods. First, whenever a patient is being videotaped there is the potential for reactivity (Keefe, 1989). Reactivity refers to the change in behavior that occurs when someone is aware of being observed. Some chronic pain patients may inhibit their display of pain behavior during a videotaped observation session, whereas others may exaggerate their behavior. Although there is no way to predict how much reactivity will occur, two steps can be taken to minimize the effects of reactivity (Hartmann & Wood, 1982). These are (1) providing patients with minimal information on the categories of behavior being observed, and (2) avoiding interaction with the patient during the observation. It should be noted that reactivity is a problem whenever a patient is observed. The degree of reactivity during a videotaped observation may not be very different from the reactivity that occurs when a physician asks a patient to carry out functional tasks during a physical examination session (Keefe & Block, 1982).

Definitions of Pain Behavior

A visitor to an inpatient pain management program was surprised that the patients failed to exhibit many observable signs that they were experiencing pain. The patients were talkative, spending most of their time in the unit's day room in recliners. They rarely displayed pain-related facial expressions or guarded movements indicative of pain.

One of the most important factors in observing pain behavior is how one defines pain behavior. The visitor, in the above example, implicitly defined pain behavior on the basis of facial expressions or guarded movements and failed to note the fact that patients had very low levels of activity and reclined most of the time. Thus, implicit assumptions about what constitutes pain behavior can determine whether an individual actually notices pain behavior occurring.

Implicit definitions of pain behavior can vary from one individual to another. Some individuals base their judgments of pain behavior on a patient's medication intake, while others focus mainly on verbal complaints or motor behaviors indicative of pain. When the term "pain behavior" is used in informal, clinical discussions, it is usually not defined in explicit terms. A patient may be described anecdotally as having a high level of pain behavior, but no indication is given about the specific behaviors that served as a basis for this impression.

Fordyce (1976) originally defined pain behaviors as those behaviors that communicate to others the fact that pain is being experienced. This definition is a general one that encompasses behaviors ranging from verbal reports of pain to measures of the frequency of doctor visits. To develop a reliable and valid observation system, one must use an operational definition that is more specific. An operational definition indicates precisely what the patient must do and what the observer must record. Thus, a good operational definition describes behavior in observable and measurable terms. It also specifies what aspect of the behavior is to be recorded, namely, frequency, duration, or intensity.

Several guidelines can be offered for developing operational definitions for pain behaviors. First, the behavior should occur with sufficient frequency that it can be observed. Behaviors that occur with very low frequency or that cannot be directly observed are generally not suitable for observation. Second, the definitions of the behavior should be written in simple, descriptive language that minimizes inference on the part of observers. This ensures that observers with different backgrounds can employ the observation methodology. It also avoids the major problems that occur when observers are attempting to judge why a patient engaged in a particular behavior. Finally, the definition should be written down in a table or manual. Written definitions are particularly useful when multiple categories of behavior are being observed. In such a case, the written definitions provide the basis for initial training of observers.

Observer Training

There is growing recognition that observer training is important in the development of a psychometrically sound observation method (Hartmann & Wood, 1982). The amount of observer training generally varies with the complexity of the observation system. Observation methods that rely on duration measures or frequency counts rarely provide intensive observer training. Time sampling and interval recording methods that require the coding of multiple categories of behavior, however, typically require a structured observer training program.

Hartmann and Wood (1982) have provided an extensive set of recommendations for training observers. The recommendations include initially giving observers an opportunity to carry out observations on an informal basis and then following this up with written materials detailing the procedures and coding categories the observers are expected to master. They also recommend having observers carry out practice coding sessions with an experienced observer. Hartmann and Wood suggest that observers reach a criterion level of reliability before starting data collection and that periodic retraining sessions be conducted to check reliability. Finally, they suggest that observers be debriefed after they finish collecting observational data to identify any problems that had occurred in coding behavior. Although Hartmann and Wood's recommendations for observer training are intended to cover general applications of behavioral observation, they appear to be quite applicable to pain behavior observation.

Assessing Reliability and Validity

If an observation method is to be truly useful in clinical or research settings it must be both reliable and valid. Reliability can be evaluated in two ways. First, one can determine *interobserver reliability* by examining the degree to which independent observers agree on the behaviors observed. A statistic that provides a good measure of interobserver reliability for dichotomous classification (e.g., presence–absence) is percentage agreement (Hartmann, 1977). The formula for calculating percentage agreement is:

$$\frac{\text{No. agreements}}{\text{No. agreements} + \text{No. disagreements}}$$

Agreements are simply the number of instances in which two observers agreed in their coding of *specific categories of behavior*, and disagreements are the number of instances in which the observers did not agree (for several alternative methods of calculating interobserver reliability, see Rudy, Turk, & Brody, Chapter 7). Percentage agreement over 80% is usually considered acceptable. If reliability falls below this level, it usually means that there are problems with the definitions of the coding categories, the coding scheme is too complex, or observer training was not sufficient.

A second way to assess the reliability of an observation method is to determine the consistency of observed behaviors across time. *Test–retest reliability* refers to the degree to which pain behavior data collected from a patient at one time are correlated with pain behavior data collected at another time. One might, for example, obtain a videotaped behavior sample from a group of chronic low back pain patients on two occasions separated by a 2-week interval. Correlational analyses could then be carried out to reveal how consistent the levels of behavior were over this time period. Given the varying nature of pain symptoms in chronic pain patients, one might expect the test-retest reliability of pain behavior observations to be in the moderate range ($r = .50$ to $r = .70$). When test–retest correlations are at the lower end of this range ($r = .50$), it suggests that there is some variability in pain behavior over time. When this occurs, there is the possibility that changes in pain behavior occurring over treatment may reflect variability in the behavior rather than actual treatment effects. One way

to deal with this problem is to incorporate control groups (e.g., waiting-list or no-treatment control groups) in behavioral treatment studies that use pain behavior as an outcome variable. This enables one to determine whether the changes in pain behavior that occur following behavioral treatment are significantly greater than the changes in pain behavior that simply occur over time with no treatment.

Several types of validity assessments are relevant in developing or evaluating pain behavior observation methods. First, one needs to examine *concurrent validity*. Concurrent validity is assessed by comparing the results of the observation method to another measure designed to measure a similar construct. For example, one might compare observation data on pain behavior to patients' scores on a self-report measure of pain behavior (Romano et al., 1988). Second, it is important to demonstrate that an observation method has adequate *construct validity*. The term "construct validity" is used to refer to the extent to which a test actually measures what it is intended to measure. One way to assess the construct validity of pain behavior observation systems is to compare trained observers' recordings of pain behavior with naive observers' estimates of the patient's pain. If the behaviors coded by trained observers truly are pain behaviors, then patients having high levels of these behaviors should be rated by naive observers as having higher levels of pain. A third type of validity is *discriminant validity*. Discriminant validity refers to the extent to which observed pain behaviors discriminate patients having pain from patients who do not. Discriminant validity of an observation system for recording pain behavior in patients having episodic facial pain, for example, could be evaluated by comparing the pain behavior of patients having facial pain at the time of observation with the pain behavior of patients who are pain free.

Although duration and frequency measures are widely utilized in behavioral observation, the reliability and validity of these observational measures have not received much research attention. The data that have been reported raise questions about the validity of one of the most common duration measures used in the chronic pain area: patient diary records of activity. Kremer, Block, and Gaylor (1981), for example, used a time sampling procedure to record data on activity level and social contact from four chronic pain patients who were undergoing intensive treatment inpatient pain treatment program. The time sampling procedure was highly reliable (interobserver reliability as determined by percentage agreement = 85%). There was a discrepancy, however, between the observational data and the data that came from patients' records of their own activity. Substantial increases in activity level and social interaction recorded by observation were not evident in the patient's own activity recordings. Sanders (1983) reported similar findings in a study that compared patients' reports of walking/standing time with records obtained from an electromechanical activity monitor that automatically recorded standing/walking time. He found that chronic low back pain patients consistently underestimated the amount of time they spent engaging in these activities. Taken together, the findings of these studies suggest that one should be cautious in interpreting selfobservation data collected from chronic pain patients.

One way to improve the accuracy of selfreport data in chronic pain patients is to provide them with training in observation methods. Fordyce (1976), for example, has long maintained that patients should be given explicit instructions in methods for diary recording before they are asked to keep daily records of their activity. It should be noted that the one study that has shown a high degree of agreement between patient records and objective measures of activity provided each patient with extensive training in the diary method before data collection (Follick, Ahern, & Laser-Wolston, 1984).

Data on the reliability and validity of direct observation methods have primarily come from recent studies that used trained observers to record pain behavior during videotaped behavior samples. In the early 1980s we carried out a series of studies evaluating the reliability and validity of an observation method for recording pain behavior in low back pain patients (Keefe & Block, 1982). The observation method was designed to measure motor pain behaviors that occur during simple daily activities. Patients were asked to engage in a series of standardized tasks (walking, sitting, standing, and reclining). The patients were videotaped as they performed these tasks, and the videotapes were subsequently scored by trained observers using an interval recording method. The cate-

gories of pain behavior recorded included guarding (stiff, interrupted, or rigid movement), bracing (pain-avoidant static posturing), rubbing of the painful area, facial grimacing, and sighing. A composite score, total pain behavior, was computed for each patient based on the sum of the number of occurrences of each pain behavior category.

Our research revealed that trained observers were highly reliable in coding the pain behavior categories. Interobserver reliability, determined using the percentage agreement formula, ranged from 93% to 99%. Although we did not assess test–retest reliability, the observation method was sensitive enough to detect changes in pain behavior that occurred following a treatment intervention (Keefe & Block, 1982). The observation method also showed evidence of good concurrent validity; patients' ratings of pain correlated significantly with total pain behavior ($r = .71, p < .01$). The construct validity of the observation method was examined by having observers with no knowledge of the pain behavior observation system independently rate patients' pain. The naive observers' ratings correlated significantly with total pain behavior ($r = .67$ to $r = .69, p < .05$). Finally, the observation method had adequate discriminant validity in that the behaviors considered to be pain behaviors were much more frequently observed in pain patients than in pain-free depressed and normal subjects.

Follick, Ahern, and Aberger (1985) developed an observation method, the Audiovisual Taxonomy of Pain Behavior, that is also designed to record pain behavior in low back pain patients. This observation method differed from that of Keefe and Block (1982) in two major ways. First, pain behaviors were elicited by tasks that were more physically demanding (e.g, exercising or bending). Second, the set of pain behavior coding categories was larger and included a total of 16 observable pain behaviors. Follick et al. (1985) found that 7 of the 16 coding categories could be reliably coded and occurred with acceptable frequency. Interobserver reliability for these categories was high (percentage agreement = 83–91%). The discriminant validity of this method was supported by the finding that four of the seven pain behavior codes accounted for 75% of the variance differentiating pain patients from normal controls.

The pain behavior observation system we

developed for low back pain patients (Keefe & Block, 1982) has been adapted for use with a number of other patient populations. Karen Anderson and her colleagues modified this system in order to apply it to rheumatoid arthritis (RA) patients (Anderson et al., 1987b). The RA observation system has seven pain behavior categories, some of which are specific to arthritis patients (e.g., rigidity, namely, excessiveness stiffness of the joint, and active rubbing—actively massaging an affected joint). Reliability checks showed that the interobserver reliability of this system was high (percentage agreement between 96% and 100%). Test–retest reliability was assessed by having patients return for a second observation. Although the average length of time between the first and second observation session was 12 days, the test–retest reliability was high ($r = .78$, $p < .001$). The RA observation method has also been found to be sensitive to changes in pain behavior following treatment (McDaniel et al., 1986). The validity of the this observation system has been supported by several findings. First, pain ratings made by naive observers were significantly correlated with total pain behavior (McDaniel et al., 1986). Second, total pain behavior was significantly correlated with a composite index of overall disease activity that included measures of grip strength, painful joint count, physician's ratings of disease activity, rheumatoid factor titers, and erythrocyte sedimentation rate (Anderson et al., 1987a). Finally, total pain behavior scores successfully discriminated RA patients from pain-free depressed and normal controls.

The UAB (University of Alabama—Birmingham) Pain Behavior Scale (Richards, Nepomuceno, Riles, & Suer, 1982) represents a departure from the observation methods discussed above in that it is designed to be completed by health professionals during daily hospital rounds. The system has 10 pain behavior categories that are rated on a 3-point scale of increasing frequency. Richards et al. (1982) reported that interrater reliability for this observation method was good (.94–.96). Test–retest reliability of the total score for 50 patients on two consecutive days was also high ($r = .89$). The convergent validity of this scale is supported by the finding that well behaviors (e.g., self-reported walking, sitting, and standing) were inversely related to the observed ratings of pain behavior. The concurrent va-

lidity of this method, however, was not found to be good. Pain behavior ratings were not significantly correlated with patients' pain ratings on the McGill Pain Questionnaire (MPQ) (Melzack, 1975) or a (0–10) pain rating scale. Feuerstein, Greenwald, Gamache, Papciak, and Cook (1985) developed a modified version of the UAB scale that introduced standardized tasks into the assessment protocol. This modified scale, based on eight behavioral categories, had a very high correlation ($r = .98$) with the original version. More important is the finding that Feuerstein et al.'s modified version of the UAB scale has demonstrated good construct validity in that it correlates well with patients' ratings of their own pain.

Another observation method designed for use in clinic settings is the Observational Scale of Behavioral Distress developed by Jay and Elliott (1984). This observation method is used to assess behavior in children undergoing painful medical procedures. Trained observers using this method have been able to reliably carry out live observations on children who experience acute pain during bone marrow aspirations. The mean interobserver reliability for this method is high ($r = .84$). A revised version of this method (Elliott, Jay, & Woody, 1987) that reduced the number of behavioral categories from 11 to 8 has also been found to have a high degree of internal consistency (Cronbach's alpha, $r = .72$). The construct validity of this observation scale also appears to be strong in that observed distress behaviors were significantly correlated with nurses' ratings of distress, patients' ratings of fear, and patients' ratings of anticipated pain from the procedure.

Taken together, recent studies provide strong support for the reliability and validity of newly developed observation methods for recording pain behavior in chronic pain patients. The methods that have shown especially good psychometric properties are those that sample pain behavior during standardized tasks.

A METHOD FOR OBSERVING PAIN BEHAVIOR IN OSTEOARTHRITIS PATIENTS

In this section we present a detailed description of a standardized method we developed for observing pain behavior in patients having osteoarthritis (OA) of the knees. The description highlights practical details for each of the basic elements of pain behavior observation.

Rationale for Observing Pain Behavior

In the mid-1980s we developed an observation method to provide descriptive data on pain behavior in patients having osteoarthritis of the knees (Keefe, Caldwell, et al., 1987). The observational method was initially designed to provide descriptive data that could be used to study how pain behavior related to patients' pain coping strategies (Keefe, Caldwell, et al., 1987). The observation method was also intended to serve as an outcome measure in a later study evaluating the effectiveness of a cognitive behavioral group therapy intervention for enhancing patients' pain coping skills (Keefe et al., 1990).

Our preliminary observations of osteoarthritis patients in clinical settings revealed two findings. First, the patients varied in their pain behavior: some displayed high levels of pain behavior, while others displayed few or no pain behaviors. Second, most patients complained of pain on movement and tended to exhibit nonverbal pain behaviors when asked to walk or to transfer from one position to another. These initial observations suggested that it might be fruitful to systematically observe pain behavior in order to identify factors, such as disease severity, chronicity of pain, or coping strategies, that might explain the variability in pain behavior among patients. Our preliminary results also suggested that a structured observation session that involved tasks designed to elicit pain behavior (e.g., walking) would be needed to sample pain behavior in osteoarthritic knee pain patients.

Sampling and Recording Pain Behavior

The method we used to sample and record pain behavior was an adaptation of that initially employed with low back pain patients. Implementing this method requires that one attend to practical issues such as setting, videotape equipment, instructions, and preparing videotape records for scoring.

Setting

One can gather observational data on pain behavior in almost any setting where there is sufficient room. We have collected observational data in an examination room, the patient's hospital room, or a physical therapy area. When using observational measures for research studies such as our osteoarthritis project, the specific setting for observation is probably less important than making sure the same setting is used within and across the patients being compared. Standardizing the setting for observation helps to reduce variability in behavior that may relate to differences in the physical environment.

The room in which observation sessions are conducted should ideally have several features. First, it needs to have an examination table, stool for stepping up onto the table, and chair without arms. Patients are asked to recline on the examination table and to use the stool to help them get into the reclining position. This task is somewhat difficult for most osteoarthritis patients having knee pain, and it tends to elicit pain behavior. Transferring in and out of a chair that does not have arms can also be somewhat physically demanding for these patients and thus provides a good opportunity for observing pain behavior. Second, the room should have an adequate space so that patients can be asked to engage in walking during the observation. A room that is at least 8–10 feet wide is required. Third, approximately 15 feet of space is needed in front of the patient so that the camera can be positioned. This camera placement enables one to keep most of the patient's body in the field of view of the camera. Finally, it is important that the room have adequate lighting and privacy.

Videotape Equipment

In gathering data on pain behavior in osteoarthritis patients, we have used a standard-sized videocamera and VHS format standard size videocassettes. If recorded at the slowest speed, a total of 15, 10 minute observation sessions can fit on one cassette. The newer minicameras are probably less intrusive, but use smaller cassettes that have less recording space on them. We use a tripod to hold the videocamera. Although most videocameras can be easily hand held, a tripod helps to steady the camera and enables the person conducting the observation to attend to other tasks such as delivering instructions and timing the session.

In our experience, four videocamera features have been particularly useful. First, a camera that has a built-in stereo audio microphone is preferred. Stereo is desirable because it enables one to record on two audio tracks. One of these tracks can be dubbed with scoring instructions, and the other can provide an audio record of the session. Second, it is best to use a camera that has the lowest LUX level possible. The lower the LUX level, the better the quality of picture in dark rooms. A camera that can take good pictures even in a poorly illuminated room enables one to have more flexibility in choosing a room in which to carry out observation sessions. Third, a zoom and wide angle lens is helpful in situations when the camera must be placed either nearer than 15 feet or farther away than 15 feet from the patient. Fourth, videocameras having graphics capabilities are particularly useful because they enable one to enter identifying information about the patient directly onto the videotape.

Instructions

In order to elicit pain behavior, we have asked osteoarthritis patients to perform a sequence of sitting, standing, walking, and reclining tasks. The tasks include a 1- and 2-minute standing period, a 1- and 2-minute sitting period, two 1-minute reclining periods, and two 1-minute walking periods. These tasks are identical to those used in our low back pain studies. We felt they were appropriate for osteoarthritis patients for several reasons. First, the tasks are common daily activities that most patients engage in. Second, a number of these tasks tend to increase arthritic pain somewhat and thus provide a means of sampling pain behavior. Finally, we felt the tasks were not so demanding that patients would be unable to do them.

The order of the tasks is randomized for each patient using a set of cue cards that are shuffled after each observation session. This randomization is designed to prevent order effects. Before the observation session starts, the individual recording the session explains to the patient the tasks to be performed. The patient is then instructed to perform the task (sitting, standing, walking, or reclining) that appears on the first cue card for the specified length of time (1 or 2 min). The patient is then asked to perform the second task for the specified time period, then the third, and so on. In order to standardize the length of the observation session, patients are given only the allotted period of time to complete a given task. If they have not

completed the task before the time period expires, they are instructed to move on to the next task.

Throughout the observation, an attempt is made to minimize conversation and contact with the patient. Thus, if the activity is a static position, the individual conducting the observation session simply verifies that the patient is within the viewfinder of the camera and then spends the remainder of the interval watching the stopwatch. If the task involves movement (walking or shifting from one position to another), then the viewfinder is used to ensure that part of the subject's movement is not cropped out of the picture. During the 10-minute observation period, inadvertent reinforcement of the patient with talking, smiling, joking, or excessive eye contact is avoided.

Preparing Videotaped Records for Scoring

The videotaped records are scored using an interval recording system. Each 10-minute videotape is divided into 30-second intervals consisting of 20-second observe, 10 second record segments. So as to standardize the timing of the observe and record segments verbal instructions to "observe" and "record" are dubbed onto the tape. If the videocamera has a stereo sound feature, one channel can be dubbed with instructions for the observers. An audiotape having twenty, 20-second observe, 10-second record prompts on it can be used for dubbing purposes.

Definitions of Pain Behavior Coding Categories

The pain behavior coding categories used for osteoarthritis patients are separated into three major groups: (1) position codes, (2) movement codes, and (3) pain behavior codes (Keefe, Caldwell, et al., 1987). The position codes include the three, mutually exclusive major body postures patients are asked to assume during the behavior sample, namely, sitting, standing, reclining. The movement codes include pacing (walking) and shifting (moving from one position to another in the vertical plane). The position and movement codes were included in the observation system so that we could study the relationship of pain behavior to the patient's body posture and dynamic movement.

The pain behavior coding categories used with osteoarthritis patients were identified by means of clinical observations and preliminary analysis of videotaped behavior samples. Five pain behaviors were exhibited by many patients and occurred with reasonable frequency: guarding, active rubbing of the knee, unloading the joint, rigidity, and joint flexing. Table 16.1 provides the operational definition for each of the pain behavior categories as well as for the position and movement categories included in the scoring system.

Observer Training

In our studies of osteoarthritis patients, we have relied on research assistants and college undergraduates to serve as observers. Observers go through a systematic training program that involves several steps. The first step involves learning the definitions of each the coding categories listed in Table 16.1. Observers study the definitions and are tested to ensure that they understand the definitions. Second, the observers are instructed in the use of a scoring sheet. Table 16.2 displays a sample scoring sheet. As can be seen, the scoring sheet provides space for each of 20 recording intervals

and groups the individual coding categories into the three major groups (position, movement, and pain behaviors). During each scoring interval, observers simply circle the specific behavior coding categories observed. We use an interval recording method in which the observer simply notes the occurrence of a behavior. Thus, each behavior code is circled only once during any interval.

The third phase of training involves practice scoring of videotapes of osteoarthritis patients. A previously trained observer (the master observer) conducts these practice sessions. The novice observers are shown several 30-second segments of a videotape and then are asked to score the patient behaviors they observe. The novices then compare their scoring with that of the master observer. After each practice session, problem areas are addressed and feedback is provided on the accuracy of coding. As the novices begin to develop their observation skills, the master observer gradually increases the number of intervals being scored. Typically, practice sessions begin with a single interval, move to 5, 10, and 15 intervals, and eventually involve scoring an entire 20-interval

TABLE 16.1. Behavioral Categories of the Osteoarthritis Pain Behavior Observation System

Position Codes	
Standing (std)	Patient in an upright position with one or both feet on the floor for at least 3 sec
Sitting (sit)	Patient resting upon buttocks for at least 3 sec. If the patient is in the process of moving to or from a reclining position, do not score as a sit. Rather, this would be included in the shift (see below)
Reclining (rec)	Patient resting in a horizontal position for at least 3 sec
Movement Codes	
Pacing (pce)	Moving two or more steps in any direction within the space of 3 sec
Shifting (sft)	Change in postion upward or downward. (Example—changing from a sitting to a reclining position or a reclining to a standing position). A shift does not include the transition from standing to walking or walking to standing since no upward or downward shift is involved
Pain Behavior Codes	
Guarding (gd)	Abnormally slow, stiff, interrupted or rigid movement while shifting from one position to another or while walking
Active rubbing (ar)	Hands moving over or grabbing the affected knee (knees) and the legs, hands must be palms down and rubbing must last 3 sec
Unloading joint (unj)	Shifting of weight from one leg to the other during a stand
Rigidity (rgd)	Excessive stiffness of the affected knee or knees during activities other than walking (during walking this would be scored as guarding)
Joint-flexing (jf)	Flexing of the affected knee or knees while in a static position (i.e., during standing or sitting). This may take place in conjunction with unloading of a joint

TABLE 16.2. Pain Behavior Scoring Sheet

Patient: _____   Observer: _____

Date: _____

Pain Location: _____

	Position				Movement	Pain behavior				
1.	std	sit	rec	pce	sft	gd	ar	unj	rgd	jf
2.	std	sit	rec	pce	sft	gd	ar	unj	rgd	jf
3.	std	sit	rec	pce	sft	gd	ar	unj	rgd	jf
4.	std	sit	rec	pce	sft	gd	ar	unj	rgd	jf
4.	std	sit	rec	pce	sft	gd	ar	unj	rgd	jf
5.	std	sit	rec	pce	sft	gd	ar	unj	rgd	jf
6.	std	sit	rec	pce	sft	gd	ar	unj	rgd	jf
7.	std	sit	rec	pce	sft	gd	ar	unj	rgd	jf
8.	std	sit	rec	pce	sft	gd	ar	unj	rgd	jf
9.	std	sit	rec	pce	sft	gd	ar	unj	rgd	jf
10.	std	sit	rec	pce	sft	gd	ar	unj	rgd	jf
11.	std	sit	rec	pce	sft	gd	ar	unj	rgd	jf
12.	std	sit	rec	pce	sft	gd	ar	unj	rgd	jf
13.	std	sit	rec	pce	sft	gd	ar	unj	rgd	jf
14.	std	sit	rec	pce	sft	gd	ar	unj	rgd	jf
15.	std	sit	rec	pce	sft	gd	ar	unj	rgd	jf
16.	std	sit	rec	pce	sft	gd	ar	unj	rgd	jf
17.	std	sit	rec	pce	sft	gd	ar	unj	rgd	jf
18.	std	sit	rec	pce	sft	gd	ar	unj	rgd	jf
19.	std	sit	rec	pce	sft	gd	ar	unj	rgd	jf
20.	std	sit	rec	pce	sft	gd	ar	unj	rgd	jf

session. Each observer is required to score a practice series of 10-minute videotaped observation sessions and show acceptable reliability with the master observer (over 85% agreement) before they are considered fully trained.

The final step of training is to conduct periodic retraining sessions. These sessions are especially important in research applications in which the goal is to obtain reliable and accurate data. Retraining sessions help to prevent the phenomenon known as observer drift. Observer drift occurs when observers unwittingly begin to modify coding category definitions after carrying out a series of observations on their own. The retraining sessions should be scheduled periodically (e.g., every 2 weeks or after scoring data from every 10 patients). In the retraining sessions, the master observer reviews coding category definitions, scoring methods, and leads the observers in practice scoring of videotapes. When scoring pain behavior in a research study such as our osteoarthritis project, it is important to keep a written log of retraining sessions to document data on interobserver reliability.

Reliability and Validity Data

In our research with osteoarthritis patients, we have carried out assessments of both the reliability and validity of the pain behavior observation method (Keefe, Caldwell, et al., 1987). Reliability has been assessed in two ways. First, we have calculated interobserver reliability by having observers independently and simultaneously score the same videotaped behavior sample. Interobserver reliability was evaluated using the percentage agreement formula for 30 of the first 87 osteoarthritic knee pain patients we studied. Our findings revealed a very high degree of interobserver reliability (percentage agreement = 93.7%). Second, in unpublished research we have evaluated the test–retest reliability of our observation method. Pain behavior observations were carried out on a group of 36 patients who, as part of a treatment outcome study (Keefe et al., 1990), were assigned to a routine medical treatment control condition. A 10-minute videotaped behavior sample was obtained prior to entry into the study (time 1), 10 weeks later (time 2), and 6 months after time 2 (time 3). Test–retest reliability was found to be acceptable. Patients' total pain behavior at time 1 correlated significantly with total pain behavior at time 2 ($r = .53$, $p < .005$) and at time 3 ($r = .53$, $p < .005$).

We have also assessed the concurrent, discriminant, and construct validity of this observation method (Keefe, Caldwell, et al. 1987). The concurrent validity of the observation method was supported by the finding that patients' ratings of pain on a 0–10 scale were significantly correlated with their total pain behavior scores ($r = .46$, $p < .0001$). The observation method also showed adequate discriminant validity in that we found that patients who were having pain at the time of observation ($n = 37$) exhibited significantly more pain behavior ($t = 2.82$, $p < .007$) than those who were pain free ($n = 14$). To assess the construct validity of the observation method, we showed a series of videotaped segments collected from 20 osteoarthritis patients to a group of 13 rheumatologists. The rheumotologists were asked to rate each patients' pain level using a 0–10 rating scale and 100-millimeter Visual Analogue Scale (VAS). The rheumatologists' ratings were found to be significantly correlated with patients total pain behavior (0–10 ratings, $r = .65$, $p < .002$; VAS ratings, $r = .64$, $p < .003$). Thus, patients who trained observers scored as having higher levels of pain behavior were viewed by rheumatologists as having more pain, while patients who were scored as having lower levels of pain behavior were viewed by rheumatologists as having less pain.

Taken together, the results of our studies with osteoarthritis patients provide strong support the reliability and validity of this observation method.

CLINICAL APPLICATIONS OF OBSERVATION: ISSUES AND RECOMMENDATIONS

There are a number of important issues that arise when one tries to incorporate behavioral observation methods into clinical practice settings. First is the issue of time. To gather data on pain behavior one must spend time observing behavior in a naturalistic setting such as a clinic, home, or lab setting. A commitment to gathering observational data usually means that a clinician will need to make adjustments in workload and/or shift priorities. Carrying out observations may mean that the practicing clinician has less time available for gathering information using other assessment methods (e.g., interviews) or for carrying out treatment procedures. One of the best ways to reduce the time demands of observation is to carry out preliminary observations before implementing data collection. These observations can help to pinpoint behaviors that can serve as the targets for behavioral observation. A patient, for example, may show one or two pain behaviors (e.g., excessive guarding or pain avoidant posturing) that are particularly important targets for assessment and treatment efforts. Preliminary observations also can help to identify time periods during the day when pain behaviors are most likely to occur. Observations on our inpatient pain unit, for example, revealed that there were two times each day when patients were especially likely to exhibit pain behavior. These were meal times and the time when patients came to the nursing station to obtain their medications. By restricting observation to key periods of the day, one can significantly reduce the costs of observation while still obtaining an adequate sample of pain behavior.

A second issue in applying observation systems in clinical settings is the need for videotape equipment. Most of the sophisticated behavioral observation systems reviewed in this chapter have utilized videocameras and recording equipment. Although this equipment is useful in training observers and providing a permanent record of the observation session, it can be expensive. We believe that videotape equipment is a helpful tool, but not a necessity, in performing observations. Research has shown that reliable and valid behavioral data can be collected without the assistance of videotape equipment (Hartmann & Wood, 1982). Live observations carried out in naturalistic settings can serve as a basis for defining pain behaviors, developing behavior sampling strategies, and training observers. Naturalistic observations are not only less expensive, they are probably less intrusive than videotaped observations. Individuals new to the field of behavioral observation should be aware that most practicing behavioral oriented clinicians rely on live, rather than videotaped, observation methods.

A third important issue in applying observation methods in clinical practice is the need for observer training. The complex and sophisticated behavioral observation methods used in research studies require extensive observer training. Individuals who gather data using these methods are recruited and trained specifically to serve as observers. In practice settings, one must usually rely on clinical staff to perform the functions of observers. Although these staff usually do not have the time for intensive observer training, they often have considerable clinical expertise, understand the concept of pain behavior, and are capable of gathering high quality observation data. Brief periods of training can be used to teach staff to use simple observation methods such as duration measures or frequency counts. With periodic reliability checks and review of recording methods, reliable and valid data on pain behavior can be obtained.

Clinical staff are sometimes resistant to carrying out behavioral observations. They may view observation as a burden that is imposed on their already busy work schedules. Although they may agree to collect data, the quality of the data may not be high. To avoid this problem, the individual staff members who are to serve as observers need to be involved in the development and implementation of any pain behavior observation system. We think it is important to involve staff in writing definitions, setting schedules for observation, and checking reliability. Observation data that are gathered should also be shared with the observers on a daily basis so that they can be used in evaluating treatment outcome. If observation methods are to be effectively integrated into a pain unit or program, they must be viewed by all as contributing to the clinical management of the patient.

Can behavioral observation methods be adapted to new clinical populations? Most of the observational methods discussed in this paper have been used to record pain behavior in patients suffering from persistent pain conditions such as low back or arthritic pain. These methods, however, need not be restricted to these populations. Jay and Elliott (1984), for example, have demonstrated that observation methods can be used to record behavior in children who are experiencing acute pain due to medical procedures. Observational methods have also been used to record pain behavior in terminal lung cancer patients (Ahles et al., 1990). When adapting existent observational systems to new pain populations, there are two important considerations. First, the tasks used to elicit pain behavior during a structured observation session must be relevant to the pain condition studied. Walking or transferring from one position to another may elicit pain behavior in low back pain patients but may be of little value in eliciting pain behavior in a patient having facial pain. Preliminary observations may be needed to determine the best strategies for eliciting and sampling pain behavior. Second, new coding categories may need to be developed. The topography of pain behaviors can vary from one clinical condition to another. Reviewing videotapes of patient behavior can be particularly useful in identifying coding categories for specific pain conditions.

A final important issue in the clinical application of observation methods is the role that pain behavior plays in the overall assessment of the pain experience. Observations of pain behavior are meant to provide one measure of the pain experience. They are designed to complement, not replace, other forms of pain assessment. Chronic pain is a complex, multidimensional phenomenon (Melzack & Wall, 1965). Thus, pain behavior observation should be one component of a comprehensive assessment that includes the use of pain perception measures, standardized psychological tests, and a variety of medical evaluations. Thus, to analyze pain behavior, observational data need to be combined with information on the underlying tissue pathology, the perception of pain, and the degree of emotional suffering (Fordyce, 1979). It is only by viewing pain behavior in its biopsychosocial context that we are likely to achieve significant advances in our ability to assess and treat chronic pain.

REFERENCES

Ahles, T.A., Coombs, D.W., Jensen, L., Stukel, T., Maurer, L.H., & Keefe, F.J. (1990). Development of a behavioral observation technique for the assessment of pain behaviors in cancer patients. *Behavior Therapy, 21,* 449–460.

Anderson, K.O., Bradley, L.A., McDaniel, L.K., Young, L.D., Turner, R.A., Agudelo, C.A., Gaby, N.S., Keefe, F.J., Pisko, E.J., Snyder, R.M., & Semble, E.L. (1987a). The assessment of pain in rheumatoid arthritis: Disease differentiation and temporal stability of a behavioral observation method. *The Journal of Rheumatology, 14,* 700–704.

Anderson, K.O., Bradley, L.A., McDaniel, L.K., Young, L.D., Turner, R.A., Agudelo, C.A., Keefe, F.J., Pisko, E.J., Snyder, R.M. and Semble, E.L. (1987b). The assessment of pain in rheumatoid arthritis: Validity of a behavioral observation method. *Arthritis and Rheumatism, 30,* 36–43.

Block, A.R., Kremer, E.F., & Gaylor, M. (1980). Behavioral treatment of chronic pain: Variables affecting treatment efficacy. *Pain, 8,* 367–375.

Cailliet, R. (1968). *Low back pain syndrome.* Philadelphia: Davis.

Connally, G.H., & Sanders, S.H. (1991). Predicting low back pain patients' response to lumbar sympathetic nerve blocks and interdisciplinary rehabilitation: The role of pretreatment overt pain behavior and cognitive coping strategies. *Pain, 44,* 139–146.

Elliott, C.H., Jay, S.M., & Woody, P. (1987). An observation scale for measuring children's distress during medical procedures. *Journal of Pediatric Psychology, 12,* 543–551.

Ferster, C.B. (1965). Classification of behavioral pathology. In L. Krasner & L.P. Ullman (Eds.), *Research in behavior modification* (pp. 6–26). New York: Holt, Rinehart, & Winston.

Feuerstein, M., Greenwald, M., Gamache, M.P., Papciak, A.S., & Cook, E.W. (1985). The Pain Behavior Scale: Modification and validation for outpatient use. *Journal of Psychopathology and Behavioral Assessment, 7,* 301–315.

Follick, M.J., Ahern, D.K., & Aberger, E.W. (1985). Development of an audiovisual taxonomy of pain behavior: Reliability and discriminant validity. *Health Psychology, 4,* 555–568.

Follick, M.T., Ahern, D.K., & Laser-Wolston, N. (1984). Evaluation of a daily activity diary for chronic pain patients. *Pain, 19,* 373–382.

Fordyce, W.E. (1976). *Behavioral methods for chronic pain and illness.* St. Louis, Mosby.

Fordyce, W.E. (1979). Environmental factors in the genesis of low back pain. In J.J. Bonica, J.E. Liebeskind, & D.G. Albe-Fessard (Eds.), *Advances in pain research and therapy* (Vol. 3, pp. 659–666). New York, Raven Press.

Fordyce, W.E., Fowler, R.S., Lehmann, J.F., & DeLateur, B. (1968). Some implications of learning in problems of chronic pain. *Journal of Chronic Disease, 21,* 179–190.

Hartmann, D.P. (1977). Considerations in the choice of interobserver reliability estimates. *Journal of Applied Behavior Analysis, 10,* 103–110.

Hartmann, D.P, & Wood, D.D. (1982). Observational methods. In A.S. Bellack, M. Hersen, & A.E. Kazdin (Eds.), *International handbook of behavior modification and therapy* (pp. 109–138). New York: Plenum Press.

Jay, S.M., & Elliott, C. (1984). Behavioral observation scales for measuring children's distress: the effects of increased methodological rigor. *Journal of Consulting and Clinical Psychology, 52,* 1106–1107.

Keefe, F.J. (1989). Behavioral measurement of pain. In C.R. Chapman and J.D. Loeser (Eds.), *Issues in pain measurement* (pp. 405–424). New York: Raven Press.

Keefe, F.J., & Block, A.R.(1982). Development of an observation method for assessing pain behavior in chronic low back pain patients. *Behavior Therapy, 13,* 363–375.

Keefe, F.J., Brantley, A., Manuel, G., & Crisson, J.E. (1985). Behavioral assessment of head and neck cancer pain. *Pain, 23,* 327–336.

Keefe, F.J., Caldwell, D.S., Queen, K.T., Gil, K.M., Martinez, S., Crisson, S., Crisson, J.E., Ogden, W., & Nunley, J. (1987). Osteoarthritic knee pain: A behavioral analysis. *Pain, 28,* 309–321.

Keefe, F.J., Caldwell, D.S., Williams, D.A., Gil, K.M., Mitchell, D., Robertson, C., Martinez, S., Nunley, J., Beckham, J.C., Crisson, J.E., & Helms, M. (1990). Pain coping skills training in the management of osteoarthritic knee pain: a comparative study. *Behavior Therapy, 21,* 49–62.

Keefe, F.J., Crisson, J.E., & Trainor (1987). Observational methods for assessing pain: A practical guide. In J.A. Blumenthal & D.C. McKee (Eds.), *Applications in behavioral medicine and health psychology: A clinician's source book* (pp. 67–94). Sarasota, FL: Professional Resource Exchange.

Keefe, F.J., & Gil, K.M. (1986). Behavioral concepts in the analysis of chronic pain. *Journal of Consulting and Clinical Psychology, 54,* 776–783.

Kremer, E., Block, A., & Gaylor, M. (1981). Behavioral approaches to chronic pain: The inaccuracy of patient self-report measures. *Archives of Physical Medicine and Rehabilitation, 62,* 188–191.

McDaniel, L.K., Anderson, K.O., Bradley, L.A., Young, L.D., Turner, R.A., Agudelo, C.A., & Keefe, F.J.(1986). Development of an observation method for assessing pain behavior in rheumatoid arthritis patients. *Pain, 24,* 165–184.

Melzack, R. (1975). The McGill Pain Questionnaire: Major properties and scoring methods. *Pain, 1,* 277–279.

Melzack, R., & Wall, P.D. (1965). Pain mechanisms: A new theory. *Science, 150,* 971–979.

Richards, J.S., Nepomuceno, C., Riles, M., & Suer, Z. (1982). Assessing pain behavior: The UAB Pain Behavior Scale. *Pain, 14,* 393–398.

Romano, J.M., Syrjala, K.L., Levy, R.L., Turner, J.A., Evans, P., & Keefe, F.J. (1988). Observational assessment of pain behaviors: Relationship to patient functioning and treatment outcome. *Behavior Therapy, 19,* 191–202.

Romano, J.M., Turner, J.A., Friedman, L.S., Bulcroft, R.A., Jensen, M.P., & Hops, H. (1991). Observational assessment of chronic pain patient–spouse behavioral interactions. *Behavior Therapy, 22,* 549–567.

Sanders, S.H. (1983). Automated versus self-monitoring of "up-time" in chronic low back pain patients: A comparative study. *Pain, 15,* 300–306.

Turk, D.C., Meichenbaum, D., & Genest, M. (1983). *Pain and behavioral medicine: A cognitive-behavioral perspective.* New York: Guilford Press.

Waddell, G., McCulloch, J.A., Kummel, E., & Venner, R.M. (1980). Nonorganic physical signs in low-back pain. *Spine, 5,* 117–125.

White, B. & Sanders, S.H. (1986). The influence of patients' pain intensity ratings of antecedent reinforcement of pain talk or well talk. *Journal of Behavior Therapy and Experimental Psychiatry, 17,* 155–159.

V

SPECIAL TOPICS

Chapter 17

The Assessment of Pain in Children and Adolescents

PATRICIA A. McGRATH, PhD
MARGARET C. BRIGHAM, PhD

Interest in the assessment and management of children's pain has increased at an unprecedented rate during the past decade. The dynamic evolution of pediatric pain as a specialty area is reflected by the numerous research articles and clinical reports that have been published in a broad spectrum of medical, nursing, pain, psychology, and health journals. In addition, the first books on the assessment and treatment of children's pain were published in the past few years (McGrath, 1990b; McGrath & Unruh, 1987; Ross & Ross, 1988; Tyler & Krane, 1990). At the most recent World Congress on Pain in 1990, the International Association for the Study of Pain approved the formation of its first Special Interest Group, a multidisciplinary consortium devoted to pain in children. The first International Symposium on Pediatric Pain was convened in 1988, with a European Congress in 1989, and a second International Symposium in 1991. The journal *Pain* recently formed an editorial panel on pediatrics, and *The Journal of Pain and Symptom Management* is hosting a special series of articles on pediatric pain.

The impetus for the present interest in pediatric pain derives from four sources. First, an increasing concern about the adequacy of pain management for newborn infants and children prompted many retrospective chart reviews that unequivocally documented underprescription and underadministration of analgesics as common problems within many clinical settings. Second, the assumption that children's pain could not be assessed was refuted, as several investigators designed reliable and valid techniques for measuring pain and distress in infants and children. Third, the refinement of more effective analgesic therapies for adults motivated comparable clinical research to evaluate new interventions for children. Fourth, and most recently, increased financial support from hospitals, governments, and pharmaceutical companies has provided a solid foundation for developing pediatric pain clinics and for sustaining much basic and clinical research on children's pain problems.

As a consequence of these converging clinical and research developments, much research is now focused on improving pain control for infants and children by determining the pharmacokinetics and pharmacodynamics of varied analgesics in infants, by expanding the use of regional anesthetic techniques to relieve surgical pain, by evaluating different analgesic regimens to select optimal doses, dosing intervals, and administration routes, by integrating nonpharmacological approaches more routinely into clinical practice, and by teaching children basic physical, behavioral, and cognitive pain-reducing strategies. Intrinsic to all these endeavors is the need to assess a child's pain accurately. Accurate pain assessment requires careful consideration of the plasticity and complexity of children's pain perception, the influence of developmental factors, and the specific type of pain experienced. An overview of these critical issues is presented in this chapter, prior to a description of the primary measurement instruments available for clinical use. Emphasis is placed on a practical approach to evaluating children's pain from a comprehensive multidimensional perspective.

THE PLASTICITY AND COMPLEXITY OF CHILDREN'S PAIN PERCEPTION

Pain for infants, children, and adolescents is a complex multidimensional perception that varies in quality, intensity, duration, location, and unpleasantness. Like adults, children can experience pain without injury or apparent injury, and they can sustain injury without experiencing pain. A child's pain is not merely an immediate and inevitable consequence of tissue damage. Moreover, the strength of the pain is not predetermined by the extent of tissue damage. Instead, a child's pain is modified by many situational, emotional, familial, and developmental factors. Even newborn infants may experience different pains from the same noxious stimulus (e.g., a heel lance) because of differences in the situation in which it is administered (e.g., how the heel is touched before lancing, whether the infant's attention is diverted during the lancing). Children's nociceptive systems have the capacity to respond differently to the same amount of tissue damage. This plasticity is a unique feature of the pain system. The neural excitation initiated peripherally by tissue damage may be influenced at many sites within the central nervous system. Diverse physical, environmental, and psychological factors can affect nociceptive processing, so that even though a child's pain is often initiated by tissue damage, the subsequent pain experienced depends on these factors in relation to the actual tissue damage.

A model depicting the role of situational, behavioral, and emotional factors on a child's pain perception is shown in Figure 17.1. A noxious stimulus initiates a sequence of neural events that may lead to pain; many factors can intervene, however, to alter the sequence of nociceptive transmission and modify a child's pain perception. Some factors are relatively stable for a child, such as sex, age, cognitive level, previous pain experience, family, and cultural background (shown in the closed box). These factors shape how children generally

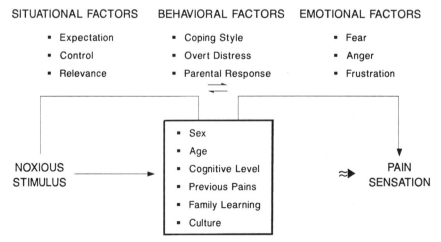

FIGURE 17.1. A model of the situational, behavioral, and emotional factors that affect a child's pain. From McGrath (1989), page 199. Copyright 1989 by the U.S. Cancer Pain Relief Committee. Reprinted by permission of Elsevier Science Publishing Co., Inc.

interpret and experience the various sensations evoked by tissue damage. In contrast, the situational, behavioral, and emotional factors (listed at the top of the figure) vary dynamically depending on each new situation or context in which a child experiences pain. Physicians, nurses, and other health professionals can alter these context-specific factors to profoundly lessen a child's pain.

The individual effects of age, sex, cognitive level, family, and culture on modifying pain are not yet known, even though we do know that these factors can influence a child's response and, perhaps, sensitivity to pain. However, the pain-modulating effects of many other factors have been well-studied. After Melzack and Wall (1965) first proposed the existence of a descending pain-modulating system as part of their gate control theory of pain, much research has been conducted to identify the critical internal and environmental factors that activate this system (Barrell & Price, 1975, 1977; Craig, 1980, 1984; Dubner, Hoffman, & Hayes, 1981; Duncan, Bushnell, Bates, & Dubner, 1987; Dworkin, Chen, Schubert, & Clark, 1984; Dworkin, Schubert, Chen, & Clark, 1986; Hayes, Dubner, & Hoffman, 1981; Hilgard, 1969; Johnson, Dabbs, & Leventhal 1970; McGrath, Brooke, & Varkey, 1981; Price, 1984; Thompson, 1981; von Graffenried, Adler, Abt, Nuesch, & Spiegel, 1978; Watkins & Mayer, 1982; Weisenberg, 1977, 1984; Weisenberg & Tursky, 1976; Zborowski, 1962). Comparable results from physiological studies on nociceptive mechanisms in monkeys and parallel psychological studies on pain perception in adults confirm that several situational, behavioral, and emotional factors modify both the neuronal responses and the pain evoked by a constant noxious stimulus. Subsequent clinical studies indicate that children's pains are modified by these same factors (McGrath, 1990b). Even when the causal relationship between an injury and a subsequent pain seems direct and obvious, the pain experienced is determined by many factors. As with adults, children's pain is often initiated by tissue damage caused by a noxious stimulus, but the consequent pain is neither simply nor directly related to the amount of tissue damage. Perhaps even more than in adults, differing pain responses to the same tissue damage are noted in children. While plasticity and complexity are critical features for all pain perception, plasticity seems an even more important feature for controlling children's pain. Therefore, children's pain may be easier to modulate by altering relevant context-specific factors than adults' pain.

Situational, behavioral, and emotional factors vary according to the context in which pain is experienced and have a powerful role in modulating pain. Situational factors refer to the particular combination of psychological and contextual factors that exist in a specific pain situation. They include a child's understanding about the pain source, expectations regarding the quality and intensity of pain sensations, ability to control or predict what will happen, focus of attention, ability to use a pain-reducing strategy, and the relevance or meaning of the pain. Situational factors naturally influence how a child behaves and feels when he or she experiences pain, so that there are reciprocal interactions among situational, behavioral, and emotional factors. Behavioral factors include a variety of specific behaviors that either precipitate pain (e.g., a child's tense posture) or occur in response to pain (e.g., a child's limitation of physical activity). Generally, the more overtly distressed a child is, the greater the pain. Some distress behaviors may be inadvertently conditioned over repeated medical procedures by parents and staff; children may act out, become nauseated prior to scheduled treatments, or become sullen and withdrawn. The presence of these behaviors, rather than positive coping and pain-reducing behaviors, inevitably increases children's pain and exacerbates their emotional distress. Children's emotional reactions to pain may vary extensively from a relatively calm acceptance to fear, anxiety, anger, depression, or frustration. In general, the more fearful and anxious a child is, the stronger and more unpleasant the pain.

Situational, behavioral, and emotional factors vary extensively not only for different children experiencing the same tissue damage, but also for the same child experiencing the same tissue damage at different times. Even though the pain source remains constant, the specific combination of situational, behavioral, and emotional factors is unique for each occurrence of pain. The gradual recognition that a child's pain is not simply and directly related to the nature and extent of tissue damage has profound implications for the assessment and management of children's pain. Clinical emphasis shifts from an exclusive focus on the source of tissue damage to a more comprehensive focus, not only on the source of tissue damage but also on the relevant situational, behavioral, and emotional factors that modulate nociceptive processing. Pain assessment is inextricably linked to pain management. Unless we assess the internal and environmental factors that modify a child's pain, our attempts to control it will necessarily be inadequate. Because the same noxious stimulus does not produce equivalent pain in all children, we cannot control pain by gearing our interventions solely to the source of tissue damage.

DEVELOPMENTAL FACTORS

From birth, infants display overt behavioral and physiological distress in response to tissue damage. The specific nature of their distress responses changes as infants mature, so that there are developmental differences in behavioral responses and pain expression for neonates, infants, toddlers, children, and adolescents (for review, see McGrath, 1990b; McGrath & Unruh, 1987; Ross & Ross, 1988; Tyler & Krane, 1990). Although it is possible to assess children's distress and pain from infancy throughout adolescence, these developmental differences influence the selection of pain measures.

At a very early age, children recognize that pain is an unpleasant sensory and emotional experience. Their understanding about pain and their descriptions of pain naturally depend on their age, cognitive level, and previous pain experience. They judge the strength and unpleasantness of pain in comparison to sensations they have already experienced. Like adults, the nature and diversity of children's previous pain experience form their frame of reference for perceiving all new pain. Children's frames of reference are constantly changing as they mature and sustain more diverse types of tissue damage. Yet, despite their changing frames of reference, all children can communicate meaningful information about their pain. However, their ability to describe their pain attributes—the quality (aching, burning, tearing, gnawing, stinging, throbbing, sharp or dull), intensity (weak to strong), duration (a few seconds to years), location (many body sites internally and on the skin surface), frequency (constant or episodic), and unpleasantness (a mild annoyance to an intolerable discomfort—develops as they ma-

ture. Children learn to describe the temporal, spatial, and qualitative aspects of all their sensations, not just their pain sensations. They learn specific words to denote different sounds, colors, tastes, and smells. Similarly, they learn a vocabulary to describe their pains.

Children's pain vocabularies evolve gradually as they mature and as they experience different types and different intensities of pain. The language that they learn to describe their own pains develops from the language that is used by their families and peers, and from characters depicted in books, on television, and in movies. Children naturally differ in the words that they use to describe their pains because of differences in their backgrounds, previous pain experiences, and learning. Yet, although the sophistication and ingenuity of their pain descriptions, like the quality and diversity of their pain experiences, vary idiosyncratically, all children understand both the intrinsic physical and emotional aspects of hurting.

It is essential to communicate with children about pain using their own terminology. Most toddlers (approximately two years of age) can communicate the presence of pain, using words learned from their parents to describe the sensations that they feel when they hurt themselves. They often use concrete examples and analogies to describe their perceptions. Gradually, children learn to differentiate and describe three levels of pain intensity using the terms that they have learned to describe the different sizes and amounts of physical objects, for example, "a little, some, a lot." By the age of five, most children can differentiate a wider range of pain intensities and they can use quantitative scales to rate their pain intensity. Children can also understand and communicate other aspects of their pain perceptions (sensory and emotional) in more abstract concepts as they mature.

Thus, administration of a pain measure requires a basic appreciation of the different developmental stages for children and their cognitive levels. Basic interviewing skills are required to ensure that children are comfortable and truly understand the questions. Questions should be spaced so that difficult or emotionally arousing items are interspersed with easier items. When children are asked to rate a specific dimension of their pain (e.g., intensity), they should first complete a brief calibration task to ensure that they understand the particular concept (e.g., rating magnitude).

This calibration task enables the clinician to assess whether a child can use the scale and make meaningful judgments about his or her perceptions.

ACUTE, CHRONIC, AND RECURRENT PAIN

Pain is a common sensation for children and adults. Most children will experience many different pains in most parts of their bodies—internally in muscles, bones, joints, teeth, and viscera, as well as externally on the skin surface. Children's pain varies extensively in quality, intensity, duration, frequency, and unpleasantness. As for adults, all children's pains are classified as acute, chronic, and recurrent in consideration of the temporal characteristics of the pain condition, the presumed etiology or source of noxious stimulation, the biological significance, the major situational, emotional, and psychological factors common to that pain type, and the recent demonstration that distinct physiological mechanisms mediate acute and chronic pain (McGrath, 1990b).

Acute pain is evoked by a well-defined noxious stimulus, has a relatively short duration, and usually provides an important protective warning signal. The pain generally diminishes progressively as an injury heals. Acute pains caused by tissue damage are the most common pains that infants, children, and adolescents experience. Children naturally sustain a diverse array of routine injuries, varying from superficial bumps, scrapes, and burns to deeper wounds that cause moderate to severe tissue damage. All children also inevitably experience other acute pains due to illness and medical and dental treatments, while some children, who require prolonged medical care, experience numerous and repeated painful procedures for several months or years. Most children do not experience prolonged physical or emotional distress from acute pain, because the pain is explicable, brief, and easily controlled by pharmacological and nonpharmacological interventions. However, children who need frequent invasive treatments may become progressively more anxious and frightened throughout their treatment regimen. The more afraid, tense, anxious, and distressed these children become, the stronger their pain becomes during procedures. These children may experience prolonged physical and emotional distress.

Chronic pain refers to pain caused by a prolonged disease, pain that lasts beyond the usual time period required for healing an injury, and pain that develops and persists without obvious physical damage. Unlike acute pain, chronic pain does not serve a protective biological function to signal tissue damage, even when it is associated with an underlying disease process such as cancer. Usually, multiple sources of noxious stimulation affect both peripheral and central mechanisms, so that the specific cause of pain is often poorly defined. Children experience prolonged physical and emotional distress as a result of their continuous pain, evidenced by fatigue, sleeplessness, irritability, restricted physical abilities, frustration, anger, and depression. Children experience chronic pain caused by arthritis, cancer, sickle cell anemia, hemophilia, neuralgia, accidental trauma, phantom limb pain, burns, and Reflex Sympathetic Dystrophy. As for adults, children's chronic pain affects the entire family and must be viewed from a broader context. Consequently, efforts to relieve chronic pain from a unidimensional perspective, in which pain is considered as synonymous with the nature and extent of tissue damage, will fail. Childhood chronic pain must be viewed from a multidimensional perspective because multiple sensory, environmental, and emotional factors are responsible for the pain, no matter how seemingly clear-cut an organic etiology may be. Treatment requires a thorough assessment of the multiple factors contributing to the pain, as well as regular measurements of pain intensity. Pharmacological, physical, and psychological pain-control strategies must be incorporated into a flexible intervention program, which is selected to meet the unique needs of each child.

Recurrent Pain Syndromes are chronic-like conditions in which otherwise healthy and pain-free children experience repeated episodes of headaches, abdominal pains, or limb pains. The episodes persist beyond a 3-month period and are not symptomatic of an underlying physical disease requiring medical treatment. Recurrent pains share some of the attributes commonly associated with acute pain and some commonly associated with chronic pain. Individual pain episodes are brief, but the syndrome is prolonged and may persist throughout a child's life. Painful episodes often are attributed to multiple causes because they develop in the absence of a well-defined single organic etiology and may be triggered by a variety of internal and environmental factors. There is no consistent biological significance for the pain. However, for some children, the pains provide a protective function and signal underlying stress, anxiety, or depression. Multidimensional assessment of the extent to which situational, behavioral, and emotional factors are the primary causes for the recurrent pain is required, because pharmacological methods alleviate the pain of an episode, but they generally do not relieve the syndrome. An integrated flexible approach combining physical, behavioral, and cognitive methods is more effective for controlling the syndrome.

Thus, pain management for all children involves strategic planning based on a careful and thorough pain assessment. The primary clinical objectives are to identify the source of noxious stimulation, assess the sensory aspects at a particular point in time (generally to facilitate diagnosis and monitor treatment efficacy), and determine the extent to which relevant factors are exacerbating the pain. The different constellation of physical, situational, emotional, and behavioral factors for acute, chronic, and recurrent pain guides the selection of specific pain measures to achieve these clinical objectives.

EVALUATING A CHILD'S PAIN

A child's pain complaint should be evaluated as carefully as any other presenting symptom. Precise information about the location, quality, intensity, and duration of a pain is required for an accurate differential diagnosis of the pain etiology and design of an appropriate treatment plan. Yet, consistent documentation of a child's pain has traditionally been neglected in most hospitals and medical practices. Hospital wards rarely have adopted notation guidelines for charting children's pain. Often notations include "voiced pain complaints," "crying and fussy," or "irritable"; they are not standardized as to terminology, recording frequency, and criteria for evaluating the presence or intensity of a child's pain.

Recently, however, the consistent evaluation and documentation of a child's pain have received increasing recognition as essential components of medical care. The present focus has evolved from debating whether children's pain should be assessed to selecting practical age-appropriate measurement instruments. Many behavioral, physiological, and self-report instruments are now available as a result of intensive research conducted throughout the past decade. (For review, see Beyer & Wells, 1989; McGrath, 1987a, 1990b; McGrath & Unruh, 1987; Ross & Ross, 1988; Tyler & Krane, 1990). Because space limitations preclude a comprehensive description of each instrument, this review focuses on the instruments available for routine clinical use. Dual emphasis is placed on the utility of available measures for assessing specific sensory aspects of pain (e.g., intensity) at discrete time points and for evaluating the pain-modulating role of situational, behavioral, and emotional factors.

The criteria for an accurate pain measure for children are similar to those required for any measuring instrument. A pain measure must be valid, in that it unequivocally measures a specific dimension of a child's pain so that changes in a child's pain ratings reflect meaningful differences in a child's pain experience. The measure must be reliable, in that it provides consistent and trustworthy pain ratings regardless of the time of testing, regardless of the age or sex of the child, and regardless of who administers the measure to the child. The measure must be relatively free from a response bias in that children use it similarly regardless of differences in how they wish to please adults or differences in how adults may administer it. The pain measure should be versatile—practical for assessing different types of pain and for use in diverse clinical settings.

Like pain measures for adults, children's pain measures may be classified as behavioral, physiological, or psychological depending on the nature of the child's response that is monitored. Behavioral measures include several observational procedures in which independent raters record the type of behaviors that children exhibit when they are in pain, as well as the frequency of their occurrence, such as the number of minutes children cry during an injection. Presumably, an objective evaluation of the nature and frequency of children's pain behaviors provides an accurate estimate of the strength of their pain experiences. Physiological pain measures include a variety of techniques that monitor the body's responses to a noxious stimulus, such as increased heart rate. The nature and extent of the body's natural pain responses might constitute an objective index for children's pain experiences. Both behavioral and physiological measures provide indirect estimates of pain becausee the presence or strength of children's pain is inferred solely from the type and magnitude of their behavioral and physiological responses to a noxious stimulus. In contrast, psychological measures can provide direct estimates for many different dimensions of pain. These include several projective and self-report methods in which children describe their understanding of pain or their subjective experiences of pain.

PAIN MEASURES AVAILABLE FOR CLINICAL USE

Behavioral Pain Measures

Most behavioral pain measures have been designed to obtain concise records of how children respond when they experience pain. Usually, a trained observer monitors children in pain (e.g., during invasive medical procedures, after surgery, or throughout specified physical activities for children with chronic pain) and documents any behaviors that suggest discomfort such as crying, flailing, grimacing, complaining about pain, and protectively guarding certain body parts. The distress behaviors commonly observed among children are subsequently identified as "pain" behaviors. Itemized behavioral checklists/scales are then developed listing the behaviors specific for each type of pain. Clinicians complete the checklist by noting which behaviors occur and how long they last. The rationale is that an objective evaluation of children's pain behaviors should provide an accurate estimate of the strength of their pain experiences. A child's pain level is calculated either by adding the number of observed behaviors or by first assigning a weighted distress value to each behavior (e.g., crying at needle insertion would have a higher distress value than grimacing) and then summing the individual values to produce a composite score. Differential weighting increases the sensitivity of a behavioral measure by establishing a priori the specific distress level represented by each behavior. The behavioral pain measures currently available for infants and children are listed in Table 17.1.

These measures monitor cries and other vocalizations, facial expressions, general body movements, or specific behaviors during invasive procedures. Cries and facial expressions

TABLE 17.1. Behavioral Pain Measures

Infant Pain Behavior Rating Scale	Procedure Behavior Checklist
Postoperative Comfort Score	Observational Scale of Behavioral Distress
Pain/Discomfort Scale	Children's Hospital of Eastern Ontario Pain Scale
Douleur Enfant Gustave-Roussy Scale	
Procedural Behavioral Rating Scale—Revised	Emergency Room Distress Behavior Checklist

have been monitored as potential pain measures for infants (Grunau & Craig, 1987; Johnston & Strada, 1986), while vocalizations and body movements have been monitored for toddlers and older children. At present, cries and facial expressions require special monitoring equipment and highly trained raters for interpretation. Because this chapter focuses on pain measures currently available for clinical practice, these measures are not reviewed (for review of cry and facial expressions as pain measures in infants, see Beyer & Wells, 1989; Johnston, 1989; McGrath, 1990b; Owens & Todt, 1984).

Three behavioral scales are available for quantifying acute pain in infants. The Infant Pain Behavior Rating Scale (IPBRS) is a time-sampling overt distress scale designed for measuring infants' vocalizations, expressive body movements, and facial expressions during injections (Craig, McMahon, Morison, & Zaskow, 1984). The IPBRS also records the nature of care infants receive (e.g., the use of praise, distraction, or soothing interventions by mothers during procedures) to provide information about the infants' social environment. This unique feature enables caregivers to identify the environmental factors that are influencing the infants' pain reactivity. The content validity of the IPBRS has been supported indirectly by research on infants' cries and facial expressions as pain measures. The interrater reliability of the scale is high and its utility is promising (Craig et al., 1984). The Postoperative Comfort Score was designed to measure infants' postoperative distress in the recovery room (Attia, Amiel-Tison, Mayer, Shnider, & Barrier, 1987). Ten behavioral responses (e.g., facial expression, quality of cry, consolability) are scored as 0, 1, or 2 to indicate increasing distress. This scale demonstrated a reduction in infants' pain as a function of relatively small doses of intraoperative opioid, supporting its validity as a useful means to quantify infant's distress (Barrier, Attia, Mayer, Amiel-Tison, & Shnider, 1989). However, further validity and reliability studies are needed to establish the limitations and generalizability of this scale. The Pain/Discomfort Scale (PDS) is used to measure infants' and children's overt responses postoperatively (Broadman et al., 1987). This scale measures responses in four behavioral categories (crying, movement, agitation, and posture) and arterial blood pressure. Behavioral responses are weighted on a 0–2 scale to represent increasing severity. Although promising, this scale also requires further validity and reliability studies.

Several behavioral checklists/scales have been used to measure children's overt distress during invasive treatments, after surgery, and to evaluate children with persistent pain (Gauvain-Piquard, Rodary, Rezvani, & Lemerle, 1987; Glebe-Gage, McGrath, & Kissoon, 1991; Jay, Ozolins, Elliott, & Caldwell, 1983; Katz, Kellerman, & Siegel, 1980, 1981; Katz, Varni, & Jay, 1984; LeBaron & Zeltzer, 1984; McGrath, Johnson, et al., 1985). Many of these behavioral rating scales yield a numeric score that represents an integrated index of a child's emotional, cognitive, and physical state. The Procedural Behavioral Rating Scale—revised (PBRS-r) is a standardized scale designed for measuring distress during cancer treatments (Katz et al., 1980, 1981). Eleven behaviors (e.g., cry, scream, physical restraint, requests for emotional support) are monitored at three specified time periods throughout a bone marrow aspiration or a lumbar puncture. The number of observed distress behaviors yields the child's pain score. Although this scale is straightforward, relatively easy to complete, and has high interrater reliability, valuable information about the intensity of each distress behavior is not recorded.

However, two scales have been developed to measure both the quality and frequency of children's overt distress during cancer treatments. The Procedure Behavior Checklist (PBCL) lists eight validated distress behaviors (LeBaron & Zeltzer, 1984). The behaviors are identical or similar to those on the PBRS-r. An observer rates the intensity of each behavior and assigns a value from 1 to 5, where 1 = very mild distress and 5 = extremely intense distress. One limitation of this scale is that the behavioral categories are not mutually exclusive, so that some distress behaviors could be assigned to more than one category. For example, muscle tension and physical resistance are defined as separate behavioral categories, but in many cases the two responses would co-occur as components of an overall reaction. This feature can compromise the interrater reliability of the scale, and may result in misinterpretation of the severity of children's distress. The Observational Scale of Behavioral Distress (OSBD) specifies the criteria for weighting eight behaviors along a 1–4 continuum to represent increasing levels of distress (Jay et al., 1983). Behaviors (e.g., information seeking, cry, flail) are monitored continuously in 15-second intervals throughout cancer procedures. Initial studies have demonstrated that the OSBD is a valid and reliable measure of children's distress (Elliott, Jay, & Woody, 1987; Jay & Elliott, 1984; Jay et al., 1983). A recent study to evaluate the efficacy of cognitive-behavior therapy and oral valium for reducing children's pain during cancer treatment, showed that children's distress scores on the OSBD were consistent with their pain ratings on a 5-item facial scale and with changes in their heart rate, further demonstrating the utility of this measure as a means of quantifying children's pain and distress during cancer treatments (Jay, Elliot, Woody, & Siegal, 1991). Each of these scales, the PBRS-r, PBCL, and OSBD are more appropriate for children aged 6 to 10 years than adolescents, because adolescents do not display the same overt distress behaviors as younger children (e.g., crying, screaming).

The behavioral scales for assessing acute procedure-evoked pain formed the basis for the design of a behavioral scale to assess acute treatment-evoked pain for children under 5 years of age receiving emergency medical care. The Emergency Room Distress Behavior Checklist monitors 14 general distress categories (e.g., screaming, altered breathing, physical resistance) (Glebe-Gage et al., 1991). The presence of each behavior is noted before and during treatment so that the pain score is simply the total of observed behaviors and not a more sensitive weighted value. At present, this scale has limited utility because the distress behaviors children exhibit during emergency treatments vary with their age, preparatory information, and the site and severity of injuries.

The Children's Hospital of Eastern Ontario Pain Scale (CHEOPS) was designed to measure postoperative pain in toddlers and children between 1 and 7 years of age (McGrath, Johnson, et al., 1985). Six behaviors (crying, facial expression, verbal expression, torso position, touch behavior, and leg position) are assigned weighted values on a 0–4 scale to reflect increasing pain. The CHEOPS scores for children's postoperative pain correlated with nurses' ratings for children's pain, but the nurses were not blind to the child's medical status, compromising the validity of their ratings (McGrath, Johnson, et al., 1985). Although interrater reliability for the CHEOPS is good, a recent study raises questions about its validity and generalizability for all postoperative pain assessment; children's postsurgical pain scores on the CHEOPS differed from their scores on self-report methods (Beyer, McGrath, & Berde, 1990). Although behavioral assessments are useful in clinics, when there is a discrepancy between behavioral pain scores and children's self-reports, health professionals should believe children's own pain ratings.

Although most behavioral scales have been developed to quantify a child's acute pain level at a particular point in time, evaluation of children's behaviors is also a valuable component in the comprehensive assessment of the multiple emotional and situational factors that may precipitate, maintain, or exacerbate children's acute, recurrent, or chronic pain. A child's general demeanor, physical activity levels, and specific coping and distress responses, as well as the responses of family and medical staff, can be monitored as part of the pain assessment. Evaluation of children's behaviors before and after invasive procedures can provide information about the role of situational, emotional, and behavioral factors for children's pain. Gauvain-Piquard et al. (1987) designed a weighted behavioral scale for measuring disease-related cancer pain in toddlers and young children (2–6 years of age). The scale consists of 7 behaviors that indicate pain, 6 behaviors that indicate depression (e.g., lack of expressiveness, social withdrawal), and 4 behaviors that indicate anxiety (e.g., moodiness, irritability). All behaviors are rated on a scale from 1 to 4 to represent increasing severity. The scale is used to record behaviors occurring during a 4-hour period when the child is not undergoing invasive treatment procedures. The revised scale shows promise as a method of evaluating factors contributing to pain and emotional distress in young children (Gauvain-Piquard et al., 1991).

In summary, many behavioral measures have been designed primarily to assess acute procedure-based pain. Behavioral scales provide a reliable, valid, quantitative index of children's overt distress. These scales enable health professionals to objectively quantify children's distress with minimal response bias and to ensure uniformity in observation periods. Such uniformity is essential for valid and reliable estimates of a child's pain, particularly when distress scores are used to monitor recovery, determine analgesic dosing, and evaluate the effectiveness of nonpharmacological pain control strategies. However, although a reduction in children's overt distress scores generally indicates reduced acute pain, caution is required. All children do not exhibit distress in direct proportion to the intensity of their pain. Behavioral pain-intensity ratings do not always correlate with self-reported pain ratings (Beyer et al., 1990; Glebe-Gage et al., 1991). Some children may behave stoically but still experience pain, whereas other children may exhibit many overt distress responses in clinics even before a scheduled treatment. The relationship between children's subjective experience of pain and their distress behaviors is significantly influenced not only by the type of pain experienced, but also by the situation in which the pain occurs. Thus, some distress behaviors that indicate the presence of pain in one situation are not appropriate indices in another situation. For example, some children may seek information and request emotional support during a bone marrow aspiration as a positive coping strategy, rather than as a distress response (McGrath, 1990b). Similarly, the absence of overt distress may reflect factors such as fatigue, depression, or conscious intention, rather than a lack of pain. Although no one behavioral scale is appropriate for all types of acute, recurrent, and chronic pain, children's behaviors provide valuable information about activities that may trigger recurrent pain episodes or exacerbate chronic pain. Therefore, behavioral assessments constitute an intrinsic component of a comprehensive pain assessment. Information should be obtained about the child's distress responses and behavioral restrictions during pain episodes (e.g., crying, withdrawal from physical activities, dependence on parental intervention), their coping behaviors, and pain-related interactions between children and families. Such an approach is analogous to that traditionally adopted for assessing chronic pain in adults, in which one goal is to evaluate behavioral limitations and identify any secondary gains. The nature of a child's behaviors in response to pain necessarily depends on the location (as well as type) of pain, so that multiple scales are required to encompass all types of pain. Thus, although behavioral assessment is a valuable tool for quantifying a child's distress during painful medical treatments, particularly for children under 5 years of age, behavioral measures are not adequate measures of pain for all children.

Physiological Pain Measures

Physiological parameters have been monitored in infants and children as potential pain measures; they include heart rate, respiration rate, blood pressure, palmar sweating, cortisol and cortisone levels, transcutaneous oxygen pressure levels, vagal tone, and endorphin concentrations (Anders, Sachar, Kream, Roffwarg, & Hellman, 1971; Beaudoin, Janes, & McAllister, 1991; Booth, McGrath, Brigham, Frewen, & Whittall, 1990; Campos, 1991; Gunnar, 1986; Gunnar, Isensee, & Fust, 1987; Harpin & Rutter, 1982, 1983; Jay et al., 1983; Johnston & Strada, 1986; Katz et al., 1982; Melamed & Siegel, 1975; Owens & Todt, 1984; Porter & Porges, 1991; Szyfelbein, Osgood, Atchison, & Carr, 1987; Szyfelbein, Osgood, & Carr, 1985). These parameters are not reviewed individually because standardized physiological pain measures are not yet available for clinical practice. Certain abrupt changes from children's baseline levels in response to noxious stimulation (such as increased heart rate and decreased respiration rate in response to heel lance) have generally been interpreted as indicating increased distress and pain. However, physiological measures, like behavioral indices, reflect a generalized and complicated overt response to some stress-inducing stimuli, rather than a specific localized response to pain. Thus, physiological responses are often positively correlated with behavioral distress and occasionally correlate with self-reports of pain, but no one physiological response constitutes an unequivocal measure of children's pain.

Physiological levels provide useful information about children's distress states, but only in the clinical situations where children are routinely monitored. As a consequence, physiological pain assessments have limited utility for evaluating acute pain and extremely limited utility for evaluating recurrent and chronic pain. Only palmar sweating (sweat produced from glands in the palms of hands in response to noxious and stressful stimuli) shows promise for many types of pain (Gedaly-Duff, 1989). In summary, physiological measures provide indirect estimates of pain, so that it is necessary to infer how much pain children experience simply from the magnitude of children's overt responses.

Psychological Pain Measures

Because precise information about the quality, intensity, location, duration, and affective dimensions of pain can be obtained only by objectively evaluating children's subjective experience, a diverse array of qualitative and quantitative psychological measures have been designed to evaluate the varied sensory, situational, and emotional aspects of children's pain. These include projective methods, in which children's attitudes or perceptions of pain are inferred from their selection of colors, their drawings, or their interpretations of cartoons and stories (Eland, 1974, 1982; Eland & Anderson, 1977; Jeans & Gordon, 1981; Kurylyszyn, McGrath, Capelli, & Humphreys, 1986; Lollar, Smits, & Patterson, 1982; Scott, 1978; Unruh, McGrath, Cunningham, & Humphreys, 1983), and self-report methods, in which children directly describe their pain and rate its intensity (Abu-Saad, 1984a, 1984b; Abu-Saad & Holzemer, 1981; Aradine, Beyer, & Tompkins, 1988; Beales, 1982; Beyer, 1984; Beyer & Aradine, 1986, 1987, 1988; Beyer & Knapp, 1986; Bieri, Reeve, Champion, Addicoat, & Ziegler, 1990; Carpenter, 1990; Eland, 1983; Gaffney, 1988; Harrison, Badran, Ghalib, & Rida, 1991; Hester, 1979; Jacox, 1980; Jeans, 1983; Jerrett, 1985; Maunuksela, Olkkola, & Korpela, 1987; McGrath, 1987a, 1987b, 1990b; McGrath & de Veber, 1986a, 1986b; McGrath, de Veber, & Hearn, 1983; Petrovich, 1957; Piquard-Gauvain, Rodary, Rezvani, & Lemerle, 1984; Pothmann & Goepel, 1984; Price, McGrath, Rafii, & Buckingham, 1983; Ross & Ross, 1984; Savedra, Gibbons, Tesler, Ward & Wegner, 1982;

Savedra, Tesler, Ward, Wegner, & Gibbons, 1981; Savedra, Tesler, Ward, Holzemer, & Wilkie, 1987; Szyfelbein et al., 1985; Tesler, Ward, Savedra, Wegner, & Gibbons, 1983; Varni, Thompson, & Hanson, 1987; Whaley & Wong, 1987; Wilkie et al., 1990). The available psychological measures for assessing children's pain are listed in Table 2.

Projective Methods

Only two structured projective measures are available for clinical use: the Eland Color Tool (Eland, 1982; Eland & Anderson, 1977) and the Pediatric Pain Inventory (PPI) (Lollar et al., 1982). The Eland Color Tool was designed to enable children to describe pain in colors, rather than words. Children choose different colors to represent different levels of "hurt." They then use the appropriate crayons to color the intensity and location of their pain on a body outline. Because of its intuitive appeal to younger children, the Eland Color Tool has practical clinical utility as a means of allowing children to describe their pain, although the validity of the measure is limited by the child's ability to match a particular level of pain with a color. The PPI consists of 24 cartoon pictures illustrating potentially painful situations in four settings: medical, recreational, common activities of daily living, and psychosocial (Lollar et al., 1982). Children describe the content of each picture, then rate the pictures according to intensity and duration of the pain depicted. Parents also complete the PPI with reference to their child's perspective. The results provide information not only about children's frame of reference for interpreting pain, but also information about potential disparities between parents' and children's perceptions. The use of cartoon drawings is a familiar and appealing method for eliciting information and establishing rapport, particularly for younger children.

Projective methods can provide relevant information about a child's subjective perceptions, including their sensory experience, frame of reference for understanding pain sensations, coping skills, and the emotional impact of the pain. These methods are useful for young children or children who are unable to express their feelings verbally. However, the primary limitation for their clinical utility is the current lack of age-appropriate guidelines for interpreting a child's responses. Further research is required to develop coding schemes that enable health professionals to accurately interpret children's perceptions and identify children at risk for increased pain because of situational and emotional factors. At present, projective measures can provide valuable information to compliment children's direct descriptions of their pain.

Rating Scales

A plethora of direct self-report methods are available as pain measures for children. As listed in Table 17.2, these include qualitative and quantitative rating scales to describe the sensory aspects of children's pain and relevant situational, emotional, and behavioral factors. Most self-report methods consist of quantitative scales to measure pain intensity in children, such as poker chip, word, number, thermometer, face, and Visual Analogue Scales (VASs). Children are asked to choose a level on the scale that best matches the intensity of their own pain (i.e., a number of poker chips, a particular word from none to strong, a level on a number or thermometer scale varying from 0 to 100, a face from a series of faces varying in emotional distress, a position on a VAS). These scales are easy to administer, requiring only a few minutes for children to rate their pain intensity. Pain intensity scales have been used extensively for children in many clinical situations.

Because children's concept of magnitude evolves as they mature, Hester (1979) developed a simple category scale for assessing pain in young children ages 4–7, whose understanding of temporal-spatial concepts is limited. Children choose the number of colored

TABLE 17.2. Psychological Pain Measures

Projective methods	
Eland Color Tool	Pediatric Pain Inventory
Rating scales	
Poker Chip Scale	Word Scale
Number Scale	Pain Thermometer
Children's Global	Facial Scale
Rating Scale	Visual Analogue Scale
Oucher Scale	
Interview methods	
Pain Diary/Log	Pediatric Pain Questionnaire
Varni-Thompson	Children's Comprehensive
Pediatric Pain	Pain Questionnaire
Questionnaire	

poker chips (from 0 to 4), representing "pieces of hurt," to match their own pain. The poker chip scale is easy to administer, appeals to younger children, and is reliable and valid. However, the scale provides only five discrete levels of pain, so that its utility is limited as a sensitive pain measure.

Although rating scales in which words are used to denote increasing levels of pain (e.g., mild, moderate, severe) are convenient to use for adults, they have not been validated for children. Caution must be used in assigning number values to words and in interpreting what children mean by their choices, because children's pain language depends on their age, cognitive level and previous pain experience (McGrath, 1990b). Children should be encouraged to describe pain in their own language as part of a clinical interview. When possible, standardized questions and age-appropriate prompts should be used to elicit qualitative and quantitative information about children's pain experiences. This format can provide reliable and valid pain descriptions, as reviewed in the following section on interview methods.

Numerical rating scales, which consist of vertical or horizontal scales, usually graduated from 0 to 10 or 0 to 100, are used frequently for older children. These scales are often presented as large "pain thermometers" in which children select a height of mercury to match their pain intensity (Szyfelbein et al., 1985). Zero is usually designated as "no pain," whereas the other endpoint is designated as "most pain possible." Although most children above 5 years old can effectively rate pain intensity on number scales, validation studies are required to ensure that a child's choice of a number or level accurately reflects his pain level.

The Children's Global Rating Scale (CGRS), designed to measure pain in young children, is a variation on typical number scales using comic book characterizations (Carpenter, 1990). The CGRS includes 5 lines, each progressively more wavy to represent increasing levels of fear and pain. The wavy lines are placed along a 1–4 vertical scale. Younger children select a wavy line to rate their pain, and older children select a number. Additional research is required to determine the CGRS's validity, reliability, and utility in clinical situations.

Several facial scales, comprised of a series of faces varying in emotional distress, have been developed (Bieri et al., 1990; Douthit, 1990; Kuttner & Lepage, 1989; LeBaron & Zeltzer, 1984; Maunuksela et al., 1987; McGrath, de Veber, & Hearn, 1985; Whaley & Wong, 1987). Children select the face that best matches their own pain and distress. Often, the faces are assigned pain values from 0, 1, 2, and so on to reflect increasing pain. As a consequence, validation studies are a critical prerequisite in the development of facial scales, because children's perceptions of the pain and distress expressed by the faces may not follow the assigned 0, 1, 2, and pain values. The Children's Anxiety and Pain Scale (CAPS) was designed to measure pain and anxiety in children aged 4 to 10 years (see Kuttner & LePage, 1989). The CAPS consists of two sets of five drawings of children's faces—one set displays increasing levels of pain and the other set displays increasing levels of anxiety. The values for faces were obtained in a rigorous manner, establishing preliminary evidence for its discriminant validity. Objective values were also obtained for the Facial Affective Scale, a series of nine faces representing different levels of unpleasantness (McGrath, de Veber, & Hearn, 1985). This scale has been studied in children with acute, recurrent, and chronic pain; results indicate that the scale is a measure of overall pain affect, not pain intensity (McGrath, 1990b). Recently, a series of studies was conducted to establish the reliability and validity of a 7-item facial scale designed to measure pain intensity (Bieri et al., 1990; Bieri et al., 1985). The authors note that although their initial research focused on pain intensity, additional research is in progress to determine whether the scale is also measuring the affective component of pain.

The Oucher Scale consists of six photographs of a young boy's face displaying different expressions of pain (Aradine et al., 1988; Beyer, 1984; Beyer & Aradine, 1986, 1987). The faces, ranked from 0 to 5 to represent increasing pain levels, are placed along a thermometer scale. The facial scale is intended for use by younger children, and the number scale can be used by older children. The scale is available commercially as a portable tool for clinical use; it is mounted on cardboard with the scale on one side and instructions on the back. Unfortunately, some practitioners have erroneously interchanged the independent facial and thermometer scales, thus compromising their validity. The values for the faces should not be determined by their position along the thermometer.

VASs are a form of cross-modality matching, in which children adjust the length of a line to match the strength of their pain perceptions. These scales provide a versatile and convenient method for assessing pain intensity in children. Generally, children over 5 years of age are able to use VAS in a reliable and valid manner to rate their pain intensity, regardless of their sex or health status. These scales have been used as a measure of pain intensity for acute, recurrent, and chronic pain (Abu-Saad, 1984a, 1984b; Berde, Lehn, Yee, Sethna, & Russo, 1991; Fradet, McGrath, Kay, Adams, & Luke, 1990; Kapelushnik, Koren, Solh, Greenberg, & de Veber, 1990; McGrath, 1987a, 1987b; McGrath, 1991; McGrath & de Veber, 1986a, 1986b; McGrath et al., 1983; McGrath & Hillier, 1992; Vandvik & Eckblad, 1990; Zeltzer et al., 1991). In addition, VASs can be used to assess many different aspects of pain, such as unpleasantness, sadness, and perceived control. As a consequence, VASs are an essential component of many structured interviews and pain questionnaires for children with recurrent or chronic pain.

Interview Methods

Children's interviews have traditionally had a minor role in pain assessment. Yet, the interview is ideally suited to the assessment of children's understanding of their pain, as well as the factors that influence it. Clinicians should conduct interviews with all children (when possible) not only to inquire about the sensory features of children's pain, but also about their associated fears, anxieties, and potential coping abilities. Table 17.3 lists the essential features of a pain assessment, including the information obtained from children, parents, health care professionals, and hospital records.

A structured format is a set of standard questions addressed to all children in a similar manner. This format ensures that all children will be interviewed in a consistent manner to obtain similar information about their pain problem and the manner in which the pain affects their lives and families. Several structured and semistructured interviews with age-appropriate questions have been designed to assess children's knowledge about pain and to

TABLE 17.3. Principal Features of Pain Assessment

Pain characteristics	Treatment factors
History	Nature of interventions
Location	Pattern of pain relief
Intensity	Criteria for determining
Quality	efficacy
Duration	
Frequency	Behavioral factors
	Child's learned pain
Situational factors	behaviors
Clinical environment	Physical activities and
Child's understanding	limitations
of pain	Family and social
Child's expectations	environment
Child's perceived	
control	Emotional factors
Relevance of disease or	Frustration
pain-inducing stimuli	Anger
	Sadness
	Fear
	Anxiety

evaluate the language they use to describe pain (Abu-Saad, 1984a, 1984b; Abu-Saad, Kroonen, & Halfens, 1990; Gaffney, 1988; Harrison et al., 1991; Ross & Ross, 1984, 1988; Savedra et al., 1982; Savedra, Tesler, Holzemer, Wilkie, & Ward, 1989; Savedra et al., 1981; Varni et al., 1987; Wilkie et al., 1990). Children can easily use many adjectives to describe the quality and location of their pain.

Pain diaries and logs are used to assist children to monitor different aspects of their pain, as illustrated by the pain log for children with recurrent headaches in Figure 17.2. Children above 5 years of age complete a separate pain log (with parental assistance as needed) for each headache they experience, so that the therapist can identify pain triggers, modify the behaviors that exacerbate pain, and evaluate specific analgesic interventions (McGrath, 1990b).

Three structured interviews and pain questionnaires have been developed for children. The Pediatric Pain Questionnaire includes eight questions about children's pain history, pain language, the colors they associate with pain, the emotions they experience with pain, their worst pain experiences, the ways they cope with pain, the positive aspects of pain, and the location of their current pain (Tesler et al., 1983).

The Varni/Thompson Pediatric Pain Questionnaire includes VASs, color-coded rating scales, and verbal descriptors to provide information about the sensory, affective, and eval-

Name: _____

Face sheet color: _____
Please complete the following questions for each
headache that you experience.

1. Day_____ Date_____

2. Time started _____ What were you doing
   when you started to get the headache?

   _____

3. Time ended _____ What did you do then?

   _____

4. How strong was your pain? That is, how much
   did it hurt?

   |_____|

5. How unpleasant was your pain? That is, how
   much did it bother you?

   |_____|

6. Which face looked that way you felt?

   _____

7. What do you think triggered this headache?

   _____

   _____

   _____

8. What did you do to relieve the pain? (if you
   took any medication, write down what and
   how much.)

   _____

   _____

FIGURE 17.2. Log completed by children to describe
the sensory features, context, triggers, and interventions
associated with headaches experienced during treatment.
From McGrath (1990a), page 297. Copyright 1990 by
Guilford Publications. Reprinted by permission.

uative dimensions of children's chronic pain, as
well as information about the child and family's
pain history, symptomatology, pain relief interventions, and socioenvironmental situations
that may influence pain. This questionnaire is
completed separately by the child, parent, and
physician (Varni et al., 1987).

The Children's Comprehensive Pain Questionnaire (CCPQ) was developed for children
with recurrent or chronic pain to provide quantitative and qualitative information about the
sensory dimensions of their pain and contributing situational, behavioral, and emotional
factors. The CCPQ includes general (open

ended) and supplied format questions, VASs,
and affective facial scales. Initial validity and
reliability studies indicate that the questionnaire provides an accurate, thorough, and objective format for assessing many dimensions of
children's pain (McGrath, 1990b).

Structured pediatric interviews are limited to
the extent that children must be able to comprehend specific questions and communicate
verbally with the interviewer. However, children should not be restricted to specific answers or response categories. The interviewer
must be trained to pursue hesitant or superficial responses in order to elicit the most accurate and thorough information about a child's
pain experience. Interviewers cannot simply
record appropriate responses on a structured
checklist. To obtain a true picture of children's
pain, interviewers must listen and guide in
order to elicit comprehensive and accurate information. Although the design and standardization of brief structured interviews, as well as
comprehensive pain questionnaires, may be
geared toward an objective assessment of symptoms, emotional reactions, and behaviors associated with children's pain problems, these
interviews must be administered by trained and
conscientious individuals.

GUIDELINES FOR SELECTING A
PAIN MEASURE

Because all pain measures are not equally appropriate for all children or for all types of pain,
the critical issue is how to select the best
available method for evaluating a child's pain.
The best available method is one that is valid,
reliable, and appropriate for the age and cognitive level of the child, and one that satisfies
specific clinical objectives. Many simple, easy
to administer pain scales provide meaningful
values that reflect a child's pain intensity and
are ideal measures for evaluating analgesic effectiveness throughout a child's treatment. But
they are not adequate measures for revealing
the nature of a child's pain experience or for
assessing the relevant situational factors that
affect pain. In contrast, lengthy structured
interviews combined with standardized pain
questionnaires are essential components of a
thorough pain assessment for children with
recurrent pain syndrome and for children with
chronic pain, but are rarely required for most

children treated for acute pain problems in hospitals and outpatient clinics.

Thus, clinicians who treat a wide range of children's health problems require a flexible pain measurement inventory comprised of both specific pain-intensity measures and more comprehensive pain assessment instruments. Only previously validated pain measures should be used in clinical practice, unless clinicians are willing to conduct the rigorous research necessary to prove that a new measure is valid and reliable. Although the specific clinical objectives, the particular medical environment, and the child's unique pain problem determine the range of possible pain measures, a child's age and cognitive level dictate the ultimate selection.

At present, we must rely on behavioral and physiological distress indices to infer the presence and severity of pain in infants. Although some behavioral checklists have been developed for infants, further study is required to demonstrate their reliability, validity, and versatility for clinical use. Yet, a quantitative index of a child's distress state could be obtained in most clinics by completing a brief behavioral checklist noting marked changes in overall body activity, facial grimacing, and crying. This type of checklist provides a gross distress index that could be completed at the same regular intervals in which a child's health status is assessed. Marked physiological changes also can signify critical variations in children's distress levels, in clinical situations where children's systems are routinely monitored. Future efforts should be expended to refine behavioral scales to facilitate convenient and objective evaluations of infants' and toddlers' distress and to revise the physiological monitoring systems currently used in hospitals so that they can signal a child's pain-induced distress. In the interim, some hospitals are developing multidisciplinary pain teams to ensure that personnel are using uniform criteria to interpret infants' distress signals. The discussion, formulation, revision, and gradual implementation of these guidelines are essential for developing practical pain measures for infants.

Although behavioral and physiological distress measures are valuable tools for inferring pain in infants, they are also valuable auxiliary tools for toddlers, children, and adolescents. The strength of these methods is that they provide a broader base of information about the factors that affect a child's pain, knowledge that is essential for optimal pain control. For example, the behavioral interactions between parents and children during invasive cancer treatments or during recurrent painful episodes must be evaluated to design a treatment program to minimize children's pain. Children's behaviors are influenced by environmental cues (the sights and sounds associated with painful treatments or interventions), familial factors (parental responses and expectations), and situational factors as well as sensory input. Caution must be used in interpreting children's pain solely from their scores on these scales because their behaviors are not passive reflections of their pain intensity. Because a child's pain behaviors naturally vary in relation to the type of pain experienced, different behavioral scales must be used for children with acute, recurrent, and chronic pain.

Self-report measures represent the gold standard in pediatric pain measurement because they are the only reliable source for obtaining information about specific dimensions of children's pain experiences. Many rating scales are available as reliable and valid measures of pain intensity. The poker chip method, best suited to children under 5 years old, asks children to choose the number of chips (0–4) that shows how much they hurt. Children 5 years of age and older can use pain thermometers, number rating scales, facial scales, and VASs quickly and easily to rate their pain. These measures are convenient and practical methods for assessing pain intensity for children experiencing acute pain. Children can complete the scales both in clinics and at home. Children should first practice the method by using the scale to rate the pain associated with some common childhood experiences such as a bruise, a finger pinch, a scraped knee, and a burn. The child's ratings should reflect different levels of pain for the different types of injuries. Simple quantitative pain scales are sufficient for most clinical situations when the objective is to measure pain intensity in otherwise healthy and pain-free children.

Both quantitative and qualitative assessment tools are required for children with recurrent or chronic pain and for children with diseases that require long-term management. Comprehensive pain assessments for these children begin with the recognition that the contributing and causative factors must be evaluated, in addition to pain intensity. A standardized assessment inventory should be developed with some pain measures that vary according to the specific pain problem (e.g., cancer, arthritis). Such flexible assessment inventories have been designed for children referred to the pain clinic at Children's Hospital of Western Ontario (McGrath, 1990b). Common pain referrals to this clinic include acute pain related to medical procedures (blood sampling, cancer treatment, growth hormone injections), acute pain evoked by injury or disease (burns, phantom limb pain, postsurgical pain), recurrent pain syndromes (headaches, abdominal pain, limb pain), chronic pain associated with disease or injury (hemophilia, arthritis, neuralgia, accidental trauma, cancer), and chronic pain associated with psychological etiology.

The current assessment inventories for these different pains evolved from a straightforward approach based on the recognition that a child's pain is plastic and complex. All pain assessments include two components: (1) an initial evaluation of the pain complaint in relation to the child and the specific factors that affect his or her pain (as illustrated in Figure 17.1), and (2) subsequent regular assessment of pain intensity using VASs and pain affect using facial affective scales. All assessments begin with a semistructured interview conducted independently with parents, child, and if appropriate, the referring physician or nurse. Children then complete brief standardized scales to obtain information about their minimum and maximum pains, their ratings of pain associated with common childhood injuries, and a simple calibration task to determine how well they can use VASs. Assessment inventories for more prolonged pain conditions also include standardized age-appropriate measures of emotion, depression, anxiety, and family interactions, as appropriate. These scales enable the therapist to understand the child's frame of reference for evaluating pain, and to design an appropriate treatment plan.

Acute pain evoked by invasive medical procedures is a relatively simple type of pain to measure because it is amenable to observational, physiological, and direct scaling techniques. However, for chronic or recurrent pain, it is not possible to consistently observe children's behavior or record their physiological responses throughout the day when their pain may fluctuate. For these children, it is necessary to incorporate measures that evaluate salient features of the child's pain experience on a continuing and long-term basis. As a conse-

quence, a combination of direct scaling approaches, along with behavioral scales that record general behaviors, such as school attendance, physical activity, and medication requirements, are preferable to the brief overt distress checklists that have been developed for treatment-evoked pain. When possible, these children should regularly complete pain diaries with intensity and affective rating scales in order to monitor variations in their pain experiences. This approach is also recommended for children who will require long-term invasive procedures, such as children with cancer, diabetes, and growth hormone deficiency.

In summary, evaluating a child's pain requires an integrated approach. Clinicians should always ask a child directly about his or her pain experience, and determine precisely the sensory characteristics to facilitate an accurate diagnosis. They should also assess relevant situational, behavioral, and emotional factors to modify their potential pain exacerbating impact, and should regularly measure a child's pain intensity to monitor the efficacy of the selected intervention. Interviews, structured questionnaires, and simple rating scales form the primary tools needed to assess pain adequately for most children above 5 years of age. For infants, toddlers, and cognitively impaired children, physicians must infer the presence and severity of pain by evaluating changes in children's behaviors and physiological states.

Acknowledgments. Dr. McGrath is supported as a Career Scientist of the Ontario Ministry of Health, National Health Research and Development Programme. The secretarial assistance of Mavis Jones is gratefully acknowledge.

REFERENCES

Abu-Saad, H. (1984a). Assessing children's responses to pain. *Pain, 19,* 163–171.

Abu-Saad, H. (1984b). Cultural group indicators of pain in children. *Maternal–Child Nursing Journal, 13,* 187–196.

Abu-Saad, H., & Holzemer, W.L. (1981). Measuring children's self-assessment of pain. *Issues in Comprehensive Pediatric Nursing, 5,* 337–349.

Abu-Saad, H.H., Kroonen, E., & Halfens, R. (1990). On the development of a multidimensional Dutch pain assessment tool for children. *Pain, 43,* 249–256.

Anders, T. F., Sachar, E. J., Kream, J., Roffwarg, H., & Hellman, L. (1971). Behavioral state and plasma cortisol response in the human newborn. *Pediatrics, 46,* 532–537.

Aradine, C.R., Beyer, J.E., & Tompkins, J.M. (1988). Children's pain perceptions before and after analgesia: A study of instrument construct validity and related issues . . . the oucher. *Journal of Pediatric Nursing, 3,* 11–23.

Attia, J., Amiel-Tison, C., Mayer, M.N., Shnider, S.M., & Barrier, G. (1987). Measurement of postoperative pain and narcotic administration in infants using a new clinical scoring system. *Anesthesiology, 67,* A532.

Barrell, J.J., & Price, D.D. (1975). The perception of first and second pain as a function of psychological set. *Perception and Psychophysics, 17,* 163–166.

Barrell, J.J., & Price, D.D. (1977). Two experiential orientations toward a stressful situation and their related somatic and visceral responses. *Psychophysiology, 14,* 517–521.

Barrier, G., Attia, J., Mayer, M.N., Amiel-Tison, C., & Shnider, S.M. (1989). Measurement of post-operative pain and narcotic administration in infants using a new clinical scoring system. *Intensive Care Medicine, 15,* S37–S39.

Beales, J.G. (1982). The assessment and management of pain in children. In P. Karoly, J.J. Steffen, & D.J. O'Grady (Eds.), *Child health psychology: Concepts and issues* (pp. 154–179). Elmsford,NY: Pergamon Press.

Beaudoin, C. A., Janes, M., & McAllister, M. (1991). The physiological responses of premature infants to heel-stick blood sampling. *Journal of Pain and Symptom Management, 6,* 193.

Berde, C.B., Lehn, B.M., Yee, J.D., Sethna, N.F., & Russo, D. (1991). Patient-controlled analgesia in children and adolescents: A randomized, prospective comparison with intramuscular administration of morphine for postoperative analgesia. *Journal of Pediatrics, 118,* 460–466.

Beyer, J.E. (1984). *The oucher: A user's manual and technical report.* Evanston,IL: Judson.

Beyer, J.E., & Aradine, C.R. (1986). Content validity of an instrument to measure young children's perceptions of the intensity of their pain. *Journal of Pediatric Nursing, 1,* 386–395.

Beyer, J.E., & Aradine, C.R. (1987). Patterns of pediatric pain intensity: A methodological investigation of a self-report scale. *Clinical Journal of Pain, 3,* 130–141.

Beyer, J.E., & Aradine, C.R. (1988). Convergent and discriminant validity of a self-report measure of pain intensity for children. *Children's Health Care, 16,* 274–282.

Beyer, J.E., & Knapp, T.R. (1986). Methodological issues in the measurement of children's pain. *Children's Health Care, 14,* 233–241.

Beyer, J.E., McGrath, P.J., & Berde, C.B. (1990). Discordance between self-report and behavioral pain measures in children aged 3–7 years after surgery. *Journal of Pain and Symptom Management, 5,* 350–356.

Beyer, J.E., & Wells, N. (1989). The assessment of pain in children. *Pediatric Clinics of North America, 36,* 837–854.

Bieri, D., Reeve, R.A., Champion, G.D., Addicoat, L., & Ziegler, J.B. (1990). The Faces Pain Scale for the self-assessment of the severity of pain experienced by children: Development, initial validation, and preliminary investigation for ratio scale properties. Pain, 41, 139–150.

Bieri,D., White, L., O'Gorman Hughes, D., Vowels, M., Newsum, M., Warren, J., & Miller, C. (1985). Communication of self perceived pain in children.

Medical Pediatric Oncology, 13, 143.

Booth, J. C., McGrath, P. A., Brigham, M. C., Frewen, T., & Whittall, S. (1990). Critically-ill neonates' distress responses during invasive medical procedures. *Pain, Supplement 5,* S28.

Broadman, L.M., Hannallah, R.S., Belman, A.B., Elder, P.T., Ruttimann, U., & Epstein, B.S. (1987). Postcircumcision pain: A prospective evaluation of subcutaneous ring block of the penis. *Anesthesiology, 67,* 399–402.

Campos, R. G. (1991). Temperament and soothing responses to pain-induced distress. *Journal of Pain and Symptom Management, 6,* 195.

Carpenter, P.J. (1990). New method for measuring young children's self-report of fear and pain. *Journal of Pain and Symptom Management, 5,* 233–240.

Craig, K.D. (1980). Ontogenetic and cultural influences on the expression of pain in man. In H.W. Kosterlitz & L.Y. Terenius (Eds.), *Pain and society* (pp. 37–52). Weinheim, West Germany: Verlag Chemie.

Craig, K.D. (1984). Emotional aspects of pain. In P.D. Wall & R. Melzack (Eds.), *Textbook of pain* (pp. 153–161). Edinburgh: Churchill Livingstone.

Craig, K.D., McMahon, R.J., Morison, J.D., & Zaskow, C. (1984). Developmental changes in infant pain expression during immunization injections. *Social Science and Medicine, 19,* 1331–1337.

Douthit, J.L. (1990). Psychosocial assessment and management of pediatric pain. *Journal of Emergency Nursing, 16,* 168–170.

Dubner, R., Hoffman, D.S., & Hayes, R.L. (1981). Neuronal activity in medullary dorsal horn of awake monkeys trained in a thermal discrimination task: III. Task-related responses and their functional role. *Journal of Neurophysiology, 46,* 444–464.

Duncan, G.H., Bushnell, M.C., Bates, R., & Dubner, R. (1987). Task-related responses of monkey medullary dorsal horn neurons. *Journal of Neurophysiology, 57,* 289–310.

Dworkin, S.F., Chen, A.C.N., Schubert, M.M., & Clark, D.W. (1984). Cognitive modification of pain: Information in combination with N_2O. *Pain, 19,* 338–351.

Dworkin, S.F., Schubert, M.M., Chen, A.C.N., & Clark, D.W. (1986). Psychological preparation influences nitrous oxide analgesia: Replication of laboratory findings in a clinical setting. *Oral Surgery, Oral Medicine, Oral Pathology, 61,* 108–112.

Eland, J.M. (1974). *Children's communication of pain.* Unpublished master's thesis, University of Iowa.

Eland, J.M. (1982). Minimizing injection pain associated with prekindergarten immunizations. *Issues in Comprehensive Pediatric Nursing, 5,* 361–372.

Eland, J.M. (1983). Children's pain: Developmentally appropriate efforts to improve identification of source, intensity and relevant intervening variables. In G. Felton & M. Albert (Eds.), *Nursing research: A monograph for non-nurse researchers* (pp. 64–79). Iowa City: University of Iowa Press.

Eland, J.M., & Anderson, J.E. (1977). The experience of pain in children. In A.K. Jacox (Ed.), *Pain: A source book for nurses and other health professionals* (pp. 453–471). Boston: Little, Brown.

Elliott, C.H., Jay, S.M., & Woody, P. (1987). An observational scale for measuring children's distress during medical proceedings. *Journal of Pediatric Psychology, 12,* 543–551.

Fradet, C., McGrath, P.J., Kay, J., Adams, S., & Luke, B.

(1990). A prospective survey of reactions to blood tests by children and adolescents. *Pain, 40,* 53–60.

Gaffney, A. (1988). How children describe pain: A study of words and analogies used by 5–14 year-olds. In R. Dubner, G.F. Gebhart, & M.R. Bond (Eds.), *Pain research and clinical management* (Vol. 3, pp. 341–347). Amsterdam: Elsevier.

Gauvain-Piquard, A., Rodary, C., Francois, P., Rezvani, A., Kalifa, C., Lecuyer, N., Cosse, M., & Lesbros, R. (1991). Validity assessment of DEGR^R scale for observational rating of 2–6-year-old child pain. *Journal of Pain and Symptom Management, 6,* 171.

Gauvain-Piquard, A., Rodary, C., Rezvani, A., & Lemerle, J. (1987). Pain in children aged 2–6 years: A new observational rating scale elaborated in a pediatric oncology unit—preliminary report. *Pain, 31,* 177–188.

Gedaly-Duff, V. (1989). Palmar sweat index use with children in pain research. *Journal of Pediatric Nursing, 4,* 3–8.

Glebe-Gage, D., McGrath, P.A., & Kissoon, N. (1991). Children's responses to painful procedures in the emergency department. In M.R. Bond, J.E. Charlton, & C.J. Woolf (Eds.), *Proceedings of the VIth World Congress on Pain* (pp. 437–442). Amsterdam: Elsevier.

Grunau, R.V.E., & Craig, K.D. (1987). Pain expression in neonates: Facial action and cry. *Pain, 28,* 395–410.

Gunnar, M. R. (1986, April). *The organization of "stress" responses in the newborn.* Paper presented at the International Conference for Infant Studies, Symposium on Stress and Coping, Los Angeles.

Gunnar, M. R., Isensee, J., & Fust, L. S. (1987). Adrenocortical activity and the Brazelton Neonatal Assessment Scale: Moderating effects of the newborn's biobehavioral status. *Child Development, 58,* 1448–1458.

Harpin, V. A., & Rutter, N. (1982). Development of emotional sweating in the newborn infants. *Archives of Disease in Childhood, 57,* 691–695.

Harpin, V. A., & Rutter, N. (1983). Making heel pricks less painful. *Archives of Disease in Childhood, 58,* 226–228.

Harrison, A., Badran, S., Ghalib, R., & Rida, S. (1991). Arabic children's pain descriptions. *Pediatric Emergency Care, 7,* 199–203.

Hayes, R.L., Dubner, R., & Hoffman, D.S. (1981). Neuronal activity in medullary dorsal horn of awake monkeys trained in a thermal discrimination task: II. Behavioral modulation of responses to thermal and mechanical stimuli. *Journal of Neurophysiology, 46,* 428–443.

Hester, N.K. (1979). The preoperational child's reaction to immunization. *Nursing Research, 28,* 250–255.

Hilgard, E.R. (1969). Pain as a puzzle for psychology and physiology. *American Psychologist, 24,* 103–113.

Jacox, A.K. (1980). The assessment of pain. In W.L. Smith, H. Merskey, & S.C. Gross (Eds.), *Pain: Meaning and management* (pp. 75–88). New York: SP Medical & Scientific Books.

Jay, S.M., & Elliott, C.H. (1984). Behavioral observation scales for measuring children's distress: The effects of increased methodological rigor. *Journal of Consulting and Clinical Psychology, 52,* 1106–1107.

Jay, S.M., Elliott, C.H., Woody, P.D., & Siegel, S. (1991). An investigation of cognitive-behavior therapy combined with oral valium for children undergoing painful medical procedures. *Health Psychology, 10,* 317–322.

Jay, S.M., Ozolins, M., Elliott, C.H., & Caldwell, S. (1983). Assessment of children's distress during painful medical procedures. *Health Psychology, 2,* 133–147.

Jeans, M.E. (1983). The measurement of pain in children. In R. Melzack (Ed.), *Pain measurement and assessment* (pp. 183–189). New York: Raven Press.

Jeans, M.E., & Gordon, D.J. (1981). An investigation of the developmental characteristics of the concept of pain. *Pain (Suppl. 1),* S11.

Jerrett, M.D. (1985). Children and their pain experience. *Children's Health Care, 14,* 83–89.

Johnson, J.E., Dabbs, J.M., Jr., & Leventhal, H. (1970). Psychosocial factors in the welfare of surgical patients. *Nursing Research, 19,* 18–29.

Johnston, C.C. (1989). Pain assessment and management in infants. *Pediatrician, 16,* 16–23.

Johnston, C.C., & Strada, M.E. (1986). Acute pain response in infants: A multidimensional description. *Pain, 24,* 373–382.

Kapelushnik, J., Koren, G., Solh, H., Greenberg, M., & de Veber, L.L. (1990). Evaluating the efficacy of EMLA in alleviating pain associated with lumbar puncture; comparison of open and double-blinded protocols in children. *Pain, 42,* 31–34.

Katz, E.R., Kellerman, J., & Siegel, S.E. (1980). Behavioral distress in children with cancer undergoing medical procedures: Developmental considerations. *Journal of Consulting and Clinical Psychology, 48,* 356–365.

Katz, E.R., Kellerman, J., & Siegel, S.E. (1981). Anxiety as an affective focus in the clinical study of acute behavioral distress: A reply to Schacham and Daut. *Journal of Consulting and Clinical Psychology, 49,* 470–471.

Katz, E. R., Sharp, B., Kellerman, J., Marston, A. R., Hershman, J. M., & Siegel, S. E. (1982). Beta-endorphin immunoreactivity and acute behavioral distress in children with leukemia. *Journal of Nervous and Mental Disease, 170,* 72–77.

Katz, E.R., Varni, J.W., & Jay, S.M. (1984). Behavioral assessment and management of pediatric pain. *Progress in Behavior Modification, 18,* 163–193.

Kurylyszyn, N., McGrath, P.J., Cappelli, M., & Humphreys, P. (1986). Children's drawings: What can they tell us about intensity of pain? *Clinical Journal of Pain, 2,* 155–158.

Kuttner, L., & LePage, T. (1989). Face scales for the assessment of pediatric pain: A critical review. *Canadian Journal of Behavioral Sciences, 21,* 198–209.

LeBaron, S., & Zeltzer, L. (1984). Assessment of acute pain and anxiety in children and adolescents by self-reports, observer reports, and a behavior checklist. *Journal of Consulting and Clinical Psychology, 52,* 729–738.

Lollar, D.J., Smits, S.J., & Patterson, D.L. (1982). Assessment of pediatric pain: An empirical perspective. *Journal of Pediatric Psychology, 7,* 267–277.

Marshall, R.E. (1989). Neonatal pain associated with caregiving procedures. *Pediatric Clinics of North America, 36,* 885–903.

Maunuksela, E.L., Olkkola, K.T., & Korpela, R. (1987). Measurement of pain in children with self-reporting and behavioral assessment. *Clinical Pharmacological Therapy, 42,* 137–141. McGrath, P.A. (1987a). An assessment of children's pain: A review of behavioral, physiological, and direct scaling techniques. *Pain, 31,* 147–176.

McGrath, P.A. (1987b). The multidimensional assessment and management of recurrent pain syndromes in children and adolescents. *Behaviour Research and Therapy, 25,* 251–262.

McGrath, P.A. (1989). Evaluating a child's pain. *Journal of Pain and Symptom Management, 4,* 198–214.

McGrath, P.A. (1990a). Pain assessment in children—a practical approach. In D.C. Tyler & E.J. Krane (Eds.), *Advances in pain research and therapy* (Vol. 15, pp. 5–30). New York: Raven Press.

McGrath, P.A. (1990b). *Pain in children: Nature, assessment and treatment.* New York: Guilford Publications.

McGrath, P.A., Brooke, R.I., & Varkey, M. (1981). Analgesic efficacy and subject expectation for clinical and experimental pain. Pain (Suppl. 1), S13.

McGrath, P.A., & de Veber, L.L. (1986a). Helping children cope with painful procedures. *American Journal of Nursing, 86,* 1278–1279.

McGrath, P.A., & de Veber, L.L. (1986b). The management of acute pain evoked by medical procedures in children with cancer. *Journal of Pain and Symptom Management, 1,* 145–150.

McGrath, P.A., de Veber, L.L., & Hearn, M.T. (1983). Modulation of acute pain and anxiety for pediatric oncology patients. *Conference Proceedings, American Pain Society,* Abstract 93.

McGrath, P.A., de Veber, L.L., & Hearn, M.T. (1985). Multidimensional pain assessment in children. In H.L. Fields, R. Dubner, & F. Cervero (Eds.), *Advances in pain research and therapy* (Vol. 9, pp. 387–393). New York: Raven Press.

McGrath, P.A., & Hillier, L.M. (1992). Phantom limb pain in children: A case study to illustrate the utility of pain logs in clinical practice. *Journal of Pain and Symptom Management, 7,* 46–53.

McGrath, P.J., Johnson, G., Goodman, J.T., Schillinger, J., Dunn, J., & Chapman, J.-A. (1985). CHEOPS: A behavioral scale for rating postoperative pain in children. In H.L. Fields, R. Dubner & F. Cervero (Eds.), *Advances in pain research and therapy* (Vol. 9, pp. 395–402). New York: Raven Press.

McGrath, P.J., & Unruh, A. (1987). *Pain in children and adolescents.* Amsterdam: Elsevier.

Melamed, B. G., & Siegel, L. J. (1975). Reduction of anxiety in children facing hospitalization and surgery by use of filmed modeling. *Journal of Consulting and Clinical Psychology, 43,* 511–521.

Melzack, R., & Wall, P.D. (1965). Pain mechanisms: A new theory. *Science, 150,* 971–978.

Owens, M. E., & Todt, E. H. (1984). Pain in infancy: Neonatal reaction to a heel lance. *Pain, 20,* 77–86.

Petrovich, D.V. (1957). The Pain Apperception Test: A preliminary report. *Journal of Psychology, 44,* 339–346.

Piquard-Gauvain, A., Rodary, C., Rezvani, A., & Lemerle, J. (1984). Establishment of a new rating scale for the evaluation of pain in young children (2–6 years) with cancer. *Pain (Suppl. 2),* S25.

Porter, F. L., & Porges, S. W. (1991). Vagal tone: An index of stress and pain in high risk newborn infants. *Journal of Pain and Symptom Management, 6,* 206.

Pothmann, R., & Goepel, R. (1984). Comparison of the Visual Analog scale (VAS) and a Smiley Analog Scale (SAS) for the evaluation of pain in children. *Pain (Suppl. 2),* S25.

Price, D.D. (1984). Dorsal horn mechanisms of pain. In R.A. Davidoff (Ed.), *The handbook of the spinal cord* (pp. 751–777). New York: Marcel Dekker.

Price, D.D., McGrath, P.A., Rafii, A., & Buckingham, B. (1983). The validation of Visual Analogue Scales as ratio scale measures for chronic and experimental pain. *Pain, 17,* 45–56.

Ross, D.M., & Ross, S.A. (1984). Childhood pain: The school-aged child's viewpoint. *Pain, 20,* 179–191.

Ross, D.M., & Ross, S.A. (1988). *Childhood pain: Current issues, research, and management.* Baltimore: Urban & Schwarzenberg.

Savedra, M.C., Gibbons, P.T., Tesler, M.D., Ward, J.A., & Wegner, C. (1982). How do children describe pain? A tentative assessment. *Pain, 14,* 95–104.

Savedra, M.C., Tesler, M.D., Holzemer, W.L., Wilkie, D.J., & Ward, J.A. (1989). Pain location: Validity and reliability of body outline markings by hospitalized children and adolescents. *Research in Nursing & Health, 12,* 307–314.

Savedra, M.C., Tesler, M.D., Ward, J.A., Wegner, C., & Gibbons, P.T. (1981). Description of the pain experience: A study of school-age children. *Issues in Comprehensive Pediatric Nursing, 5,* 373–380.

Scott, R. (1978). "It hurts red": A preliminary study of children's perception of pain. *Perceptual and Motor Skills, 47,* 787–791.

Szyfelbein, S. K., Osgood, P. F., Atchison, N. E., & Carr, D. B. (1987). Variations in plasma beta-endorphin and cortisol levels in acutely burned children. *Pain (Suppl. 4),* S234.

Szyfelbein, S.K., Osgood, P.F., & Carr, D.B. (1985). The assessment of pain and plasma beta-endorphin immunoactivity in burned children. *Pain, 22,* 173–182.

Tesler, M.D., Ward, J.A., Savedra, M.C., Wegner, C., & Gibbons, P. (1983). Developing an instrument for eliciting children's description of pain. *Perceptual and Motor Skills, 56,* 315–321.

Thompson, S.C. (1981). Will it hurt less if I can control it? A complex answer to a simple question. *Psychological Bulletin, 90,* 89–101.

Tyler, D.C., & Krane, E.J. (Eds.). (1990). *Advances in pain research and therapy* (Vol. 15). New York: Raven Press.

Unruh, A., McGrath, P.J., Cunningham, S.J., & Humphreys, P. (1983). Children's drawings of their pain. *Pain, 17,* 385–392.

Vandvik, I.H., & Eckblad, G. (1990). Relationship between pain, disease severity and psychosocial function in patients with juvenile chronic arthritis (JCA). *Scandinavian Journal of Rheumatology, 19,* 295–302.

Varni, J.W., Thompson, K.L., & Hanson, V. (1987). The Varni/Thompson Pediatric Pain Questionnaire: I. Chronic musculoskeletal pain in juvenile rheumatoid arthritis. *Pain, 28,* 27–38.

von Graffenried, B., Adler, R., Abt, K., Nüesch, E., & Spiegel, R. (1978). The influence of anxiety and pain sensitivity on experimental pain in man. *Pain, 4,* 253–263.

Watkins, L.R., & Mayer, D.J. (1982). Organization of endogenous opiate and nonopiate pain control systems. *Science, 216,* 1185–1192.

Weisenberg, M. (1977). Pain and pain control. *Psychological Bulletin, 84,* 1008–1041.

Weisenberg, M. (1984). Cognitive aspects of pain. In P.D. Wall & R. Melzack (Eds.), *Textbook of pain* (pp. 162–172). Edinburgh: Churchill Livingstone.

Weisenberg, M., & Tursky, B. (1976). *Pain: New perspec-*

tives in therapy and research. New York: Plenum Press.

Whaley, L., & Wong, D.L. (1987). *Nursing care of infants and children*. St. Louis: Mosby.

Wilkie, D.J., Holzemer, W.L., Tesler, M.D., Ward, J.A., Paul, S.M., & Savedra, M.C. (1990). Measuring pain quality: Validity and reliability of children's and adolescents' pain language. *Pain, 41,* 151–159.

Zborowski, M. (1962). Cultural components in responses to pain. *Journal of Social Issues, 8,* 16–30.

Zeltzer, L., Regalado, M., Nichter, L.S., Barton, D., Jennings, S., & Pitt, L. (1991). Iontophoresis versus subcutaneous injection: A comparison of two methods of local anesthesia delivery in children. *Pain, 44,* 73–78.

Chapter 18

Assessment of Pain in the Elderly

STEPHEN W. HARKINS, PhD
DONALD D. PRICE, PhD

The content of "old age" is culturally determined. Its onset is not precisely definable in any given individual. Even with retirement options, there is no rite of passage or developmental event that marks transition from "late middle-age" to "old age." Unlike developmental stages earlier in life, particularly those under rather restricted genetic control, developmental events in the later years of life are highly variable and reflect the life history of the individual or the history of environmental events interacting with genetic factors. While aging actually begins at conception, the term is used frequently in English to refer to processes which begin at some later point in adult life. Technically, the term senescence should be used to refer to the biological changes of later life which increase the probability of death. "Senescence" is a process that is detrimental to the individual in that it is associated with decreased vitality. It is progressive, irreversible, and species specific.

One of the central challenges in the study of aging, per se, in the later years of adult life is differentiation of age dependent biological changes from chronic illnesses and disease processes, because the probability of chronic health problems increase with age. This distinction is often blurred and is confounded by the fact that definitions of "normal,"

"abnormal," and "successful" aging are often dependent upon the view of the writer. It is also unclear whether the increasing number of individuals who are surviving into the sixth, seventh, and eighth decades of life are indeed more healthy, as healthy, or less healthy than past generations of older individuals. Similar questions can be raised concerning quality of life in relation to pain. Recurrent and chronic pain are likely major sources of reduced quality of life and increased depression in the elderly.

Similar to the sociocultural determinants of what constitutes the content of "old age," the content of "pain" is strongly influenced by social history, cultural expectations, and individual differences. The human pain experience is not solely mediated by specific sensory processes but is strongly influenced by meaning of the pain to the individual and effectiveness of personal and social coping resources (Melzack & Wall, 1965; Price, 1988; Turk & Rudy, 1988). It is now recognized that the human pain experience is not solely due to sensory or nociceptive events but involves a complex interaction of sensory, affective, cognitive, and behavioral processes (Melzack & Wall, 1965) some of which are influenced not only by cultural background and sociocultural history (e.g., birth cohort) but also may be selectively or interactively influenced by chronological or physiological age.

Algerian sheep herders and Nepalese Porters, for example, are quite able to discriminate among painful cutaneous shocks, but are remarkably unwilling to label these shocks as "painful" (Clark & Clark, 1980). Beecher (1959) noted that different meanings of pain influenced requests for medication in wounded soldiers in battle compared to civilian surgical patients. Soldiers whose wounds permitted escape from battle tended to deny pain associated with even extensive wounds or reported so little pain that they did not require analgesics as frequently as civilian, postsurgical patients who actually had less tissue damage. Postsurgery, the civilians' requests for medication were strikingly more frequent than in the wounded soldiers whose wounds represented escape from combat.

> These data state in numerical terms what is known to all thoughtful clinical observers: There is no simple, direct relationship between the wound per se and the pain experienced. The pain is in a very large part determined by other factors, and of great importance here is the significance of the wound, i.e. reaction to the wound. (Beecher, 1959, p. 165)

Age, in the later years of life, likely influences the meaning of both old, recurrent pains as well as new pains. This possibility is relatively unexplored.

Pain is a symptom and can be a disease in its own right. It is a subjective experience that may be defined by a group or an individual as pathological, a source for concern and fear, and yet be seen by others as a relatively tolerable part of everyday adult life. Pains that are new in the middle aged individual but which have a long history in the older adult (e.g., osteoarthritis of some duration) may not differ in intensity but may well be associated with quite different levels of pain-related suffering and distress. More familiar pains (at least of this type) are likely to be associated with less emotional suffering and distress unless they produce limitations in activities of daily living.

In the face of the variability in the very concepts of the content of "old age" and of "pain" it is interesting that many lay individuals, as well as health care and allied health professions specialists, consider that old age is associated with a loss of pain sensibility and perception. The idea that the elderly person often displays decreased sensitivity to pain is ubiquitous. The misconception of significant loss of pain sensation with normal aging is, in part, based on inappropriate or poorly operationalized methods of assessment of what constitutes both "old age" and the human pain experience.

PRESBYALGOS AS A SENSORY PROCESS

If older adults experience pain as less intense than younger adults this might be termed "presbyalgos" (*Presby*—old; *Algos*—pain; Harkins, 1988; Harkins, Kwentus, and Price, 1990). Considering the magnitude of age related changes in vision and audition, it is not surprising that many individuals expect old age to be related to losses in the processes of nociception. Well-documented age-related changes do occur in vision, audition, olfaction, some skin senses, and some aspects of gustation. Presbycusis (*cusis*—hearing) and presbyopia (*opia*—vision) begin as subtle changes in the mid- to late 40s and early 50s. Presbycusis is associated with a loss of sensitivity for sound that is bilaterally symmetrical, progressive, irreversible, and greater for higher than lower frequencies. It is greater in men than women and is often associated with noise exposure history (see Olsho, Harkins, & Lenhardt, 1985). Presbyopia refers to a loss of accommodation, a decrease in near point vision, with increasing age and certain other changes including longer time for adaptation to light changes, decreased pupil size, and yellowing of the lens (see Kline & Schieber, 1985). Documented age related differences in olfaction include reduced sensitivity to odors and ability to identify odors (Doty, 1989) but not necessarily memory for odors (Wood & Harkins, 1987). Less stricking differences have been observed for age differences in taste sensitivity (Bartoshuk, et al., 1986; Bartoshuk, 1989). Older individuals are less able to identify certain food substances compared to younger individuals (Schiffman, 1977), and this may reflect impairment in retrieval of taste and odor names from long-term memory for tastes rather than loss of sensory processes. Age in the later years of life is also associated with an increase in threshold, but not dynamic response, of higher frequency mechanoreceptor and does not seem to influence low frequency receptors in the skin (Verillo, 1979).

Reasons to Expect Age Changes in Pain Perception

If age in the later years of life does produce a decrease in pain sensitivity, or presbyalgos, this could be due to multiple physiological processes. Older age may be associated with a decrease in nociceptor density and this could produce a decrease in sensitivity to noxious stimuli with increasing age, but no convincing evidence exists, to our knowledge, for lower numbers of these processes in older compared to younger adults. There also may be changes in central coding for pain with increasing age. Evidence exists that cerebral-evoked potentials to experimental pain (noxious laser stimulation) are reduced in amplitude and increased in latency in older compare to younger adults (Gibson, et al., 1991). Such findings might be interpreted as evidence that age dulls the senses of pain perception. Age differences in response to experimental pain does not, however, clearly support the presence of presbyalgos (Harkins & Warner, 1980).

Methodological Issues

The literature on age and pain is uniquely concerned with age differences and not age changes. All experimental and most clinical studies of pain in the later years of life are cross-sectional in design. There are no longitudinal studies of pain in adults. Cross sectional studies confound age at time of measure with birth cohort and, therefore, sociocultural history. Cross sectional studies measure groups of different ages at the same point in time and provides information on "age" differences. Age differences in pain perception assessed by cross-sectional study may well reflect response bias differences in labeling events as "pain." Elevated pain threshold, for example, in the old adult compared to the younger individual, might reflect a bias against reporting an event as painful. Several studies have reported that older individuals withhold responses in studies of sensory threshold in order to reduce uncertainty. Such cautiousness would produce artificially elevated pain thresholds. Similar biases likely influence report of clinical and chronic pain.

Research on effects of age on pain needs to give more explicit attention ot assessment of the multiple stages and dimensions of pain processing (cf. Price & Harkins, Chapter 8). In particular, consideration should be given as to whether age has effects on nociceptive sensory processing, the immediate unpleasantness that attends painful stimuli, cognitive processes related to more complex emotional responses associated with pain (i.e., suffering), behavioral expressions related to pain, and differences in meaning of specific acute, recurrent, and chronic pains across the life span. Study of these issues can be complicated by the problem that age is associated with illness producing cognitive impairment (i.e., dementia of the Alzheimer's type, multi-infarct dementia, parkinsonism) which influences ability to accurately report these various subjective dimensions of pain. The effects of age on the various dimensions of the human pain experience (Melzack, 1973) have yet to be systematically evaluated.

Demography: Some Brief Notes

The number of chronic health problems increases with age, and many of these problems are associated with discomfort, pain, and suffering. It has been argued that health problems in the elderly are being compressed more and more into the very last years of life (Fries, 1980; Fries, Green, & Levine, 1989), but this is questionable. It is more likely that the number of individuals with significant morbidity associated with pain is actually increasing. Estimates are that over 80% of individuals 65 years of age and older suffer from at least one major chronic health problem. Many of these health problems are associated with recurrent discomfort and pain. The level of unnecessary suffering in these individuals is not known.

If pain perception changes with age, that is, if presbyalgos exists, this would be of considerable importance because, as noted above, pain is a major symptom of numerous acute and chronic diseases. Knowledge of atypical symptom presentation in special patient populations is also of critical importance in the diagnostic process. The very nature of the increasing number of older adults requires attention to possible age effects on pain perception.

Preliminary data from the 1990 Census indicate that there are some 31.2 million persons 65 years of age and older in the United States. This represents approximately 12.6% of the total population. Individuals age 75 years of age and over number some 13 million (5.3% of the total population) and are the group most likely to suffer multiple chronic health problems and be in need of support services, including long-term care. In 1980 there were approximately 1.4 million persons in long-term care facilities, and this increased to some 1.8 million in 1990 (a 24.2% increase). Individuals over 75 are more likely to be "frail" and require support services. Recurrent and chronic pain in this segment of our population likely has a major impact on quality of life.

EXPERIMENTAL STUDY OF PAIN IN THE ELDERLY

It is unlikely that clinically significant age changes occur in sensory processes involved in pain perception in the vast majority of those 65 years of age and older. This statement is, however, open to question because laboratory studies of age differences in pain perception are somewhat ambiguous.

Pain in the Laboratory

Studies conducted in the controlled setting of the laboratory presumably permit inferences to be drawn concerning individual differences in pain perception. For the most part these psychophysical studies have focused on sensory-discriminative responses to nociceptive stimuli. Relatively simple and intuitively pleasing psychophysical endpoints, such as threshold and tolerance, or more complex procedures designed to measure accuracy of detection or discrimination (e.g., Sensory Decision Theory indices of accuracy and response bias) have been employed in the laboratory study of pain in the elderly. The results of these studies are important in that they influence thinking about how the older adults perceive a painful event, willingness to accept pain as a symptom in these individuals, and the manner in which clinical pain is managed in the old adult.

Table 18.1 summarizes a number of laboratory studies which contrast younger and older individuals' responses to experimental pain. As is apparent, the findings are contradictory. Among eleven studies using painful radiant- or contact-heat procedures, six report increased pain sensory thresholds and/or pain reaction thresholds in older adults that indicate an age-related decrease in pain sensitivity. Three

TABLE 18.1. Laboratory Studies of the Effect of Age on Psychophysical Indices of Pain Sensitivity

Stimulus	Source Reference	Psychophysical Endpoints and Findings
Thermal:		
Radiant heat	Schumacher et al. (1940)	Sensory thresholds *No age effects*
	Hardy et al. (1943)	Sensory thresholds *No age effects*
	Chapman & Jones (1944)	Sensory thresholds *Higher in elderly* Reaction thresholds *Higher in elderly*
	Chapman & Jones (1944)	Sensory thresholds *higher in elderly* Reaction thresholds *Higher in elderly*
	Birren et al. (1950)	Pain sensory thresholds *No age effects* Pain reaction thresholds *No age effects*
	Sherman & Robillard (1964a, 1964b)	Sensory thresholds *Higher in elderly* Reaction thresholds *Higher in elderly*
	Procacci et al. (1970, 1974)	Sensory thresholds *Higher in elderly*[a]
	Clark & Mehl (1971)	Sensory thresholds *Higher in 55-year-olds compared to younger adults*
Contact heat	Kenshalo (1986)	Sensory thresholds *No age effects*
	Harkins, Price, & Braith (1989)	Magnitude matching *Slight age effects*[a]
Electrical shock:		
Cutaneous	Collins & Stone (1966)	Sensory threshold *Lower in elderly* Tolerance *Lower in elderly*
	Tucker et al. (1989)	Sensory threshold *Higher in elderly*
Tooth	Mumford (1965)	Sensory threshold *No age effects*
	Mumford (1968)	Sensory threshold *No age effects*

(continued)

TABLE 18.1. *(Continued)*

Stimulus	Source Reference	Psychophysical End- points and Findings
	Harkins & Chapman (1976)	Sensory threshold *No age effects* Discrimination accuracy *Lower in elderly* Response bias (criteria) *Age effects: Variable*
	Harkins & Chapman (1977a)	Sensory threshold *No age effects* Discrimination accuracy *Lower in elderly* Response bais (criteria) *Age effects: Variable*
Pressure:		
Achilles tendon	Woodrow et al. (1972)	Tolerance *Lower in elderly*
Cold: pressor	Walsh et al. (1989)	Tolerance (time) Males: *Lower with increasing age* Females: *Minimal increase with increasing age*

[a]See text and Figure 18.1.

additional studies using radiant heat report no age differences. One study employing contact heat reported some age effects, but these effects, although statistically significant, were so slight as to be considered clinically nonsignificant. One other study employing contact heat stimuli reported no age differences (see Table 18.1).

Three studies employing tooth shock indicate no age difference in pain threshold. One study employing cutaneous shock found lower pain sensory threshold and lower pain tolerance in older individuals. Another study, using pressure delivered to the Achilles tendon reported lower pain tolerance in older compared to younger individuals. These latter two studies suggest greater pain sensitivity (or wisdom) in the older compared to younger adult.

Thus, the psychophysical studies of age differences in pain intensity perceptions are ambiguous; some indicate an age-associated decrease in sensitivity to pain; some indicate no

age effects; several indicate increased sensitivity to pain in the laboratory with advancing age. Such results, likely, reflect errors in conceptualization of age as a variable in pain research and the facts that different psychophysical procedures and endpoints, as well as different techniques for pain induction in the laboratory, measure different phenomena. As we have previously suggested, the variability among results in the experimental studies of age difference in pain measured in the laboratory is the results of differences in means use to induce pain, differences in the psychophysical procedures used, as well as differences in criteria used for subject inclusion and screening (Harkins, 1988; Harkins et al., 1990; Harkins & Warner, 1988).

In two studies employing discrimination of very mild, painful electrical shocks delivered to teeth, we reported that elderly subjects were less accurate than younger individuals in discriminating between the shocks. In these studies two shocks slightly greater than pain threshold were delivered to healthy unfilled teeth. Subjects were not told that there were only two shocks. Responses were made on a six-point response scale ranging from "nothing" to "moderate pain" and reaction times were recorded. There were no age differences in reaction time, indicating the elderly had sufficient time to formulate their responses. Table 18.2 summarizes partial results of these studies (Harkins & Chapman, 1976, 1977a, 1977b).

Age groups did not differ on pain threshold.

TABLE 18.2. Summary of Results of Two Studies of Age Differences in Pain Perception[a]

	Age	Threshold (μA)	Discrimination ability
Young ($n = 20$) (SD)	22.9 2.3	7.1 4.3	1.21 0.53
Elderly ($n = 20$) (SD)	67.3 16.8	8.0 5.8	0.62 0.39
t-test ($df = 1,38$)		0.61	4.05[b]

[a]Stimuli were two electrical shocks delivered to healthy, unfilled teeth. Shocks were set to be slightly above pain threshold (low shock at 1 μA and higher shock at 3 μA above threshold). Young and elderly groups were composed of 10 men and 10 women each.
[b]$p < .01$.

They did, however, differ on ability to discriminate between the two tooth shocks. The index of discrimination ability in Table 18.2 is based on Sensory Decision Theory (SDT), a psychophysical procedure useful in studies of detection and discrimination. SDT assumes that the observer's threshold is never absolute and that discrimination between two suprathreshold stimuli is probabilistic. In the present case, the results indicate that the elderly are less accurate in discriminating between the two shocks than are the younger individuals. These results were interpreted to reflect an age related deficit in processing nociceptive events (Harkins & Chapman, 1976, 1977b). This was suggested to be central rather than peripheral because the age groups did not differ on pain threshold.

In these studies subjects responded on a 6-point rating scale after each tooth shock. Proper controls were performed so that a warning stimulus was presented and, as noted, ample time was given in which to respond so that the older individuals were not under a time pressure. An important fact, however, is that the requirement of decisions on a 6-point rating scale requires considerable memory for the sensory intensity of prior stimuli and memory for the prior rating of the perceived intensity, making the task a rather difficult procedure with considerable time delay between prior events to be "matched" on the rating scale. Individuals who do not accurately remember the category used to rate a stimulus of a given sensory intensity will have a reduction in their measure of sensory discrimination. As a result of cognitive factors, they will appear, in this type of task, to have reduced ability to discriminate between noxious stimuli. Such an age related difference in discrimination accuracy would likely reflect age differences in "fluid" cognitive facilities as much as age differences in pain sensitivity. Fluid cognitive capacity is well documented as decreasing with increasing age (Labouvie-Vief, 1985).

Task demands can place the older adult at a distinct disadvantage compared to the younger individual in laboratory experiments. The results in Table 18.2 likely reflect age differences in ability to accurately perform a complex and lengthy psychophysical task that included numerous factors in addition to perception and report of nociceptive stimuli (Coppola & Gracely, 1983; Gracely, 1989).

There is no "ideal" or best method for assessment of pain in the laboratory or for that matter in the clinic. When the objective is to determine individuals' differences in pain sensitivity and performance abilities, it is likely that the simpler the demand of the experimental task, the better. The cold pressor task which evaluates tolerance to pain resulting from immersion of a limb in cold water has minimal performance demand on the subject. Walsh, Schoenfeld, Ramamurthy and Hoffman (1989) noted that increasing age was associated with *lower* cold presser tolerance in males but slight increases in females (see Table 18.1).

In a study employing six levels of contact thermal stimuli and direct magnitude estimation procedures, Harkins, Price, and Martelli (1986) reported minimal effects of age on pain ratings of intensity and unpleasantness. The contact heat stimuli were from 43°C to 51°C pulses presented to the ventral surface of the forearm. The stimuli lasted for 5 seconds from the adapting baseline of 34°C. Each of the six temperatures were presented twice in two separate sessions. In one session, subjects were instructed to rate the sensory intensity of heat pulses on a 150-cm Visual Analogue Scale (VAS) labeled "no sensation" on the leftmost endpoint and "the most intense sensation imaginable" on the rightmost endpoint of the scale. In separate sessions the subject was instructed to rate the unpleasantness of the heat pulses on VASs labeled "not bad at all" (left endpoint) and "the most intense bad feeling imaginable" (right endpoint). Considerable effort was taken to instruct the subjects with regard to the procedures as well as to the differences between the pain intensity and unpleasantness rating dimensions. Partial results from this study are shown in Figure 18.1.

As shown in Figure 18.1 the young ($n = 21$; mean age 25), middle aged ($n = 10$; mean age 53), and the elderly ($n = 13$; mean age 72) produced magnitude estimation ratings on VASs for the intensity of the contact heat stimuli that are quite similar. A significant age by temperature interaction was observed for several intensities, and this was due to the oldest group rating some lower temperatures as less intense and some higher temperatures as more intense compared to the younger groups. Visual inspection of the data in Figure 18.1, however, shows that the age by stimulus intensity interaction is a weak effect. It accounted

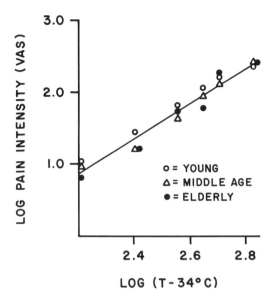

FIGURE 18.1. Psychophysical functions for intensity of contact heat pulses (43 to 51°C; 5-sec duration; from an adapting temperature of 34°C) plotted against VAS ratings of pain intensity in healthy young (mean age 25), middle-age (mean age 53) and older (mean age 73 years) volunteers. When plotted in base *e* log–log coordinates, the points are well fit by a single regression line for all three groups of subjects. The results indicate that age groups are more similar than different for intensity ratings of nociceptive heat pulses delivered to volar surface of the forearm. From Harkins, Price, and Martelli (1986). Copyright 1986 The Gerontological Society of America. Reprinted by permission.

for less than 1% of the variability in pain ratings and is not likely of a magnitude to be significant in how pain presents as a clinical symptom.

The direct scaling procedures employed in the study shown in Figure 18.1 offers a methodological advantage in that the rating is of the stimulus at the time of stimulation (see Price and Harkins, Chapter 8). There are only minimal performance and intellectual burdens placed on the participants. The results shown in Figure 18.1 have been successfully replicated by others (Kenshalo, 1986).

Many of the studies summarized in Table 18.1 suffer from one or more conceptual or methodological limitations. They present no evidence for age changes, only results suggestive of age differences. They confound age at time of measures with birth cohort effects. They suffer from poor specification of subject selection procedures and criteria, and provide

scant information on instructions and training procedures. Most suffer from small numbers of subjects and questionable psychophysical endpoints.

Nevertheless, a simple tally of the findings of the studies summarized in Table 18.1 indicates that most of the studies support no or slight age differences in pain perception (ten studies). Five indicate elevated threshold in older participants, and one found elevated threshold in middle-aged individuals (Clark & Mehl, 1971). Interestingly, several studies observed *reduced* tolerance in the elderly for cutaneous shock (Collins & Stone, 1966), pressure (Woodrow, Friedman, Siegelaub, & Collen, 1972), and cold pressor pain (Walsh et al., 1989).

How we interpret these experimental studies is important. As noted above, results of experimental studies influence our thinking of pain as a symptom, its role in diagnostic assessment, and how we proceed with treatment. The studies summarized (Table 18.1) indicate that *age in the later years of life likely does not result in a clinically significant decrease in pain perception* in older individuals physically and mentally able to find their way to the laboratory (or the pain clinic). This may not be true of frail older adults presenting with atypical symptoms at the Emergency Room or in the primary care clinic for that matter. Other factors may influence the accuracy of pain assessment in the acutely ill or demented older individual, and clinical assessment of pain in the geriatric patient with atypical symptom presentation presents a diagnostic challenge. But age, per se, as a biological phenomenon, appears to have essentially no impact on the sensory or perceived unpleasantness of pain and this contrasts strikingly with the well-documented changes in most sensory systems as discussed above. This is not to suggest that pain in the elderly is not associated with significant physical, social, and psychological morbidity. In fact, the limited information available on recurrent, persistent, and chronic pain prevalence suggests that pain is a major source of unnecessary suffering and limitation in activities of daily living in the elderly.

Pain Prevalence in the Elderly

Population based studies indicate that pain occurs with considerable frequency in older adults. The experimental studies of pain in the laboratory, although somewhat contradictory, indicate that age in the later years of life is not a major factor reducing pain sensibility. That is, age is not an analgesic. Studies of prevalence of pain in various surveys indicate, as might be expected, an increase in recurrent or persistent pain in older adults (Valkenburg, 1988). Crook, Rideout and Browne (1984), in a telephone survey of 372 families, found that morbidity rate for persistent pain increased with age, and persons with persistent pain used health care services (as indicated by both increased physician and hospital visits) more frequently than did those with acute (temporary) pain. In their study, Crook, et al (1984) define "persistent" pain as pain that often was troublesome and that occurred within the past 2 weeks. Pain that was not often troublesome but that had occurred in the past 2 weeks was defined as "temporary." Interestingly, some individuals viewed recurrent pain problems (e.g., arthritis) as temporary, not as episodes of a persistent or chronic condition. Crook et al. (1984) computed age-specific morbidity rates for persistent pain. The overall estimate was 139 cases of persistent pain per 1,000 population independent of age. Rates were age dependent as shown in Figure 18.2. Persistent pain was estimated at 76 per 1,000 in individuals between 10 and 30 years of age and increased to 400 per 1,000 in those over 81 years of age. Origin of pain was unknown or spontaneous in onset in approximately 70% of the sample and was associated with an accident in 26% of those

reporting persistent pain. Further, parental history for persistent pain was positive in 60% of those reporting persistent pain.

In a survey of 3,097 rural individuals 65 years of age and older, Lavsky-Shulan et al. (1985) found that low back pain was reported by approximately 24 percent of the women and 18 percent of the men in the study. Report of low back pain decreased with increasing age in both men and women, likely reflecting increased mortality and institutionalization rates with increasing age in this older sample. Pain may be an unrecognized factor related to mortality and increased likelihood of admission to long-term care facilities in the elderly. Presence of low back pain was also associated with reductions in physical activities. While several indices of activities of daily living have been shown to be reliable and valid for use with the geriatric population, there is no such index for identification of pain specific limitations in activities of daily living.

The Nuprin Pain Report (Sternbach, 1986) involved a telephone survey similar to that of Crook et al. (1984) and evaluated pain in a representative sample of the adult population of the continental United States. Information on prevalence and severity of different kinds of pain was evaluated in 1,254 persons, 179 of whom were 65 years of age and older. Younger adults were more likely than older adults to report experiencing pain associated with headaches, backaches, muscles, stomach, and teeth.

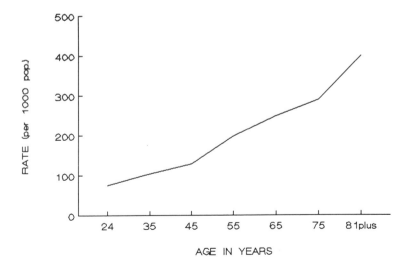

FIGURE 18.2. Rates of "persistent" pain in a telephone survey of community dwelling individuals. Note the increase in prevalence of persistent pain problems with increasing age. (Persistent pain was defined as a pain that was often troublesome and that had occurred during the past two weeks.) Based on data presented in Crook et al. (1984).

Some 71 percent of those 65 and above reported joint pain, whereas 41 percent of those 18 to 24 reported such pain as present.

Harkins (1988) presented data summarized from some 88,000 patients making approximately 500,000 visits to five family practice sites in the Commonwealth of Virginia (Marsland, Wood, & Mayo, 1976). Medical visits associated with conditions likely to be accompanied by significant pain such as arthritis, angina of effort, and fractures of the spine, pelvis, and ribs increased with age. Pain conditions typically evaluated at the multidisciplinary pain clinic, such as headaches and back pain, peaked in the 3rd and 4th decades and decreased with increasing age.

Information on musculoskeletal pain in relation to age is available in the National Health and Nutrition Examination Survey: Follow-up Survey of 1982–1984 which sampled the noninstitutionalized population of the United States. This survey included information on musculoskeletal pain problems in individuals between the ages of 32 and 86. Table 18.3 presents the percentage of individuals reporting significant musculoskeletal pain during the week prior to the interview. Interestingly, the relative percentages, although lowest (36%) in the youngest group (mean age 36.8 years) and highest in the oldest group (54% of those with a mean age 81.8 years), are quite similar in the middle years to the later years of life. The nature of the questions asked influences these types of survey results, and it is likely that the type of musculoskeletal pain problem is age sensitive but this is not apparent in this particular analysis of these data.

In this survey, individuals with pain were

TABLE 18.3. Percentage of Individuals Reporting Musculoskeletal Pain During Past Week and VAS Pain Ratings for Various Age Groups

Age	SD	N	Percentage reporting pain (%)	Percentage reporting pain (N)	Pain VAS Ratings
36.8	1.7	13.92	36	(502)	26.6
44.4	2.9	2312	42	(981)	29.5
54.2	2.9	2030	48	(979)	33.8
64.2	2.8	1512	51	(777)	35.5
75.2	2.8	1573	50	(779)	35.7
81.8	1.6	622	54	(337)	37.8

Note. From National Center for Health Statistics, NHANES Follow-Up Survey (1982–1984). Original tabulations from public use tapes.

also asked to rate the intensity of their pain over the past week on a VAS. These VAS pain ratings are shown for each of the age groups in Table 18.3. Pain-VAS ratings increased with increasing age, suggesting that musculoskeletal pain increases in severity, as well as frequency, with increasing age. The high frequency of such pain in the older segment of our population suggests that persistent, recurrent, and chronic pain may represent significant assessment and treatment challenges in the elderly.

CHRONIC PAIN AND AGE

Chronic pain is likely quite similar in most respects in both younger and older adults. Nevertheless, the older segments of our population are underrepresented in utilization of the expertise present in multidisciplinary pain clinics. Figure 18.3 presents the age distribution for 174 consecutive patients evaluated and treated at a multidisciplinary pain clinic. Less than 8% of the sample exceeded 65 years of age and the older-elderly, those in their late 70s or older, were essentially absent from this clinic sample. Informal surveys of pain clinics suggest that the age distribution illustrated in Figure 18.3 is not atypical.

The "old-old" in our population are increasing the most percentagewise and have the greatest risk of chronic health problems, many

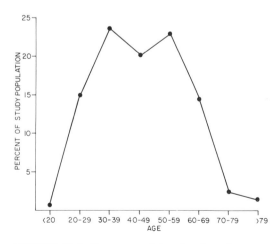

FIGURE 18.3. Percentage of chronic pain patients as a function of age who were evaluated and treated at a multidisciplinary chronic pain clinic in an 18 month period. From Harkins, Kwentus, and Price (1984). Copyright 1984 Raven Press. Reprinted by permission.

of which are associated with significant pain and suffering. The old-old are characterized as those in their mid-70s and older, many of whom are frail and require aid in activities of daily living and supportive services for health reasons. The rather striking absence of our oldest adults in the clinics best equipped to reduce unnecessary pain and suffering may reflect a number of prejudices and myths. Included is acceptance of pain on the part of the older individual. The myth that pain is a normal consequence of growing older is a powerful force. Furthermore, the health care delivery system suffers from varying degrees of frank ageism and ignorance resulting in a referral bias against the older adult. In fact, there is no convincing evidence that age, per se, in the later years of life is a factor in treatment outcome for most older pain patients, although some have suggested that age is the major predictor of treatment outcome for certain conditions (Graff-Radford & Nalibof 1988). It is likely that age per se is not the major factor in outcome in such cases. Rather, poor treatment outcome will be correlated with comorbidity and frailty. In the oldest-old, those who are active, vital, and otherwise basically healthy, treatment for pain is likely to be as positive as in younger-old adults (Keefe & Williams, 1990; Middaugh, Levin, Lee, Barchie, & Roberts, 1988; Puder, 1988; Sorkin, Rudy, Hanlon, Turk, & Stieg, 1990).

Only a few studies to date have evaluated chronic pain in older patients. In general, the results indicate more similarities than differences. Tait, Chibnall, and Margolis (1990) report no relation between "extent" of chronic pain and age. They define pain extent in terms of body area reported as painful. Sorkin et al. (1990) report that differences appear less important than similarities in chronic pain patients who are old (mean age of 72.5) versus those who are younger (mean age of 27.7 years). This parallels the conclusion of Harkins et al. (1986) with regard to the effects of age on report of experimental pain. Sorkin et al. found no differences in acceptance of treatment by older, chronic pain patients or dropout rates compared to younger patients. Older patients were found to have a lower ratio of cognitive to physical coping skills but no difference in use of prescription analgesics compared to younger patients.

Sorkin et al. (1990) also observed no age group differences on subscales of the West Haven–Yale Multidimensional Pain Inventory (MPI) (Kerns, Turk, & Rudy, 1985; see also Kerns & Jacobs, Chapter 14) or the Pain Experience Scale (PES) (Turk & Rudy, 1988). Moreover, patient groups did not differ on depression as assessed by the Center for Epidemiology Studies Depression Scale (CES-D) (Radloff, 1977), although the depression scores were elevated in both the elderly (mean score of 27.7) and the younger pain patients (mean 24.3). These scores are indicative of significant potential depression in both groups, and this finding is particularly interesting because emerging information, as discussed below, indicates that pain may be a major source of depression, limitation of activities, and psychosocial morbidity in older individuals.

Sorkin et al. (1990) concluded that there is no support from their studies to suggest "that older age should be viewed as a contraindication for multidisciplinary pain management despite negative [age] stereotypes and greater physical pathology" (p. P67) in older compared to younger pain patients. Middaugh et al. (1988) support their conclusion. They also present evidence that older and younger chronic pain patients are quite similar. They evaluated patients' responses to a multidisciplinary chronic pain rehabilitation program. They assessed multiple indices that were likely to be related to pain, including ratings of pain intensity, health-care utilization, activity tolerance, medication usage, somatization, depression and anxiety. At initial evaluation, the older group ($n = 17$; ages 55 to 78) evidenced greater health-care utilization (four times greater) and higher medication use (about two times greater) than in younger patients ($n = 20$; 29 to 48 years of age. At posttreatment follow up (approximately 1 yr), the older group benefited as much or more than the younger group on most of the responses dimensions assessed at entry into the study. Similar positive treatment results in older chronic pain patients were reported by Puder (1988). In an evaluation of a 10-week cognitive-behavioral group therapy program for chronic pain, Puder (1988) studied 69 patients who ranged in age from 27 to 80 years. Treatment resulted in a decrease in the impact of pain on activities and use of medications as well as an increase in ability to cope with pain. Age, per se, was not related to treatment outcome.

Sorkin et al. (1990) also found no age differences in pain severity based on the MPI Pain

Severity index. In our own analysis of this issue, we have observed no statistically significant adult age differences in report of either intensity or unpleasantness of chronic pain as measured by VAS ratings in a pilot study. These results are shown in Figure 18.4. Pain intensity (sensory) is plotted in this figure on the *x* axis and unpleasantness is plotted on the *y*-axis. Individuals were requested to rate the intensity and the unpleasantness of their chronic pain at its lowest, usual, and highest levels over the past week. While there was a tendency for the older group (mean age 69; age range 59 to 79 years of age) to rate their chronic pain as less intense than the younger group (mean age 37; age range 26 to 50 years) these differences were not significant. Similarly, there was a tendency for the elderly to report their pain as less unpleasant, but again these rating differences for pain as its lowest, usual, or highest were not significantly different from younger individuals.

Further study is required to determine if the lack of statistical significance between the age groups is due to the small sample sizes resulting in a Type II error. More importantly, however, is the fact that young and elderly chronic pain patients are consistent in their ratings of pain intensity relative to pain unpleasantness on the

VASs. Thus, ratings of chronic pain by both groups fall on the similar regression lines for the sensory-affective relationship. These preliminary data of ratings of chronic pain in older pain patients combined with the VAS ratings of experimental pain shown in Figure 18.1 indicate that direct magnitude scaling procedures are likely to be valuable tools for pain assessment in the noncognitively impaired elderly pain patients.

VAS ratings were also made by these patients of their emotions related to the chronic pain problem. These emotion or pain-related mood ratings are shown in Figure 18.5. Younger patients experienced greater negative emotions associated with their chronic pain compared to

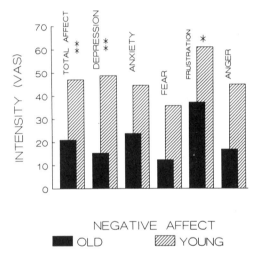

FIGURE 18.5. Ratings of pain related emotions in chronic pain patients. Old and young chronic pain patients (as in Figure 18.4) rated the level of depression, anxiety, frustration, anger, and fear specifically associated with their pain problem. Age groups differed on total negative affectivity (Total Affect; average of the five individual pain moods) and on the individual ratings of depression and frustration related to their chronic pain. Ratings were made on 150-mm visual analogue scales (VASs) for each emotion. VASs were labeled "No depression" (or fear, etc.) on the left end of the scale and "The most extreme depression imaginable" (or other emotion) on the right most end. Care was taken to ensure that individuals were rating their emotions specifically related to their chronic pain problem. These results indicate that domain specific affect related to chronic pain may differ with chronological age in adults and this likely is due to age differences in birth cohort (and therefore psychological and social history) and expectations. These differences in negative affectivity specifically related to chronic pain are not likely due to age differences in quantity or quality of the chronic pain.

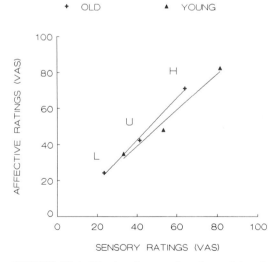

FIGURE 18.4. Visual analogue scale ratings of chronic pain sensory intensity and unpleasantness in young (mean age 37) and elderly (mean age 69) patients. Sensory intensity ratings are plotted on the *x*-axis against unpleasantness ratings plotted on the *y*-axis. Pain ratings are for chronic pain at its lowest (L), usual (U), and highest (H) over the past week. No significant group differences were observed.

older patients. The reduced level of pain-related negative affect in the elderly compared to the younger patients may reflect the lower levels of pain seen in Figure 18.4 for the older patients. Even though not statistically significant, the group differences in pain sensory intensity and unpleasantness ratings (shown in Figure 18.4) may have a disproportional effect and explain the group differences in pain-related suffering as seen in Figure 18.5. Alternatively it is possible that chronic pain has different meanings to the two groups resulting in different levels of "suffering" reflecting, in part, age group differences in prior pain experiences, expectations, and response biases.

In summary, it appears that pain intensity and unpleasantness are quite similar for both younger and older chronic pain patients but that chronic related emotions and suffering are more intense in the latter.

CHRONIC PAIN AND DEPRESSION IN OLDER ADULTS

The results presents in Figure 18.5 should not be overinterpreted. They are based on a study specifically designed to screen subjects for affective disorders. Care was taken to include only patients judged on the basis of scores on personality inventories and psychiatric examination to be free from affective disorder. Such a sample is biased and is not likely to be representative of the adult chronic pain population at large. The lower negative affectivity in older pain patients compared to younger patients shown in Figure 18.5 is not consistent with the findings of Sorkin et al. (1990), who employed the MPI (Kerns, Turk, and Rudy, 1985) and observed that elderly chronic pain patients did not differ from younger chronic pain patients on any dimension of the MPI affective distress and interference. Sorkin et al.'s patients, however, appeared to be moderately to severely depressed, and this could account for the differences from findings illustrated in Figure 18.5. The relation among depression and pain in the later years of life has yet to be adequately evaluated, and it is therefore highly recommended that history of affective disorder and current affective state be assessed concurrently with pain assessment in the geriatric pain patient. Some evidence exists that pain is a powerful moderator of both decreased positive affect, increased depression, and reduced activities of daily living in older individuals. Moss, Cawton, and Glicksman (1991) found that pain 1 year, 6 months, and 1 month prior to death was the major factor in determining presence and level of depression in older adults.

In residential, long-term care facilities for the elderly, only a few studies have attempted to evaluate the effects of pain on depression, activities of daily living, or psychosocial impairment. The nursing home population represents a particularly challenging opportunity for gerontological research in general and for evaluations of the impact of pain and pain control methods on quality of life in the older adult. In these settings particular attention must be paid to the mental status of the resident and the limitations on quantitative assessment due to cognitive impairment.

Currently some 50 to 60% of older residents in nursing homes and long-term care settings suffer some form of progressive dementia, the most frequent being dementia of the Alzheimer's type. Stroke related cognitive impairments (multi-infarct dementia) represent the second most frequent form of dementia in the elderly. The impact of progressive dementia on accuracy of symptom report represents a major challenge for pain assessment and management. No systematic studies of pain in the cognitively impaired older adult exist. Indeed, no systematic studies of pain in residents in long-term care facilities and nursing homes exist. Although there are no systematic studies of pain in the long-term care setting, several recent surveys indicate that pain is a major source of suffering, limitation of activities, depression, and psychological morbidity in nursing home residents. Roy and Thomas (1986) report that 87% of 132 elderly residents in a nursing home ($n = 97$) or from a day care program for the elderly ($n = 35$) reported having a problem with pain. A significant positive relationship between depression and pain intensity was observed in both samples. While a large percentage (84%) of those reporting pain were receiving analgesics, the authors suggest that there is an inclination to underestimate pain prevalence, its intensity, and its impact on the older nursing home resident. In all probability, pain complaints in the elderly, particularly those in long-term care settings, are frequently viewed by staff as efforts to gain attention or somatic expressions of depression. This is unfortunate.

The view of pain presenting as a symptom of

masked depression has been questioned and largely discredited (Feinman, 1985). It may well be that a significant amount of depression and restriction in daily physical and social activities in the nursing home resident and the older adult in the community may be due to pain. Parmelee, Katz and Lawton (1991) also observed a significant relation between pain and depression in nursing home residents. Greater pain was associated with greater levels of depressive symptoms.

In a sample of 133 middle-aged and elderly persons (apparently community dwelling individuals) Williams and Schulz (1988) found that level of depression was directly related to pain severity even after controlling for income, social support, physical dependency, and age. They imply the causal relation is that of pain influencing symptoms of depression and not pain as a symptom of masked depression.

Ferrel, Ferrell, and Osterweil (1990) point out that pain is understudied in geriatric medicine in general and this is particularly true in the nursing home setting. In an evaluation of 97 nursing home residents they report that approximately 71% suffer from at least one pain, a figure similar to that reported by Roy and Thomas (1986). Of those with pain, 34% reported it as continuous and 66% as intermittent. Cause of pain included low back (40%), arthritis of appendicular joints (24%), pain associated with a previous fracture (14%), and neuropathies (11). However, they found little correlation between pain, depression, mental status, or basic activities of daily living. This finding is consistent with a pilot study we recently conducted in which no relation was observed between depression (scores on the CES-D, Radloff, 1977) and the McGill Present Pain Intensity scale in 19 residents in a veterans medical center long-term care facility. Thus, it appears that the relations among presence of chronic pain, its severity, depression, and impact on activities of daily living and social activities are unclear for both ambulatory, community-dwelling elderly, and residents in long-term care facilities. Development of appropriate pain assessment instruments for this population is necessary. This will require sensitivity, creativity, and perseverance to clarify the nature of the impact of pain in the later years of life on quality of life. Such information will act to reduce suffering, decrease morbidity, and increase quality of life for many older individuals currently untreated or inappropri-

ately treated for chronic and recurrent painful conditions.

TREATMENT OF GERIATRIC CHRONIC PAIN

Pain assessment, not treatment, is the major focus of this chapter. Treatment without accurate assessment is doomed to failure at best and iatrogenic consequences at worse. In treatment planning for the geriatric pain patient attention must be focused not only on age-related changes in pharmacodynamics and kinetics of analgesics but also on coexisting health problems and medication usage. Aggressive intervention and treatment of long-standing pain problems in the frail elderly individual may be more detrimental to the patient than the pain. Fortunately, age changes in pharmacokinetics and dynamics of analgesics are fairly well identified (see Harkins et al., 1990). Table 18.4 summarizes some aspects of pharmacological management of pain in the geriatric patient. Management of specific painful conditions as well as description of atypical presentation of pain as a symptom in acute disorders has increasingly been the subject of topical reviews in the geriatric literature (see recent issues of the *Journal of the American Geriatrics Society, Geriatrics,* and similar clinical journals).

Clinics designed specifically to address the unique needs of the geriatric pain patient population are needed and will likely emerge as this need is recognized. Such clinics would also serve as a resource for education, diagnosis, and treatment of atypical pain symptom presentation in the acutely ill elderly patient as well as a site for treatment of recurrent and chronic pain in the elderly. Such a clinic needs to be multidisciplinary in nature with clinical expertise in pain management and in geriatrics. The model for such a clinic has been described by Helme, Katz, Neufeld, Lachal, and Corran (1989). They describe a multidisciplinary pain management clinic specifically directed for the geriatric population that was established in 1986 in Melbourne. Based on review of their first 100 cases, they report a 50% improvement in their elderly pain patients. The authors note that

the recognition of multiple pathology influences management decision, the particular limitations and side-effects of drugs used in this age group, and the need to consider the contribution of

TABLE 18.4. Drugs Used in Treatment of Pain in the Elderly[a]

Drug	Dosage Considerations	Adverse Effect in the Elderly	Special Characteristics
Narcotic analgesic	Reduce dosage in elderly to ½–¼ that of younger patients	Nausea, vomiting, urinary retention Respiratory depression with excessive doses, especially in patients with COPD or sleep apnea	More useful for acute pain than chronic pain and for moderate to severe pain not responsive to nonnarcotic analgesics
	Clearance reduced in elderly	Constipation more frequent in elderly; bowel regime needed concurrently	More useful for dull pain than for sharp or colicky pain
	Fixed time interval preferred to ad lib or PRN dosing	Mood alterations, psychomimetic effects and delerium more frequent; sedation but later tolerance	PCA dosing home infusion for terminal pain
Antidepressants	Low doses to avoid side effects	In elderly, constipation/postural hypotension/urinary retention more frequent; more sensitive to anticholinergic effects, delerium conduction/arryth cardiovascular effects as well as sedation, drowsiness OD potential, ↓ seiz. threshold	Drug of choice for chronic deafferentation pain Amitriptyline and trazodone have independent analgesic action useful in nondepression patients Relief in days
Carbamazepine	100 mg bid, increase very slowly to tolerance (max 800 mg/day)	Nausea, vomiting or sedation may limit compliance, ataxia, lethargy, confusion Bone marrow (very rare) depression, hepatic failure, rash (can be SJ), CNS depression may limit use	Effective for trigeminal neuralgia and for denervation neuropathy
Mixed Agonists/ Antagonists	Dezocine Nubain Butorphanol Pentazocine Nalbuphine	Psychomimetic effects including hallucinations, vivid dreams	Never give to patients getting opiate agonists or will displace pure agonists from muricytos and lead to withdrawal
Benzodiazepines	Increased half life in the elderly. Lorazepam and Oxazepam have shorter half lives and are easily metabolized by elderly.	Sedation, drowsiness and decreased cognitive performance may persist for some time after drugs are withdrawn. Amnestic effects	Education and counseling should be preferred means of reducing anxiety. More useful in patients with musculoskeletal pain. May paradoxically increase pain in some
Nonsteroidal Anti-inflammatories	Higher serum levels in elderly because of lowered albumin binding	Salt and water retention GI bleeding Allergic reactions Blood dyscrasia platelet dysfunction Renal dysfunction	Should be administered with meals. Should be monitored in patients who are anticoagulated. Since ibupropen and aspirin are nonprescription, patients should be cautioned against excess use
Toradol (Ketorolac)	First IV/IM NSAID	Same as above	Many drug interactions. Especially good in bone pain
Phenothiazine	Low doses for pain Questionable efficacy? Over-sedation generally the most common reason for pain relief.	Sedation Constipation Orthostasis Urinary retention Tardive dyskinesia Extrapyramidal syndromes	Denervation pain Thalamic pain Synergistic with antidepressants Tardive dyskinesia a special risk in elderly

(continued)

TABLE 18.4. *(Continued)*

Drug	Dosage Considerations	Adverse Effect in the Elderly	Special Characteristics
Corticosteroids	Use in dose required to treat underlying medical condition (i.e. arthritis, polymyalgia rheumatica, etc.) QOD dosing, best for decreased SE's if possible	Osteoporosis Hypothalamic-pituitary suppression Decreased resistance to infection Diabetes mellitus NA/H_2O retention Myopathy GI upset Euphoric mood	Not to be used for symptomatic treatment but as needed for medical indication For cancer pain—lyse tumor cells and relieve nerve and spinal cord compression secondary to tumors Produce euphoria and increased appetite
Topical ointment capsaicin	Two strengths (1) 0.025% for post-herpetic neuralgia (2) 0.075% for diabetic neuropathy pain Apply 4 times/day Delayed effect (up to six weeks)	Burning sensation	Benefits in 70–80% of patients for post-herpetic neuralgia Modifies substance P, resulting in decreased nociceptive input to cord

*a*Modified from Harkins, Kwentus, and Price (1990).

home, social and family factors in the management plan make the pain clinic for the elderly a particularly useful recourse for the practicing physician. (p. 30)

The geriatric pain clinic is an idea whose time has come and Dr. Helme, Director of the National Research Institute of Gerontology and Geriatric Medicine of Australia, and associates have recognized this need.

The importance of the multidisciplinary approach is particularly clear in assessment of pain in the older adults with a cognitive impairment. It has been suggested that organic brain syndrome or dementia can contribute significantly to the pain experience in the older adults. That is, pain may be the presenting symptoms in older patients with dementia (Hendler, 1981). There is conflicting evidence, however, of a direct link between dementia and pain in the elderly (Taylor, Mailis, Vanderlinden, & Shoichet, 1988). It is likely, due to a lack of understanding of how to assess pain in individuals with memory disorders associated with illnesses such as dementia of the Alzheimer's type, and that many older cognitively impaired individuals experience unnecessary pain and suffering. The multidisciplinary geriatric pain clinic would be the appropriate resource for systematic study of these issues.

CONCLUSION

Pain assessment in the older adult requires recognition of several facts. First, there is no single, ideal pain assessment method, in general, and this is also true for pain assessment in special populations such as the elderly. In the laboratory care must be take to use psychophysical endpoints and nociceptive stimuli which are not likely to place the older adult at a disadvantage due to cognitive or performance demands. In the clinic, pain assessment strategies which work with younger patients are likely to work equally well for assessment of geriatric pain, if the patients are not suffering cognitive limitations due to a dementing illness. Secondly, several dimensions, in addition to those typically recognized to influence pain (Melzack & Wall, 1965; Price, 1988) must be considered. These additional dimensions include (1) comorbidity; (2) mental status; (3) pain independent functional status and activities of daily living; (4) specification of pain-dependent limitations in instrumental activities of daily living; (5) current affect, mood, and emotional disorders including possible drug and alcohol abuse; (6) history of affective disorder and addition; and (7) history of health-care utilization. Appropriate multidisciplinary assessment guidelines for geriatric pain are not available. Until they are, a good dose of common, sense absent of ageism and gerontophobia are recommended (Butler & Gastel, 1980).

REFERENCES

Bartoshuk, L. M. (1989). Taste: Robust across the life span? *Annals New York Academy of Science, 561,* 65–75.

Bartoshuk, L. M., Rifkin, B., Marks, L. E., and Bars, P. (1986). Taste and aging. *Journal of Gerontology, 41,* 51–57.

Beecher, H. K. (1959). *Measurement of subject responses: Quantitative effects of drugs.* New York: Oxford University Press.

Birren, J. E., Shapiro, H. B., & Miller, J. H. (1950). The effect of salicylate upon pain sensitivity. *Journal of Pharmacology and Experimental Therapeutics, 100,* 67–71.

Butler, R. N., & Gastel, B. (1980). Care of the aged: Perspectives on pain and discomfort. In L. K. Y. Ng & J. J. Bonica (Eds.), *Pain and discomfort* (pp. 297–312). Amsterdam: Elsevier/North Holland.

Chapman, W. P., & Jones, C. M. (1944). Variations in cutaneous and visceral pain sensitivity in normal subjects. *Journal of Clinical Investigation, 23,* 81–91.

Clark, W. C., & Clark, S. B. (1980). Pain responses in Napalese porters. *Science, 209,* 440–442.

Clark, W. C., & Mehl, L. (1971). Thermal pain: A sensory decision theory analysis of the effect of age and sex on d', various response criteria, and 50 percent pain threshold. *Journal of Abnormal Psychology, 78,* 202–212.

Collins, G., & Stone, L. A. (1966). Pain sensitivity, age and activity level in chronic schizophrenics and in normals. *British Journal of Psychiatry, 112,* 33–35.

Coppola, R., & Gracely, R. H. (1983). Where is the noise in SDT pain assessment? *Pain, 17,* 257–266.

Crook, J., Rideout, E., & Browne, G. (1984). The prevalence of pain complaints in a general population. *Pain, 18,* 299–314.

Doty, R. L. (1989). Influence of age and age-related diseases on olfactory function. *Annals of the New York Academy of Science, 561,* 76–86.

Feinmann, C. (1985). Pain relief by antidepressants: Possible modes of action. *Pain, 23,* 1–8.

Ferrell, B. A., Ferrell, B. R., & Osterweil, D. (1990). Pain in the nursing home. *Journal of the American Geriatrics Society, 38,* 409–414.

Fries, J. F. (1980). Aging, natural death, and the compression of morbidity. *New England Journal of Medicine, 300,* 130–135.

Fries, J. F., Green, L. W., & Levine, S. (1989). Health promotion and the compression of morbidity. *Lancet, 4,* 481–483.

Gibson, S. J., Gorman, M. M., & Helme, R. D. (1991). Assessment of pain in the elderly using event-related cerebral potentials. In M. R. Bond, J. E. Charlton, & C. J. Woolf (Eds.), *Proceedings of the VIth World Congress on Pain* (pp. 527–533). Amsterdam: Elsevier.

Gracely, R. H. (1989). Pain psychophysics. In C. R. Chapman & J. D. Loeser (Eds.), *Issues in pain management* (pp. 211–229). New York: Raven Press.

Graff-Radford, S. B., & Nalibof, B. D. (1988). Age predicts treatment outcome in postherpetic neuralgia. *Clinical Journal of Pain, 4,* 1–4.

Hardy, J. D., Wolff, H. G., & Goodell, H. (1943). The pain threshold in man. *American Journal of Psychiatry, 99,* 744–751.

Harkins, S. W. (1988). Pain in the elderly. In R. Dubner, F. G. Gebhart, & M. R. Bond (Eds.), *Proceedings of the Vth World Congress on Pain* (pp. 355–357). Amsterdam: Elsevier.

Harkins, S. W., & Chapman, C. R. (1976). Detection and decision factors in pain perception in young and elderly men. *Pain, 2,* 253–264.

Harkins, S. W., & Chapman, C. R. (1977a). Age and sex differences in pain perception. In B. Anderson & B. Matthews (Eds.), *Pain in the trigeminal region* (pp. 435–441). Amsterdam: Elsevier/North Holland.

Harkins, S. W., & Chapman, C. R. (1977b). The perception of induced dental pain in young and elderly women. *Journal of Gerontology, 32,* 428–435.

Harkins, S. W., Kwentus, J., & Price, D. D. (1984). Pain and the elderly. In C. Benedetti, C. R. Chapman & G. Moricca (Eds.), *Advances in pain research and therapy* (Vol. 7, pp. 103–212). New York: Raven Press.

Harkins, S. W., Kwentus, J., & Price, D. D. (1990). Pain and suffering in the elderly. In J. J. Bonica (Ed.), *Management of pain* (2nd ed., pp. 552–559). Philadelphia: Lea & Febiger.

Harkins, S. W., Price, D. D., & Braith, J. (1989). Effects of extraversion and neuroticism on experimental pain, clinical pain, and illness behavior. *Pain, 36,* 209–218.

Harkins, S. W., Price, D. D., & Martelli, M. (1986). Effects of age on pain perception: Thermonociception. *Journal of Gerontology, 41,* 58–63.

Harkins, S. W., & Warner, M. H. (1980). Age and pain. In C. Eisdorfer (Ed.), *Annual review of gerontology and geriatrics* (Vol. 1, pp. 121–131). New York: Springer Publishing Company.

Helme, R. D., Katz, B., Neufeld, S., Lachal, J., & Corron, H. T. (1989). The establishment of a geriatric pain clinic: A preliminary report of the first 100 patients. *Australian Journal of Ageing, 8,* 27–30.

Hendler, N. (1981). Exaggerated pain because of cognitive impairment. In N. Hendler (Ed.), *Diagnosis and nonsurgical management of chronic pain* (pp. 33–36). New York: Raven Press.

Keefe, F. J., & Williams, D. A. (1990). A comparison of coping strategies in chronic pain patients in different age groups. *Journal of Gerontology, 45,* P161–P165.

Kenshalo, D. R., Sr. (1986). Somesthetic sensitivity in young and elderly humans. *Journal of Gerontology, 41,* 732–742.

Kerns, R. D., Turk, D. C., & Rudy, T. E. (1985). The West Haven–Yale Multidimensional Pain Inventory (WHYMPI). *Pain, 23,* 345–356.

Kline, D. W., & Schieber, F. (1985). Vision and aging. In J. E. Birren & R. W. Schie (Eds.), *Handbook of the psychology of aging* (2nd ed., pp. 296–331). New York: Van Nostrand Reinhold.

Labouvie-Vief, G. (1985). Intelligence and cognition. In J. E. Birren & K. W. Schaie (Eds.), *Handbook of the psychology of aging* (pp. 500–530). New York: Van Nostrand Reinhold.

Lavsky-Shulan, M., Wallace, R. B., Kohout, F. J., Lemke, J. H., Morris, M. C., & Smith, I. M. (1985). Prevalence and functional correlates of low back pain in the elderly: The Iowa 65+ Rural Health Study. *Journal of the American Geriatrics Society, 33*, 23–28.

Marsland, D. W., Wood, M. B., & Mayo, F. (1976). *Content of family practice: A statewide study in Virginia and its clinical, educational, and research implications.* New York: Appleton-Century-Crofts.

Melzack, R. (1973). *The puzzle of pain.* New York: Basic Books.

Melzack, R., & Wall, P. D. (1965). Pain mechanisms: A new theory. *Science, 150*, 971–979.

Middaugh, S. J., Levin, R. B., Lee, W. G., Barchie, S. I., & Roberts, J. M. (1988). Chronic pain: Its treatment in geriatric patients. *Archives of Physical Medicine and Rehabilitation, 69*, 1021–1026.

Moss, M. S., Lawton, M. P., & Glicksman, A. (1991). The role of pain in the last year of life of older persons. *Journal of Gerontology, 46*, 51–57.

Mumford, J. M. (1965). Pain perception threshold and adaptation of normal human teeth. *Archives of Oral Biology, 10*, 957–968.

Mumford, J. M. (1968). Pain perception in man on electrically stimulating the teeth. In A. Soulairac, J. Cahn, & J. Charpentier (Eds.), *Pain* (pp. 224–229). London: Academic Press.

Olsho, L. W., Harkins, S. W., & Lenhardt, M. L. (1985). Aging and the auditory system. In J. E. Bitten & K. W. Schaie (Eds.), *Handbook of the psychology of aging* (pp. 332–377). New York: Van Nostrand Reinhold.

Parmelee, P. A., Katz, I. R., & Lawton, M. P. (1991). The relation of pain to depression among institutionalized aged. *Journal of Gerontology, 46*, P15–P21.

Price, D. D. (1988). *Psychological and neural mechanism of pain.* New York: Raven Press.

Procacci, P., Bozza, G., Buzzelli, G., & Della Corte, M. (1970). The cutaneous pricking pain threshold in old age. *Gerontology Clinics, 12*, 213–218.

Procacci, P., Della Corte, M., Zoppi, M., Romano, S., Maresca, M., & Voegelin, M. (1974). Pain threshold measurement in man. In J. J. Bonica, P. Procacci, & C. Pagoni (Eds.), *Recent advances in pain: Pathophysiology and clinical reports* (pp. 105–147). Springfield, IL: Chas C. Thomas.

Puder, R. S. (1988). Age analysis of cognitive-behavioral group therapy for chronic pain outpatients. *Psychology and Aging, 3*, 204–207.

Radloff, L. S. (1977). The CES-D Scale: A self-report depression scale for research in the general population. *Applied Psychological Measurement, 1*, 385–401.

Roy, R., & Thomas, M. (1986). A survey of chronic pain in an elderly population. *Canadian Family Physician, 32*, 513–516.

Schiffman, S. (1977). Food recognition by the elderly. *Journal of Gerontology, 32*, 586–592.

Schumacher, G. A., Goodell, H., Hardy, J. D., & Wolff, H. G. (1940). Univormity of the pain threshold in man. *Science, 92*, 110–112.

Sherman, E. D., & Robillard, E. (1964a). Sensitivity to pain in relationship to age. In P. F. Hansen (Ed.), *Age with a future: Proceedings of the Sixth International Congress of Gerontology, Copenhagen, 1963* (pp. 325–333). Philadelphia: Davis.

Sherman, E. D., & Robillard, E. (1964b). Sensitivity to pain in relationship to age. *Journal of the American Geriatrics Society, 12*, 1037–1044.

Sorkin, B. A., Rudy, T. E., Hanlon, R. B., Turk, D. C., & Stieg, R. L. (1990). Chronic pain in old and young patients: Differences appear less important than similarities. *Journal of Gerontology: Psychological Sciences, 45*, P64–P68.

Sternbach, R. A. (1986). Survey of pain in the United States: The Nuprin Pain Report. *Clinical Journal of Pain, 2*, 49–53.

Tait, R. C., Chibnall, J. T., & Margolis, R. B. (1990). Pain extent: Relations with psychological state, pain severity, pain history, and disability. *Pain, 41*, 295–301.

Taylor, A. E., Mailis A., Vanderlinden, R. G., & Shoichet, R. (1988). Early dementia presenting as chronic intractable pain. *Clinical Journal of Pain, 4*, 129–133.

Tucker, M. A., Andrew, M. F., Ogle, S. J., et al. (1989). Age associated change in pain threshold measured by transcutaneous neuronal electrical stimulation. *Age and Aging, 18*, 241–246.

Turk, D. C., & Rudy, T. E. (1988). Toward an empirically derived taxonomy of chronic pain patients: Integration of psychological assessment data. *Journal of Consulting Clinical Psychology, 56*, 233–238.

Valkenburg, H. A. (1988). Epidemiological considerations of the geriatric populations. *Gerontology, 34*(Suppl 1), 2–10.

Verrillo, R. T. (1979). Changes in vibrotactile thresholds as a function of age. *Sensory Processes, 3*, 49–59.

Walsh, N. E., Schoenfeld, L., Ramamurthy, S., & Hoffman, J. (1989). Normative nodel for cold pressor test. *American Journal of Physical Medicine and Rehabilitation, 68*, 6–11.

Williams, A. K., & Schulz, R. (1988). Association of pain and physical dependency with depression in physically ill middle-aged and elderly persons. *Physical Therapy, 68*, 1226–1230.

Wood, J. B., & Harkins, S. W. (1987). Effects of age, stimulus selection, and retrieval environment on odor identification. *Journal of Gerontology, 42*, 584–588.

Woodrow, K. M., Friedman, G. D., Siegelaub, A. B., & Collen, M. F. (1972). Pain tolerance: Differences according to age, sex, and race. *Psychosomatic Medicine, 34*, 548–556.

Chapter 19

Measurement of Acute Pain States

C. RICHARD CHAPMAN, PhD
GARY W. DONALDSON, PhD
ROBERT C. JACOBSON, PhD

Acute pain is a constellation of unpleasant sensory and emotional processes occurring over time. Nociception enhanced by inflammation causes most acute pain, but clinically significant pain often recruits somatic and sympathetic reflex activity and elicits neuroendocrinologic response. In patient care, acute pain problems are usually prolonged periods of distress characterized by fluctuating intensity and punctuated by exacerbating events (e.g., postoperative pain). The only exceptions to this are fleeting episodes of procedural pain such as venipuncture and bone marrow aspiration. In general, therefore, the concept of acute pain connotes a complex profile of somatically focused distress and arousal. In this chapter we introduce the psychological concept of *state* and examine acute pain within this framework. We demonstrate how this perspective facilitates measurement and discuss statistical tools that pertain to analysis of pain states.

STATE AND MEASUREMENT

A state is a situation-specific, organized pattern of perception and response defined within a window of time; it encompasses the individu-al's perceptual orientation, vigilance, activity level, and behavior. States are intrinsically multidimensional because they characterize central nervous system functioning and incorporate sensory, emotional, and cognitive processes. Consequently, behavioral scientists generally reserve the term state for a complex, situation-specific phenomenon. Familiar examples include anxiety, fear, hypervigilance, and grief. In describing the concept of emotion broadly, Lazarus, Kanner, and Folkman (1980) defined emotions as "complex, organized states . . . consisting of cognitive appraisals, action impulses, and patterned somatic reactions" (p. 198). They emphasized that these three components are always experienced as a whole. This precedent suggests that acute pain can be described as a state. Consistent with Lazarus et al. (1980) we view acute pain as including sensory awareness as well as patterned somatic reactions, cognitive appraisals, and action impulses.

Lazarus et al. (1980) highlighted another important property of states in their description of emotion: States are determined in part by the environments in which they occur, both physical and social. They described emotions as products of person-environment transactions, with transactions having implication for the individual's well-being. Negative feeling states like fear would thus arise from situations in which a transaction is harmful or threatening. Acute pain, as a state, is also a product of the interaction of the individual with the environment. We find it useful to describe acute pain as a product of the interaction between the brain and the environment, where "environment encompasses the somatic, social, and physical surround.

Measurement approaches for the assessment of a state may include subjective report such as the State-Trait Anxiety Inventory (Spielberger, Goursuch, & Luschene, 1970), live or videotaped observation such as coding of facial expression for the study of emotion (LeResche & Dworkin, 1984), objective measurement of physiologic response such as profiles of neuroendocrine changes over time (Moore & McQuay, 1985), or a combination of such these options. States have many features and so they offer many possibilities for measurement.

It follows from the above considerations that the concept of state implies both a specific situation and a window of time. In this respect a state is roughly analogous to a scene in a play. A scene on stage requires a situation, and it continues for some length of time. Anticipated events in the scene may be preceded by anticipatory arousal. The scene may contain a number of discrete events, elicit complex sensations and emotions, and provoke elaborate cognitive appraisals.

Imagine a performance of Shakespeare's *Julius Caesar,* and consider specifically Act III, Scene 2, which takes place in the forum immediately after the assassination. One might measure emotional arousal in the plebeians with behavioral observation methods (e.g., recording vocal loudness in decibels or frequency of body movements). It will not be enough to examine a single plebeian statement; we must view the entire scene. The emotions of the plebeians at the start of the scene stem from concern and uncertainty. They are appeased by the speech of Brutus, but then Mark Anthony enters with Caesar's body. Masterfully, he turns the feelings of the crowd to grief and in so doing achieves control of them. Finally, he incites them to indignation and riotous vengeance. Emotional arousal increases monotonically and probably exponentially as this scene progresses. Sampling one or two plebeian utterances at arbitrary points will not allow us to detect and characterize this pattern. Moreover, we are at the mercy of measurement error when we do so; we may capture a sample that badly misrepresents the overall emotional tone of the scene. We can gather numbers and generate data by arbitrary sampling, but we have not measured the emotional arousal of the plebeian crowd properly until we have characterized the context and view the arousal as a process across time.

An investigator who sets out to quantify the pain of a patient recovering from surgery faces a similar challenge: measuring the pain state as a whole rather than capturing and quantifying one or another brief event that occurs within the state. Just as it helps us to know the plot of the play when we want to assess some feature of a single scene, it is invaluable to understand the circumstances of the patients we study. In addition, we need to conceptualize the process that we study. The surgeon who looks in on his patient once a day between operation and discharge to ask about pain collects little real information about the pain experience. However, if the patient's chart has recorded the patient's pain level every two waking hours, the surgeon can easily judge whether analgesic dosage is adequate. The profile of a pain state carries far more information, and leads to more accurate appraisal, than an isolated score.

STATISTICAL CHARACTERIZATION OF STATES

The measurable features of a state are variables that change in magnitude across time, as Figure 19.1 demonstrates. One may quantify a state in much the same way that evoked potential researchers quantify electrical brain activities. The fundamental steps are (1) to identify one or more features of the phenomenon and (2) to assign numbers to those features. Like evoked potentials, states have measurable characteristics such as onset, duration, periodicity, peak magnitude, and peak latency. Most, and perhaps all, of these features can usefully characterize a headache, the pain of labor for childbirth, or the pain of sickle cell crisis. Given that one can score a pain in a reliable and valid way (e.g., attach numbers to pain magnitude consistently and accurately), measurement of that pain as a state is straightforward.

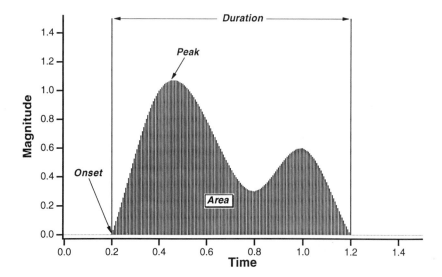

FIGURE 19.1. Measurable features of a pain state. Like a waveform, a pain state possesses a quantifiable characteristic such as onset, duration, periodicity, and peaks with magnitudes and latencies. The shaded area represents total pain over time.

Features of Pain

An investigator needs to score one or more aspects (features) of a pain in order to construct a profile of a pain state. The simplest and most common approach is to collapse all of the dimensions of pain into a single measure that one obtains from the patient's subjective report. The Visual Analogue Scale (VAS) is perhaps the most familiar approach, but several other viable options exist (Chapman & Syrjala, 1990; see also Jensen & Karoly, Chapter 9, and Price & Harkins, Chapter 8). Although the VAS clearly oversimplifies pain by forcing a multidimensional phenomenon into a single dimension, it is a solid measure that minimizes patient burden.

More complex tools exist for subjective report, and one can apply them when the nature of the pain and the patient population permit. The McGill Pain Questionnaire (MPQ) represents this option and is the best known of several multidimensional testing instruments (c.f., Choinière, Melzack, Rondeau, Girard, & Paquin,1989; see also Melzack & Katz, Chapter 10). The more complex instruments can yield multidimensional scaling: that is, they can permit an investigator to quantify several features of pain simultaneously.

One can also identify objective features of pain states or combine objective and subjective methods. For example, an investigator could obtain blood samples repeatedly following sur-

gery and quantify plasma beta endorphin or any of a number of other neurohumoral variables (see Moore & McQuay, 1985, for an example). Or one could measure facial expression through facial action coding (LeResche, 1982). As with subjective report methods, the investigator can choose between quantifying a single indicator or multiple indicators. In contrast to subjective approaches, however, the responder burden does not necessarily increase with multiple objective indicators. A single blood sample can yield a single measure of plasma beta endorphin or several neurohumoral measures such as beta endorphin, ACTH, cortisol, norepinephrine, and epinephrine, all with no additional demand upon the patient.

Of course, practical considerations limit opportunities for measuring pain comprehensively as a state. Ideally, a researcher would like to capture the complexity of acute pain in all its psychophysiologic richness, but patients in pain, by definition, experience significant distress. Most pain measurement tools require subjective report from patients. Consequently, the very thing the researcher wishes to measure impedes the ability of patients to cooperate energetically and wholeheartedly in the measurement process. Moreover, pain measurement assumes valid subjective reporting, and some patients have limited skills for performing complex self-assessment and reporting tasks. In most cases, therefore, an investigator must work out an optimal balance between the measurement opportunities inherent in a particular pain state and the responder burden that pain measurement imposes upon patients.

Repeated Measurement and Time

Because a state by definition involves a time window, the length of that window (the duration of the pain state) figures prominently in pain measurement. In the dental setting an acute pain might last only a few minutes, whereas a burn trauma patient might have weeks or months of acute pain. The first step in measuring a pain state, therefore, is attaining a thorough, phenomenologic understanding of the natural course of the state.

Normally, the duration of a pain state is the duration of the pain complaint, but exceptions occur. Because the pain state is situation specific, one might elect to limit the duration of a state under study to some specified time when the situation surrounding the patient changes. For example, a burn trauma patient might have acute pain for 28 days. However, this patient is in hospital only 24 days, and the home environment differs markedly from the hospital environment. The investigator also finds it quite difficult to collect data in a controlled manner after the patient has left the hospital. In this case, it may be expeditious to define the pain state in terms of the hospital stay, even though the patient leaves the hospital with some residual pain. In general, however, most investigators attempt to define the duration of a pain state in terms of the sensory duration of the pain.

Conceptualizing acute pain as a state or process mandates repeated measurement. Although the standard approach to acute pain measurement may allow for only a single measure, a single time point cannot, by definition, reveal anything about how a state has changed. Even if we assume that patients begin an episode of pain at roughly the same level, we cannot assume that they will all progress at the same rate. Measurement at a single time may answer some questions about therapeutic interventions, on the average, assuming monotonic change in all patients; it is insufficient to answer any question about how any particular patient changed between tissue insult and healing.

By definition, measurement of change in a pain state requires at least two measures. Although the conventional pre–post design is perhaps the modal approach to evaluating therapeutic efficacy, two points provide an inadequate basis for characterizing individual change. With only two time points, change is the difference, but no degrees of freedom remain to evaluate error or variability of the estimate. Moreover, two time points permit inference only about linear change, but most acute pain syndromes exhibit nonlinear trends. Three time points allow quadratic trend estimation; four time points, cubic trends; several time points allow estimation of complicated nonlinear trends.

How many time measurements ensure reasonable approximations? This is a question of temporal precision. It depends on the complexity of the underlying model response pattern and the reliability of the pain measure. The more complex the anticipated pain course, the more the time points required to describe it adequately. The more reliable the pain measure, the fewer time the points needed to estimate a trend of given complexity. Subjective reports contain a good deal of "noise," not because patients cannot judge their own perceptions, but because they cannot translate the multidimensional pain experience into a numerical score consistently. (Indeed, perfect consistency—as in a score that increased by one point on each occasion—would arouse suspicion that someone had fabricated the data.) Additional measurements can help filter noise, leaving a smoother trend with less unsystematic variation.

Smoothing Data

We smooth a series of pain measures from a patient (a time series) in order to obtain a "filtered" pain score with less random variability than the raw data. The simplest way to do this is by averaging a number of temporally adjacent scores. The variability of the summary depends on the number of scores included and the correlations among them. Assuming equal variances and correlations among the measurement occasions, the formula for the variance of a mean formed from m scores is

$$\frac{1}{m} \sigma^2 (1 + 2\rho)$$

where σ^2 is the variance of the individual scores and ρ is the correlation among scores.

Table 19.1 shows how common choices for

TABLE 19.1. Variance of the Mean of Temporally Adjacent Scores

Number of Components (m)	Correlation (ρ) among components								
	0	0.1	0.2	0.3	0.4	0.5	0.6	0.7	0.8
2	0.50	0.60	0.70	0.80	0.90	1.00	1.10	1.20	1.30
3	0.33	0.40	0.47	0.53	0.60	0.67	0.74	0.81	0.89
4	0.25	0.30	0.35	0.40	0.45	0.50	0.65	0.70	0.75
5	0.20	0.24	0.28	0.32	0.36	0.40	0.44	0.48	0.52

m and typical values for ρ determine the variance of a mean score (if your value for ρ is greater than .7, smoothing your data achieves little). Each entry in the table is the multiplying factor of the original variance for individual scores; values greater than 1.0 yield a higher variance for the mean scores while values less than 1.0 generate lower variances for the mean scores.

Table 19.1 can guide practical decisions about how many time points to measure. First, characterize the complexity of the model response for the acute pain under study. Roughly speaking, this can be the number of humps or bends in the average curve plus 2 (e.g., for an inverted "U" shape the complexity would be 3—1 point for the hump plus 2 points on either side). Second, add at least 1 to this number to allow for those patients who display a more complicated pattern than the average. Third, use previous data, theoretical knowledge, or your best guess to estimate the typical between-occasion correlation for your data. Fourth, look down the appropriate column of Table 19.1 until you find a noteworthy variance reduction (50% is reasonable). Fifth, look across the row to find the required number of measurements per point in the model pattern. Finally, multiply this number by the complexity determined in step two, obtaining the estimated number of time points you will need to smooth most individual pain profiles adequately.

To take an example, assume we want to characterize individual patterns for oral mucositis pain following bone marrow transplantation. The characteristic profile for this pain is quadratic, with a shape like an inverted "U." For step one, then, we would have a complexity of 3. To allow for patients with more complicated patterns, we increase this to 4. From previous experience, we know that .5 is a typical day-to-day correlation for this kind of pain report, so we look down the middle

column to learn that 4 measures per period will reduce mean pain variance by 50%. This value times the complexity of 4 equals 16, so we would need at least sixteen time points to characterize these pains; more, of course, would be better, because this would allow us to smooth even more accurately.

Choosing a Smoother

The rules of thumb described above work well with many methods for smoothing data. Most fit one of two classifications: time series approaches that assume equal measurement intervals and 1 measure per occasion, and regression approaches that treat time as a quantitative variable.

Time series approaches to smoothing generally require that one specify a constant window length. Usually, the window length will be the value of m determined above, but this is not essential. An average score is obtained for each window, and these average values are plotted and used in subsequent analyses. The windows can generate either stationary averages or moving averages.

If each window corresponds to particular time points, then the smoother replaces the original scores with a reduced number of summary scores corresponding to the new time windows. Fixed windows generate data conformable for traditional statistical applications, such as repeated measures analysis of variance. Although the scores from fixed windows can be plotted and interpreted as change scores, their discrete character renders them unsuitable as indicators of a smooth process. Smoothing also has the salutary effect of decreasing the proportion of missing data by replacing individual missing scores with window averages. Fixed windows generate snapshots taken with a wide-angle lens.

Imagine, on the other hand, allowing the

windows to slide to the right one point at a time along the time axis. If we obtain an average for each of these sliding windows, a fairly smooth curve is built up from the overlapping averages. These curves are easily plotted and interpretable as smoothly changing processes. The individual points on the curve are no longer independent, and are thus not subject to usual statistical analyses, but the curve as a whole can be analyzed with quantitative methods appropriate for dose-response curves or other smooth mathematical functions.

Moving window smoothers can work with means or medians. Running medians give less weight to individual extreme scores. Running means, although more sensitive to outliers, do a better job of tracking data that are close to normal in distribution. Some smoothers combine means and medians in multiple steps. The smoother T4253H (Velleman & Hoaglin, 1981), for example, successively applies running medians of window length 4, 2, 5, and 3; computes the residuals from this smooth; applies the smoother to the residuals; then smooths the two smooths. This is a very useful robust smoother; it is implemented as a single command in the SPSS/PC+ statistical package.

Although time series approaches assume equal measurement intervals, *regression approaches* treat time as a conventional independent variable and obtain smoothed nonlinear regressions. Equal intervals are not required, and multiple measures per occasion are allowed. Missing or unbalanced data pose no particular problems for regression approaches.

Theoretical smoothing fits the data with mathematical functions of known degree. Often, the functions are lower-order polynomials, but one can also fit exponential, logarithmic or other functions with a sensible theoretical rationale. Patients will vary in how well a particular function fits their data; statistically efficient analyses incorporate this goodness-of-fit information in estimating trend coefficients (Donaldson & Moinpour, 1992). Empirical regression smoothers use a moving window on the independent variable (time), obtaining conditional expectations for the outcome. Most such smoothers allow the user to choose the width of the window, thus controlling the tension or flexibility of the obtained fit. Some regression smoothers also allow the user to adjust weights within the window. As with time series approaches, regression smoothers vary in their degree of robustness (insensitivity to extreme scores). *Lowess* (Cleveland, 1979, 1981, 1985) is rather robust, downweighting extreme points. Smoothing by distance-weighted least-squares, or DWLS (McLain, 1974), is not as robust as *Lowess* but tends to give smoother curves. The *supersmoother* algorithm (Friedman, 1984) chooses three sets of overlapping weights based on multiple cross-validation.

Both time series and regression smoothers will faithfully yield transformed data that appear systematic. Even random data will drift up and down, and all smoothers will capitalize on random variation to yield a "trend" that looks systematic. One should therefore take care not to overinterpret smoothed data; real data and random data will look equally "smooth" after transformation.

FOUR PAIN SYNDROMES

To clarify the concept of pain as a state we compare and discuss four acute pains: postoperative pain, burn trauma pain, the pain of renal calculus, and the pain of oral mucositis. Each has a representative profile, as revealed in Figures 19.2–19.5, which consists of VAS data for pain intensity.

Figure 19.2 profiles postoperative pain for a group of patients. There are hundreds of reports of postoperative pain in the literature; however, in nearly all cases study patients have received medication or other treatment so that the natural course of the pain is uncertain. Chapman and Cox (1977) studied unmedicated renal transplant patients. The kidney recipients in this study received no postoperative pain medication. Figure 19.2 illustrates the mean pain scores for 11 of their subjects. For such patients postoperative pain comes on rapidly; the patient awakens from the anesthetic and experiences severe pain, even while at rest. Over several days the resting pain declines monotonically and exponentially, not disappearing until after discharge from hospital. Note that, because the data in Figure 19.2 are mean scores for the sample, they obscure the marked variability that appears within each individual's data set. For the individual, purposeful movement including pulmonary toilet, sitting up, and ambulation all cause spikes of pain exacerbation. The course of any individual's pain is never as smooth as the mean for the group suggests.

Figure 19.3 depicts data from 1 of 42 burn

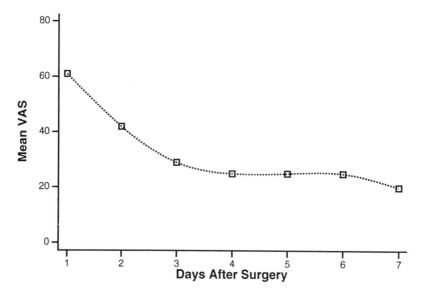

FIGURE 19.2. Mean daily pain scores over one week for 11 postoperative patients.

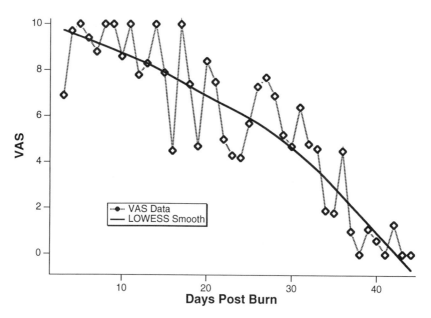

FIGURE 19.3. Changes in pain report (0–10 VAS) for a burn trauma patient. The dotted line depicts changes in raw scores. The solid line represents the data following transformation by smoothing. These data illustrate that seemingly erratic scores may vary about a consistent trend.

patients studied by Choinière et al. (1989). The investigators instructed patients to report pain using a VAS at its worst during the past 24 hours; they collected data during morning hours. Note the marked day-to-day variation in pain magnitude as well as the consistent trend that the smoothing procedure has extracted from the data. There are many reasons for such

variation in pain scores. Burn trauma patients suffer from a resting pain upon which the pain of dressing change is superimposed once or twice each day. Repeated experiences with de-bridement condition emotional response in many burn patients so that they experience intense fear at every new dressing change, even before the noxious stimulation occurs. This accentuates the emotional aspects of debridement pain. With healing, patients must stretch contracted joints, and this too imposes spikes of intense pain upon background pain levels. The pain of rehabilitation exercises, stretching joints, and ambulation tracks that of debridement in intensity fluctuation, but is typically at roughly half the magnitude of dressing change pain. Pain reports from such patients must reflect a complex mixture of painful events.

The ideal temporal precision for measuring pain by subjective report may be unattainable because pain, like a fractal, seems to expand in elaborate detail with every new increase in focus. Figure 19.4 relates the experience of one of the authors with a renal calculus. Kidney stones create bouts of intense visceral, often nauseating, pain interrupted by periods of comfort and normality. This pain pattern is nonmonotonic, episodic but unpredictable, and it ends abruptly after a particularly intense period with the passage of the stone. The small windows illustrate what might happen (a hypothetical experiment) if an investigator repeatedly increased the temporal precision of pain measurement.

Obtaining one measure per day yields relatively coarse temporal precision. If we expand one arbitrarily selected day to yield a pain profile over 24 hours, we see that marked variability appears across this smaller time window. Expanding a single 1-hour time point from the 24-hour window, we find that the pain varies markedly, even within this 1 hour.

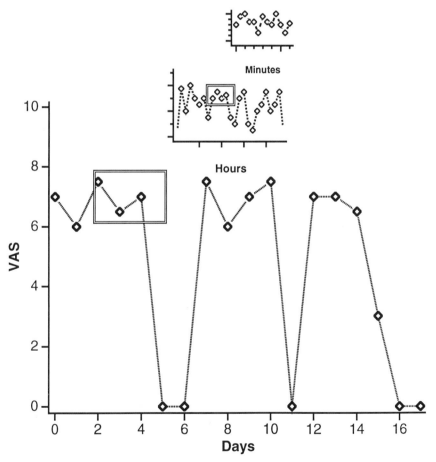

FIGURE 19.4. Increasing temporal precision in pain measurement cannot eliminate instability in pain report. These data, shown as hypothetical VAS scores ranging from 0 to 10, are derived from the memory of one author. They represent pain associated with a renal calculus. The small box on the large plot of pain change over days identifies a single day. The smaller graph immediately above it opens this day into 24 hours and displays variability across hours. The small box identifies a single hour. The third and smallest graph expands that hour into 60 minutes and displays change in pain over minutes. The repeated pattern of variability across time scales illustrates the fractal nature of pain perception.

It is no surprise, then, that pain measures obtained at an arbitrary point each day will demonstrate "jitter" about a consistent trend (as shown in Figure 19.3). In the hypothetical case of this renal calculus patient, increasing the temporal precision of the measures does not yield much advantage over a daily pain report, and the costs in man hours and patient responder burden would be prohibitive.

The oral mucositis pain of patients who suffer chemoradiotherapy toxicity during bone marrow transplantation comes on gradually and monotonically, peaks, and then declines monotonically, as Figures 19.5a and b illustrate. Patients receive aggressive chemotherapy and total body irradiation in preparation for bone marrow transplantation, and the oral pain they experience reflects a time-limited toxicity. Day "0" in marrow transplantation indicates the date of the actual transplantation of bone marrow from a donor. The preparative, toxic treatments occur within the preceding 10 days, and oral mucositis comes on gradually. The pain follows the course of and roughly reflects the severity of the patient's oral pathology (Schubert, Williams, Lloid, Donaldson, & Chapko, in press). We show both untransformed scores and a "smoothed" representation of the patient's data produced by the Lowess smoothing algorithm (Cleveland, 1985). The areas under the smoothed and unsmoothed curves are nearly identical; only the fluctuations have been removed.

Figure 19.5a shows smoothing with tension set at 0.5, which indicates that the smoothing window includes 50% of the data points. Figure 19.5b depicts the same patient's data with a smooth set at 0.1. The inset figures show the discrepancy between smoothed and untransformed data sets; that is, the residuals formed by subtracting the smoothed data from the raw scores. Such residuals should be randomly distributed about zero with no temporal pattern. In these cases autocorrelation (correlation between adjacent data points) appears, particularly for the heavier smooth in Figure 19.5a, suggesting that the transformation has not captured all the systematic variation. Examination of post-smooth residuals for serial correlation can point to local bias in the smooth and suggest unanticipated factors that may have biased the clinical measurement process.

Figure 19.5a illustrates one of the limitations of smoothing procedures. Although the smoothed graph simplifies the trend of the data and minimizes the influence of extreme scores, it clips the peaks and thereby loses such key information as the patient's maximal pain score. Moreover, it imputes pain where the patient did not report pain in the days preceding "0." Using less stringent smoothers or adjusting the "tension" on the Lowess smoother (as 19.5b demonstrates) can increase increase agreement with daily reports, but at the expense of parsimony. Smoothers are not panaceas; they express an alternative opinion of reality that is in some respects more credible and in other respects less credible than the raw data. An investigator must use such tools thoughtfully.

MODEL RESPONSE PATTERNS

Regardless of the type of pain under study, one can plan to quantify it according to the predominant pattern of response or trend that characterizes that pain. Thus, we could form a model for oral mucositis pain based on a quadratic (inverted "U") trend or characterize postoperative pain as a declining monotonic function. Statistical transformations such as logarithmic or square root transforms may help force some difficult response patterns into forms that facilitate scoring. For oral mucositis pain, for example, we could measure the area under the curve or the maximum amplitude of the curve at its peak. For postoperative pain, we could quantify the duration, rate of decrease, or area under the curve. The essential point is that one apply a model—an ideal type— to each individual subject, scoring the individual response pattern, not according to its own prominent features but according to features that characterize the ideal type.

A marked discrepancy typically exists between the model for a pain and the data for the individual case. This need not concern us unduly; patients differ in many respects, including degree of tissue trauma, rate of healing, and in constitutional factors such as age and sex. The only necessary criterion for measurement is that the individual pattern should fit the broad concept represented in the model. For example, scores from all postoperative pain patients should show a monotonically decreasing function. If we cannot classify a patient's response pattern in accordance with our

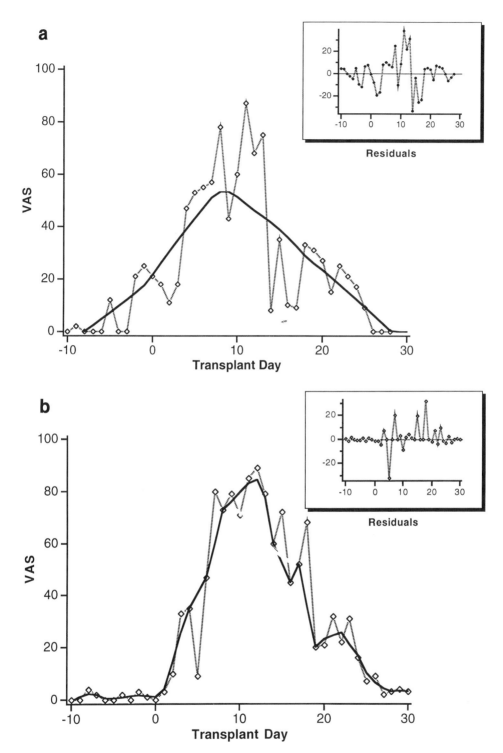

FIGURE 19.5. Changes in oral pain across days in bone marrow transplantation patients. The dotted lines indicate raw scores. The solid lines indicate the "smooths" produced by the Lowess transformation algorithm. The insets display the residuals formed by subtracting the smooths from the raw scores. **a:** We set tension at .5 to impose a strong smoothing effect. **b:** We restricted tension to .1 to preserve some features of the day-to-day variability.

model, then our assumptions about the measurement of that patient's pain are untenable.

By measuring pain as a state, we can evaluate the homogeneity of a sample of patients. Suppose for, example, that we study 100 bone marrow transplantation patients, recording their VAS pain scores daily. Imagine that some of these patients, let us say seven, do not show a quadratic trend and instead demonstrate a second peak in oral mucositis or a failure to decline in pain report within the standard time window. This suggests the operation of some process that we do not understand.

By carefully checking patient records, we might well find that these patients suffered acute graft-versus-host-disease (GVHD) following bone marrow transplantation. Oral mucositis is often a symptom of this complication. When GVHD onset coincides with the normal healing period of oral mucositis caused by chemoradiotherapy toxicity, the result can be prolonged oral pathology and pain. Once we have ascertained that GVHD has compromised our assumptions for the seven patients, we can decide whether or not to drop them from the sample; of course, this judgment depends on the specific goals of the study at hand. The important point is that we need not proceed with analysis on the basis of unquestioned assumptions about homogeneity in our sample. Ability to validate one's measurement assumptions is clearly an asset for clinical research projects.

STATE VERSUS STANDARD APPROACH

If we elect to use a conventional rather than a state approach to acute pain, we will normally measure a patient in acute pain one or more times following the onset of pain. For example, we might measure the postoperative pain of ambulatory surgery patients by telephone interview conducted within an hour or so of the patient's return home. Or we might ask sickle cell crisis patients for VAS estimates of pain intensity when they first appear at the emergency room. Such approaches are common practice. In essence, the investigator takes a "snapshot" of the pain; that is, he or she characterizes it at a single point in time.

State concepts force us to envisage pain as a process characterized within a specified time window by its size and unique shape. Measurement consists of scoring features of this process

rather than of sampling one or more discrete points. In practice, of course, numerous discrete points are used to approximate a continuous process. Because the state approach gathers and uses far more information, it will yield more reliable measurement. On the other hand, the state approach requires more intensive and thorough data collection, and this costs more in data collection manpower, responder burden, and database management. As our renal calculus examples illustrates, one cannot glean all of the detail in subjective pain report by increasing temporal precision, and we can offer no explicit guidelines for how much detail in repeated measurement is enough. Each study has a unique cost–benefit ratio that determines the frequency of repeated measurement. In most cases the advantages of state measurement justify the costs and effort that state analysis entails.

THERAPEUTIC ENDPOINT AND STATE

Therapeutic "endpoint" in studies of analgesic interventions is a potentially misleading concept if one takes the term literally, for it implies that a single point in time can define outcome. If acute pain is a state, no optimal single moment exists at which one should measure the effects of an intervention. Rather, analgesic effect depends on treatment-related changes in the pain state as a whole. An opioid infusion might reduce the area under the curve or the peak amplitude of the curve characterizing a pain state. A nonsteroidal anti-inflammatory drug might reduce the duration of a pain state as well as its area. By identifying state properties rather than raw pain scores as markers of therapeutic effect, an investigator increases both the quality of measurement and his ability to draw meaningful clinical inferences from the study outcome.

Measurement of a single point in the course of an acute pain state is fraught with peril, as we have shown above. Unexplained variation in single pain scores over time can produce false positive and false negative outcomes. The state itself, however, may show treatment effect clearly in peak magnitude, rate of pain reduction, time of pain offset (duration), or in area. Using state concepts, one measures the process of therapeutic resolution of pain rather than a therapeutic endpoint. Measurement of pain as a state thus offers advantages for the study of treatment effects.

CONCLUSIONS

We have introduced the concept of state as an approach to pain measurement and demonstrated its potential applications for several types of acute pain using the conventional VAS to demonstrate the state concept. State measurement requires repeated measures and in this sense it is inherently multivariate. One could conduct doubly multivariate measurement by using more than one measure of pain and collecting scores repeatedly and systematically across time. Although complexity increases, adding additional variables to the approach we have described does not change the basic principle: analysis of pain states (as opposed to single "snapshots" of acute pain) takes advantage of more information and therefore yields stronger scientific inference. In addition, state analysis allows an investigator to examine and characterize individual differences more powerfully than conventional approaches permit. By examining such differences, researchers can validate otherwise untestable assumptions about their samples and glean insights about the nature of the pain state under study.

Acknowledgments. A grant from the National Cancer Institute (CA-38552) supported this work. The authors thank Drs. Melzack, Choinière and their colleagues for providing the raw scores used for Figure 19.3.

REFERENCES

Chapman, C.R., & Cox, G.B. (1977). Anxiety, pain and depression surrounding elective surgery: A multivariate comparison of abdominal surgery patients with kidney donors and recipients. *Journal of Psychosomatic Research, 21,* 7–15.

Chapman, C.R., & Syrjala, K.L. (1990). Measurement of pain. In J.J. Bonica (Ed.), *The management of pain in clinical practice* (2nd ed., pp. 580–594). Lea & Febiger: Philadelphia.

Choinière, M., Melzack, R., Rondeau, J., Girard, N., & Paquin, M.J. (1989). The pain of burns: characteristics and correlates. *Journal of Trauma, 29,* 1531–1539.

Cleveland, W.S. (1979). Robust locally weighted regression and smoothing scatter plots. *Journal of the American Statistical Association, 74,* 829–836.

Cleveland, W.S. (1981). LOWESS: A program for smoothing scatter plots by robust locally weighted regression. *The American Statistician, 35,* 54.

Cleveland, W.S. (1985). *The elements of graphing data.* Monterey, CA: Wadsworth Advanced Books and Software.

Donaldson, G.W., & Moinpour, C. M. (1992). Strengthened estimates of individual pain trends in children following bone marrow transplantation. *Pain, 48,* 147–155.

Friedman, J.H. (1984). *A variable span smoother* (Tech. Rep. No. 5). Laboratory for Computational Statistics, Dept. of Statistics, Stanford University, Stanford, CA.

Lazarus, R.S., Kanner, A.D., & Folkman, S. (1980). Emotions: A cognitive-phenomenological analysis. In R. Plutchik & H. Kellerman (Eds.), *Emotion: Theory, research and experience* (pp. 189–218). San Diego: Academic Press.

LeResche, L. (1982). Facial expressions in pain: A study of candid photographs. *Journal of Nonverbal Behavior, 7,* 46–56.

LeResche, L., & Dworkin, S. (1984). Facial expressions accompanying pain. *Social Science Medicine, 19,* 1325–1330.

McLain, D.H. (1974). Drawing contours from arbitrary data points. *Computer Journal, 17,* 318–324.

Moore, R.A., & McQuay, H.J. (1985). Neuroendocrinology of the postoperative state. In G. Smith & B.G. Covino (Eds.), *Acute pain* (pp. 133–154). London: Buttersworth.

Schubert, M.M., Williams, B.E., Lloid, M.E., Donaldson, G.D., & Chapko, M.K. (in press). Clinical assessment scale for the rating of oral mucosal changes associated with cancer therapy: Development of an oral mucositis index. *Cancer.*

Spielberger, C.D., Goursuch, R.L., & Lushene, R.E. (1970). *The State-Trait Anxiety Inventory.* Palo Alto, CA: Consulting Psychologists Press.

Velleman, P.F., & Hoaglin, D.C. (1981). *Applications, basics, and computing of exploratory data analysis.* Boston: Duxbury Press.

Chapter 20

Assessment of Patients with Headaches

FRANK ANDRASIK, PhD

Recurrent headache is a widespread problem among people of all ages. For example, a recent large-scale epidemiologic investigation reported that 57% of male and 76% of female adolescent and young adults experienced one or more headache episodes within the past month (Linet, Stewart, Celentano, Ziegler, & Sprecher, 1989). Migraine prevalence was found to be 3.0% for males and 7.4% for females. Adverse effects of headache were high, with 8% of males and 14% of females missing all or part of planned activities (work or school) due to headache. The Nuprin Pain Report (Sternbach, 1986) projected that approximately 157 million days of productive work activity are lost to headache each year for full-time employees and 638 million days if part-time employees and homemakers are included. In 1984, headache accounted for about 18 million outpatient physician visits (Ries, 1986). Interestingly, only 15% of males and 28% of females contacted by Linet et al. (1989) had sought medical consultation for headache management during the preceding year, suggesting the majority of sufferers decide to "tough it out" on their own, presumably resorting to over-the-counter preparations and home remedies as necessary. Headache is fairly prevalent in young children, gradually increases with age, such that by age

15 approximately 20% report recurrent complaints, and often persists throughout life (Bille, 1962, 1981; Sillanpaa, 1983a, 1983b). Jay and Tomasi (1981) reported that 22% of the children they saw at a hospital pediatric unit were referred for reasons related to recurrent headache.

HEADACHE ASSESSMENT

Headache, like other pain disorders covered in this volume, is largely subjective, absent of reliable objective markers, and multidetermined, calling for a comprehensive, multifactorial assessment approach. This section addresses the following aspects of assessment: psychological needs of the headache patient, the importance of a physical/neurological evaluation, various classification and diagnostic considerations, and an overview of the biopsychological model of headache as a guiding framework for assessment.

Psychological Needs of Headache Patients: Headache through the Eyes of Patients

By the time a patient is motivated to seek treatment, headache complaints may be embedded within strong emotional reactions. Chief among these are frustration, anger at the headache, oneself, or others, tension and nervousness, depression, helplessness, and fear (Barnat & Lake, 1983). It is important for the practitioner to be cognizant of the fears, concerns, and questions patients bring with them to the first interview and to realize that these may be at variance with the clinician's thinking. Results from Packard's (1979) survey of the expectations of patients and physicians at the initial interview are instructive. When asked to list what they sought most from the initial visit, an explanation for what was causing the headache was mentioned foremost by patients (by about one-half). Physicians, on the other hand, stated they believed patients most wanted pain relief (mentioned by two-thirds). Thus, patients and physicians held markedly opposed views about chief needs to be addressed in the initial evaluation. Only a minority of patients felt it might be helpful to have additional medical consultations (eye examinations, laboratory test, etc.). Neither patient nor physician described psychological evaluation as important, indicating the need for tact when considering this type of referral. Packard (1979) aptly summarized the significance of these findings:

> If we believe patients are mainly seeking pain relief, that will be our goal. However, if the patient is mainly concerned about knowing what is wrong, or about his eyes, or simply wants a doctor who is willing to follow him for his headaches, our pill may well be doomed to failure and we may miss our greatest opportunity of providing relief: a simple explanation and reassurance (p. 373)

Thus, patience, reflective listening, support, and education merit high priorities at the initial visit.

Medical Evaluation

It is imperative that patients be evaluated for the presence of permanent structural defects or diagnosable physical conditions other than a primary headache disorder. Neurological examination and select laboratory evaluations are seen as essential components of the initial workup of the headache patient and should be arranged early on. Nonphysician practitioners are urged to refer all potential patients to a physician who is experienced with headache prior to accepting the patient into treatment. With many cases, a close collaboration needs to be maintained with the physician throughout treatment. Even after arranging a medical evaluation, the nonphysician therapist must be continually alert for evidence of a developing underlying physical problem. Table 20.1 contains a list of some "danger signs" that may suggest a need for immediate referral to a physician.

TABLE 20.1. "Danger Signs" in Headache Pain Patients that May Suggest the Need for Immediate Referral to a Physician[a]

1. Headache is a new symptom for the individual in the past 3 months, or the nature of the headache has changed markedly in the past 3 months.
2. Presence of any sensory or motor deficits preceding or accompanying headache other than the typical visual prodromata of migraine with aura. Examples include weakness or numbness in an extremity, twitching of the hands or feet, aphasia, or slurred speech.
3. Headache is one sided and has always been on the same side of the head.
4. Headache is due to trauma, especially if it follows a period of unconsciousness (even if only momentary).
5. Headache is constant and unremitting.
6. For a patient reporting tension-type headache-like symptoms:
   a. Pain intensity has been steadily increasing over a period of weeks to months with little or no relief.
   b. Headache is worse in the morning and becomes less severe during the day.
   c. Headache is accompanied by vomiting.
7. Patient has been treated for any kind of cancer and now has a complaint of headache.
8. Patient or significant other reports a noticeable change in personality or behavior or a notable decrease in memory or other intellectual functioning.
9. The patient is over 60 years of age, and the headache is a relatively new complaint.
10. Pain onset is sudden and occurs during conditions of exertion (such as lifting heavy objects), sexual intercourse, or "heated" interpersonal situation.
11. Patient's family has a history of cerebral aneurysm, other vascular anomalies, or polycystic kidneys.

Note: From Andrasik and Baskin (1987), page 327. Copyright 1987 Plenum Press. Reprinted by permission.
[a]List developed in consultation with Lawrence D. Rodichok, M.D. Diagnoses have been modified to be compatible with the new system proposed by the International Headache Society (1988).

TABLE 20.2. Classification of Headache

1. Migraine
   1.1 Migraine without aura
   1.2 Migraine with aura
   1.5 Childhood periodic syndromes that may be precursors to or associated with migraine
2. Tension-type headache
   2.1 Episodic tension-type headache
       2.1.1 Episodic tension-type headache associated with disorder of pericranial muscles
       2.1.2 Episodic tension-type headache unassociated with disorder of pericranial muscles
   2.2 Chronic tension-type headache
       2.2.1 Chronic tension-type headache associated with disorder of pericranial muscles
       2.2.2 Chronic tension-type headache unassociated with disorder of pericranial muscles
3. Cluster headache and chronic paroxysmal hemicrania
   3.1 Cluster headache
       3.1.1 Cluster headache periodicity undetermined
       3.1.2 Episodic cluster headache
       3.1.3 Chronic cluster headache
4. Miscellaneous headaches unassociated with structural lesion
5. Headache associated with head trauma
   5.1 Acute posttraumatic headache
       5.1.1 with significant head trauma and/or confirmatory signs
       5.1.2 with minor head trauma and no confirmatory signs
   5.2 Chronic posttraumatic headache
       5.2.1 with significant head trauma and/or confirmatory signs
       5.2.2 with minor head trauma and/or confirmatory signs
6. Headache associated with vascular disorders
7. Headache associated with nonvascular intracranial disorder
8. Headache associated with substances or their withdrawal
   8.1 Headache induced by acute substance use or exposure
       8.1.1 Nitrate/nitrite-induced headache
       8.1.2 Monosodium glutamate–induced headache
       8.1.3 Carbon monoxide–induced headache
       8.1.4 Alcohol-induced headache
       8.1.5 Other substances
   8.2 Headache induced by chronic substance use or exposure
       8.2.1 Ergotamine-induced headache
       8.2.2 Analgesics abuse headache
       8.2.3 Other substances
   8.3 Headache from substance withdrawal (acute use)
       8.3.1 Alcohol withdrawal headache (hangover)
       8.3.2 Other substances
   8.4 Headache from substance withdrawal (chronic use)
       8.4.1 Ergotamine withdrawal headache
       8.4.2 Caffeine withdrawal headache
       8.4.3 Narcotics abstinence headache
       8.4.4 Other substances
   8.5 Headache associated with substances but with uncertain mechanism
       8.5.1 Birth control pills or estrogens
       8.5.2 Other substances
9. Headache associated with noncephalic infection
10. Headache associated with metabolic disorder
11. Headache or facial pain associated with disorder of cranium, neck, eyes, ears, nose, sinuses, teeth, mouth, or other facial or cranial structures
12. Cranial neuralgias, nerve trunk pain, and deafferentation pain
13. Headache nonclassifiable

Note: From Headache Classification Committee of the International Headache Society (1988), pp. 13–17. Copyright 1988 Scandinavian University Press. Reprinted by permission.

Headache Classification and Diagnosis

Experts have grouped headaches into 13 different categories (see Table 20.2), with categories 1, 2, 3, 5, and 8 being the most likely to present for treatment at pain specialty clinics/centers (thus, some of the subtypes are listed for these five specific categories). Draft diagnostic criteria recently proposed for these 5 particular headache types are listed in Table 20.3 (Headache Classification Committee of the International Headache Society, 1988).

This classification system and proposed criteria depart markedly from those available previously (Ad Hoc Committee on the Classification of Headache, 1962). The new system came about from efforts to incorporate heretofore unacknowledged headache types (headaches associated with substances or their withdrawal and with trauma), to apply advances in etiological understanding, to reclassify certain subtypes (cluster now being recognized as a separate diagnostic entity), and to sharpen overall inclusion and exclusion criteria in the hopes of improving diagnostic accuracy. Accu-

TABLE 20.3. Headache Diagnostic Criteria

1.0   Migraine

1.1   Migraine without aura

A. At least 5 attacks fulfilling B–D
B. Headache attacks lasting 4–72 hours (2–48 hours for children below age 15), untreated or unsuccessfully treated
C. Headache has at least two of the following characteristics:
  1. unilateral location
  2. pulsating quality
  3. moderate or severe intensity (inhibits or prohibits daily activities)
  4. aggravation by walking stairs or similar routine physical activity
D. During headache at least one of the following:
  1. nausea and/or vomiting
  2. photophobia and phonophobia
E. At least one of the following:
  1. History, physical, and neurological examinations do not suggest 1 of the disorders listed in groups 5–11 (see Table 20.1)
  2. History and/or physical, and/or neurological examinations do suggest such disorder, but is ruled out by appropriate investigations
  3. Such disorder is present, but migraine attacks do not occur for the first time in close temporal relation to the disorder

1.2   Migraine with aura

A. At least 2 attacks fulfilling B
B. At least 3 of the following 4 characteristics:
  1. One or more fully reversible aura symptoms indicating focal cerebral cortical and/or brain stem dysfunction
  2. At least 1 aura symptom develops gradually over more than 4 minutes or 2 or more symptoms occur in succession
  3. No aura symptom lasts more than 60 minutes. If more than 1 aura symptom is present, accepted duration is proportionally increased
  4. Headache follows aura with a free interval of less than 60 minutes. It may also begin before or simultaneously with the aura
C. Same as Migraine without aura, criteria E

2.0   Tension-Type

2.1   Episodic tension-type headache

A. At least 10 previous headache episodes fulfilling criteria B–D. Number of days with such headache <180/year (<15/month)
B. Headache lasting from 30 minutes to 7 days
C. At least 2 of the following pain characteristics:

  1. Pressing/tightening (nonpulsating) quality
  2. Mild or moderate intensity (may inhibit, but does not prohibit activities)
  3. Bilateral location
  4. No aggravation by walking stairs or similar routine physical activity
D. Both of the following:
  1. No nausea or vomiting (anorexia may occur)
  2. Photophobia and phonophobia are absent, or one but not the other is present.
E. Same as Migraine without aura, criteria E

2.1.1   Episodic tension-type headache associated with disorder of pericranial muscles

A. Fulfills criteria for 2.1
B. At least one of the following:
  1. Increased tenderness of pericranial muscles demonstrated by manual palpation or pressure algometer
  2. Increased EMG level of pericranial muscles at rest or during physiological tests

2.1.2   Episodic tension-type headache unassociated with disorder of pericranial muscles

A. Fulfills criteria for 2.1
B. No increased tenderness of pericranial muscles. If studied, EMG of pericranial muscles shows normal levels of activity

2.2   Chronic tension-type headache

A. Average headache frequency ≥ 15 days/month (180 days/year) for ≥ 6 months fulfilling criteria B–D listed below
B. Same as criteria B, episodic tension-type headache
C. Both of the following:
  1. no vomiting
  2. No more than 1 of the following: nausea, photophobia, or phonophobia
D. Same as Migraine without aura, criteria E

2.2.1   Chronic tension-type headache associated with disorder of pericranial muscles

A. Fulfills criteria for 2.2
B. Same as criteria B for 2.1.1

2.2.2   Chronic tension-type headache unassociated with disorder of pericranial muscles

A. Fulfills criteria for 2.2
B. Same as criteria B for 2.1.2

3.1   Cluster headache

A. At least 5 attacks fulfilling B–D
B. Severe unilateral orbital, supraorbital, and/or temporal pain lasting 15–180 minutes untreated

(continued)

TABLE 20.3. *(Continued)*

C. Headache is associated with at least 1 of the following signs which have to be present on the pain-side:
  1. Conjunctival injection
  2. Lacrimation
  3. Nasal congestion
  4. Rhinorrhea
  5. Forehead and facial sweating
  6. Miosis
  7. Ptosis
  8. Eyelid edema
D. Frequency of attacks from 1 every other day to 8 per day.
E. Same as criteria E, for 1.1

5.2   Chronic posttraumatic headache

5.2.1 With significant head trauma and/or confirmatory signs

A. Significance of head trauma documented by at least 1 of the following:
  1. Loss of consciousness
  2. Posttraumatic amnesia lasting more than 10 minutes
  3. At least 2 of the following exhibit relevant abnormality: clinical neurological examination, x-ray of skull, neuroimaging, evoked potentials, spinal fluid examination, vestibular function test, neuropsychological testing
B. Headache occurs less than 14 days after regaining consciousness (or after trauma, if there has been no loss of consciousness).
C. Headache continues more than 8 weeks after regaining consciousness (or after trauma, if there has been no loss of consciousness).

5.2.2 With minor head trauma and no confirmatory signs

A. Head trauma that does not satisfy 5.2.1.A
B. Headache occurs less than 14 days after injury
C. Headache continues more than 8 weeks after injury

8.2   Headache induced by chronic substance use or exposure

A. Occurs after daily doses of a substance for ≥ 3 months.
B. A certain required minimum dose should be indicated
C. Headache is chronic (15 days or more a month)
D. Headache disappears within 1 month after withdrawal of the substance

8.2.1 Ergotamine-induced headache

A. Is preceded by daily ergotamine intake (oral ≥ 2 mg, rectal ≥ 1 mg)
B. Is diffuse, pulsating, or distinguished from migraine by absent attack pattern and/or absent associated symptoms

8.2.2 Analgesics abuse headache

A. One or more of the following:
  1. ≥ 50 g aspirin a month or equivalent of other mild analgesics
  2. ≥ 100 tablets a month of analgesics combined with barbiturates or other nonnarcotic compounds
  3. One or more narcotic analgesics

mulated evidence suggests diagnostic precision has been improved considerably (Weeks, 1992). These criteria are being continuously reviewed, with a revised draft planned in 1993.

The revised classification system upholds traditional etiological distinctions between migraine headache and tension-type headache, although some argue the two are simply manifestations of similar underlying physiological processes (Raskin, 1988; Saper, 1986). As research unfolds, migraine is being found to be marked by biochemical imbalances, neurotransmitter/receptor dysfunction, and neuronal suppression, in addition to the peripheral vascular abnormalities once thought to be the key causal factor (Saper, 1986). The frequent failure to find evidence of muscle abnormalities and the clinical observation that the particular symptom pattern of tension-type symptoms has a direct bearing on outcome led the authors

of the new classification system to categorize tension-type patients along two dimensions, leading to four specific subtypes: those who do and do not evidence pericranial muscle tension crossed by those whose symptoms are either episodic or chronic (with the chronic variety being the most treatment resistant).

Recent developments in psychophysiological assessment may lead to further improvements in diagnosing and judging the merits of continued adherence to a muscular abnormality model for tension-type headache. Use of a bilateral frontal-posterior neck electrode placement, a muscle scanning protocol, or a dynamic approach (with recordings taken during movement and postural changes as well as rest) show promise in assessment (Ahles, King, & Martin, 1984; Ahles et al., 1988; Hudzinski & Lawrence, 1988, 1990). More detailed discussion of psychophysiological assessment approaches that may be helpful with headache patients may be found in the chapter by Flor, Miltner, and Birbaumer (Chapter 11).

It has been pointed out that a substantial portion of individuals currently diagnosed as tension-type headache who have no appreciable muscle tension component may in actuality be migraine headaches "transformed" to now resemble tension headache (Mathew, Reuveni, & Perez, 1987). It is also likely that a sizable percentage of chronic tension-type headaches may be resulting in part from the iatrogenic effects of certain medications. Distinctions between migraine and tension headache remain in part because of their differential responses to pharmacological agents (see Diamond, 1990; Diamond & Dalessio, 1986; Mathew, 1990; Raskin, 1988, for guidelines for medical management).

A new diagnostic entity concerns "headaches associated with substances or their withdrawal." Research suggests that two types of medication commonly prescribed for headache patients, namely, analgesics (Kudrow, 1982; Rapoport, 1988; Worz, 1983) and ergotamine preparations (Saper, 1987; Saper & Jones, 1986; Worz, 1983), can lead to "rebound" headaches if overused. The term "rebound" refers both to the worsening of the headache as the medication wears off and to the fact that the patient goes through a marked exacerbation after abrupt discontinuation of the medication (withdrawal-like phenomenon). It is this sequence of symptoms that "seduces" patients into taking ever-increasing amounts of medication, establishing a vicious cycle. Saper (1987) describes the typical course of ergotamine abuse, which is summarized in Table 4.

Kudrow (1982) tracks a similar course in tension-type headache patients—a patient takes increasing amounts of analgesics, which subsequently increases pain symptomatology and then render the headache refractory to treatments that formerly would have been of benefit. Kudrow conducted an empirical test by randomly assigning analgesic abusers to one of four conditions in a 2 × 2 contingency table (see Table 20.5). Patients were either withdrawn from or allowed to continue analgesics and simultaneously were assigned either to placebo or amitriptyline (the most commonly prescribed prophylactic drug for this form of headache). He found that mere withdrawal from analgesics led to measurable improvement, withdrawal combined with a proven medication led to the greatest improvement, and, perhaps most importantly, that allowing patients to continue analgesics at an abusively high level markedly interfered with the effectiveness of the medication (effectiveness was reduced by approximately 60%).

Clinicians working with headache patients need to be familiar with criteria for medication abuse, to inquire carefully about current and past medication consumption, and to arrange, in close collaboration with a physician, a medication reduction/detoxification plan for patients suspected of experiencing medication rebound headache. Ergotamine withdrawal can be difficult to accomplish on an outpatient basis and may require a brief hospital stay. Saper reports that within 72 hours of ergotamine withdrawal patients may experience their most intense headache, which may last up to 72 hours (often necessitating a 6–7 day hospital stay). Saper suggests that dosage days per week are the more critical variable in determining if ergotamine is being abused. He suggests any patient consuming ergotamine on more than 2 days per week is a candidate for medication withdrawal. Kudrow had analgesic abusers withdraw on their own (in the absence of therapist contact) and encountered high rates of dropout in the process. Regular therapist contact and support, concurrent provision of appropriate prophylactic medication as necessary, and beginning

TABLE 20.4. Clinical Features and Evolution of Ergotamine Dependency Syndrome

History:	Intermittent migraine or mixed migraine-tension headache
Ergotamine:	Insidious increase to greater than 2 dosage days per week
Headache:	Parallel increase in migraine frequency
Ergotamine:	Use becomes irresistible and predictable
Headache:	Becomes refractory to other appropriate treatment
Ergotamine:	Patient demands increasing amounts of medicine
Ergotamine:	Withdrawal following discontinuation
Other:	Concurrent symptoms of depression, sleep disturbance, and loss of well-being

TABLE 20.5. Treatment Outcome

	Amitriptyline	Placebo
Analgesics withdrawn	72%	43%
Analgesics continued	30%	18%

From Kudrow (1982).

instruction in behavioral coping skills may help patients to be more successful in completing a needed medication washout period.

Three other types of headache (cluster, menstrual migraine, and posttraumatic) deserve special mention because of their varied outcomes to treatment. For the typical migraine and tension-type headache (uncomplicated by medication overuse and episodic in nature), both pharmacological and nonpharmacological approaches appear to be of similar effectiveness (see Andrasik, 1986; Blanchard & Andrasik, 1985; Holroyd & Andrasik, 1982; for descriptions and discussions of relaxation, biofeedback, and cognitive-behavioral/stress coping treatment procedures). Attempts to treat patients diagnosed as cluster or menstrual migraine (the latter defined as headaches occurring 3 days prior to, during, or 3 days following menses) chiefly by nonpharmacological treatments have proven to be largely unsuccessful (Blanchard, Andrasik, Jurish, & Teders, 1982; Solbach, Sargent, & Coyne, 1984; Szekely et al., 1986). An exception to the refractory nature of menstrual migraine to nonpharmacological treatment was found in a recent article (Gauthier, Fournier, & Roberge, 1991). Given the mixed results, statements about the efficacy of nonpharmacological approaches for menstrual migraine must remain equivocal.

Nonpharmacological approaches may still be of value to some cluster and menstrual migraine patients, however, in helping them cope better with the distress often resulting from having to endure repeated, intense attacks of these types of headache. Finally, patients whose headaches occur following trauma typically experience a multitude of problems that make treatment particularly difficult (Barnat, 1986). A coordinated, interdisciplinary approach, similar to that found in place at most comprehensive pain centers, is typically required (Duckro, Tait, Margolis, & Silvermintz, 1985; McGrady, Bernal, Fine, & Woerner, 1983; Muse, 1986). Inpatient headache specialty units have sprouted across the country to handle complicated cases, such as the medication abuser, and posttraumatic headache (see Table 20.6 for a listing of typical inpatient admission criteria).

A Biopsychological Framework for Headache Assessment

The biopsychological model of headache states that the likelihood of any individual experi-

TABLE 20.6. Criteria for Admission to Headache Inpatient Unit

1. Prolonged, unrelenting headache, with associated symptoms, such as nausea and vomiting, that, if allowed to continue, would pose a further threat to the patient's welfare.
2. Status migraine.
3. Dependence on analgesics, caffeine, narcotics, barbiturates, and tranquilizers.
4. Habituation to ergots; ergots taken on a daily basis, when stopped, cause a rebound headache.
5. Pain that is accompanied by serious adverse reactions or complications from therapy; continued use of such therapy aggravates pain.
6. Pain that occurs in the presence of significant medical disease; appropriate treatment of headache symptoms aggravates or induces further illness.
7. Chronic cluster that is unresponsive to treatment.
8. Treatment requiring copharmacy with drugs that may cause a drug interaction and necessitating careful observation within a hospital environment (MAOI's and Beta-blockers).
9. Patients with probably organic cause to their headaches requiring appropriate consultations and perhaps neurosurgical intervention.

Note: From Freitag (1986), page 210. Copyright 1986 Williams & Wilkins. Reprinted by permission.

encing headache depends upon the specific pathophysiological mechanisms that are "triggered" by the interplay of the individual's physiological status (e.g., level of autonomic arousal), environmental factors (e.g., stressful circumstances, certain foods, alcohol, toxins, hormonal fluctuations), the individuals's ability to cope with these factors (both cognitively and behaviorally), and consequential factors that may serve to reinforce, and thus increase, the individual's chances of reporting head pain (Waggoner & Andrasik, 1990). The main determinant for the resulting headache is the pathophysiological biological response system that is activated. Psychological factors do not play a causal role per se. Rather, psychological factors contribute to headache as (1) trigger factors, (2) maintaining or exacerbating factors (to illustrate, ask the patient which is worse, onset of a headache when the patient is refreshed and rested or when work and family frustrations are at a peak), and (3) as sequelae to continued head pain and subsequent life disruption.

The prolonged presence of headache begins to exert a psychological toll on the patient over time, such that the patient becomes "sick and tired of feeling sick and tired." The negative thoughts and emotions arising from the repeated experience of headache thus can become further stressors or trigger factors in and of themselves (referred to as "headache-related distress"), serving at that point both to help maintain the disorder and to increase the severity and likelihood of future attacks. Pointing out the direct and indirect psychological influences on headache may make it easier for the patient to understand and accept the role of psychological factors and can often facilitate referral for adjunctive psychological/psychiatric care when needed. This model points out the various areas to address when interviewing headache patients.

Initially, the interviewer should inquire about any obvious precipitants. Gallagher (1990) provides a comprehensive discussion of the major suspected triggers for vascular headaches (such as diet, tension, hormonal fluctuations, irregular sleep, and hunger). The patient may need to undergo a period of systematic record keeping before triggers become apparent. A more involved form of monitoring is that performed in cognitive-behavioral or stress-coping training approaches. In this treatment, patients are taught intensive self-monitoring skills to enable them to identify the covert and overt events that precede, accompany, and follow stressful or headache-eliciting transactions. Patients seek to identify the sensations, feelings, thoughts, and behaviors associated with stressful events and headache attacks. As the patient becomes adept at self-monitoring, the therapist assists the patient in identifying relationships between situational variables (criticism from significant other), thoughts ("I can't do anything right"), and emotional, behavioral, and symptomatic responses (depression, withdrawal, and headache).

Table 20.7 summarizes one day of recording by a patient undergoing cognitive-behavioral therapy (Holroyd & Andrasik, 1982). This patient's diary provides fertile ground for hypotheses for intervention. Headache onset, it is noted, was preceded by resentment and anxiety over work demands and the apparent sexual overtures of a fellow employee, as well as by nausea and sensations of tingling and lightheadedness. The patient appears unable to take actions that might resolve these conflicts or to manage the emotional distress and tension these situations arouse. It is speculated that her inner dialogue of conflict undermines her ef-

forts to cope more effectively with the situation. Not all self-monitoring yields such rich assessment data, and most headache sufferers experience at least some of their headaches as appearing without warning. These headaches are dealt with by attempting to modify the psychological correlates of headache and altering factors in the patient's life that may increase vulnerability to headache even when they do not occur in close proximity to the headache attacks themselves.

The psychological status of the patient deserves special attention in order to identify conditions (formal thought disorder, certain personality disorders) that might interfere with treatment and need to be handled prior to treatment of the headache per se or that may otherwise compromise treatment. For example, studies have consistently shown that patients displaying only minor elevations on a scale commonly used to assess depression (Beck Depression Inventory) have a diminished response to self-regulatory treatments (Blanchard et al., 1985; Jacob, Turner, Szekely, & Eidelman, 1983) and even abortive medication (Holroyd et al., 1988). Other variables (anxiety, scales 1, 2, and 3 of the MMPI) have been suggested as predictive of response to certain treatments, but they have yet to undergo cross-validation and, thus, are of uncertain value.

The relationship between stress and headache has long been noted in the literature (Henryk-Gutt & Rees, 1973; Howarth, 1965). Stress-induced migraine may occur not at the peak of stress, but during a period of relaxation immediately following stress (April 16 for tax accountants, at the end of the term for teachers). Stress probably interacts with other precipitants to increase vulnerability to migraine, without necessarily precipitating any particular migraine episode. It is important to realize that a patients' stress experience is idiosyncratic; stress rests within the individual's cognitive interpretive framework. That is, what determines whether any given event is stressful is more a function of how the patient appraises the event.

Lazarus and Folkman (1982) distinguish two types of appraisal: primary—whether a given event is judged to be significant to the patient's well-being, and secondary—whether the patient possesses the available resources or options to respond successfully to the event. What is appraised as significant by one patient

TABLE 20.7. Sample from Self-Monitoring Record of Events Associated with Onset of Headache

Time	Situation	Physical sensations	Thoughts	Feeling (0–100)	Behavior
8:00 AM	Breakfast, husband says I look "scattered"	—	Worry about getting to work on time (e.g., If I'm late Mr._____ will notice)	Anxiety (25) Hurt (20)	Rush through breakfast, leave dishes in sink
10:00 AM	Given too many technical letters to type	Upset stomach from coffee, tense muscles	Everybody assumes I'm superwoman. No one takes account of other demands on my time	Anxiety (30) Annoyance (20)	Rushed typing, curt on telephone, take extra long break to calm down
12:00 noon	Jerry (fellow employee and supervisor) asks me to lunch. Talks suggestively about recent divorce	Lightheaded, tingling sensations in head and face, nausea	Jerry in on the make. I don't like fending him off—so why am I here. Am I seductive?	Anxiety (50) Awkwardness (40) Is that a feeling?	Try and offer sympathy but resent ulterior motive. Probably curt
2:00 PM	Spencer gives me long report with 5 tables to be done by 5:00	Headache—back of neck	F--- him—he didn't even ask what else I had to do. Fantasize Spencer stuck in elevator. No time to relax	Anger (60) Anxiety (60)	Typing report—distractedly
4:00 PM	Report completed	Headache worsening, nausea	If I could quit ruminating and was more organized I would get more work done	Anger (40) Anxiety (50)	Give report for correction. Complain to Susan. Type letters

Note: From Holyroyd and Andrasik (1982), page 303. Copyright 1982 Academic Press Inc. Reprinted by permission.

may not be by another. For any given headache sufferer, stress is likely operating in one or more ways and in concert with other various biologic influences. Take as an example, the headache sufferer who is able to drink a glass or two of red wine and escape headache when feeling "on top of the world," but is not able to do so when overworked, eating on the run, and so on. Therapists need to recognize that major stressful life events are not always the main culprit. Rather, more recent evidence indicates that everyday "ups and downs" or "hassles" are sufficient to engage biologic headache mechanisms (Andrasik et al., 1982; Holm, Holroyd, Hursey, & Penzien, 1986; Levor et al., 1986). More discussion of psychological and cognitive aspects may be found in the chapters by Bardley, Haile, and Jaworski (Chapter 12) and DeGood and Shutty (Chapter 13).

Fordyce (1976) has pointed out how pain complaints can be maintained by environmental consequences; Fowler (1975) has applied this perspective to headache patients. A patient is most likely to "learn" pain behavior when (1) pain behavior is positively reinforced or rewarded or (2) "well" behavior is insufficiently reinforced, punished, or aversive (see Keefe & Williams, Chapter 16). Therapists can unwittingly become a part of the learned pain behavior process in several different ways. Attention from others is a near universal reinforcer; the sympathetic ear of a therapist can be especially powerful. Medication prescribing practices can foster untoward learning effects as well. Palliative medications are often prescribed on an "as-needed" basis, accompanied by the caution, "Take this only when you really need it; it is powerful and may be addicting." When instructed in this manner, many patients will delay taking the medication until their pain becomes barely tolerable or near maximum level. If the medication effectively relieves the headache, medication taking behavior has become strongly reinforced and is likely to become more frequent in the future (based on principles of learning theory).

A final trap can occur when treating patients whose headache severity has markedly compromised their day-to-day functioning (a common occurrence with posttraumatic headache). Such patients are typically instructed, "Do only what you can" or continue activities "until the pain becomes unbearable." The patient begins an activity, experiences increased pain, and then stops. Stopping the activity reduces discomfort and makes the patient less likely to engage in activity in the future. Consequently, therapists need to probe for environmental conditions that may be serving to maintain headache pain behavior and to be aware of how he or she may subtly begin to contribute to the headache problem itself.

The way out of these traps is to lessen (gradually) attention given to pain symptoms, encourage and reinforce efforts to cope with head pain (ask, "How are you trying to manage your headaches?" rather than, "How is your headache today?"), encourage the inactive patient to set daily goals and stick to them despite the pain level, and arrange for needed analgesic medications to be taken on a time-contingent, as opposed to a pain-contingent, basis. Fordyce (1976) presents a detailed format for questions to ask of patients and family members being treated for chronic pain, which are also appropriate to consider when evaluating headache patients.

When significant cognitive deficits or diminished cognitive capacities are observed or suspected (such as the case of posttraumatic headache), it may be helpful to conduct a structured neuropsychological screening to determine if referral to a clinical neuropsychologist is warranted. Penzien, Rains, and Holroyd (in press) recommend use of the Cognitive Capacities Screening Examination (Jacobs, Bernhard, Delgado, & Strain, 1977) or the Mini-Mental State (Folstein, Folstein, & McHugh, 1975) for this purpose. There seems to be little utility to use of these measures on a routine basis in a headache practice. When tested in such a setting, only 2 of 88 patients scored in the range suggesting significant organic involvement (Lawson et al., 1988).

MEASUREMENT OF HEADACHE PAIN

The Headache Diary/Log

Pain is a private event and no method yet exists that can reliably objectify any headache parameters. By default, subjective ratings of head pain, sampled throughout the day, have come to be regarded as the "gold standard." In early research on headache (Budzynski, Stoyva, Adler, & Mullaney, 1973), patients completed self-monitoring records like the one depicted in Figure 20.1 on a daily basis. The recording grids were typically reproduced on a $3'' \times 5''$ index card and patients were asked to make hourly determinations of their head pain on a graded intensity scale and also to record any medications consumed. Because change in headache can occur along varied dimensions (change in frequency, length, or severity), data from the records were summarized in various ways: (1) frequency—number of discrete headaches over a specified interval; (2) duration—length of time between headache onset and offset; (3) peak intensity—highest intensity value for a given period, which allows the therapist to determine if the "edge" is being taken off headaches; (4) headache index/activity—a composite measure that incorporates all dimensions, calculated by summing all intensity values (which would yield a value of 53 for the sample record); and (5) medication consumption—number of pills taken for headache, a behavior "motivated" by pain.

Simple pill counts become problematic when patients take more than one medication or switch medications during treatment or when comparison across patients is desired. Coyne, Sargent, Segerson, and Obourn (1976) had medical experts rate the potency for various analgesic preparations used to control migraine. We added to this list and grouped the medications by potency values that ranged from 1 to 7 (see Table 20.8). A Medication Index can be obtained by multiplying and then summing the number of pills taken by their respective potency value. These measures are typically summarized weekly, plotted on graph paper, and shown to the patient to demonstrate progress.

It is important to monitor medication consumption for several reasons. First is to be on guard for excessive use that may be triggering rebound headache. Second, many patients specifically request nonpharmacological treatment

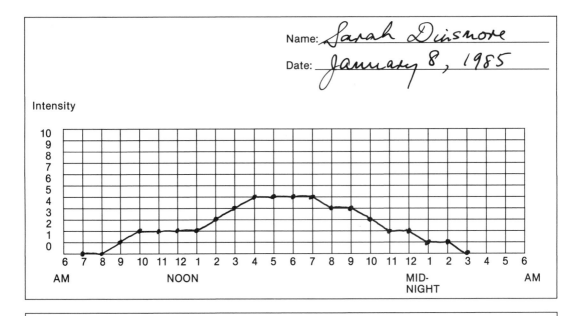

Name: *Sarah Dinsmore*

Date: *January 8, 1985*

Intensity

0 No Headache

2 Slightly painful—I only notice it when I focus my attention on it.

4 Mildly painful—I can ignore it most of the time.

6 Moderately painful—I continually notice it but I can continue what I am doing.

8 Very painful—I can only perform tasks which require little concentration.

10 Extremely painful—It makes it virtually impossible to do anything.

Medication: Each time medication is taken for headache please indicate amount, type, and dosage level.
Example: 1-Valium, 5 mg.

1. *2 - Tylenol*   3. *1 - Tyl + Codeine* 5. *1 - Tyl + Codeine*

2. *3 - Tylenol*   4. *2 - Tylenol*   6. *2 - Tylenol*

FIGURE 20.1. Front (*top panel*) and back side (*bottom panel*) of a sample headache diary. From Andrasik and Burke (1987), pages 49–50. Copyright 1987 Professional Resource Exchange (Sarasota, FL). Reprinted by permission.

because of a desire to reduce or eliminate their need for medication. Systematic measures are necessary to evaluate progress toward this goal. Finally, concurrent tracking of pain parameters and medication allows the therapist to determine if observed improvements in pain level are due in part to increased use of medications or enhanced compliance to a prescribed prophylactic regimen.

Several modifications to the intensive, hourly recording format have been proposed in order to improve compliance and accuracy.

Epstein and Abel (1977), when observing patients, noted most did not record continuously; rather, they would periodically fill in these recordings later by recall. Their modified procedure asked patients to make ratings only four times per day: wakeup/breakfast, lunch, evening meal, and bedtime. These events tend to occur at fairly regular times during a patient's day and are times that are easily discriminated. Collins and Martin (1980) compared this reduced demand format to a bihourly monitoring schedule and found they yielded

TABLE 20.8. Relative Potency of Headache Drugs on a Seven-Point Scale

1	2	3	4	5	6	7
APC[a]	Darvon[a]	Cafergot[a]	Codeine[a]	Demerol[a]	Dialudid[a]	Morphine[a]
Alka Seltzer[a]	Fiorinal[a]	(Cafregon)[a]	Empirin Compound			
Anacin[a]	Darvocet N[a]	Cynergen[a]	with Codeine #3[a]			
Aspirin[a]	Dolene	Flexeril	Leratine[a]			
Bufferin[a]	Soma	Librium	Ponstel[a]			
Cope[a]		Valium	Talwin*			
Empirin[a]		Triavil	Percodan			
Excedrin[a]		Inderal	Tylenol III			
Midrin[a]		Tranxene	(with Codeine)			
Nervine[a]		Ergostat	Empracet			
Norgesic[a]		Tofranil	Tylenol IV			
Parafon[a]		Elavil	(with Codeine)			
Persistin[a]		Propranol				
Phenaphen[a]		Sansert				
Robaxisal[a]		Ergottar				
Sinutab[a]		Zomax				
Tylenol[a]		Dilantin				
Vanquish[a]		Sinequan				
Coricidin D		Endep				
Corincider		Seconal				
Arthritic						
Ascription						
Actifed						
Phenilin						
Motrin						
Idenal						
Dimetapp						
Sudafed						
Percogesic						
Rondec						

Note: From Blanchard and Andrasik (1985), page 52. Copyright 1985 Pergamon Press. Reprinted by permission.
[a]These items were included in the original scale published by Coyne et al. (1976).

fairly equivalent results. Epstein and Abel additionally asked patients to record situational variables and methods used to manage pain. They also attempted to evaluate possible extra-laboratory indications of headache by conducting clinical interviews or engaging in telephone conversations with persons in the patient's natural environment (spouse, personal physician, etc.), hoping to find information that would provide additional insights for treatment planning and progress assessment.

Although a time-sampling format (such as four times per day) is less demanding for patients and is likely to yield more reliable and valid data, it does have some shortcomings. When using this type of approach, it is not possible to obtain true measures for frequency and duration of headache. If either of these are of prime interest to the therapist, then the format would have to be altered. Chronic or unwavering pain lends itself quite nicely to either format, but the clinician might want to

make alterations for individuals with infrequent, but discrete, prolonged migraine attacks. In the latter case, the patient could make ratings repeatedly throughout an attack or, alternatively, could note the time of onset and offset and then perform a single rating of peak headache intensity. This would allow the therapist to keep track of all key parameters. We have used this procedure successfully in an investigation of self-regulatory treatment for pediatric migraineurs (Andrasik, Burke, Attanasio, & Rosenblum, 1985). If patients resist recording on multiple occasions throughout the day, then a single recording at the end of the day is most advisable. Occasionally a patient's symptoms will display "reactivity" when being recorded systematically and worsen because of this increased symptom focus. These type reactions are typically short-lived, but if they persist many alternatives can substitute.

A critical concern with any type of daily monitoring record is the level of patient compliance. In an analog sample of college students, approximately 40% of subjects evidenced some degree of noncompliance; the most common form of noncompliance involved subjects recalling and completing ratings at a later time (Collins & Thompson, 1979). Reviewing pain records regularly, socially praising efforts to comply (yet refraining from punishing noncompliance), and having the patient mail records to the office when gaps between appointments are large may help emphasize the importance of and facilitate accurate record keeping.

It is not unusual for clinicians to have their patients monitor headache on a systematic basis during treatment but to conduct follow-up evaluations by interview or questionnaire completion. Several studies have examined correspondence between these two approaches: prospective, daily monitoring versus retrospective, global determinations (Andrasik et al., 1985; Andrasik & Holyroyd, 1980; Cahn & Cram, 1980). Very different results emerge, with the latter believed to yield biased *overestimates* of improvement. The clinician needs to be aware of bias when it is necessary to alter measures midstream and not be lulled into uncritical acceptance of biased global reports of benefit.

Alternative or Supplementary Approaches

A number of supplementary and/or alternative approaches are being pilot tested at present, and three may be easily adopted by the practitioner: (1) measurement of multiple aspects of pain, (2) social validation of patient improvement, and (3) measurement of pain behavior or behavior motivated by pain.

The experience of pain is complex and includes several dimensions or aspects, such as sensory, affective, and evaluative (see Jensen & Karoly, Chapter 9, Price & Harkins, Chapter 8, and Melzack & Katz, Chapter 10). The sensory component, for example, includes stimulus attributes such as intensity, location, and quality of the pain, and the affective (or reactive) component involves a patient's emotional reaction to the pain, fears about what the pain may signal, and concerns about ability to cope in a socially acceptable manner. Research suggests that the headache diary as typically used is sensitive primarily to the sensory (or intensity) dimension and is not all that effective for

tapping into the affective dimension (Andrasik, Blanchard, Ahles, Pallmeyer, & Barron, 1981). We adapted Tursky's (1976) idiographic multidimensional measurement technique for separating the two dimensions of pain (sensory and affective) in the aforementioned study (Andrasik et al., 1981). Although effective, Tursky's procedure requires considerable patient time for administration and therapist time for scoring, which restricts its utility for everyday clinical application. Items contained in the McGill Pain Questionnaire (Melzack, 1975; Melzack & Katz, Chapter 10) are similarly designed to access varied components of pain, and these items may be more practical for use by therapists. Price, McGrath, Rafii, and Buckingham (1983) successfully piloted a procedure for assessing the sensory and affective aspects of chronic pain by use of Visual Analog Scales (VASs) (see Jensen & Karoly, Chapter 9). Their approach could be adapted for use with headache patients and repeated at various times during the day. In their procedure, the VASs were anchored as follows: "no sensation" and "the most intense sensation imaginable" for the sensory dimension and "not bad at all" and "the most intense bad feeling possible for me" for measuring the affective dimension.

The clinical utility of considering multiple aspects of the pain experience is illustrated by the following. When using standard headache diary measures alone, it is not uncommon for a patient to complete treatment with no appreciable change being reflected in pain ratings. Upon interview, such patients often describe marked improvement, most notable in the level of distress now experienced. Although it is possible that such comments result from efforts/demands to please the therapist, it seems more likely that even though the sensory aspects of pain have not changed, significant change has occurred in the affective realm. In support, patients may report: "Even though my head hurts just as much, I don't let it bother me so." "It still hurts a lot, but I can cope with it better now." Failure to incorporate aspects other than the sensory dimension may lead to a loss of much clinically important information.

Another approach we have found useful is based on the notions of social validity (Kazdin, 1977; Wolf, 1978). In a supporting investigation, we administered a brief questionnaire to a significant other identified by the patient (parent, spouse, child, roommate) upon completion of treatment and asked that these forms be completed and returned to us without conferring with the patient (Blanchard, Andrasik, Neff, Jurish, & O'Keefe, 1981). One part of the questionnaire asked the significant other to rate the degree of change in the patient's headache activity since the patient entered treatment. Ratings were made on a 100-mm VAS, which was anchored at the leftend by "unchanged" and at the other by "extremely improved or completely cured." Measuring the distance between the leftmost end of the scale to the point indicated by the significant other yielded a percentage improvement score (ranging from 0 to 100%). Ratings provided by significant others correlated modestly ($r = .44$) with actual diary ratings completed by the patients, suggesting some usefulness to this approach. When the line of best fit was plotted for data collected from 62 patients, it was noted to intercept the *y*-axis above the 0 point; the point at which patient diaries reflected 0% improvement, ratings by significant others reflected about 30% improvement. Based on this, it is possible that the data provided by significant others are positively biased or that the significant others may be reacting to another aspect of pain (such as the affective component). Statisticians who reviewed this paper offered yet another possible explanation. They pointed out that measurement biases could be operating because the two measures that were compared had different endpoints (significant other ratings could not reflect deterioration, whereas the diary measures could). If clinicians decide to use this type of approach, it is recommended that the description for the left-most end of the VAS be modified to read something like "markedly worse" and that "no change/no improvement" be centered midway between the two end-points.

Philips (1983a, 1983b) has pointed out the limitations of measurement approaches that rely solely on subjective reports of headache sufferers. The fundamental problem is that physiological, subjective, and behavioral aspects are not perfectly correlated. Attention to all dimensions is needed to provide the most helpful assessment. Philips and Hunter (1981) reported on the preliminary development of a behavioral checklist for use with headache patients, which was subsequently refined by Philips and Jahanshahi (1986). The revised checklist is composed of 49 items, with items designed to yield three different subscores (avoidance behavior, verbal and nonverbal complaints, and help-seeking behavior) and a total score. In their 1986 study several psychometric properties were investigated (test–retest reliability, factor structure, and construct validity). One-week test–retest coefficients were acceptable for all scores except help-seeking behavior ($r = .53$). Thirteen, rather than the hypothesized three factors emerged, and they, along with item loadings, are presented in Table 20.9. Of particular note is the predominance of avoidance factors. The last two factors contain only one item each, which suggests caution in their use. Construct validity was supported.

Philips and Jahanshahi (1986) point out the practical use of this revised checklist: calculation of the factor scores permits more precise specification of the type of pain behavior emitted by the patient, which then can be used for planning treatment. For example, patients scoring high on verbal and nonverbal complaint factor scores may be especially prone to secondary gain and may require certain environmental modifications. Those scoring high on the medication factor may be more prone to problems from medication rebound. It is important to remember that the scale as used by Philips and Jahanshahi is completed by patients themselves and, thus, constitutes *self-report* of behavior (not actual behavior). Several of the factors could be adapted to permit actual behavior observations, with information provided by treatment staff, significant others, and so on.

Quality of Life and Functional Impairment

It is only recently that researchers have begun to assess the impact of different chronic conditions on a patient's functioning and well-being. Osterhaus and Townsend (1991) administered an updated version of a quality-of-life scale used in the Medical Outcomes Study (Stewart et al., 1989) to over 500 migraineurs. When the obtained data were compared to data previously collected on various other medical disorders (hypertension, diabetes, arthritis, myocardial infarction, and gastrointestinal disorders), it was found that the personal impact of migraine was more serious for several of the indices. Overall, results showed that although migraineurs functioned better physically, their

TABLE 20.9. PA2 Varimax-Rotated Factor Matrix Including only Items with Loadings >0.30[a]

Factor 1. Social avoidance (21.9%)			Factor 6. Stimulation avoidance (42.6%)		
Item 44.	Avoid discos/dances	0.76	Item 34.	Avoid loud noise	0.63
Item 32.	Avoid party-going	0.71	Item 33.	Lie down/rest/sleep	0.50
Item 36.	Avoid cinema	0.68	Item 12.	Avoid bright lights	0.30
Item 26.	Avoid pub-going	0.53	Item 15.	Avoid going to work	0.27
Item 31.	Avoid travel in cars	0.51			
Item 48.	Avoid having visitors	0.50	Factor 7. Nonverbal complaint (45.7%)		
Item 29.	Avoid visiting	0.49			
Item 27.	Avoid sex	0.41	Item 47.	Grimace, frown, pull face	0.60
			Item 30.	Sigh, moan, cry out	0.54
Factor 2. Housework activities (27.2%)			Item 37.	Change posture	0.46
			Item 10.	Grip, rub, stroke site of pain	0.36
Item 11.	Avoid heavy housework	0.69			
Item 42.	Avoid light housework	0.61	Factor 8. Verbal complaint (48.5%)		
Item 24.	Avoid shopping	0.54			
Item 38.	Avoid odd jobs in house	0.50	Item 21.	Tell friend	0.67
Item 45.	Slow down in physical movements	0.48	Item 43.	Tell acquaintance	0.62
Item 5.	Avoid cooking	0.47	Item 6.	Tell someone in family	0.54
Item 25.	Limp, drag yourself	0.38			
			Factor 9. Self-help strategies A (51.2%)		
Factor 3. Daily mobility avoidance (31.6%)			Item 40.	Have alcohol	0.51
			Item 35.	Go swimming	0.49
Item 2.	Avoid lifting objects	0.70	Item 13.	Sit on hard chair	0.30
Item 3.	Avoid public transportation	0.56			
Item 8.	Avoid walking stairs	0.54	Factor 10. Self-help strategies B (53.8%)		
Item 7.	Avoid restaurants	0.53			
Item 49.	Avoid carrying	0.48	Item 41.	Have back massaged	0.50
Item 16.	Avoid bending	0.41	Item 4.	Apply heat	0.37
Item 46.	Avoid stretching	0.34			
			Factor 11. Medication (56.1%)		
Factor 4. Activities avoidance (35.6%)			Item 1.	Take prescribed pill	0.57
Item 18.	Avoid gardening	0.64	Item 28.	Take unprescribed pill	0.51
Item 23.	Avoid cleaning car	0.54			
Item 22.	Avoid time on hobbies	0.44	Factor 12. Cry (58.4%)		
			Item 14.	Cry	0.44
Factor 5. Daily exercise avoidance (39.2%)					
			Factor 13. Distract (60.5%)		
Item 20.	Avoid standing	0.53			
Item 19.	Avoid walking	0.46	Item 17.	Distract yourself by reading etc.	0.57
Item 39.	Avoid spending time with cohabiters	0.40			
Item 9.	Avoid gentle exercise	0.38			

Note: From Philips and Jahanshahi (1986), page 120. Copyright 1986 Pergamon Press. Reprinted by permission.
[a]The cumulative percentage of variance is given in parentheses.

behavioral functioning was at a level well below their physical capabilities. A number of scales are currently available for assessing functional impairment, but nearly all are targeted for chronic, stable conditions and are of questionable value for recurrent, episodic disorders such as headache. A potentially more useful measure currently under development is the Recurrent Illness Impairment Profile, which addresses functional impairment in the social, behavioral, cognitive, and recreational domains (Wittrock, Penzien, Mosley & Johnson, 1991). Preliminary trials have revealed high internal consistency and split-half reliability, high test–retest

reliability for all but one aspect, and evidence in support of construct validity.

SUMMARY

Headache is multidetermined, requiring a comprehensive, multifactorial assessment approach. The headache assessor needs to be mindful of a patient's need for information, understanding, and reassurance. Thus, patient education and information exchange become an important part of the assessment process early on. Assessment begins with a thorough physical and neurological evaluation to rule out permanent structural defects or diagnosable physical conditions other than a primary headache disorder. Clinicians need to remain on alert status for a developing physical problem and to maintain close medical collaboration throughout treatment to monitor such problems and to obtain assistance with medication management and modification as needed. Determination of specific headache type is necessary to determine the proper medication approach, to identify patients whose headaches may be occurring in part to medication abuse, to identify headache types that have been found to be resilient to nonpharmacological approaches alone (cluster headache and menstrual migraine), and to decide when a comprehensive, multidisciplinary approach or even hospitalization is most needed (posttraumatic headache).

A biopsychological model points out the need to search for trigger, environmental, coping, and reinforcement factors that may be linked to headache. Assessment of the psychological status of the patient deserves special attention in order to identify conditions that might preclude direct treatment of headache at the moment (significant psychiatric problem or personality disorder) or complicate current treatment and compromise progress (depression, for example). Identification of stress factors, both major and minor, are often helpful in suggesting targets for intervention. A minority of patients may require specialized neuropsychological assessment.

Finally, various approaches to measurement are recommended. The main approach ("gold standard") at present involves use of daily headache pain diaries, from which multiple parameters may be obtained (headache frequency, duration, intensity, and overall index and medication consumption). More recent approaches concern measurement of separate aspects of the pain experience (reactive as well as sensory component), validation by contact with significant others, assessment of pain behaviors or behaviors assumed to be motivated by pain, and determination of the impact upon nonheadache variables, such as quality of life and functional impairment.

Although headache is a disorder of a long-standing nature, it is only recently that researchers have begun to explore various assessment dimensions in a rigorous fashion. Readers are referred to other recent reviews for additional discussion of developments in headache assessment (Andrasik & Burke, 1987; Lake, 1981; Philips, 1983a, 1983b; Thompson, 1982; Thompson & Figueroa, 1983).

REFERENCES

Ad Hoc Committee on Classification of Headache. (1962). Classification of headache. *Journal of the American Medical Association, 179,* 717–718.

Ahles, T., King, A., & Martin, J.E. (1984). EMG biofeedback during dynamic movement as a treatment for tension headache. *Headache, 24,* 41–44.

Ahles, T.A., Martin, J.B., Gaulier, B., Cassens, H.L., Andres, M.L., & Shariff, M. (1988). Electromyographic and vasomotor activity in tension, migraine, and combined headache patients: The influence of postural variation. *Behaviour Research and Therapy, 26,* 519–525.

Andrasik, F. (1986). Relaxation and biofeedback for chronic headaches. In A.D. Holzman & D.C. Turk (Eds.), *Pain management: A handbook of psychological treatment approaches* (pp. 213–239). New York: Pergamon.

Andrasik, F., & Baskin, S. (1987) Headache. In R.L. Morrison & A.S. Bellack (Eds.), *Medical factors and psychological disorders: A handbook for psychologists.* (pp. 325–349). New York: Plenum.

Andrasik, F., Blanchard, E.B., Ahles, T.A., Pallmeyer, T., & Barron, K.D. (1981). Assessing the reactive as well as the sensory component of headache pain. *Headache, 21,* 218–221.

Andrasik, F., Blanchard, E.B., Arena, J.G., Teders, S.J., Teevan, R.C., & Rodichok, L.D. (1982). Psychological functioning in headache sufferers. *Psychosomatic Medicine, 44,* 171–182.

Andrasik, F., & Burke, E.J. (1987). Assessment of headaches. In J.A. Blumenthal & D.C. McKee (Eds.), *Applications in behavioral medicine and health psychology: A clinician's source book* (pp. 39–65). Sarasota, FL: Professional Resource Exchange.

Andrasik, F., Burke, E.J., Attanasio, V., & Rosenblum, E.L. (1985). Child, parent, and physician reports of a child's headache pain: Relationships prior to and following treatment. *Headache, 25,* 421–425.

Andrasik, F., & Holroyd, K.A. (1980). Reliability and concurrent validity of headache questionnaire data. *Headache, 20,* 44–46.

Barnat, M.R. (1986). Post-traumatic headache patients I: Demographics, injuries, headache and health status. *Headache, 26,* 271–277.

Barnat, M.R., & Lake, A.E., III. (1983). Patient attitudes about headache. *Headache, 23,* 229–237.

Bille, B. (1962). Migraine in school children. *Acta Paediatrica Scandinavica, 51,* 1–151.

Bille, B. (1981). Migraine in childhood and its prognosis. *Cephalalgia, 1,* 71–75.

Blanchard, E.B., & Andrasik, F. (1985). *Management of chronic headaches: A psychological approach.* New York: Pergamon.

Blanchard, E.B., Andrasik, F., Evans, D.D., Neff, D.F., Appelbaum, K.A., & Rodichok, L.D. (1985). Behavioral treatment of 250 chronic headache patients: A clinical replication series. *Behavior Therapy, 16,* 308–327.

Blanchard, E.B., Andrasik, F., Jurish, S.E., & Teders, S.J. (1982). The treatment of cluster headache with relaxation and thermal biofeedback. *Biofeedback and Self-Regulation, 7*, 185–191.

Blanchard, E.B., Andrasik, F., Neff, D.F., Jurish, S.E., & O'Keefe, D.M. (1981). Social validation of the headache diary. *Behavior Therapy, 12*, 711–715.

Budzynski, T.H., Stoyva, J.M., Adler, C.S., & Mullaney, D.J. (1973). EMG biofeedback and tension headache: A controlled outcome study. *Psychosomatic Medicine, 35*, 484–496.

Cahn, T., & Cram, J.R. (1980). Changing measurement instrument at follow-up: A potential source of error. *Biofeedback and Self-Regulation, 5*, 265–273.

Collins, F.L., & Martin, J.E. (1980). Assessing self-report of pain: A comparison of two recording procedures. *Journal of Behavioral Assessment, 2*, 55–63.

Collins, F.L., & Thompson, J.K. (1979). Reliability and standardization in the assessment of self-reported headache pain. *Journal of Behavioral Assessment, 1*, 73–86.

Coyne, L., Sargent, J., Segerson, J., & Obourn, R. (1976). Relative potency scale for analgesic drugs: Use of psychophysical procedures with clinical judgments. *Headache, 16*, 70–71.

Diamond, S. (1990). (Ed.). *Migraine headache prevention and management.* New York: Marcel Dekker.

Diamond, S., & Dalessio, D.J. (1986). *The practicing physician's approach to headache* (4th ed.). Baltimore: Williams & Wilkins.

Duckro, P.N., Tait, R., Margolis, R.B., & Silvermintz, S. (1985). Behavioral treatment of headache following occupational trauma. *Headache, 25*, 328–331.

Epstein, L.H., & Abel, G.G. (1977). An analysis of biofeedback training effects for tension headache patients. *Behavior Therapy, 8*, 37–47.

Folstein, M.F., Folstein, S.E., & McHugh, P.R. (1975). "Mini-Mental State": A practical method for grading the cognitive state of patients for the clinician. *Journal of Psychiatric Research, 12*, 189–198.

Fordyce, W.E. (1976). *Behavioral methods for chronic pain and illness.* St. Louis: Mosby.

Fowler, R.S. (1975). Operant therapy for headaches. *Headache, 15*, 1–6.

Freitag, F.G. (1986). Headache clinics and inpatient units for treatment of headache. In S. Diamond & D.J. Dalessio (Eds.), *The practicing physician's approach to headache* (4th ed., pp. 200–213). Baltimore: Williams & Wilkins.

Gallagher, R.M. (1990). Precipitating cause of migraine. In S. Diamond (Ed.), *Migraine headache prevention and management* (pp. 31–44). New York: Marcel Dekker.

Gauthier, J.G., Fournier, A., & Roberge, C. (1991). The differential effects of biofeedback in the treatment of menstrual and nonmenstrual migraine. *Headache, 31*, 82–90.

Headache Classification Committee of the International Headache Society. (1988). Classification and diagnostic criteria for headache disorders, cranial neuralgias, and facial pain. *Cephalalgia, 8*, (Suppl. 7), 1–96.

Henryk-Gutt, R., & Rees, W.C. (1973). Psychological aspects of migraine. *Journal of Psychosomatic Research, 17*, 141–153.

Holm, J.E., Holroyd, K., Hursey, K.G., & Penzien, D. (1986). The role of stress in recurrent tension headaches. *Headache, 26*, 160–167.

Holroyd, K.A., & Andrasik, F. (1982). A cognitive-behavioral approach to recurrent tension and migraine headache. In P.C. Kendall (Ed.), *Advances in cognitive-behavioral research and therapy* (Vol. 1, pp. 275–320). New York: Academic Press.

Holroyd, K.A., Holm, J.E., Hursey, K.G., Penzien, D.B., Cordingley, G.E., Theofanous, A.G., Richardson, S.C., & Tobin, D.L. (1988). Recurrent vascular headache: Home-based behavioral treatment vs. abortive pharmacological treatment. *Journal of Consulting and Clinical Psychology, 56*, 218–223.

Howarth, E. (1965). Headache, personality, and stress. *British Journal of Psychiatry, 111*, 1193–1197.

Hudzinski, L.G., & Lawrence, G.S. (1988). Significance of EMG surface electrode placement models and headache findings. *Headache, 28*, 30–35.

Hudzinski, L.G., & Lawrence, G.S. (1990). EMG surface electrode normative data for muscle contraction headache and biofeedback therapy. *Headache Quarterly, 1*, 224–229.

Jacob, R.G., Turner, S.M., Szekely, B.C., & Eidelman, B.H. (1983). Predicting outcome of relaxation therapy in headaches: the role of "depression." *Behavior Therapy, 14*, 457–465.

Jacobs, J.W., Bernhard, M.R., Delgado, A., & Strain, J.J. (1977). Screening for organic mental syndromes in the medically ill. *Annals of Internal Medicine, 86*, 40–46.

Jay, G.W., & Tomasi, L.G. (1981). Pediatric headaches: A one year retrospective analysis. *Headache, 21*, 5–9.

Kazdin, A.E. (1977). Assessing the clinical or applied importance of behavior change through social validation. *Behavior Modification, 1*, 427–452.

Kudrow, L. (1982). Paradoxical effects of frequent analgesic use. In M. Critchley, A. Friedman, S. Gorini, & F. Sicuteri (Eds.), *Headache: Physiopathological and clinical concepts. Advances in Neurology* (Vol. 33, pp. 335–341). New York: Raven Press.

Lake, A.E., III. (1981). Behavioral assessment considerations in the management of headache. *Headache, 21*, 170–178.

Lawson, P., Kerr, K., Penzien, D.B., Hursey, K.G., Ray, S.E., Arora, R., Marcus-Mendoza, S., & Holm, J.E. (1988, November). *Caveats in using mental status examinations: Factors that may influence performance.* Paper presented at the annual meeting of the Association for Advancement of Behavior Therapy, New York.

Lazarus, R.S., & Folkman, S. (1984). Coping and adaption. In W.D. Gentry (Ed.), *The handbook of behavioral medicine* (pp. 282–325). New York: Guilford Press.

Levor, R.M., Cohen, M.J., Naliboff, B.D., McArthur, D., & Heuser, G. (1986). Psychosocial precursors and correlates of migraine headache. *Journal of Consulting and Clinical Psychology, 54*, 347–353.

Linet, M.S., Stewart, W.F., Celentano, D.D., Ziegler, D., & Sprecher, M. (1989). An epidemiologic study of headache among adolescents and young adults. *Journal of the American Medical Association, 261*, 2211–2216.

Mathew, N.T. (1990). *Neurologic clinics: Headache.* Philadelphia: Saunders.

Mathew, N.T., Reuveni, U., & Perez, F. (1987). Transformed or evolutive migraine. *Headache, 27*, 102–106.

McGrady, A.V., Bernal, G.A.A., Fine, T., & Woerner, M.P. (1983). Post traumatic head and neck pain, a multimodal treatment approach. *Journal of Holistic Medicine, 5*, 130–138.

Melzack, R. (1975). The McGill Pain Questionnaire:

Major properties and scoring methods. *Pain, 7,* 277–299.

Muse, M. (1986). Stress-related, post-traumatic chronic pain syndrome: Behavioral treatment approach. *Pain, 25,* 389–394.

Osterhaus, J.T., & Townsend, R.J. (1991, June/July). *The quality of life of migraineurs: A cross sectional profile.* Paper presented at the 5th International Headache Congress, Washington, DC.

Packard, R.C. (1979). What does the headache patient want? *Headache, 19,* 370–374.

Penzien, D.B., Rains, J.C., & Holroyd, K.A. (in press). Psychological assessment of the recurrent headache sufferer. In C.D. Tollison & R.S. Kunkel (Eds.), *Headache: Diagnosis and interdisciplinary treatment.* New York: Urban Schwarzenberg.

Philips, C. (1983a). Assessment of chronic headache behavior. In R. Melzack (Ed.), *Pain measurement and assessment* (pp. 155–163). New York: Raven Press.

Philips, C. (1983b). Chronic headache experience. In R. Melzack (Ed.), *Pain measurement and assessment* (pp. 97–103). New York: Raven Press.

Philips, C., & Hunter, M. (1981). Pain behaviour in headache sufferers. *Behaviour Analysis and Modification, 4,* 257–266.

Philips, H.C., & Jahanshahi, M. (1986). The components of pain behaviour report. *Behaviour Research and Therapy, 24,* 117–125.

Price, D.D., McGrath, P.A., Rafii, A., & Buckingham, B. (1983). The validation of Visual Analog Scale as ratio scale measures for chronic and experimental pain. *Pain, 17,* 45–56.

Rapoport, A.M. (1988). Analgesic rebound headache. *Headache, 28,* 662–665.

Raskin, N.H. (1988). *Headache* (2nd ed.). New York: Churchill Livingstone.

Ries, P.W. (1986). Current estimates from the national health interview survey, United States, 1984. *National Center for Health Statistics: 1986.* Vital and Health Statistics, Series 10, No. 156 (DHHS Publication No. PHS 86-1584). Washington, DC: U.S. Government Printing Office.

Saper, J.R. (1986). Changing perspectives on chronic headache. *Clinical Journal of Pain, 2,* 19–28.

Saper, J.R. (1987). Ergotamine dependency: A review. *Headache, 27,* 435–438.

Saper, J.R., & Jones, J.M. (1986). Ergotamine dependency. *Clinical Neuropharmacology, 9,* 244–256.

Sillanpaa, M. (1983a). Changes in the prevalence of migraine and other headaches during the first seven school years. *Headache, 23,* 15–19.

Sillanpaa, M. (1983b). Prevalence of headache in prepu-berty. *Headache, 23,* 10–14.

Solbach, P., Sargent, J., & Coyne, L. (1984). Menstrual migraine headache: Results of a controlled, experimental, outcome study of nondrug treatments. *Headache, 24,* 75–78.

Sternbach, R.A. (1986). Survey of pain in the United States: The Nuprin Pain Report. *Clinical Journal of Pain, 2,* 49–53.

Stewart, A.L., Greenfield, S., Hays, R.D., Wells, K., Rogers, W.H., Berry, S.D., Mcglynn, E.A., & Ware, J.E. (1989). Functional status and well-being of patients with chronic conditions. *Journal of the American Medical Association, 262,* 907–913.

Szekely, B., Botwin, D., Eidelman, B.H., Becker, M., Elman, N., & Schemm, R. (1986). Nonpharmacological treatment of menstrual headache: Relaxation biofeedback behavior therapy and person-centered insight therapy. *Headache, 26,* 86–92.

Thompson, J.K. (1982). Diagnosis of headache pain: An idiographic approach to assessment and classification. *Headache, 22,* 221–232.

Thompson, J.K., & Figueroa, J.L. (1983). Critical issues in the assessment of headache. In M. Hersen, R.M. Eisler, & P.M. Miller (Eds.), *Progress in behavior modification* (Vol. 15, pp. 81–111). New York: Academic.

Tursky, B. (1976). The development of a pain perception profile: A psychophysical approach. In M. Weisenberg & B. Tursky (Eds.), *Pain: New perspectives in therapy and research* (pp. 171–194). New York: Plenum Press.

Waggoner, C.D., & Andrasik, F. (1990). Behavioral assessment and treatment of recurrent headache. In T.W. Miller (Ed.), *Chronic pain* (Vol. 1, pp. 319–361). Madison, CT: International Universities Press.

Weeks, R.E. (1992, March). *Controversies in the diagnostic classification of headache: Toward a clinically meaningful, reliable system.* Paper presented at the annual meeting of the Association for Applied Psychophysiology and Biofeedback, Colorado Springs, CO.

Wittrock, D.A., Penzien, D.B., Mosley, T.H., & Johnson, C.A. (1991). The Recurrent Illness Impairment Profile: Preliminary results using the headache version. *Headache Quarterly, 2,* 138–139.

Wolf, M.M. (1978). Social validity: The case for subjective measurement or how applied behavior analysis is finding its heart. *Journal of Applied Behavior Analysis, 11,* 203–214.

Worz, R. (1983). Analgesic withdrawal in chronic pain treatment. In K. A. Holyroyd, B. Schlote, & H. Zenz (Eds.), *Perspectives in research on headache* (pp. 137–144). Toronto/Lewiston, NY: Hogrefe.

Chapter 21

How to Assess Cancer Pain

CHARLES S. CLEELAND, PhD
KAREN L. SYRJALA, PhD

Poorly controlled pain has such deleterious effects on the cancer patient and the patient's family that its proper management should have the highest priority in the routine care of the patient with cancer. Not only do mood and quality of life deteriorate in the presence of pain, but pain has adverse effects on such measures of disease status as appetite and activity. Pain of severe intensity may be a primary reason why both patients and their families decide to abandon treatment, or even why patients decide to actively end their lives. The fear of uncontrolled pain is a key motivator behind a growing movement to legalize euthanasia for terminally ill patients.

There is strong evidence that the majority of patients can obtain pain relief if adequate treatment is provided. Studies of the World Health Organization's (1986) guidelines for cancer pain relief indicate that 70 to 90% of patients are relieved if this simple protocol for oral analgesics and adjuvant medications is followed (Takeda, 1987; Ventafridda, Tamburini, Caraceni, DeConno, & Naldi 1987). When oral analgesics are not effective, a variety of supplemental pain management techniques can provide control. It is estimated that approximately 95% of patients could be free of significant pain (Foley, 1985). Unfortunately, despite the current availability of treatment,

several studies document widespread undertreatment of pain. One analysis of 11 published reports of cancer pain treatment covering nearly 2,000 patients in nonhospice settings estimates that 50–80% did not have adequate pain control (Bonica, 1985). In another analysis (Cleeland, 1991) patients were asked about how much relief they received from their pain treatment. Less than half of the patients sampled reported that their pain was effectively managed.

Although there are multiple barriers to good pain control for the patient with cancer, inadequate assessment is the most obvious. Unrecognized pain will not be treated, and pain whose severity is underestimated will not be treated aggressively enough. In a recent study, 1,177 Eastern Cooperative Oncology Group (ECOG)-affiliated physicians responded to a survey designed to determine their knowledge of cancer pain management and the methods they use to manage pain (Von Roenn, Cleeland, Gonin, & Pandya, 1991). Together, these physicians reported treating over 70,000 cancer patients in the previous 6 months. Only 50% of these physicians felt that pain management was good or very good in their own practice setting. The respondents ranked a list of potential barriers to optimal cancer pain management in the order in which the barrier was perceived to impede pain management in their own practic settings. By far the most frequently identified barrier was lack of pain assessment; 76% of respondents rated pain assessment as one of the top four barriers to good pain management. Patient reluctance to report pain, intimately related to inadequate assessment, was the next most frequently cited barrier, identified among the top four by 62%.

Why is assessment so often inadequate? Appropriate models of assessment and tools to aid its accomplishment are available for the majority of situations where assessment is needed. Despite the recognition that pain assessment is important, formal pain assessment is rarely practiced in most cancer care settings. It is rarely practiced for a number of reasons: health care providers do not have the time to fully assess pain and its impact; health care providers do not have the skills necessary to adequately assess pain and pain treatment effects. Pain assessment is not a standard part of patient appointments, so that other priorities supplant symptom evaluation. When assessment is conducted, it is often nonstandard and brief, generating little information that would be useful in developing a pain treatment plan. Studies of agreement between providers and patients on the severity of pain uniformly demonstrate only modest correlations (Cleeland, 1984), and correlations are reduced even more when patients with moderate to severe pain are studied (Grossman, Sheidler, Swedeen, Mucenski, & Piantadosi, 1991). It is often up to patients to volunteer that they have pain, or that the pain treatment they are receiving is not effective, yet several studies have shown that patients are reluctant to be assertive in reporting their pain (Dar, Beech, Barden, & Cleeland, 1992; Hodes, 1989). When providers do ask about pain, they rarely attempt to quantify the severity of the pain or to document its characteristics and determinants. Even more rare is any attempt to assess the impact that pain is making on the emotional or functional status of the patient and the family.

In this chapter we examine some of the methodological and practical issues in the assessment of cancer pain and its impact. We describe a "minimal data set" of information needed for treatment planning, and suggest how pain questionnaires might be used to improve assessment. Although our focus is on the clinical assessment of pain, we describe how similar pain assessment procedures can be used

in such areas as clinical trials, quality assurance, and prevalence surveys. While we will deal solely with the type of data that can be obtained by questionnaires, interview, and observation of the patient, pain that is at least moderate in severity calls for the addition of a careful neurologic exam and appropriate medical diagnostic procedures. A recent retrospective survey (Gonzales, Elliot, Portenoy, & Foley, 1991) found that two-thirds of patients referred for pain assessment had new (and often treatable) pathology diagnosed as a result of neurological evaluation and follow-up.

Regardless of etiology, pain can be defined from several different theoretical perspectives, each of which may dictate specific assessment techniques. Within the field of cancer pain, we are concerned with the clinical management or clinical research applications of assessment. For these uses, our information sources center on patients' subjective reports of their pain and of functional impairment caused by the pain. Behavioral observation also has a role in cancer patient management, primarily when patients are not able to provide self-report (Chapko, Syrjala, Bush, Jedlow, & Yanke, 1991). In clinical research, behavioral observation can be similarly of value when self-report is not possible or as a method for establishing reliability and validity of pain assessment by using multiple indicators of the pain construct (see Keefe & Williams, Chapter 16, and Craig, Prkachin, & Grunau, Chapter 15).

PREVALENCE OF CANCER PAIN

Cancer is a generic term, applied to a variety of different diseases that have in common a distortion of cell development, leading to unregulated proliferation of cell growth that in turn results in invasion and metastases. The primary site and cell type of a cancer dictates many of its features including rate of development, response to anticancer therapies, common sites of metastatic spread of disease, and the course, severity, and quality of pain. Using requirements for analgesics while in the hospital as a criterion for inclusion, Foley (1979) found that 85% of patients with primary bone tumors and 52% of patients with breast cancer had pain requiring analgesics other than aspirin or acetaminophen, in contrast to 20% with lymphomas and only 5% with leukemias. Of those cancer patients who seek specialized pain treatment, less than 10% will have pain not related to their disease or its treatment (Foley, 1985).

Pain will eventually effect the majority of patients with cancer. Significant pain is rarely a problem before metastatic disease is present. Only 5–10% of patients with nonmetastatic disease report persistent disease-related pain (Daut & Cleeland, 1982). Clinicians have long been aware that the majority of cancer patients with advanced cancer will need careful pain management. It is estimated that 60–80% of such patients will have significant pain (Cleeland, 1984, 1985; Portenoy, 1989).Less attention has been paid to the problem of pain for patients prior to the end stage of disease. Once the disease has metastasized, 20–40% of both hospitalized patients and outpatients report pain of a severity that impairs function (Cleeland, 1984). Both the presence and severity of pain are dictated by several factors, including the primary site of the disease and metastatic location. Many cancers that were painless at onset become associated with a high prevalence of pain as the disease progresses. Breast disease is an excellent example of this. Although rarely painful in the early stages, half of those affected report pain after metastatic spread of their disease (Foley, 1979; Spiegel & Bloom, 1983).

Of the patients who achieve a cure, a substantial percentage have indefinite periods of treatment-related pain, although the prevalence of posttreatment pain has not been well studied. Because patients now live longer with their disease, greater numbers of patients have to face potentially longer periods of coping with pain from their cancer.

PHYSICAL BASIS OF CANCER PAIN

Pain in cancer patients can be due to diverse causes (Payne, 1990). Furthermore, multiple pain sources often coexist. Because treatment is determined by the etiology of the pain, establishing the physical cause of the pain is an important goal of assessment. In a study of patients referred to a multidisciplinary cancer pain clinic, the vast majority had pain due to multiple etiologies (Banning, Sjogren, & Henriksen, 1991). In this study, pain due to growth of the tumor included (in decreasing frequency) visceral pain, bone pain, soft tissue invasion, and nerve or nerve plexus pressure or

infiltration. Other studies have found that bone pain is the most frequent etiology of pain (Foley, 1979). Additional patients will have pain caused by treatment (Chapman, Kornell, & Syrjala, 1987). By necessity, cancer treatment is destructive, whether in the form of surgery, chemotherapy, or radiation therapy. Pain is often the product of these destructive procedures. Some treatment-related pain is time-limited, while in other cases a more permanent treatment-related pain syndrome such as peripheral neuropathy may develop. Although pain generally becomes worse with progress of the disease, pain can also improve if the disease is responsive to anticancer therapies, such as chemotherapy or radiotherapy. Pain treatment (and assessment) needs to be sensitive to these dynamic changes in pain expression.

An important distinction needs to be made between primary nociceptive pain (pain caused by stimulation of pain receptors) and neuropathic or deafferentation pain (painful sensations that are caused by injury to peripheral or central nervous system structures). Because nociceptive pain responds to different pharmacological interventions than does deafferentation pain, this distinction is critical for both clinical management and for the design of clinical trials. Either the trial should examine pain of one particular type, or pain mechanism should be a stratification variable.

THE CONTEXT OF CANCER PAIN ASSESSMENT

Historically, most pain assessment procedures were developed for patients with pain due to nonmalignant causes. Pain assessment evolved along with the development of multidisciplinary pain clinics that, for the most part, treated patients with reasonably stable pain complaints. These patients commonly reported pain as their primary health problem. Functional impairments are associated in large measure with the pain problem. The assessment of pain due to cancer requires some reorientation, dictated by the nature of the disease, the particular psychological context of having cancer, the types of pain that cancer causes, and the dynamic and progressive nature of both the disease itself and the treatment of that disease concurrent with our treatment of the pain.

Because most pain assessment procedures

have evolved from the needs of patients with chronic stable pain, it is important to point out some major differences between the majority of patients seen in more traditional pain clinics and those seen in cancer treatment settings. Patients seen in typical multidisciplinary pain clinics most often complain freely of pain, and some treatment programs are designed to reduce the frequency of these pain complaints in these patients because of the negative social consequences of persistent pain reporting. A common, currently controversial goal in the treatment of chronic stable pain is a reduction in reliance on potent opioid analgesics. Opioid analgesics (such as morphine), however, are often required to manage pain due to cancer or its treatment (World Health Organization, 1986). As the oncologists cited above recognized, patients with cancer frequently underreport pain and pain severity. Patients with cancer often do not want to be labeled as complainers, do not want to distract their caregiver from attending to the cancer, or are afraid that their pain means that their cancer is getting worse (Hodes, 1989). Patients are often concerned about having to take potent opioids because they fear that they will become addicts, will be thought of as addicts, will loose control, or will have unmanageable side effects. They are also often concerned that if they have adequate control of pain now that they will become tolerant to the effects of analgesics when their disease progresses (Cleeland, 1989; Dar, Beech, Barden, & Cleeland, 1992).

A second major treatment goal for the traditional pain clinic is an increase in patient function and a decrease in negative emotional states. Those who have experience working with patients who have chronic stable pain have come to expect that the typical patient with persistent pain has major life adjustment problems. Many of those patients are depressed, and it is easy to see how depressed mood may perpetuate their pain. However, a reorientation of these expectations is necessary when working with cancer patients in pain. Only a minority of them will report having significantly depressed mood (Shacham, Dar & Cleeland, 1984). For those who are depressed, their mood often improves markedly when adequate pain control is established. When pain (and not disease) limits function in cancer patients, significantly improved function will frequently accompany pain relief.

TARGETS OF PAIN ASSESSMENT

For the cancer patient, what do we need to know about the pain in order to plan treatment? First, we need to know how severe it is. The World Health Organization's Cancer Pain Relief method uses a determination of pain *severity* as the primary item of information in specifying treatment (World Health Organization, 1986). The analgesics to be used in the WHO method change in type and increase in potency as pain increases in severity. But severity is not the only information obtained by subjective report that guides treatment. Models of treatment that use a wide range of therapies (such as adjunctive medications, behavioral interventions, or neuroablative procedures) demand more of subjective report data than pain intensity alone. Patients need to be able to report the *quality* of their pain. They do this by using various descriptors, such as "burning," "shooting," or "cramping." We need to obtain information about the *temporal pattern* of the pain; is it constant, or episodically more severe. Are the episodes spontaneous or do they occur with specific movements? Information on pain quality and temporal pattern, together with information on the *location* of the pain, are helpful in determining the physical basis or mechanism of the pain. Information on the physical mechanism of the pain will be useful for choosing among a wide range of analgesic and adjunctive drugs available. It will also help to determine whether nondrug options, including stimulatory, ablative and cognitive-behavioral measures, should be considered. Finally, most patients have already been treated for pain. We need information about the previous *pain treatment history*— what worked and for how long.

An adequate pain assessment will go beyond information on pain characteristics and physical mechanisms. Comprehensive treatment plans also need to be based on information about the *impact* of the pain on the patient and the patient's family. We need information about how pain interferes with patient functioning. Does pain interfere with sleep, appetite, activity, sociability, and mood? If so, perhaps treatment of pain in isolation will restore these areas of functioning. On the other hand, pain may have persisted so long that additional treatment options, such as the use of antidepressant medications or behavioral interventions, need to be exercised.

Using pain assessment instruments minimizes many patient reporting biases and assists health care professionals (HCPs) in obtaining complete information. Using pain scales that assign a metric to pain intensity and interference makes pain more of an "objective" symptom, more like other signs and symptoms such as blood pressure and heart rate. By making pain "objective," standard questions allow patients to feel freer to report its presence, severity and also to report when treatment is not working. Patients are often less concerned about acknowledging the failure of a treatment on a questionnaire than responding to questions put to them by staff who care for them. "How is your medication working?" provokes a response of "fine" or "ok" from a patient who wants to please, whereas "Rate your pain from 0 to 10" does not require the patient to judge the success or failure of the HCP's treatment. Using pain questionnaires or pain measurement scales also can serve to minimize *staff biases* in recognizing when pain is present or in estimating its severity (Cleeland, 1989a). Using standard pain measurement tools reduces staff time in the assessment process. Finally, assigning a metric to pain allows for monitoring the effectiveness of pain treatment.

Working within the typical limitations of a cancer treatment setting, pain assessment needs to be focused on those aspects of pain that will lead to differential treatment decisions. Rarely will there be the professional time or patient acceptance or endurance to complete the type of assessment typically done in multidisciplinary pain clinics. It may be helpful to think of cancer pain assessment in a decision analysis model. Some branches of the decision tree need not be followed if appropriate screening does not indicate a treatment need. We have broken the assessment procedure into three levels. Although we would consider a minimal satisfactory assessment to include screening at all levels, we have assigned level one the highest priority.

LEVEL ONE: ASSESSING PAIN SEVERITY

Standard assessment of the multidimensional aspects of cancer pain makes it clear that pain severity is the primary factor determining the impact of pain on the patient. It is also the factor that drives the urgency and energy of the treatment process. It is more important to know the severity of the pain than to know that the patient does or does not have pain. Many adults, both with and without cancer, function quite effectively with a background level of pain that does not seriously impair or distract them. As pain severity increases, however, it passes a threshold beyond which it cannot be ignored. At this point, it becomes disruptive to many aspects of the patient's life. At very high levels, pain becomes a primary focus of attention and prohibits most non-pain-related activity. Figure 21.1 presents the steps involved in the assessment of pain severity.

Pain Severity Scales

Several ways of scaling the severity or intensity of pain and associated symptoms have been advocated. It is important to keep in mind that the particular clinical or research application will dictate the type of scale that is appropriate. Verbal Descriptor Scales (VDSs) have the longest history in pain research (Lasagna, 1980). The patient is asked to pick a category, such as "none," "mild," "moderate," "severe," and "excruciating," that best describes severity. Pain relief can be categorized in a similar way, such as "none," "slight," "moderate," "lots," and "complete." More recently, Visual Analogue Scales (VASs) have become quite popular in research comparing the effectiveness of analgesic drugs (Wallenstein, 1984). Using the VAS, the patient makes a judgment of how much of the scale, usually a straight line, is equivalent to (or analogous with) the severity of the pain. One end of the line represents no pain and the other some concept such as "pain as bad as you can imagine." Numerical Rating Scales (NRSs) measure pain severity by asking the patient to select a number from 0 to 10 (an 11-point scale) to represent how severe their pain is. The numbers can be arrayed along a horizontal line, with 0 on the left and labeled "no pain" and 10 on the right, labeled "pain as bad as you can imagine." Because pain due to cancer can be quite variable over a day, patients can be asked to rate their pain rate their pain at the time of responding to the questionnaire, and also at its "worst," "least," and "average" over the past 24 hours (see Jensen & Karoly, this volume).

In clinical settings, these three scales of severity approach equivalency (Jensen, Karoly & Braver, 1986) so that ease of administration

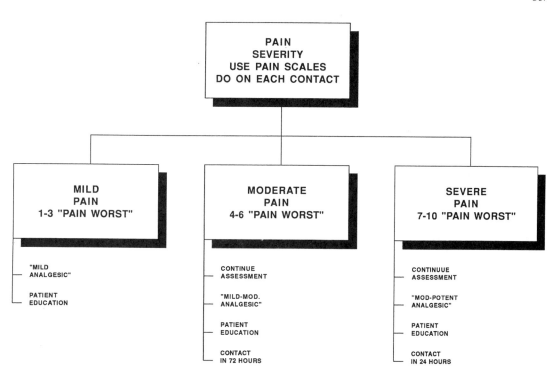

FIGURE 21.1. Assessment of cancer pain.

becomes more of a factor in scale selection. All three measures are highly intercorrelated, although the NRS and VAS are most highly correlated with each other (Syrjala, 1987). In clinical trials, the NRS has been found to be more reliable than the VAS, especially with less educated patients (Ferraz et al., 1990). With very sick patients, oral versions of the NRS are easily administered, although the written form is acceptable to most patients.

Pain Questionnaires

There are several pain measurement instruments that incorporate pain severity scales and other questions related to pain that can be used to standardize pain assessment. Three such instruments are short enough to be considered for routine clinical use with cancer patients. VASs have recently been adapted for more routine clinical use in the Memorial Pain Assessment Card (MPAC) (Fishman et al., 1987). The MPAC consists of three VASs, for pain intensity, pain relief, and mood, and one Verbal Descriptor (categorical) Scale. A short form of the McGill Pain Questionnaire (SF-MPQ) has been developed (Melzack, 1987).

The main component of the SF-MPQ consists of 15 descriptors (11 sensory, 4 affective) which are rated on an intensity scale as 0 = none, 1 = mild, 2 = moderate, or 3 = severe. Three pain scores are derived from the sum of the intensity rank values of the words chosen for sensory, affective, and total descriptors. The SF-MPQ also includes the Present Pain Intensity (PPI) index of the standard MPQ and a VAS. The Brief Pain Inventory (BPI) (Cleeland, 1989a), a refinement of the Wisconsin Brief Pain Questionnaire (Daut & Cleeland, 1982), was designed to assess pain in cancer patients (see Appendix 21.A and 21.B). Using 0 to 10 NRSs, the BPI asks patients to rate the severity of their pain at its "worst," "least," "average," and at the time the rating is made— "now." Using NRSs, with 0 being "no interference" and 10 being "interferes completely," the BPI asks for ratings of how much pain interferes with mood, walking, other physical activity, work, social activity, relations with others, and sleep. The BPI asks patients to represent the location of their pain on a pain drawing, and asks other questions about duration of pain relief and cause of pain, and provides a list of descriptors to help the patient describe pain quality. A short form of this scale has recently been developed for daily pain monitoring and for use in clinical trials.

Simple pain scales make it possible to assess pain on each outpatient contact with the patient and at least once every 24-hour period for a patient in the hospital (or more frequently if pain is identified as a problem). Because pain in cancer is often progressive, sometimes rapidly so, pain assessment is a recursive procedure, and the model presented should be thought of as being repeated until optimal pain control is achieved. For the sake of the Level One diagram, we have defined "mild," "moderate," and "severe" pain as ranges of patient response to a numeric rating of pain at its "worst."

Mild pain (1–3 "worst pain") will most probably call for a "mild" analgesic (acetaminophen or a nonsteroidal anti-inflammatory) and education about the need to report pain when it occurs, when it gets worse, or if it is not relieved by current treatment.

Moderate pain (4–6 "worst pain") will call for a more aggressive analgesic program and mandates Levels Two and Three of the assessment process. A physical-neurological examination is also indicated. Because pain at this level impairs a patient's function, a follow-up contact should be made within 72 hours to assess the efficacy of the pain treatment provided. For patients at home, this will require a phone call. When pain is *severe* (7–10 "worst pain") the steps are similar, except that the analgesic program needs to be even more aggressive and follow-up contact (reassessment) needs to occur more quickly, within 24 hours after the initial assessment is made.

Patient education is usually not thought of as part of the assessment process. For cancer patients with moderate to severe pain, however, it is critical to recognize the reluctance they may have to report pain and to contact their HCPs if they do not get pain relief. We have already mentioned some of the factors that lead to this reluctance. Patients have to be active partners in their pain assessment and treatment. They need to be made aware that many myths about addiction, rapid development of tolerance, and unmangeable side effects associated with opioid analgesics do not apply to the majority of cancer patients. They have to be reassured that, in most instances, pain relief can be obtained and that it is part of the HCP's role to provide that relief.

LEVEL TWO: ASSESSING PAIN CHARACTERISTICS

Information about aspects of the pain other than its severity will help to refine treatment plans. Much of this information can also be gathered through the use of standard questionnaires, which guide the patient's subjective reports of these additional characteristics. Further information will need to be obtained by clinical interview. The essential elements of Level Two are presented in Figure 21.2.

Pain Location

Aiding the patient in describing the location(s) of the pain they are experiencing is an essential part of pain assessment. This is most easily accomplished by asking the patient to provide a graphic representation of the location of pain. The patient is given a front and back view of a human figure and asked to shade the area of pain. Some pain questionnaires, including the BPI, include a human figure drawing for the patient to use. This item can provide a wealth of information about possible physical mechanisms contributing to the pain. It may also help to determine why pain is a greater problem with particular movements or positions. For example, patients may draw the pain in the distribution of a particular nerve, suggesting that the mechanism of pain is tumor impingement on that nerve. As disease progresses, patients may indicate pain at several locations.

Temporal Pattern of the Pain

Not all cancer pain remains at a constant level over a 24-hour period, and it is important to capture the temporal pattern of pain. Some patients will have significant exacerbation of their pain with movement, especially if the pathological process responsible for the pain is influenced by movement (pain in the back or in or near a joint) or position. Other types of pain (usually deafferentation pain) may have periods when pain spontaneously becomes more intense. These periodic increases in pain, either movement-caused or spontaneous, are often referred to as "breakthrough pain" (Portenoy & Hagen, 1990). It is becoming standard practice to include additional analgesia for the patient to take during these episodes, or even before episodes if it is possible to anticipate

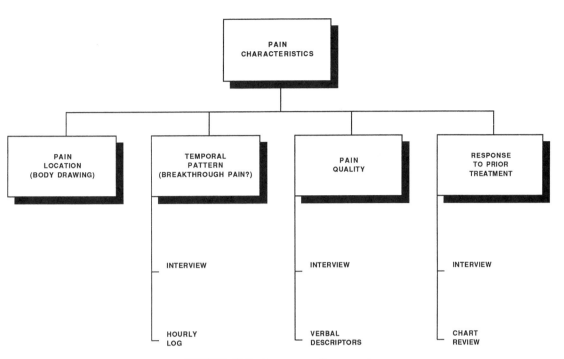

FIGURE 21.2. Assessment of cancer pain.

when they will occur. For some patients, however, the presence of breakthrough pain may indicate only that the dose or potency of the routine analgesic prescribed for pain management is inadequate. The temporal pattern of pain is often clearly described by the patient in interview. It may be necessary, however, to have patients rate their pain in a log book on an hourly basis for a 24-hour period to determine its pattern.

Pain Quality

Pain of different etiologies produces differences in the patient's subjective report of the quality of the pain. For example, pain caused by destruction of nerve pathways may be described as "numb," "pins and needles," "burning," or "shooting." Pain from tumor destruction of tissue is often described as "aching." Establishing the quality of the pain is an important part of the pain assessment, especially because the type of description used by the patient is an essential part of establishing the physical basis of the pain, which will, in turn, determine the types of therapies to be used. For example, pain due to destruction of nerve pathways is less responsive to the opioid

medications, but may be relieved by other types of medications, such as antidepressants or anticonvulsants.

People often find it difficult to spontaneously describe their pain. Word lists of potential descriptors help the patient portray pain quality. Some questionnaires, including the BPI and the SF-MPQ, include lists of words for the patient to select from.

Response to Prior Treatment

The patient's response to prior pain treatment and prognosis are additional variables that need to be considered in both patient management and in clinical research. Patients whose pain has been refractory to prior appropriately aggressive pain treatment attempts present especially difficult management problems and may require alternate routes (epidural, intrathecal, subcutaneous) of analgesic administration. Such patients will obviously require greater clinical attention and should be treated separately in designs for clinical trials. Prognosis will often be related to pain treatment choices. For example, neuro-ablative techniques (destroying the pain pathway) may be a treatment choice, but are not indicated for patients with a longer prognosis. These invasive techniques present a risk for functional impairment. The effectiveness of these treatments is also of limited duration (weeks or months) (Cleeland et al., 1986).

LEVEL THREE: ASSESSING PAIN IMPACT

Level Three of our suggested outline of pain assessment (see Figure 21.3) measures the degree to which pain interferes with areas of the patient's life, and the degree to which other symptoms interact with pain to disrupt the patient's functioning. The suggested assessment steps are again tailored to elicit information that will lead to specific treatment recommendations. Whenever pain is moderate to severe or pain is concurrent with other symptoms, an effective intervention for pain control should be based on evaluation of more than pain severity and pain mechanism. As examples, if a patient suffers from nausea and vomiting, an oral opioid may exacerbate nausea and may therefore require an antiemetic a half-hour before the opioid or, alternatively, the patient may need a nonoral route of administration. If a patient has relatively good pain control, but

only if laying down, treatment may be inadequate. A review of only pain severity and mechanism might inappropriately indicate adequate treatment had been prescribed. As these examples demonstrate, Level Three assessments for chronic cancer pain can provide valuable information even when pain, on initial screening, appears mild.

Quality of Life

The BPI provides a synopsis of areas of pain interference with functioning. Although this information is valuable and may be adequate in many cases, it does not indicate the extent to which functioning or quality of life is impaired by nonpain factors. Extensive work has been conducted over the past decade to define and test measures of quality of life (QOL) related to cancer (Cella & Tulsky, 1991; Ferrell, 1989; Moinpour et al., 1989; Spilker, 1990). The results of these efforts can now benefit the clinician or researcher by vastly reducing the patient burden demanded to measure separately each of the constructs that may interact with pain assessment and treatment. In their development of these scales, investigators have attempted to identify problems specific to pa-

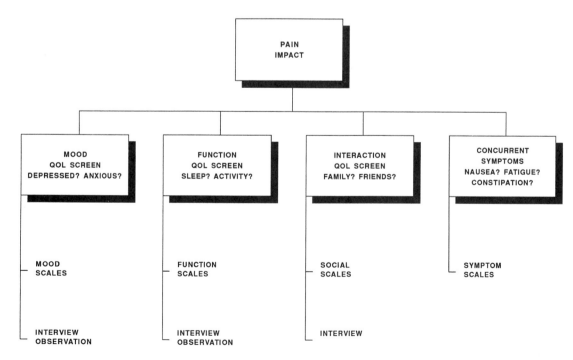

FIGURE 21.3. Assessment of cancer pain.

tients with cancer, recognizing that the nature of the disease requires that measures be extremely brief and focused.

Although it is beyond the scope of this chapter to review the entire field of instruments available to measure QOL, several measures have been selected for review. The measures described below include evaluation of physical functioning, psychological status, social relationships and, in most cases, symptoms. These domains have been identified repeatedly as minimum requirements for adequate QOL assessment (Aaronson, 1991; Cella & Tulsky, 1991; Moinpour & Hayden, 1991; Schipper, 1991). These domains also coincide with those listed under Level Three of our pain assessment model: mood, functioning, social interaction, and concurrent symptoms. The measures cover these areas in very concise form, taking less than 15 minutes to complete.

Reviews of QOL assessment recognize the importance of a generic screening tool, combined with a disease-specific module (Aaronson, 1991). In assessing pain, the extended pain evaluation with, for instance, the BPI, could constitute the disease-specific module while the scales described below complete the generic module. An ideal measure will have received adequate testing for reliability, validity, responsiveness to change, and feasibility with cancer patients. In fact, these measures are relatively new and each has a weakness in one area or another at this time. However, they each have strengths that warrant their consideration.

The EORTC-QLQ, developed through the European Organization for Research and Treatment of Cancer (Aaronson, Bullinger, & Ahmedzai, 1988), has 28 items plus two global QOL items. Disease or problem specific items are intended to be added to the scale. The measure has questions on physical abilities, symptoms, mood, cognitive function, social interactions, and finances. This scale shows promise; however, psychometric properties of the scale are still being documented (Cella & Tulsky, 1991). Advantages of the scale include its careful, conceptually based construction and its conciseness. It will hopefully be available for wider use soon.

The Functional Living Index–Cancer (FLIC) is one of the earlier developed and more widely used measures of QOL (Schipper, Clinch, McMurray, & Levitt, 1984). The scale has 22 items, with 13 subscales. The construction of the instrument was thoughtful, with good face validity and with robust physical and psychological factors. Some of the other factors are less stable as one might expect of one item scales. The FLIC seems to work well for ambulatory patients, but is less well adapted for more ill or hospitalized patients who may have difficulty comprehending or responding properly to the format (Cella & Tulsky, 1991; Ganz et al., 1988).

The Short Form Health Survey: Medical Outcomes Study (MOS) has 20 items scored in sections of physical functioning, role functioning, social functioning, mental health, health perceptions, and one item on pain (Stewart, Hays, & Ware, 1988). This measure, developed by the Rand Corporation, is reliable and valid and has been tested on diverse populations (Cella & Tulsky, 1991; Stewart, Hays, & Ware, 1988). The brevity of the scale must be kept in mind so that areas of potential problem are pursued in more detail with supplemental measures. The scale was chosen by the Southwest Oncology Group (SWOG) as the base QOL measure for their clinical trials. They then add the Symptom Distress Scale (McCorkle, 1987, discussed below) and a disease-specific section (Moinpour et al., 1989). Again, where pain is the focus of evaluation, the MOS could be combined with the Symptom Distress Scale and the BPI to evaluate patients with moderate to severe pain. If psychological functioning is impaired on the MOS, the clinician can evaluate further with mood measures or an interview.

One of these QOL measures will provide a good screening tool to determine need for further evaluation. In the areas of psychological functioning and concurrent symptoms, one of these scales alone is unlikely to be sufficient to determine treatment needs, but it should be adequate to identify the need for further follow-up.

Mood

The majority of cancer patients adjust to the stresses of the disease and its symptoms without diagnosable anxiety, depression or other psychiatric disorders (Derogatis et al., 1983; Schachman, 1984). However, patients with pain report significantly more depression and anxiety than those without pain (Ahles, Blanchard, & Ruckdeschel, 1983; Derogatis et al., 1983). Among the many symptoms possible during the course of cancer, mood disorders can be among the most difficult to identify, even though pharmacological and behavioral treatments are readily available. A difficulty in recognizing mood disruptions results from the similarity of presentation of some mood symptoms and common disease-related somatic complaints such as fatigue, weight loss, sleep disruption, decreased activity, and loss of concentration. When pain is chronic, the risk of mood disturbance is likely to increase. An assessment of mood is not adequately accomplished with any of the QOL measures or the BPI; therefore, we recommend an assessment of mood whenever pain is moderate to severe or chronic and concurrent with other somatic symptoms.

The Profile of Mood States (POMS) is one of the more commonly used measures of mood or affect in cancer patients (McNair, Lorr, & Droppleman, 1971). The scale is of value because it is relatively easy for patients to understand and complete. In addition, the scale is sensitive to change over a brief period of time, making it ideal for studying responsiveness to treatment. However, the 65-item standard version is lengthy for ill patients to complete. Consequently, a shorter version has been advocated for cancer patients (Cella et al., 1987). This version has only 11 items and can be completed quickly. The reliability of the short measure is maintained for the total score of overall distress. Although the longer version of the POMS has six factors, these factors are highly intercorrelated, and therefore one distress factor is probably adequate (Cella et al., 1987; Shumaker, Anderson, & Czajkowski, 1990). In our own research with 259 bone marrow transplant patients, we used a shortened POMS in which we selected the three items that loaded highest on each of the six factors. Internal consistency remained high for the total mood disturbance score (alpha .92) and the six factors (alphas ranged from .82 to .92). As with other researchers, we found these factors highly intercorrelated, suggesting that a single score was more appropriate than separate depression, anxiety, anger, vigor, fatigue, and confusion scores.

Measures of anxiety and depression tend to correlate rather highly, as found with the POMS. Many well-standardized, psychometrically sound measures are available to measure mood. For assessing anxiety, the State-Trait Anxiety Inventory (STAI) is most widely used

(Spielberger, 1983). The State and Trait forms are highly correlated; thus, one is advised not to administer both. Because the Trait form correlates with other measures of distress such as depression, the State version may be best to use if a measure that discriminates for levels of anxiety is wanted (Shumaker, 1990). The Beck Depression Inventory (BDI) (Beck et al., 1961) is one of the more commonly used of the several, psychometrically solid measures of this construct. The 21 items on this scale are relatively easy to complete; however, the physical symptoms of depression overlap rather heavily with common symptoms of cancer (e.g., fatigue, weight loss, loss of concentration). The clinician or researcher needs to look closely at the content of the items endorsed by the patient in addition to the overall score.

In our experience, assessment of mood in cancer patients with pain requires a focus on the affective components of mood disturbance, with somewhat more cautious evaluation of cognitive and behavioral components and with awareness, but not emphasis, on somatic components. It can be difficult, if not impossible, to be certain of the etiology of somatic symptoms; thus, empirical approaches are sometimes needed. In other words, first treat the pain, then evaluate for other pharmacological or organic contributors, and then treat the psychological symptoms, even if medication or disease progression contributes to the symptoms.

Although the POMS, STAI, and BDI have all been used with medical populations and all measure general mood disturbance, the Brief Symptom Inventory (BSI), measures a broader range of psychological disruption. The BSI is a shortened, 53-item form of the Symptom Checklist 90 and has nine subscales: depression, anxiety, hostility, phobic anxiety, paranoid ideation, somatization, obsessive-compulsive, interpersonal sensitivity, and psychoticism (Derogatis & Spencer, 1982). The total score, or Global Severity Index, correlates relatively well with the other measures of mood disturbance discussed above. If a more detailed measure of functioning is needed, without the length of a form such as the Minnesota Multiphasic Personality Inventory (MMPI), the BSI format is relatively less burdensome. It provides useful information and is easily understood by cancer patients. Of these various mood measures, the POMS is the easiest for nonpsychologists or psychiatrists to use. The other measures require some training in the structure of the scale, scoring, norms and cut-off scores for levels of mild, moderate, and severe disturbance.

Function

If a more extended measure of physical functioning is needed, beyond those provided by the QOL measures cited above, the Sickness Impact Profile (SIP) is probably the best constructed and validated of those available (Bergner, Bobbitt, Carter, & Gilson, 1981; Bergner, Bobbitt, & Pollard, 1976; Cella & Tulsky, 1991). This measure has been used with cancer patients, but is not cancer specific (Syrjala, Donaldson, Schubert, Goldberg, & Chapko, 1990). The SIP has 136 items which are relatively easy to complete for patients who can concentrate. The items are scored in 12 subscales, with three global functioning scales. Because this measure has physical, psychological, and social subscales, it could substitute for other mood or social interaction measures. The restrictions on its use include its length, the lack of cancer-specific problems as a focus, and the low sensitivity of the items for ambulatory patients who may have subtle or very specific areas of dysfunction.

Social Interaction

Social relationships are acknowledged to be very important for the functioning and well-being of cancer patients (Dunkel-Schetter, 1984; Wortman, 1984). Nonetheless, social support has been one of the most difficult areas for investigators to measure (Moinpour et al, 1989). In our experience, cancer patients tend to rate their supports very positively, resulting in a ceiling effect for measurement. In addition, "support" alone is probably not adequate as a construct for measurement. We need to know the social "environment," not just the availability of emotional, informational, or assistance supports. The Family Relations Index, a brief form of the Family Environment Scale (Moos & Moos, 1986), provides a measure of family functioning style that may inform the clinician of the family's level of conflict, cohesiveness, and expressiveness as perceived by the patient. This scale has been shown to relate to physical or psychological outcome in cancer patients (Bloom & Spiegel, 1984; Syrjala, Chapko, Cummings, Sullivan, & Carr, 1988).

As cancer patients live longer and are subjected to more aggressive treatment courses, they require greater care from their support systems. The Caregiver Impact Scale is a 14-item measure of the extent to which the key caregiver experiences responsibility for "objective" burdens (events and activities) and "subjective" burdens (feelings, attitudes, and emotions).

For more abbreviated evaluation of social interactions, the QOL measures and the BPI described above each has several items on impact of pain, disease, or general health on relationships. None of these measures provides detailed information on social networks or perceived support. The SIP, described above, has a social interaction scale that provides added information about social activities. The recent study indicating the positive effect of support groups, not only in reducing pain and distress for breast cancer patients, but in predicting longer survival, emphasizes that social interaction is an important, if not yet clearly measurable construct for cancer patients (Spiegel, Bloom, Kraemer, & Gottheil, 1989).

Concurrent Symptoms

Patients with both cancer and pain are liable to have other symptoms that need management and complicate the treatment picture. The disease itself, especially as it advances, will produce fatigue, weakness, cachexia, and may produce cognitive deficits if the central nervous system becomes involved. Cancer treatment will often produce nausea and vomiting, fatigue, and tissue damage which themselves produce pain or other unpleasant alterations in somatic sensations (Chapko, Syrjala, Schilter, Cummings, & Sullivan, 1989). The negative side-effects of analgesics and adjuvant pain management drugs are numerous, especially if aggressive side-effect prophylaxis and treatment are not included in treatment plans. The most common negative side effects of analgesic treatment include constipation, nausea, fatigue, and sedation. These other symptoms, regardless of their etiology, can negatively affect mood and function, as can pain itself. As disease advances, or during periods of aggressive treatment, it is often difficult to identify the source of these concurrent symptoms.

Many such symptoms can be treated, either

pharmacologically or behaviorally. Other symptoms may be present for limited periods of time during active anticancer treatment or until the patient develops tolerance for the analgesics and other symptom control drugs being used. At a minimum, a checklist of potential concurrent symptoms, such as the Symptom Distress Scale (McCorkle, 1987), needs to be included at this level of assessment. Having the patient rate the severity of these symptoms provides a more adequate assessment of their impact. As with pain, it is important to evaluate these symptoms over time in order to monitor changes in severity and response to treatment.

Interview Assessment of Pain Impact

The clinician can approach the gathering of information on physical, emotional, and social functioning from an interview format as well as through standardized, subjective report forms. Some of the forms, particularly the QOL scales, the BDI and the STAI, can be read to the patient. Alternatively, psychological disturbance can be assessed through a clinical interview focused on psychiatric diagnosis using DSM-III-R criteria (APA, 1987). The advantages of an interview are that some patients will be more compliant or perceive less burden with this format. In addition, an area in which a patient indicates no disruption does not have to be pursued. The danger is, of course, the converse. An area may be missed because either the interviewer or the patient determines no problem exists, thus short-circuiting the evaluation. Suicidal ideation is a risk for patients with severe uncontrolled pain and can best be assessed in an interview.

Observation of Pain Impact

Observation measures within the field of cancer have historically focused on global measures of functioning. The most well known of these is the Karnofsky Performance Status (Karnofsky, Abelmann, Craver, & Burchenalet, 1984), but other, similar 5- or 10-point global assessments are available (Lanksy et al., 1988; Morrow et al., 1981; Spitzer et al., 1981; Zubrod et al., 1960). These scales have good interrater reliabilities, but are not useful for specifying difficulties or determining treatment needs. Their primary value seems to be as outcomes for clinical trials. Observer ratings are also available for more specific activities of daily living (Selby et al., 1984; Spector, 1990) or for well behaviors (Chapko et al., 1991). These measures are less pychometrically well described. We would suggest these only in cases where patients are unable to provide their own self-report or in combination with self-report.

Pain Assessment in Children with Cancer

Pain assessment in children with cancer is even more neglected than in adults with cancer. Assessment is often more difficult because the assessment has to be tailored to the developmental stage of the child. There is a growing consensus, however, that age-appropriate assessment techniques exist that are reasonably well validated. Appropriate care of such children must include a plan for the assessment and management of all forms of cancer-related pain. A recent panel has drawn up a list of recommendations or guidelines for the assessment of pain in children (McGrath et al., 1990). The panel concluded that developmentally appropriate pain intensity measures be used with children above the age of 3, and that children over the age of 6 be given standard (Numeric, Visual Analogue) scales. Categorical scales were felt to be more difficult for children to use. Although behavioral observations should not be used in lieu of self-report, these observations are critical in pain assessment of children younger than 2 years of age or in children who do not have the ability to report their pain due to disability or disease. The panel identified certain behaviors (such as crying, clinging, reduction in normal activity, social withdrawal, sleep disturbance) that should be considered as clues that a child is experiencing pain. The three levels of assessment outlined in this chapter should work equally well for children, with the provisions recommended by the panel. The panel suggested that a Pain Problem List be formulated for every child with cancer. The goal of this list is to identify problems amenable to treatment, and to be sure that the multiple sources and dimensions of pain are addressed. The list is suggested to be a subsection of the patient's problem list as part of the medical record.

OTHER APPLICATIONS OF PAIN MEASUREMENT

Cancer pain measurement methods form the basis of several applications in addition to routine clinical assessment, including studies of the epidemiology of cancer pain, efforts to assure the quality of pain management, and the conduct of clinical trials examining the effectiveness of cancer pain treatments. A review of each of these areas will illustrate the application of pain measurement and assessment techniques.

Epidemiology of Cancer Pain

Attempts to estimate the numbers of cancer patients with pain and to determine the impact and severity of this pain are relatively recent. We have stressed the importance of assessing pain severity. The use of pain rating scales has allowed the development of an operational definition of what "significant" pain is, at least for patients with cancer. Most people face mild pain periodically (some on a daily basis) with little interference in their daily lives. As pain becomes more severe, it interferes with more domains of the patient's daily functioning. It is possible to define "significant pain" as pain that is rated at the midpoint or higher on conventional pain severity scales because, at this point, patients report that pain interferes substantially with their daily function (Cleeland, 1989a). By using this operational definition, we can estimate the percentage of cancer patients who will have significant pain, and we can also relate this pain not only to disease status but also to the type and adequacy of pain management the patient is receiving.

Studies using pain severity rating scales published in the past 10 years have documented that "significant pain," as we have just defined it, is a problem for large numbers of patients with metastatic cancer (Daut & Cleeland, 1982; Donovan & Dillon, 1987; Greenwald, Bonica, & Bergner, 1987; Peteet, Tay, Cohen, & MacIntyre, 1986; Portenoy, 1989). These studies have forced us to re-evaluate the association between disease stage and the onset of pain due to cancer. In the past, pain was typically associated with end-stage cancers, but we now realize that significant pain can be present for long periods of time, with 20–40%

of patients with metastatic disease having pain at this level. It is difficult to estimate the number of patients in the United States who will have significant pain in any given year. We know how many patients die of cancer each year and that approximately 70% of them will have had significant pain. It is much harder to estimate the numbers of patients alive today with metastatic cancer who will survive the year. For this group, if the most conservative estimate of 20% with significant pain is used, then there are thousands of additional patients with disease-related pain that impairs several areas of their functioning. Even if we exclude cancer survivors with persistent posttreatment pain, the numbers of patients with cancer or cancer survivors who have significant pain will be in the hundreds of thousands. These prevalence studies have helped to demonstrate that cancer pain is a national health problem of the highest priority, and have influenced health policy planning world-wide (World Health Organization, 1986).

Cancer patients respond differentially to similar courses of pain treatment. Clinical staging systems have been developed for all major cancers. These staging systems are the basis for estimates of prognosis and response to treatment, important for both the epidemiology of cancer and the assessment of treatment outcome. A staging system for cancer pain would be useful for an epidemiology of cancer pain as well as for outcome studies and clinical trials of pain therapies. One such system has been proposed (Bruera, MacMillan, Hanson, & MacDonald, 1989). This system attempts to rate prognosis for pain treatment on several variables, including pain mechanism, characteristics of pain, previous analgesic response, cognitive function, psychological distress, tolerance, and past history of drug or alchohol abuse. Preliminary evidence suggests that some or all of these variables will be helpful in predicting response to standard pain therapies.

Pain Measurement for Quality Assurance

Because pain is so debilitating, poorly treated pain should be considered a quality assurance issue. Patients should be guaranteed the best possible pain management. Pain assessment tools provide a method for monitoring pain in the clinic or hospital setting. Quality assurance depends on indicators of performance that can be monitored easily. If quality assurance is to encompass pain relief, a major first step will be the introduction of pain measures into routine practice, coupled with charting of the results on a routine basis. Once this is done, it is quite reasonable to establish an "incident" of poorly controlled pain that calls for review. An incident might be defined as the presence of significant pain, defined as pain that is rated at the midpoint or higher on an accepted pain rating scale. Numerical scales seem best suited for easy tracking of pain for this purpose.

Williamson (1971) has suggested that quality assurance monitoring could be programmed to trigger corrective educational measures. He has argued that education for health practice change must be based on an evaluation encompassing both outcomes and process. Only when outcome data indicate deficiencies is process evaluation warranted and educational intervention mandated. His strategy begins with a standard of care that can be reasonably operationalized, such as a given percentage of patients with significant pain. Each institution would set a maximum acceptable level for this percentage. If outcome data were worse than this level, process evaluation and education would be invoked. The outcome evaluation process would then be repeated to determine the extent of improvement.

Clinical Trials Applications

A major barrier to cancer pain management has been a lack of traditional controlled clinical trials in cancer pain management. Most of our information about the effectiveness of analgesics has come from the single-dose acute analgesic assay model (Wallenstein, 1984). In this model, a test drug and a standard drug are studied in randomized, double-blind crossover design. Subjects are assessed by trained research personnel (usually research nurses) immediately before and at specified times after the administration of the test or standard drug. On the second day of the study, the subject receives the other drug. These elegant single-institution studies have provided the basis for judging the comparative effectiveness of various analgesics. One argument advanced for this study model is that pain assessment is tightly controlled by the use of trained observers highly familiar in instructing patients in making pain ratings. Inherent in this model is the suspicion that multi-institutional studies done without these trained observers would produce information with so much observer-based errors as to be of little use.

There are many important clinical questions that cannot be answered by the single-dose assay. For instance, in cancer pain it is important to judge the efficacy of analgesics over repeated administrations. Some pharmacological interventions may take several days to reach maximum effectiveness, and the latency of their effectiveness may vary from patient to patient. Nonpharmacological interventions for pain control, including physical therapy, behavioral therapy, and temporary and permanent disruption of pain pathways do not lend themselves to evaluation by this model. Finally, it is increasingly apparent that optimal cancer pain management may involve the simultaneous applications of different pain control methods (Cleeland et al., 1986). These questions could be addressed in multi-institutional clinical trials if it can be demonstrated that pain could be measured using simple assessment tools following easily understood protocols specifying the principles of pain measurement.

Support for the feasibility of clinical trials using this type of measurement comes from several sources. First, most of the cancer pain prevalence and severity studies cited above have followed this model. Simple pain rating scales, either Visual Analogue (Greenwald et al., 1987) or Numeric (Daut & Cleeland, 1982; Donovan & Dillon, 1987), were given to patients by observers who were minimally trained in pain assessment. These studies have demonstrated that pain ratings obtained in this way vary in a logical fashion with such characteristics as disease progression, extent of metastases, and appropriateness of pain treatment. Second, clinical trials of pain relief measures in other diseases using simple pain scales in multi-institutional trials have demonstrated reliable discrimination between more and less effective treatments (Bombardier et al., 1986; Parr, Darekar, Fletcher, & Bulpitt, 1989).

Clinical trials in cancer pain management generate the need for some special considerations. Because cancer pain is progressive, often rapidly so, planning for the duration of the trial must consider the possibility that worsening disease progression will obscure real differences in the treatments being contrasted. Analgesics, especially the more potent ones like morphine, will produce side effects readily apparent to the patient, especially patients who have a history of taking analgesics. When such drugs are studied, it may be appropriate to include a so-called active placebo, a drug that is similar in its side-effect profile to the study drug but has minimal or no analgesic action. Such active placebos are more difficult to construct for the evaluation of nondrug therapies, such as the blocking of pain pathways or behavioral treatments.

CONCLUSION

Although most patients with cancer-related pain should be able to get pain relief, many are poorly managed. Inadequate pain assessment is often the reason. In the typical cancer care setting, caregivers rarely have training in pain assessment or have the time for the type of assessment typical of multidisciplinary pain clinics. Patients may be too ill to endure lengthy assessment procedures or may not complain about their pain. Recognizing these constraints, we have presented three levels of assessment. Steps at each level are designed to lead to treatment decisions. Where possible, the assessment is structured around questionnaires designed for the patient with cancer.

These questionnaires minimize patient and health professional biases and simplify the assessment process. Some steps of the assessment only need to be followed if screening suggests a potential treatment need. An assessment based on questionnaires will often need to be supplemented by interview of both patient and family, observation, and, when pain is more severe, medical-neurological examination. Proper assessment based on subjective report needs the full cooperation of the patient, yet cancer patients may be reluctant to complain of pain or other symptoms. To be full partners in the pain assessment, patients need education about their right to symptom relief, together with the nature and risks of their pain treatment. Cancer pain is dynamic and ever changing. Although sometimes pain improves for periods with tumor regression, more often, pain becomes progressively worse, requiring more aggressive use of pain therapy. Once a patient develops pain, assessment needs to be repeated frequently. The steps presented in the model have additional applications outside of clinical assessment. They can be used effectively in studies of the epidemiology of cancer pain, in quality assurance, and in clinical trials examining the effectiveness of pain treatments.

Acknowledgments. Preparation for this chapter was supported by grants CA26582 (Cleeland) and CA 38552 (Syrjala) from the US Public Health Service.

APPENDIX 21.A*

Brief Pain Inventory

Date: __ / __ / __

Name: _____ _____ _____
    Last   First   Middle Initial

Phone: (__) _____   Sex: ☐ Female   ☐ Male

Date of Birth: __ / __ / __

1) Marital Status (at present)

1. ☐ Single   3. ☐ Widowed

2. ☐ Married   4. ☐ Separated/Divorced

2) Education (Circle only the highest grade or degree completed)

Grade	0	1	2	3	4	5	6	7	8	9
	10	11	12	13	14	15	16	M.A./M.S.		

Professional degree (please specify)

3) Current occupation _____
(specify titles; if you are not working, tell us your previous occupation)

4) Spouse's Occupation _____

5) Which of the following best describes your current job status?

☐ 1. Employed outside the home, full-time
☐ 2. Employed outside the home, part-time
☐ 3. Homemaker
☐ 4. Retired
☐ 5. Unemployed
☐ 6. Other

6) How long has it been since you first learned your diagnosis ? [____] months

7) Have you ever had pain due to your present disease?

1. ☐ Yes   2. ☐ No   3. ☐ Uncertain

*Copyright 1991 Charles S. Cleeland.

APPENDIX 21.A *(continued)*

8) When you first received your diagnosis, was pain one of your symptoms?

    1. ☐ Yes   2. ☐ No   3. ☐ Uncertain

9) Have you had surgery in the past month?   1. ☐ Yes   2. ☐ No

10) Throughout our lives, most of us have had pain from time to time (such as minor headaches, sprains, and toothaches). Have you had pain other than these everyday kinds of pain during the last week?

    1. ☐ Yes   2. ☐ No

IF YOU ANSWERED YES TO THE LAST QUESTION, PLEASE GO ON TO QUESTION 11 AND FINISH THIS QUESTIONNAIRE. IF NO, YOU ARE FINISHED WITH THE QUESTIONNAIRE. THANK YOU.

11) On the diagram, shade in the areas where you feel pain. Put an X on the area that hurts the most.

Front   Back

Right   Left   Left   Right

APPENDIX 21.A *(continued)*

12) Please rate your pain by circling the one number that best describes your pain at its worst in the last week.

0	1	2	3	4	5	6	7	8	9	10

No
Pain

Pain as bad as
you can imagine

13) Please rate your pain by circling the one number that best describes your pain at its least in the last week.

0	1	2	3	4	5	6	7	8	9	10

No
Pain

Pain as bad as
you can imagine

14) Please rate your pain by circling the one number that best describes your pain on the average.

0	1	2	3	4	5	6	7	8	9	10

No
Pain

Pain as bad as
you can imagine

15) Please rate your pain by circling the one number that tells how much pain you have right now.

0	1	2	3	4	5	6	7	8	9	10

No
Pain

Pain as bad as
you can imagine

16) What kinds of things make your pain feel better (for example, heat, medicine, rest?)

_____

_____

17) What kinds of things make your pain worse (for example, walking, standing, lifting?)

_____

_____

18) What treatments or medications are you receiving for your pain?

_____

_____

19) In the last week, how much relief have pain treatments or medications provided? Please circle the one percentage that most shows how much relief you have received.

0%	10%	20%	30%	40%	50%	60%	70%	80%	90%	100%

No
Relief

Complete
Relief

APPENDIX 21.A *(continued)*

20) If you take pain medication, how many hours does it take before the pain returns?

☐ 1. Pain medication doesn't help at all.

☐ 2. One hour.

☐ 3. Two hours.

☐ 4. Three hours.

☐ 5. Four hours.

☐ 6. Five to twelve hours.

☐ 7. More than twelve hours.

☐ 8. I do not take pain medication.

21) Circle the appropriate answer for each item.
I believe my pain is due to:

Yes ☐ No ☐ 1. The effects of treatment (for example, medication, surgery, radiation, prosthetic device).

Yes ☐ No ☐ 2. My primary disease (meaning the disease currently being treated and evaluated).

Yes ☐ No ☐ 3. A medical condition unrelated to primary disease (for example, arthritis)

22) For each of the following words, check yes or no if that adjective applies to your pain.

Aching	☐ Yes	☐ No
Throbbing	☐ Yes	☐ No
Shooting	☐ Yes	☐ No
Stabbing	☐ Yes	☐ No
Gnawing	☐ Yes	☐ No
Sharp	☐ Yes	☐ No
Tender	☐ Yes	☐ No
Burning	☐ Yes	☐ No
Exhausting	☐ Yes	☐ No
Tiring	☐ Yes	☐ No
Penetrating	☐ Yes	☐ No
Nagging	☐ Yes	☐ No
Numb	☐ Yes	☐ No
Miserable	☐ Yes	☐ No
Unbearable	☐ Yes	☐ No

APPENDIX 21.A *(continued)*

23) Circle the one number that describes how, during the past week, **pain** has interfered with your:

A. General Activity

0	1	2	3	4	5	6	7	8	9	10

Does not interfere — Completely interferes

B. Mood

0	1	2	3	4	5	6	7	8	9	10

Does not interfere — Completely interferes

C. Walking ability

0	1	2	3	4	5	6	7	8	9	10

Does not interfere — Completely interferes

D. Normal work (includes both work outside the home and housework)

0	1	2	3	4	5	6	7	8	9	10

Does not interfere — Completely interferes

E. Relations with other people

0	1	2	3	4	5	6	7	8	9	10

Does not interfere — Completely interferes

F. Sleep

0	1	2	3	4	5	6	7	8	9	10

Does not interfere — Completely interferes

G. Enjoyment of life

0	1	2	3	4	5	6	7	8	9	10

Does not interfere — Completely interferes

APPENDIX 21.B*

Brief Pain Inventory (Short Form)

Date: ___/___/___   Time: _____

Name: _____ _____ _____
                    Last   First   Middle Initial

1) Throughout our lives, most of us have had pain from time to time (such as minor headaches,sprains,and toothaches). Have you had pain other than these everyday kinds of pain today?

      1.   Yes   2.   No

2) On the diagram, shade in the areas where you feel pain. Put an X on the area that hurts the most.

Right   Left   Left   Right

3) Please rate your pain by circling the one number that best describes your pain at its worst in the last 24 hours.

  0   1   2   3   4   5   6   7   8   9   10
No   Pain as bad as
Pain   you can imagine

4) Please rate your pain by circling the one number that best describes your pain at its least in the last 24 hours.

  0   1   2   3   4   5   6   7   8   9   10
No   Pain as bad as
Pain   you can imagine

5) Please rate your pain by circling the one number that best describes your pain on the average.

  0   1   2   3   4   5   6   7   8   9   10
No   Pain as bad as
Pain   you can imagine

6) Please rate your pain by circling the one number that tells how much pain you have right now.

  0   1   2   3   4   5   6   7   8   9   10
No   Pain as bad as
Pain   you can imagine

APPENDIX 21.B *(continued)*

7) What treatments or medications are you receiving for your pain?

_____

8) In the last 24 hours, how much relief have pain treatments or medications provided? Please circle the one percentage that most shows how much relief you have received.

0%	10%	20%	30%	40%	50%	60%	70%	80%	90%	100%
No										Complete
Relief										Relief

9) Circle the one number that describes how, during the past 24 hours, pain has interfered with your:

A. General Activity

0	1	2	3	4	5	6	7	8	9	10
Does not										Completely
interfere										interferes

B. Mood

0	1	2	3	4	5	6	7	8	9	10
Does not										Completely
interfere										interferes

C. Walking ability

0	1	2	3	4	5	6	7	8	9	10
Does not										Completely
interfere										interferes

D. Normal work (includes both work outside the home and housework)

0	1	2	3	4	5	6	7	8	9	10
Does not										Completely
interfere										interferes

E. Relations with other people

0	1	2	3	4	5	6	7	8	9	10
Does not										Completely
interfere										interferes

F. Sleep

0	1	2	3	4	5	6	7	8	9	10
Does not										Completely
interfere										interferes

G. Enjoyment of life

0	1	2	3	4	5	6	7	8	9	10
Does not										Completely
interfere										interferes

REFERENCES

Aaronson, N.K. (Ed.). (1991). *Quality of life research in cancer clinical trials: A need for common rules and language.* Proceedings of an International Symposium held at St. Mary Medical Center, Long Beach, CA. Williston Park, NY: Dominus.

Aaronson, N.K., Bullinger, M., & Ahmedzai, S. (1988). A modular approach to quality-of-life assessment in cancer clinical trials. *Recent results in cancer research* III (pp. 231–249). Berlin: Springer-Verlag.

Ahles, T.A., Blanchard, E.B., & Ruckdeschel, J.C. (1983). The multidimensional nature of cancer-related pain. *Pain, 17,* 277–288.

American Pain Society. (1989). *Principles of analgesic use in acute pain and chronic cancer pain.* Skokie, IL: Author.

Bannin, A., Sjogren, P., & Henricsen, H. (1991) Pain causes in 200 patients referred to a multidisciplinary cancer pain clinic. *Pain, 45,* 45–48.

Beck, A.T., Rush, A.J., Shaw, B.F., & Emery, G. (1979). *Cognitive therapy of depression.* New York: Guilford Press.

Beck, A.T., Ward, C.H., Mendelson, M., et al. (1961). An inventory for measuring depression. *Archives of General Psychiatry, 4,* 561–571.

Bergner, M., Bobbitt, R.A., Carter, W.B., & Gilson, B.S. (1981). The Sickness Impact Profile: Development and final revision of a health status measure. *Medical Care, 19,* 787–806.

Bergner, M., Bobbitt, R.A., & Pollard, W.E. (1976). Sickness Impact Profile: Validation of a health status measure. *Medical Care, 14,* 57–61.

Bloom, J., & Spiegel, D. (1984). The relationship of two dimensions of social support to the psychological well-being and social functioning of women with advanced breast cancer. *Social Science and Medicine, 18,* 831–837.

Bombardier, C., Ware, J., Russell, I.J., Larson, M., Chalmers, A., & Read, J.L. (1986). Auranofin therapy and quality of life in patient with rheumatoid arthritis. *American Journal of Medicine, 81,* 565–578.

Bonica, J.J. (1985). Treatment of cancer pain: Current status and future needs. In H.L. Fields et al. (Eds.), *Advances in pain research and therapy* (Vol. 9, pp. 589–616). New York: Raven Press.

Bruera, E., MacMillan, K., Hanson, J., & MacDonald, R.N. (1989). The Edmonton staging system for cancer pain: Preliminary report. *Pain 37,* 203–209.

Cella, D.F., Jacobson, P.B., Orav, E.J. et al. (1987). A brief POMS measure of distress for cancer patients. *Journal of Chronic Disease, 40,* 939–942.

Cella, D.F., & Tulsky, D.S. (1991). *Measuring quality of life today: Methodological aspects.* Proceedings of a International Symposium held at St. Mary Medical Center, Long Beach, CA. Williston Park, NY: Dominus.

Chapko, M.K., Syrjala, K.L., Bush, N., Jedlow, C., & Yanke, M.R. (1991). Development of a behavioral measure of mouth pain, nausea, and wellness for patients receiving radiation and chemotherapy. *Journal of Pain and Symptom Management, 6,* 15–23.

Chapko, M.K., Syrjala, K.L., Schilter, L., Cummings, C., & Sullivan, K. (1989). Chemoradiotherapy toxicity during bone marrow transplantation: Time course and variation in pain and nausea. *Bone Marrow Transplant, 4,* 181–186.

Chapman, C.R., Kornell, J.A., & Syrjala, K.L. (1986).

Painful complications of cancer diagnosis and therapy. In: C.H. Yarbro, & D.B. McGuire (Eds.), *Cancer pain: Nursing management* (pp. 46–67). Orlando, FL: Grune & Stratton.

Cleeland, C.S. (1984). The impact of pain on the patient with cancer. *Cancer, 58,* 2635–2641.

Cleeland, C.S. (1985). Measurement and prevalence of pain in cancer. *Seminars in Oncology Nursing, 1,* 87–92.

Cleeland, C.S. (1987). Impact of pain on the patient with cancer. *Cancer 58,* 2635–2641.

Cleeland, C.S. (1989a). Measurement of pain by subjective report. In C.R. Chapman & J.D. Loeser (Eds.), *Issues in pain measurement.* New York: Raven Press.

Cleeland, C.S. (1989b). Pain control: Public and physicians' attitudes. In C.S. Hill, Jr., & W.S. Fields (Eds.), *Advances in pain research and therapy* (Vol. 16, pp. 81–89). New York: Raven Press.

Cleeland, C.S. (1990). Assessment of pain in cancer: Measurement issues. In K.M. Foley, J.J. Bonica, & V. Vendatridda (Eds.), *Advances in pain research and therapy* (Vol. 16, p. 16). New York: Raven Press.

Cleeland, C.S. (1991). Research in cancer pain: What we know and what we need to know. *Cancer, 67* (Supplement), 823–827.

Cleeland, C.S., Rotondi, A., Brechner, T., Levin, A., MacDonald, N., Portenoy, R., Schutta, H., & McEniry, M. (1986). A model for the treatment of cancer pain. *Journal of Pain and Symptom Management, 1,* 209.

Dar, R., Beach C., Barden, P., & Cleeland, C.S. (1992). Cancer pain in the marital system: A study of patients and their spouses. *Journal of Pain and Symptom Management,* February 1992.

Daut, R.L., & Cleeland, C.S. (1982). The prevalence and severity of pain in cancer. *Cancer, 50,* 1913–1918.

Derogatis, L.R., Morrow, G.R., Fetting, J., Penman, D., Piasetsky, S., Schmale, A.M., Henrichs, M., & Carnicke, C.L.M., Jr. (1983). The prevalence of psychiatric disorders among cancer patients. *Journal of the American Medical Association, 249,* 751–757.

Derogatis, L.R., & Spencer, P.M. (1982). *Administration and procedures: BSI manual—I.* Clinical Psychometric Research.

Donovan, M.I. & Dillon, P. (1987). Incidence and characteristics of pain in a sample of hospitalized cancer patients. *Cancer Nursing, 10,* 85–92.

Dunkel-Schetter, C. (1984). Social support and cancer: Findings based on patient interviews and their implications. *Journal of Social Issues, 40,* 77–98.

Ferraz, M.B., Quaresma, M.R., Aquino, L.R., Atra, E., Tugwell, P., & Goldsmith, C.H. (1990). Reliability of pain scales in the assessment of literate and illiterate patients with rheumatoid arthritis. *Journal of Rheumatology, 7,* 1022–1024.

Ferrell, B.R., Wisdom, C., & Wenzl, C. (1989). Quality of life as an outcome variable in the management of cancer pain. *Cancer, 63* (Suppl. 11), 2321–2327.

Fishman, B., Pasternak, S., Wallenstein, S.L., Houde, R.W., Holland J.C., & Foley, K.M. (1987). The Memorial Pain Assessment Card: A valid instrument for the evaluation of cancer pain. *Cancer, 60,* 1151–1158.

Foley, K.M. (1979). Pain syndromes in patients with cancer. In J.J. Bonica & V. Ventafridda (Eds.), *Advances in pain research and therapy* (Vol. 2, pp. 59–75). New York: Raven Press.

Foley, K.M. (1985). Treatment of cancer pain. *New England Journal of Medicine, 313,* 84–95.

Ganz, P.A., Haskell, C.M., Figlin, R.A., LaSota, N., & Siau, J. (1988). Estimating the quality of life in a clinical trial of patients with metastatic lung cancer using the Karnofsky performance status and the Functional Living Index-Cancer. *Cancer, 61,* 849–856.

Gonzales, G.R., Elliott, K.J., Portenoy, R.K. & Foley, K.M. (1991). The impact of a comprehensive evaluation in the management of cancer pain. *Pain, 47,* 141–144.

Greenwald, H.P., Bonica, J.J., & Bergner, M. (1987). The prevalence of pain in four cancers. *Cancer, 60,* 2563–2569.

Grossman, S.A., Sheidler, V.R., Swedeen, Mucenski, J. & Piantadosi, S. (1991). Correlation of patient and caregiver ratings of cancer pain. *Journal of Pain and Symptom Management, 6,* 53–57.

Hodes, R.L. (1989). Cancer patients' needs and concerns when using narcotic analgesics. In C.S. Hill & W.S. Fields (Eds.), *Advances in pain research and therapy* (Vol. 11, pp. 91–99). New York: Raven Press.

Jensen, M.P., Karoly, P., & Braver, S. (1986). The measurement of clinical pain intensity: A comparison of six methods. *Pain, 27,* 117–126.

Karnofsky, D.A., Abelmann, W.H., Craver, L.F., & Burchenal, J.H. (1984). The use of the nitrogen mustards in the palliative treatment of carcinoma. *Cancer, 1,* 634–656.

Lansky, S.B., List, M.A., Ritter-Sterr, C., Logemann, J., & Willis, M. (1988). Performance parameters in head and neck patients. *Proceedings of the American Society of Clinical Oncology, 7,* 156.

Lasagna, L. (1980). Analgesic methodology: A brief history and commentary. *Journal of Clinical Pharmacology, 20,* 373–376.

McCorkle, R. (1987). The measurement of symptom diseases. *Seminars in Oncology Nursing, 3,* 248–256.

McGrath, P.J., Beyer, J., Cleeland, C.S., Eland, J., McGrath, P.A., & Portenoy, R. (1990). American Academy of Pediatrics Report of the Subcommittee on Assessment and Methodologic Issues in the Management of Pain in Childhood Cancer. *Pediatrics, 86*(5 Pt. 2), 814–817.

McNair, D.M., Lorr, M., & Droppleman, L.F. (1971). *EITS Manual for the Profile of Mood States.* San Diego: Educational Testing Service.

Melzack, R. (1987). The short-form McGill Pain Questionnaire. *Pain, 30*(2), 191–197.

Moinpour, C.M., Feigl, P., Metch, B., Hayden, B.A., Meyskens, F.L. Jr., & Crowley, J. (1989). Quality of life end points in cancer clinical trials: Review and recommendations. *Review, 81,* 485–495.

Moinpour, C.M., & Hayden, K.A. (1991). *Quality of life assessment in Southwest Oncology Group trials.* Proceedings of an International Symposium held at St. Mary Medical Center, Long Beach, CA. Williston Park, NY: Dominus.

Moos, R.H., & Moos, B.S. (1986). *Family Environment Scale—manual* (2nd ed.). Palo Alto, CA: Consulting Psychologists Press.

Morrow, G.M., Feldstein, M., Adler, L.M., Derogatis, L.R., Enelow, A.J., Gates, C., Holland, J., Melisaratos, N., Murawski, B., Perman, D., Schmale, A., Schmitt, M., & Morse, I. (1981). Development of brief measures of psychosocial adjustment to medical illness applied to cancer patients. *General Hospital Psychiatry, 3,* 79–81.

Parr, G., Darekar, B., Fletcher, A. & Bulpitt, C. (1989).

Joint pain and quality of life: Results of a randomised trial. *British Journal of Clinical Pharmacology, 27,* 235–242.

Payne, R. (1990). Pathophysiology of cancer pain. In K.M. Foley et al. (Eds.), *Advances in pain research and therapy* (Vol. 16). New York: Raven Press.

Peteet, J., Tay, V., Cohen, G. & MacIntyre, J. (1986). Pain characteristics and treatment in an outpatient cancer population. *Cancer, 57,* 1259–1265.

Portenoy, R.K. (1989). Cancer pain: Epidemiology and syndromes, *Cancer, 63,* 2298.

Portenoy, R.K., & Hagen, N.A. (1990). Breakthrough pain: Definition, prevalence and characteristics. *Pain, 41,* 273–281.

Portenoy, R.K., Lipton, R.B., & Foley, K.M. (1987). Back pain in the cancer patient: An algorithm for evaluation and management. *Neurology, 37,* 134–138.

Schipper, H. (1991). *Guidelines and caveats for quality of life measurement in clinical practice and research.* Proceedings of an International Symposium held at St. Mary Medical Center, Long Beach, CA. Williston Park, NY: Dominus.

Schipper, H., Clinch, J., McMurray, A., & Levitt, M. (1984). Measuring the quality of life of cancer patients: The Functional Lifing Index-Cancer: Development and validation. *Journal of Clinical Oncology, 2,* 472–483.

Selby, P.J., Chapman, J.A.W., Etazadi-Amoli, J., Dalley, D., & Boyd, N.F. (1984). The development of a method for assessing the quality of life of cancer patients. *British Journal of Cancer, 50,* 13–22.

Shacham, S., Dar, R., & Cleeland, C.S. (1984). Relationship of mood state to the severity of clinical pain. *Pain, 18,* 21.

Shumaker, S.A., Anderson, R.T., & Czajkowski, S.M. (1990). Psychological tests and scales. In B. Spilker (Ed.), *Quality of life assessments in clinical trials* (pp. 95–113). New York: Raven Press.

Spector, W.D. (1990). Functional Disability Scales. In B. Spilker (Ed.), *Quality of life assessments in clinical trials.* New York: Raven Press.

Spiegel, D., & Bloom, J. (1983). Group therapy and hypnosis reduce metastatic breast carcinoma pain. *Psychosomatic Medicine, 45,* 333.

Spiegel, D., Bloom, J.R., Kraemer, H.C., & Gottheil, E. (1989). Effect of psychosocial treatment on survival of patients with metastatic breast cancer. *Lancet, 2,* 14.

Spielberger, C.D. (1983). *Manual for the State-Trait Anxiety Inventory (Form Y).* Palo Alto CA: Consulting Psychologists Press.

Spilker, B. (Ed.). (1990). *Quality of life assessments in clinical trials.* New York: Raven Press.

Spitzer, R.L., & Williams, J.B.W. (Eds.) (1987). *Diagnostic and Statistical Manual of Mental Disorders* (3rd ed.—rev.). Washington, DC: American Psychiatric Association.

Spitzer, W.O., Dobson, A.J., Hall, J., Chesterman, E., Levi, J., Shepherd, R., Battista, R.N., & Catchlove, B.R. (1981). Measuring the quality of life of cancer patients: A concise QL-Index for use by physicians. *Journal of Chronic Disease, 34,* 585–597.

Stewart, A.L., Hays, R.D., & Ware, J.E. (1988). The MOS Short-form General Health Survey: Reliability and validity in a patient population. *Medical Care, 26,* 724–735.

Syrjala, K.L. (1987). *The measurement of pain: Cancer pain management.* Orlando, FL: Grune & Stratton.

Syrjala, K.L., Chapko, M.K., Cummings, C., Sullivan, K.M., & Carr, J.E. (1988). *Physical and psychosocial functioning in the first year after bone marrow transplantation (BMT): A prospective study.* Presented at the Society of Behavioral Medicine Annual Scientific Sessions Ninth Annual Meeting, Boston.

Syrjala, K.L., & Chapman, C.R. (1984). Measurement of clinical pain: A review and integration of research findings. In C. Benadetti, C.R. Chapman, & G. Moricca (Eds.), *Advances in pain research and therapy* (Vol. 7, pp. 71–101). New York: Raven Press.

Syrjala, K.L., Cummings, C., & Donaldson, G.W. (in press). Hypnosis or cognitive behavioral training for the reduction of pain and nausea during cancer treatment: A controlled clinical trial. *Pain.*

Syrjala, K.L., Chapko, M.K., Cummings, C., Sullivan, K.M., & Carr, J.E. (1988). *Physical and psychosocial functioning in the first year after bone marrow transplantation (BMT): A prospective study.* Presented at the Society of Behavioral Medicine Annual Scientific Sessions Ninth Annual Meeting, Boston.

Takeda, F. (1987). Management of cancer pain—WHO cancer control programme. In *Quality of life in cancer patients* (pp. 61–69). Tokyo: Diamond Planning Services.

Ventafridda, V., Tamburini, M., Caraceni, A., DeConno, F., & Naldi, F. (1987). A validation study of the WHO method for cancer pain relief. *Cancer, 59,* 850–856.

VonRoenn, J.H., Cleeland, C.S., Gonin, R., & Pandya, K. (1991). *Results of a physician attitude toward cancer pain and its management survey by ECOG.* Presented at the American Society of Clinical Oncology meeting, Houston, TX.

Wallenstein, S. (1984). Measurement of pain and analgesia in cancer patients. *Cancer, 53* (Suppl. 10), 2260–2264.

Williamson, J.W. (1971). Evaluating quality of patient care: A strategy relating outcome and process assessment. *Journal of the American Medical Association, 218,* 564–569.

World Health Organization (1986). *Cancer pain relief.* Geneva: Author.

Wortman, C.B. (1984). Social support and the cancer patient: Conceptual and methodological issues. *Cancer, 53* (Suppl. 10), 2339–2360.

Zubrod, C.G., Schneiderman, M., Frei, E., et al. (1960). Appraisal of methods for the study of chemotherapy of cancer in man: Comparative therapeutic trial of nitrogen mustart and triethylene thiosphoramide. *Journal of Chronic Disease, 11,* 7–33.

VI
METHODOLOGICAL ISSUES

Chapter 22

Epidemiological and Survey Methods: Chronic Pain Assessment

MICHAEL VON KORFF ScD

Reports of the National Institutes of Health (1986) and of the National Academy of Sciences (Osterweis, Kleinman, & Mechanic, 1987) have called for increased epidemiological research concerning chronic pain conditions. This challenge cannot be met without adequate attention to the problems of pain assessment in epidemiological research. To date, the principal contributions of epidemiology to pain research have been the estimation of prevalence rates and cross-sectional analysis of factors associated with the presence of anatomically defined pain symptoms. Based on this limited exposure to epidemiology, it is not surprising that many pain researchers regard measurement issues in epidemiology as largely concerning the conduct of morbidity surveys. This chapter does consider issues of pain assessment that arise in conducting morbidity surveys, but also considers pain measurement issues relevant to a wider range of epidemiological research.

A theme of this chapter is that population-based studies of chronic pain reveal a broad spectrum of severity. Although epidemiologic studies have described the prevalence of most common chronic pain conditions, less is known about the extent to which these conditions are associated with mild, moderate, or severe dysfunction. Epidemiology provides concepts and methods for describing the spectrum and the course of chronic pain in populations, and methods of identifying factors that influence variation in risks of developing or maintaining chronic pain and associated dysfunction. Special attention is paid to brief methods of assessing pain dysfunction suitable for use in epidemiological and survey research. These assessment methods provide a means of describing the severity of chronic pain conditions in populations and tracking their course across time.

EPIDEMIOLOGIC PERSPECTIVES

Definition and Uses of Epidemiology

Epidemiology is the study of the distribution and determinants of health states in populations (Lilienfeld & Lilienfeld, 1980). As a discipline, epidemiology provides a scientific basis for public health efforts to prevent and control disease and disability on a population basis. The contributions of epidemiology to scientific and public health research, summarized by Morris (1975), include:

1. Establishing the dimensions of morbidity and mortality as a function of person, place, and time.
2. Quantifying risks of developing morbidity as a function of host, agent, and environmental factors.
3. Identifying and defining syndromes and diseases.
4. Describing the full clinical spectrum of specific syndromes, diseases, and conditions.
5. Describing the natural history of disease in terms of onset, duration, recurrence, complications, disability, and mortality.
6. Identifying factors that influence or predict clinical course.
7. Identifying causes of disease, disability, and mortality.
8. Evaluating methods of disease prevention and control.

Population, Dynamic, and Ecologic Perspectives

Epidemiologic study of pain involves the application of three general perspectives (Dworkin, Von Korff, & Le Resche, 1992):

1. A population perspective—the occurrence of pain and associated dysfunction is studied on a population basis. When pain is studied on a population basis, a wide spectrum of pain expression and pain dysfunction is observed. Most adults experience some form of (often mild) recurrent pain condition, a significant minority experience intense-persistent pain, whereas relatively few experience substantial pain-related disability (Von Korff, Dworkin, & Le Resche, 1990). Epidemiology provides methods for studying this variation in the occurrence and severity of pain conditions in populations. The population perspective does not imply that epidemiological studies always employ random samples drawn from defined populations, only that the ultimate objective is to understand the distribution and determinants of illness on a population basis.

2. A developmental perspective—pain (like most illness and disease) is changing and dynamic rather than fixed and static. The study of

the development of pain conditions and their expression across the life span of a population are important endeavors. Studies of the pattern of development or variation of a pain condition across time provide a basis for learning about the nature and determinants of the condition.

3. An ecologic perspective—pain and related dysfunction are the result of integrated action of agent, host, and environmental factors. From this perspective, factors that initiate pain are analogous to disease agents. An agent is a proximal and necessary (but usually not sufficient) cause of disease or illness. Intrinsic modulation of pain perception, appraisal, and emotional response to pain is influenced by host factors. A host factor is a characteristic intrinsic to an organism that influences susceptibility. And social processes influencing the learning of cognitive and behavioral responses to noxious stimulation and social norms governing pain behavior (e.g, the sick role) constitute environmental factors. An environmental factor is an extrinsic circumstance that influences exposure to agents or that modifies host susceptibility. Thus, the ecologic model (like the biopsychosocial model) views pain as a dynamic and multifactorial process characterized by integrated action of biologic, psychologic and social factors.

A Dynamic Population Model of Chronic Pain

Epidemiologic research seeks to study chronic pain in populations as a dynamic process characterized by the integrated action of agent, host, and environmental factors. A major challenge is to devise methods and models of measurement able to achieve this goal.

One possible approach to conceptualizing change in chronic pain status is the dynamic population model depicted in Figure 22.1. In any given time period, persons may be pain free; experiencing acute, recurrent or persistent pain without chronic dysfunction; or experiencing a persistent pain condition with chronic dysfunction. Since chronic pain is characterized as much by change as by stability, transitions among these states over time are to be expected. The major aims of epidemiologic research concerning chronic pain and associated dysfunction can be defined in terms of this dynamic population model. These aims include: characterizing and defining chronic pain

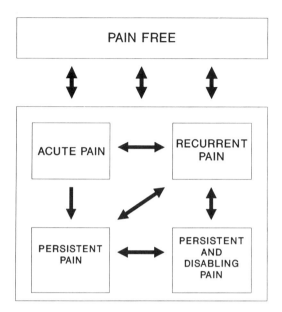

FIGURE 22.1. A dynamic population model of chronic pain. From Von Korff, Dworkin, and Le Resche (1990). Copyright 1990 Elsevier Science Publishers. Reprinted by permission.

states across the severity spectrum; estimating the probability of being in a particular state in a given time period; estimating transition probabilities among states over time; and identifying factors predicting or controlling those probabilities (Von Korff, Dworkin, & Le Resche, 1990). Thus, chronic pain in populations may be viewed as a dynamic process with flows among a defined set of pain states, and probabilities governing the transition rates among those states. A comprehensive treatment of the application of population flow models to chronic disease epidemiology is provided by Manton and Stallard (1988). Graham, Collins, Wugalter, Chung, and Hansen (1991) describe relevant approaches to analyzing dynamic categorical data that could be employed to model this sort of dynamic process.

EPIDEMIOLOGIC METHODS

Epidemiologic Measures and Their Relevance to Pain Research

Epidemiologists have developed various measures of disease occurrence and risk that can be used to measure the distribution, determinants, and natural history of disease in a dynamic population. The most important types of epidemiological measures of occurrence, risk, and natural history that are applicable to pain research include the following:

Measures of pain prevalence quantify the proportion of a population with a condition at a given point in time (point prevalence rate), the proportion of persons affected by the condition during a defined period of time (period prevalence rate), or the proportion of a population affected over their lifetime (lifetime prevalence rate). The numerator of a prevalence rate is the number of persons with the condition in the defined time period, and the denominator is the number of persons in the population or the population sample being studied.

Measures of incidence quantify the probability or rate of onset of a condition among persons with no prior history. An incidence rate is the ratio of the number of onset events divided by the observed number of person years the individuals under study were at risk of developing the condition. An incidence probability is the ratio of the number of persons developing the condition during a defined time period to the number of persons observed over the time period. Kleinbaum, Kupper, and Morgenstern (1982) provide a thorough discussion of incidence and prevalence measures.

Natural history measures quantify different aspects of clinical course such as the incubation period (Cobb, Miller, & Wald, 1959) or the interval between exposure to a risk factor and onset of the condition; episode duration; the likelihood of recovery or relapse; the likelihood of death (case-fatality rates, mortality rates, and mortality ratios); and the likelihood of becoming disabled.

Measures of relative risk quantify differences in onset rates or in prevalence rates comparing persons differing in a risk factor. The most important measure of relative risk in epidemiologic research is the odds ratio, which is the ratio of the odds of having the condition under study among persons with a risk factor to the odds of having the condition among persons lacking the risk factor (Lilienfeld & Lilienfeld, 1980).

Risk factors may be *initiators*—factors that set in motion a causal process; *promoters*—factors that enhance or potentiate a causal process already initiated (Hopkins & Williams, 1986);

or *detection factors*—factors that have no causal effect but that increase the likelihood of a case being identified (Kleinbaum et al., 1982). Empirical differentiation of initiators, promoters, and detection factors is often difficult.

Measures of prognosis quantify future risks of progression or remission of a condition as a function of current status and prognostic variables of interest.

Relationships between prevalence, incidence, and duration—the clinical course of chronic pain is frequently episodic (Von Korff, Dworkin, Le Resche, & Kruger, 1988). It has been shown that the steady-state prevalence of a chronic episodic condition is approximated by the product of its incidence rate, the average duration of episodes, and the average number of episodes over the course of the illness (Von Korff & Parker, 1980). This steady-state equation provides a basis for understanding the different ways in which prevalence rates could differ between two population groups. If two groups differ in prevalence rate of a chronic pain condition, it may be because the group with the higher rate was more likely to develop the condition, had longer episodes, was more likely to relapse, or some combination of those factors. Two groups with the same prevalence rate of a pain condition might be found to have a different schedule of incidence rates that were, in turn, counterbalanced by differences in mean episode duration in the opposite direction. Thus, clinical and epidemiologic research seeking to understand the determinants of pain conditions needs to identify strategies that differentiate factors influencing onset rates, factors influencing episode duration, and factors influencing recurrence rates.

Epidemiologic Study Designs

Lilienfeld and Lilienfeld (1980) suggest classifying epidemiologic study designs in terms of several characteristics: (1) *observational* (relying on naturally occurring variation in risk factors) or *experimental* (introducing exposure to protective factors or treatments by design); (2) *individual* (the person is the unit of observation) or *ecological* (a social group, community, state, or nation is the unit of analysis); and (3) relying on *cross-sectional* data collection or *longitudinal* data collection. Major epidemiologic study designs, and where they fit in the Lilienfeld schema, are briefly summarized:

Cross-sectional Surveys (Observational, Individual, Cross-sectional)

The methods of the sample survey have been well developed over the past 40 years. A sampling frame is established enumerating persons or sampling units in a defined population of interest. A probability sample is selected from the sampling frame using methods that may be relatively simple (e.g., a simple random sample) or complex (e.g., a multistage cluster sample). The methods of probability sampling are fully treated in a number of texts (Cochran, 1977; Kish, 1965).

Information to determine the presence or absence of chronic pain conditions and concerning possible risk factors is collected by interview usually conducted either in person or via telephone. The interview typically follows a standardized questionnaire administered by a trained interviewer with response categories precoded. Unlike clinical pain assessment, the survey interview usually must ascertain whether a pain condition of interest has been present before any further questions about intensity, persistence, interference, and other aspects of the pain condition may be asked. In some instances, a two-phase survey design can be employed to permit clinical examination and diagnostic evaluation of a subsample of persons included in the sample survey (Dworkin, Von Korff, Le Resche, & Truelove, 1988). Selection of the second phase sample is typically based on responses to the initial screening interview.

In general, sample surveys are most useful for estimation of prevalence rates of a condition and description of its distribution by self-reported or clinically measured characteristics of subjects. Survey-based analysis of the association of risk factors with a pain condition generally takes advantage of naturally occurring variation of risk factors in the sample, although a sample design may be devised to yield comparisons of special interest. The measurement of risk factor status usually relies on self-report information about the subject's current status, the subject's recollection of risk factor status in the past, simple objective measurements that can be made in a field setting such as the subject's home (e.g., weight or blood pressure), and/or collection of medical or other records data. Eaton and Kessler (1985) and Rose, Blackburn, Gillum, and Prineas (1982) provide comprehensive reviews of how modern survey research methods can be applied in the study of specific chronic conditions. A useful review of the use of cross-sectional surveys in public health research is provided by Abramson (1985).

Panel Surveys (Observational, Individual, Longitudinal)

A sample survey with longitudinal data collection is often referred to as a panel survey. Panel surveys can be useful for examining individual change over time. Cook and Ware (1983) define longitudinal study as research in which the same individuals are observed on more than one occasion. Rogosa, Brandt, and Zimowski (1982) observe that, "Certainly, two waves are better than one, but two waves of data poorly define the individual time paths and often are not sufficiently rich to yield satisfactory answers to important questions about change and growth" (p. 729).

In theory, panel surveys permit analysis of three kinds of effects of time: aging effects, cohort or period effects, and time effects (Nessleroade & Baltes, 1979). In practice, distinguishing these types of time effects is challenging. Cook and Ware (1983) provide definitions of the different types of time effects. Cohort and period effects represent the contribution of the past history or unique experience of a cohort to their series of measurements. A time effect represents the effect of the passage of time per se between measurements, while age effects reflect the passage of time with respect to the chronological age of subjects. For example, the decrease in headache prevalence with increasing age might be due to a beneficial impact of aging on the occurrence of headaches or a result of younger cohorts experiencing increases in the incidence, duration, or recurrence of headaches relative to older cohorts. Longitudinal designs can sometimes shed light on the relative merits of such alternative explanations.

Measurement issues in longitudinal research are significant. Rogosa et al. (1982) observe that,

> [M]any crucial aspects of the measurement of change have been overlooked, obscured and misunderstood in previous investigations. As a result, many current recommendations about the measurement of change are unsound. . . . An explicit definition of individual change is required for the measurement of individual change. Consequently, statistical models for the individual time paths provide the foundation for the estimation of change. (p. 726)

Case-Control Studies (Observational, Individual, Cross-sectional)

In studies of the etiology of chronic disease, the case-control design has been the most extensively used epidemiological method over the past 20 years. It is a cost-efficient method of obtaining a comparison of the association of a putative risk factor with disease onset. Because of a large number of threats to the validity of case-control studies, the use of this design has not been without controversy (Feinstein, 1979). However, the successes of the case-control method in identifying causal processes later confirmed by more rigorous methods have been well documented. A thorough treatment of the methods of the case-control study is provided by Schlesselman (1982), and a useful synopsis of the methods is provided by Greenberg and Ibrahim (1985).

The elements of a case-control study include (1) a sample of recent onset cases of the condition of interest, (2) a sample of controls selected in a way that does not introduce sampling bias with respect to risk factors relative to cases, and (3) measurements made on cases and controls using the same methods. The resulting data are analyzed via contingency table analysis. In the simplest case, a two-by-two table is constructed in which the columns represent persons with or without the condition under study. The rows represent persons with or without the putative risk factor. The odds ratio, a measure of the relative frequency of the risk factor in cases and controls, provides an estimate of the relative risk of developing the condition among cases relative to controls. The relative risk is the incidence rate among persons with the risk factor divided by the incidence rate among persons without the risk factor. Multivariate extensions of contingency table analysis have been developed that employ logistic regression or log-linear analysis to estimate adjusted odds ratios (Bishop, Fienberg, & Holland, 1978; Breslow & Day, 1980).

Prospective Studies (Observational, Individual, Longitudinal)

A prospective study is a longitudinal design that starts with cohorts not affected by the condition of interest to compare subsequent risks of onset of the condition comparing persons with versus without a risk factor of interest. These cohorts are then followed over time to identify onsets of the illness, or other endpoints of the study (e.g., recurrence of the condition, chronicity, death, disability). A prospective design requires surveillance of the cohorts to detect endpoints occurring over the follow-up period, and reasonably precise dating of the occurrence of the endpoint. Stratification of the cohorts by risk factor status at the outset, or as the study progresses, provides a basis for inference about the relationship of the risk factor to the risk of subsequent occurrence of the endpoint. A retrospective (also referred to as nonconcurrent or historical) cohort study permits longitudinal investigation of a risk factor with disease experience through the use of historical records of exposure to a risk factor and subsequent disease experience. For example, records documenting the distance survivors were from the hypocenter of the atom bomb explosion in Hiroshima have been used to study the impact of differing levels of radiation exposure on the incidence of leukemia and the incubation period from exposure to onset of disease (Cobb et al., 1959).

The analysis of data from a prospective (or retrospective) cohort study is based on comparison of the rates of occurrence of the endpoint (number of morbidity or mortality events in relation to person years of experience) among persons with versus without exposure to the putative risk factor. Kleinbaum et al., (1982) provide a thorough discussion of the design of prospective studies. Feinlab and Detels (1985) review the different variations of cohort study designs used in epidemiological research. The life table provides a nonparametric approach to statistical analysis of data from a prospective study (Gross & Clark, 1975). The analysis of prospective study data has been advanced considerably by the development of parametric and multivariate methods of survival analysis (Cox & Oakes, 1984; Kabfleisch & Prentice, 1980; Singer & Willett, in press).

Given the potential difficulties in interpretation of cross-sectional and case-control studies of chronic pain, prospective and retrospective cohort study designs may have an important role to play in understanding the onset of chronic pain, as well as factors producing disability. In order to design a cohort study, information about incidence rates is needed. For conditions with low incidence rates, larger cohorts and more years of follow-up are required to yield adequate statistical power to detect differences between persons exposed and unexposed to a risk factor than for conditions with a higher incidence rate. The lack of reliable incidence rate data for most chronic pain conditions is an impediment to the proper design of cohort studies.

Preventive and Clinical Trials (Experimental, Individual, Longitudinal)

Epidemiology is a practical science whose fundamental objective is to produce knowledge relevant to disease prevention and control. Repeatedly, epidemiological methods have yielded methods of disease prevention or control before etiologic mechanisms were understood (Morris, 1975). The clinical trial is a rigorous means of evaluating methods of disease control, while the preventive trial evaluates the effectiveness of methods of disease prevention. Preventive and clinical trials are prospective cohort studies in which exposure to a disease prevention or disease control measure is randomly allocated. Hill (1971) provides a classic discussion of the need for randomization in the evaluation of interventions and the essential concepts of the randomized trial. Meinert (1986) provides a comprehensive treatment of the design, conduct, and analysis of randomized clinical trials from an epidemiologic perspective.

The ecologic and biopsychosocial models of chronic pain posit dynamic interaction among risk factors producing chronic pain, as well as feedback relationships between a person's response to pain and risk factors for pain dysfunction. For example, when a person reduces social role performance due to chronic pain, that individual's social environment is likely to change in response that, in turn, may affect the behavioral response of the person in pain. In this sort of bidirectional causal relationship, it can be difficult to determine whether host or environmental factors are more important in determining patient outcomes. Experimental designs may be more important in quantifying the strength of effects of causal factors in pain research than in other areas of epidemiology where direction of causation is generally clear (e.g., exposure to radiation causes cancer, with no reciprocal effect).

Ecological Studies (Observational, Ecological, Cross-sectional)

In this type of study, a morbidity rate is typically compared among different social areas (Morgenstern, 1982). For example, studies comparing the rates of work disability due to back pain across countries are ecological studies.

Community Trials (Experimental, Ecological, Longitudinal)

This form of study involves intervention with a social unit (a community, a worksite, a clinic). The unit assigned to the intervention or control condition is the aggregate, not the individual. There is a growing literature on the design, implementation, and analysis of this form of ecological study (Altman, 1986; Farquhar, 1978)

Measurement Biases in Epidemiologic Research

This section reviews measurement biases relevant to pain research that have been identified and/or studied for different forms of epidemiologic research.

Sources of bias in survey research have been extensively studied (Bradburn, Rips & Shevell, 1987; Cannel, 1977; Converse & Traugott, 1986) and include measurement bias in questionnaires, a variety of reporting biases, as well sampling biases such as undercoverage (persons missed by the sampling method) and nonresponse (persons refusing interview or not contacted).

Recall bias is a significant issue in epidemiologic research concerning pain because it is often necessary to ask subjects whether they have experienced an anatomically defined pain condition over some defined period of time (e.g., 2 weeks, 6 months, 1 year). Means, Nigam, Zarrow, Loftus, and Donaldson (1989), in a monograph on autobiographical memory for health-related events, make a distinction between semantic memory and episodic memory. Semantic memory is conceptually structured information resistant to interference from other memory traces. Episodic memory is a temporally ordered set of autobiographical events that can be more difficult to retrieve. It is important, both from a substantive and a methodologic standpoint, to know what features of a chronic pain condition (e.g., persistence, intensity, interference, meaning, disability) lead to encoding of the pain condition as a semantic or as an episodic memory. If more severe, disabling, and longer lasting pain conditions are more likely to be encoded as semantic memory, then the accuracy of recall of severe chronic pain conditions experienced in the past 3, 6, or 12 months may be adequate. Less persistent and severe pain problems may be more likely to be forgotten.

Unlike pain assessment in a clinical setting in which the pain condition is often the presenting complaint, in an epidemiologic survey it is often necessary to ask subjects about whether they have experienced pain at a given anatomical site. It is not possible to ask follow-up questions about intensity, persistence, and disability until the subject has reported the presence of the pain condition of interest. In pain surveys conducted to date, subjects have been asked whether they have experienced an episode of an anatomically defined pain condition in time periods of 2 weeks (Crook, Rideout & Browne, 1984), 6 months (Von Korff et al., 1988), and 1 year (Sternbach, 1986). Other differences in these studies do not permit conclusions about the magnitude of the effect on prevalence rates of asking about shorter versus longer reporting periods. Comparison of the results of these surveys does suggest that asking subjects site-specific questions about the presence of pain conditions (see Von Korff and Sternbach survey results) yields higher prevalence rates than asking questions about the presence of a pain condition without mentioning an anatomical site (see Crook survey results).

Research by the National Center for Health Statistics provides estimates of the probability of recall of selected chronic conditions known to have been present in the prior year because they were treated (Madow, 1973). For example, diabetes, sinusitis, and hypertension were recalled by more than 80% of treated cases, while asthma, headache, and arthritis were recalled by more than 60% of treated cases. This research showed that the agreement of self-report and medical records data increased with the number of visits for a chronic condition and was higher if the subject had received medicines for the condition of interest.

Based on research showing that memory for doctors visits decays rapidly with increasing time since the visit (Cannel, 1977), an important issue is how long a recall period should be employed in asking subjects about chronic pain conditions. There are trade-offs for short versus long reporting intervals (Drury, 1989; Von Korff & Dworkin, 1989). A short reporting period, all else being equal, should minimize forgetting of pain conditions if the subject is not experiencing pain at the time of the interview. However, a very short reporting interval may tend to underrepresent persons with acute or recurrent pain conditions relative to those with persistent pain due to the phenomena of length-biased sampling (Shepard & Neutra, 1977). That is, among all persons experiencing a pain condition during a given interval (e.g., 1 year), persons with persistent pain would be more likely to be identified with a short (e.g., 2 week) recall period than persons with acute or recurrent pain. In addition, a short reporting interval may not afford a sufficient time period for questions regarding the subject's characteristic pattern of pain (worst and average intensity, number of disability days, number of days in pain, etc.).

Prior research has shown that survey questions about pain intensity, interference, disability days, and persistence for a 6-month reporting period predict past and future use of health care and pain medications measured by automated data sources (Von Korff et al., 1990), and predict chronic pain status at 1 year follow-up (Von Korff & Dworkin, 1989) and 3-year follow-up (Von Korff, Ormel, Keefe, & Dworkin, in press). These results support the validity of a 6-month reporting period for pain ratings. A short reporting period may not yield as reliable an estimate of a subject's characteristic chronic pain status because of the large within-subject variability in pain status over time. For example, in assessing chronic pain status it may be more informative to know that a subject has experienced back pain on 90 days in the prior 6 months relative to knowing a subject has experienced pain on 7 days in the prior 2 weeks, even though 2-week recall may be more accurate than 6-month recall.

In a study of high utilizers of health care who had made a health-care visit for back pain within the prior year (Von Korff, 1991), it was found that recall was high (88%) if the visit had occurred within the prior 6-months, but was lower (73%) if the visit had occurred more than 6-months before the interview. Persons with multiple visits were more likely to recall their back pain episode (92%) than persons with a

single visit (69%). Depressed persons were more likely to recall their back pain episode (91%) than nondepressed persons (74%), particularly among persons whose visit was more than 6 months before the interview (88% vs. 57%). This suggests that a mid-range recall period (3–6 months) may be preferable to longer or shorter recall periods. A three to six month reporting interval is long enough to afford useful information on the characteristic pattern of pain and to reduce length-biased sampling. At the same time, a 3- to 6-month reporting period may be short enough to reduce forgetting and recall biases related to affective distress.

Other cognitive processes are relevant to the recall of pain in survey research, but have not been adequately studied for pain report. *Forward telescoping* is a tendency for respondents to report events that occurred before the reference period as having occurred during the reference period. This may be particularly problematic in studies estimating first onset rates of pain conditions. If subjects tend to report first onset as more recent than it actually was, incidence rate estimates could be substantially inflated. There is evidence that this phenomena occurs for recall of first onset of mental disorders (Simon & Von Korff, in press).

Using personal *landmark events* to improve recall of the course of a chronic pain condition may be a useful interviewing strategy (Means et al., 1989). For example, if subjects were being questioned about the offset of a pain condition over a 6-month recall period, showing the subject a time line with salient personal events (birthdays, Christmas, going on vacation, etc.) may improve the subject's ability to accurately recall when the pain condition remitted.

Regression to the Mean

When the sampling frame for an epidemiologic (or clinical) study is patients seeking treatment for a pain complaint, the phenomena of regression to the mean needs to be taken into account. Patients seek treatment for a pain complaint when its severity flares up or exceeds its characteristic severity (Von Korff, Wagner, Dworkin, & Saunders, 1991). Thus, subjects sampled at time of entering treatment have been self-selected by exceeding their pain threshold for treatment seeking. Because of the phenomena of regression to the mean, persons sampled at time of seeking care can be expected to have reduced pain levels at a later point in time with or without treatment (Whitney & Von Korff, in press). Statements about the average improvement in pain conditions among persons who have sought treatment, or inference about the effectiveness of treatments based on uncontrolled research, must take into account within subject regression to the mean to their characteristic pain level. This phenomena of regression to the mean is of substantive as well as methodologic interest, as it may lead providers and patients to reach false conclusions about the efficacy of worthless treatments administered during a pain flare-up.

In addition to the sources of bias encountered in surveys, investigators conducting longitudinal studies need to be aware of additional sources of bias including loss to follow-up, missing data, and measurement biases introduced by repeated measurement. Missing data and losses to follow-up can substantially reduce sample size in a longitudinal survey, particularly if observations are made on more than two occasions. Such losses are generally not at random; thus, they may introduce an important source of bias. Measures that may be biased by repeated measurement or that may "drift" over time also present problems in longitudinal studies, as do unreliable measures.

There are a series of measurement biases that are particularly relevant in case-control studies. These potential biases have been summarized by Sackett (1979). Among the most important are *prevalence-incidence bias* or bias introduced by studying prevalent rather than incident cases when inference about onset risks is desired. In the case of chronic pain, this might lead to confusing factors affecting duration or recurrence with factors influencing onset risk. *Admission rate* (Berkson's) *bias* can occur in studies in which cases are identified in a treatment setting and the putative risk factor is associated with the probability of being treated in the facility where the cases are identified. This potential bias should be of concern to any investigator wishing to study etiologic factors for chronic pain among cases ascertained in a pain clinic because of the highly selected nature of persons utilizing such facilities. Research suggests that patients who seek treatment for a pain complaint have more intense and persistent pain, and more recent onset of their pain condition, than persons with the same pain complaint who have not recently sought treatment (Von Korff et al., 1991).

Recall bias of risk factors may occur if the presence of the pain condition leads to selective recall of events possibly associated with onset. Persons with a chronic pain problem may search for an explanation of their pain that may jog their memories about injuries or other possible risk factors that would be forgotten by a person without chronic pain. This potential bias might be overcome, in some instances, by using objective sources of information to assess risk factor history, such as the medical record or records maintained by an employer. *Family information bias* may occur in studies of familial aggregation of chronic pain. Persons with a pain condition may be more aware of the occurrence of similar conditions in relatives than persons without that pain condition (Sackett, 1979).

RELIABILITY AND GENERALIZABILITY

A recurring theme in the preceding material is that epidemiologic and survey research on chronic pain typically requires assessment of the characteristic level and pattern of pain expression over a period of time, rather than assessment of an individual's pain status only at a particular point in time. Determining a person's characteristic chronic pain status is made difficult by the large across time variability in individual pain status, and the diverse sources of variation in pain measurement.

Variation in pain measurement may be due to the measurement method such as the scale or questions used (see Jensen & Karoly, Chapter 9), the scaling of responses, the length of the recall period, method of prompting for condition or anatomical site, and the method of administration (e.g., personal interview, self-administered questionnaire, telephone interview). Additional variation may be due to the timing of measurement: the number of times pain status is measured, time of day, day of week, and timing of measurement in relation to milestones in the natural history of the condition or treatment seeking. And the context of measurement may also contribute to variation (e.g., work, home, health-care, or research settings). These different sources of variation lead to a series of questions about pain measurement in field research:

> What measurement methods and modes of administration are reliable and valid?

When and where should pain status be assessed?

On how many different occasions and at what intervals does pain status need to be assessed to obtain a stable estimate of an individual's characteristic chronic pain status?

Although a great deal of attention has been paid to the question of assessing the reliability and validity of alternative methods of assessing chronic pain, the remaining issues (mode of administration, timing and setting of administration, number of measurements and their spacing required to reliably determine characteristic pain status) have received less attention. To the extent these other issues have been addressed, they are typically considered one at a time, rather than assessing all sources of variation in pain measurement within a common conceptual and analytic framework.

Generalizability Theory

Generalizability theory (Shavelson & Webb, 1991), developed by Chronbach et al. (1972), provides a unified conceptual and methodological approach to considering multiple sources of variation in measurement (see also Rudy, Turk, & Brody, this volume). This approach may be particularly relevant to evaluation of pain measurement in epidemiologic and survey research. Llabre et al.. (1988), who applied generalizability theory to the evaluation of the measurement of blood pressure, have summarized key concepts:

In generalizability theory, a particular measurement is viewed as a sample from a larger universe of possible measurements that could have been taken for an individual. This universe is called the universe of admissible observations and is characterized by many dimensions called facets. A facet is a potential source of variability in the measurements. For example, in assessing blood pressure the facets may include the occasion when the measurement is taken, the device used, or the setting involved. Each specific instance of a facet is called a condition. Thus, the office, the home, or the workplace are specific conditions of a source of variability in blood pressure measurement, the setting facet. The mean of all measurements for one person across all conditions and all facets is the universe score for that person. In the context of generalizability theory, the question of the reliability of blood pressure measurements has to

do with the extent to which a single reading or a composite of multiple readings is representative of the universe score for a person. (p. 98)

For example, their application of generalizability theory to blood pressure measurement showed that, in the laboratory, only one reading was needed to generalize across the same day for the same instrument. At least one replication with each of two instruments was needed to generalize across instruments in the laboratory. Six or more readings were needed to generalize across the same day in work or home settings. To generalize across days, one or two readings from each of two days were required for systolic blood pressure and readings from each of three days were required for diastolic blood pressure.

The application of this type of factorial approach to evaluating methods of pain measurement in epidemiologic and survey research is likely to be more productive than trying to identify a single "best" pain measurement instrument for epidemiological or for survey research. Moreover, the question of the number and spacing of observations required to obtain a generalizable estimate of an individual's chronic pain status is an important issue for future research. It is possible that the number and spacing of observations may be more important in increasing the generalizability of assessment of chronic pain status than the specific method of measurement employed (Dworkin et. al., 1992).

VALIDITY

Several criteria are relevant to evaluation of the validity of a measure of chronic pain status for use in epidemiologic research including:

1. How strongly is the assessment associated with other concurrent measures of chronic pain status made by the same method (e.g., self-report)?
2. How strongly is the assessment associated with other concurrent indicators of chronic pain dysfunction made by other methods (e.g., pain behavior data from medical records, employment records, or observation)?
3. How strongly does the assessment predict chronic pain status at some future point in time as determined by the same method of

assessment, by the same method of data collection but a different method of assessment, and by a different method of data collection and assessment?

4. To what extent is the method of assessment able to differentiate subjects across the full spectrum of chronic pain dysfunction observed in general population samples, primary care samples and tertiary care (pain clinic) samples?

There is more known about the validity of self-report assessment of chronic pain status (as defined by criteria 1–4) than is known about the generalizability of chronic pain assessment (as defined in the preceding section). In work directly relevant to defining the spectrum of chronic pain in epidemiologic and survey research, Turk and Rudy (1987, 1988) have advanced multiaxial classification of chronic pain (see Turk & Rudy, this volume). They developed a taxonomy of chronic pain based on Multidimensional Pain Inventory (MPI) data (Kerns, Turk, & Rudy, 1985; see Kerns & Jacob, Chapter 16). They identified three pain profiles: adaptive coping, interpersonal distress, and dysfunctional chronic pain. Dysfunctional chronic pain is a profile of severe pain, functional disability, psychological impairment, and low perceived life control. They, and others, have shown that MPI data are reliable and have concurrent validity in classifying pain clinic patients as dysfunctional or not. The assessment method has been shown to have concurrent validity for several different anatomical pain sites including back pain, headache, and temporomandibular disorder pain.

Using a different set of items to assess pain dysfunction, but drawing on Turk and Rudy's concepts of dysfunctional chronic pain, Von Korff et al. (1990) evaluated the validity of grading chronic pain status in a general population sample. In this research, dysfunctional chronic pain was defined as severe and persistent pain accompanied by 7 or more days in the prior 6 months when the subject was unable to carry out usual activities due to pain. They found that 2.7% of the population sample and 15.7% of a sample of persons from the same population seeking treatment for temporomandibular disorder (TMD) pain met these criteria for dysfunctional chronic pain. In both samples, dysfunctional chronic pain was associated with psychological impairment, unfavor-

able self-assessment of global health status, and frequent use of health-care visits and pain medications as assessed by computerized health-care data. The predictive validity of the graded classification of dysfunctional chronic pain was also assessed among the TMD pain patients (Von Korff & Dworkin, 1989). Among patients meeting criteria for dysfunctional chronic pain at baseline, 42.3% also met criteria again 1 year later. In contrast, 11.8% of patients with severe and persistent pain at baseline, and 5.2% of patients with recurrent pain at baseline, met study criteria for dysfunctional chronic pain 1 year later.

As part of the development of study measures for the Medical Outcomes Survey, Sherbourne (1992) evaluated the concurrent validity of a global pain assessment scale whose items were consistent with Turk and Rudy's construct of dysfunctional chronic pain. She reported high internal consistency (alpha = 0.83). The scale was strongly associated ($r > 0.50$) with concurrent measures of physical functioning, physical role limitations, self-rated health status, and health distress. It was moderately associated ($r > 0.30$) with concurrent measures of emotional role limitations, sleep disturbance, cognitive functioning, psychological distress and well-being, and resistance to illness.

In primary care samples of back pain, headache and TMD pain patients, Von Korff, Ormel, Keefe, and Dworkin (in press) used a method analogous to Guttman scaling to develop an approach to graded classification of dysfunctional chronic pain. The graded classification of chronic pain was based on items measuring characteristic pain intensity, interference with usual activities, family and social activities, work activities, and disability days due to pain. Evaluation of concurrent validity found that the graded classification of chronic pain dysfunction showed a strong and monotonically increasing relationship with unemployment rate, a Pain Impact Scale score, depression, unfavorable ratings of health status, frequent use of narcotic analgesics in the prior month, and frequent pain-related doctors visits. Applying the same criteria for grading chronic pain dysfunction to the population sample employed in earlier research (see above) and followed up 3 years later, they found that chronic pain dysfunction at baseline strongly predicted chronic pain status at 3 year follow-up.

These results provide strong support for the validity of Turk and Rudy's (1987) construct of dysfunctional chronic pain in pain clinic, primary care, and general population samples. Available data suggest that the construct can be applied to different anatomically defined pain conditions, that it has concurrent and predictive validity across several different methods of assessment, and that measures of chronic pain dysfunction are associated with important psychological and behavioral correlates of chronic pain assessed by self-report and by medical records data.

BRIEF MEASURES OF CHRONIC PAIN DYSFUNCTION

This section provides the items, response scales, and scoring rules for three brief methods of assessing dysfunctional chronic pain.

The items for a brief screening version of the MPI (Kerns et al., 1985) are presented in Table 22.1A.* Items for the Medical Outcomes Survey-Pain Index (MOS-PI) developed by Sherbourne (1992) are provided in Table 22.2. Eight of the 12 items were adapted from items in the Wisconsin Brief Pain Questionnaire (Daut, Cleeland, & Flanery, 1983). Patients not reporting pain in the prior 4 weeks are skipped out of the remaining items. Methods of scoring the MOS-PI are described elsewhere (Sherbourne, 1992). Items for grading chronic pain status (GCPS) are provided in Table 22.3A. The pain intensity items in this scale were formatted to permit administration by personal interview, by telephone interview, or by self-administration. The average of the three pain intensity items is used to measure characteristic pain intensity (Dworkin et al., 1990). The activity limitation days item and interference with usual activities rating item were drawn from prior epidemiologic research reported by Von Korff et al. (1988). The two interference items rating change in social and in work activities were adapted from the MPI (Kerns et al., 1985). An overall disability score is calculated from the three interference items

*The items for this scale were provided for this chapter by Thomas Rudy, who also provided information on cut-points, sensitivity, and specificity of the scale for identifying dysfunctional chronic pain patients as defined by the full set of MPI items (see Table 22.1B).

TABLE 22.1A. Screening Questions for Dysfunctional Chronic Pain from the Multidimensional Pain Inventory

1. Rate your level of pain at the present moment.

					VERY INTENSE	
NO PAIN					PAIN	
0	1	2	3	4	5	6

2. How much has your pain changed the amount of satisfaction or enjoyment you get from taking part in social and recreational activities?

					EXTREME	
NO CHANGE					CHANGE	
0	1	2	3	4	5	6

3. During the past week how tense or anxious have you been?

NOT AT ALL					EXTREMELY	
0	1	2	3	4	5	6

4. How much has pain changed your ability to take part in recreational and other social activities?

					EXTREME	
NO CHANGE					CHANGE	
0	1	2	3	4	5	6

5. During the past week how well do you feel you've been able to deal with your problems?

					EXTREMELY	
NOT AT ALL					WELL	
0	1	2	3	4	5	6

6. On the average, how severe has your pain been during the past week?

					EXTREMELY	
NOT AT ALL					SEVERE	
0	1	2	3	4	5	6

7. During the past week, how successful were you in coping with stressful situations in your life?

NOT AT ALL					EXTREMELY	
SUCCESSFUL					SUCCESSFUL	
0	1	2	3	4	5	6

8. During the *past week,* how irritable have you been?

NOT AT ALL						
IRRITABLE					EXTREMELY	
0	1	2	3	4	5	6.

Note: From Kerns, Turk, and Rudy (1985).

and the activity limitation days item. Classification criteria for grading chronic pain status are provided in Table 22.3B. The classification criteria were based on the results of item response analyses indicating that the intensity and interference items formed a hierarchical (Guttman) scale (Von Korff et al., in press). The cut-points for the scoring were chosen both on the bases of prior empirical research

TABLE 22.1B. Scoring Rules for Identifying Dysfunction Chronic Pain with a Screening Version of the Multidimensional Pain Inventory

Pain Severity (PS) = Q1 + Q6
Interference (I) = Q2 + Q4
Life Control (LC) = Q5 + Q7
Affective Distress (AD) = Q3 + Q8

Based on analysis of 1,000 pain clinic cases classified as dysfunctional or not based on application of the multivariate classification algorithm to the full set of MPI items, the following scoring rules were recommended (Rudy, personal communication):

1. Classify each scale as indicating a dysfunctional response if the following criteria are met: PS> = 9; I> = 10; LC< =6; AD > = 8.
2. To maximize the sensitivity of screening (95%) while maintaining acceptable specificity (69%), classify the subject as dysfunctional if two or more of the scales yield a dysfunctional score.
3. For approximately equal sensitivity (84%) and specificity (82%), classify the subject as dysfunctional if Pain Severity (PS) *or* Interference (I) yield a dysfunctional score *AND* Life ControL (LC) *OR* Affective Distress (AD) yield a dysfunctional score.

and to facilitate grading chronic pain status of primary care patients by the clinician during the initial visit.

If any of these scales were used in a prevalence survey, it would be necessary to determine whether a subject had a pain problem before the detailed questions could be asked. Two approaches to this problem have been used in prior research. One is to ask a general question about whether a pain problem has been present in the reference period of interest. The MOS-PI exemplifies this approach. A similar approach has been used by Crook, Rideout, and Browne (1984). A second approach is to ask about anatomically defined pain conditions. The latter approach has been used by Von Korff et al. (1988) and by Sternbach (1986) for multiple pain sites, and by all epidemiologic surveys concerning a single anatomically defined pain condition. Asking a filter question about pain at a specific anatomical site yields substantially higher reporting rates than a general question about pain without reference to anatomical site. However, in research in which filter questions are asked about multiple anatomical sites, provision needs to be made for asking follow-up questions for each pain site elicited, or for having the subject chose a single

"worst" pain condition. When a 6-month reference period is used with filter questions covering multiple pain sites, at least one-third of an adult sample can be expected to report multiple pain conditions (Dworkin et al., 1990).

Review of the three brief scales indicate many similarities and some differences. All three ask questions about characteristic pain intensity (pain right now, average pain, and/or worst pain). All three scales include items concerning pain-related interference with activities (pain-related activity limitation days and/or ratings of interference with activities). The MPI Short Scale and the MOS-PI also include items concerning the psychological effects of pain. The GCPS scale did not include items about psychological impacts, but it has been shown to strongly predict psychological impairment (Von Korff et al., in press). It is likely that all three scales are moderately to strongly correlated, and that all three would classify similar patients as dysfunctional.

Given the similarities among the three scales, what are the advantages and disadvantages of each? The MPI has been used extensively in pain clinic populations and provides multidimensional information about pain status. A researcher using MPI scales in epidemiologic work would be able to determine the extent to which cases were as severe as dysfunctional pain clinic cases. There are also site-specific normative data available for the MPI. Disadvantages of this scale are that it has not been evaluated in general population or primary care samples. Longer term prognostic data for the MPI are not yet reported.

The MOS-PI is part of a larger assessment battery that assesses a number of aspects of functioning and well-being. Because it briefly covers a large number of areas using items that have generally been found to predict health outcomes and behaviors, the MOS is becoming widely adopted in health services research applications. Normative data are available for general medical patients, but population, pain clinic, and site-specific normative data are not available. The short- or long-term prognostic value of the MOS-PI has not yet been reported.

The items used to grade chronic pain status have been evaluated in a large population survey with a 3-year follow-up and in large samples of primary care pain patients. It has

TABLE 22.2. Medical Outcomes Survey Pain Index

1. Did you experience any bodily pain in the past 4 weeks?	No (SKIP OUT)	1
	Yes	2
2. During the *past 4 weeks*, how often have you had pain or discomfort?	Once or twice	1
	A few times	2
	Fairly often	3
	Very often	4
	Every day or almost every day	5
3. When you had pain during the *past 4 weeks*, how long did it usually last?	A few minutes	1
	Several minutes to an hour	2
	Several hours	3
	A day or two	4
	More than two days	5

4. During the *past 4 weeks*, how much did pain interfere with the following things?

	NOT AT ALL	A LITTLE BIT	MODERATELY	QUITE A BIT	EXTREMELY
a. Your mood	1	2	3	4	5
b. Your ability to walk or move about	1	2	3	4	5
c. Your normal work (including both work outside the home and housework)	1	2	3	4	5
d. Your recreational activities	1	2	3	4	5
e. Your enjoyment of life	1	2	3	4	5

5. During the *past 4 weeks*, how many days did pain interfere with the things you usually do? (Your answer may range from 00 to 28 days)   Number of days

—— ——

6. Please circle the one number that best describes your pain on the *average* over the past 4 weeks.

PAIN AS BAD
AS YOU CAN
NO PAIN   IMAGINE
1 2 3 4 5 6 7 8 9 10 11 12 13 14 15 16 17 18 19 20

7. Please circle the one number that best describes your pain *at its worst* over the past 4 weeks.

PAIN AS BAD
AS YOU CAN
NO PAIN   IMAGINE
1 2 3 4 5 6 7 8 9 10 11 12 13 14 15 16 17 18 19 20

Note: From Sherbourne (1992). Copyright 1992 RAND. Reprinted by permission.

not yet been evaluated in a pain clinic population. Its prognostic value at 3-year follow-up has been reported for a general population sample. Site-specific normative data have been reported for primary-care back pain, headache, and TMD pain patients. The questions and response scoring were designed to be suitable for administration as a paper and pencil questionnaire, by personal interview, or by telephone interview. The scale could be used to provide a continuous measure of pain dysfunction, but its intended use is grading the level of pain dysfunction into ordered categories. The hierarchical criteria for grading chronic pain

status are simple, easy to communicate, and may be replicable using other measures of pain intensity and interference.

In the absence of research comparing the measurement properties of these three brief measures of pain dysfunction, it would be reasonable to assume that they have roughly equal reliability and validity. Each of the measures has strengths and weaknesses that need to be considered in deciding on an approach to measuring the severity of pain dysfunction in epidemiologic and survey research. The organizing construct of chronic dysfunctional pain appears to provide a useful approach to the

TABLE 22.3A. Questions for a Graded Classification of Chronic Pain

1. How would you rate your [ANATOMICAL SITE] pain on a 0 to 10 scale at the present time, that is right now, where 0 is "no pain" and 10 is "pain as bad as could be"?

									PAIN AS BAD
NO PAIN									COULD BE
0	1	2	3	4	5	6	7	8	9	10

2. In the past 6 months, how intense was your worst pain rated on a 0 to 10 scale where 0 is "no pain" and 10 is "pain as bad as could be"?

									PAIN AS BAD
NO PAIN									COULD BE
0	1	2	3	4	5	6	7	8	9	10

3. In the past 6 months, on the average, how intense was your pain rated on a 0 to 10 scale where 0 is "no pain" and 10 is "pain as bad as could be"? [That is, your usual pain at times you were experiencing pain.]

									PAIN AS BAD
NO PAIN									COULD BE
0	1	2	3	4	5	6	7	8	9	10

4. About how many days in the past 6 months have you been kept from your usual activities (work, school or housework) because of [ANATOMICAL SITE] pain?

DISABILITY DAYS

_____ _____ _____

5. In the past 6 months, how much has [ANATOMICAL SITE] pain interfered with your daily activities rated on a 0 to 10 scale where 0 is "no interference" and 10 is "unable to carry on any activities"?

									UNABLE TO
									CARRY ON ANY
NO INTERFERENCE									ACTIVITIES
0	1	2	3	4	5	6	7	8	9	10

6. In the past 6 months, how much as [ANATOMICAL SITE] pain changed your ability to take part in recreational, social and family activities where 0 is "no change" and 10 is "extreme change"?

									EXTREME
NO CHANGE									CHANGE
0	1	2	3	4	5	6	7	8	9	10

7. In the past 6 months, how much has [ANATOMICAL SITE] pain changed your ability to work (including housework) where 0 is "no change" and 10 is "extreme change"?

									EXTREME
NO CHANGE									CHANGE
0	1	2	3	4	5	6	7	8	9	10

Note: Adapted from Dworkin et al. (1990), Von Korff et al. (1988), and Kerns et al. (1985).

TABLE 22.3B. Scoring Rules and Classification Criteria for Grading Chronic Pain Status

Scoring

Characteristic pain intensity is a 0 to 100 score derived from questions 1–3:

Mean (pain right now, worst pain, average pain) × 10

Disability score is a 0 to 100 score derived from questions 5–7:

Mean (daily activities, social activities, work activities) × 10

Disability points

Add the indicated points for disability days (Question 4) and for disability score.

Disability days (0–180)		Disability Score (0–100)	
0–6 days	0 points	0–29	0 points
7–14 days	1 point	30–49	1 point
15–30 days	2 points	50–69	2 points
31 + days	3 points	70 +	3 points

Classification

Pain free	
Grade 0	No pain problem (prior 6 months)
Low disability	
Grade 1	Characteristic pain intensity
Low intensity	less than 50, and less than 3 disability points
Grade II	Characteristic pain intensity
High intensity	of 50 or greater, and less than 3 disability points
High disability	
Grade III	3–4 disability points,
Moderately limiting	regardless of characteristic pain intensity
Grade IV	5–6 disability points
Severly limiting	regardless of characteristic pain intensity

assessment of severity that yields brief and reliable measures that perform well in both concurrent and prospective prediction, and that yield valid and reliable measurement in general population, primary care, and pain clinic samples.

SUMMARY

This review has considered issues of pain measurement in epidemiologic and survey research within the context of the major objectives, perspectives, and methodologic approaches of epidemiology. Measurement in epidemiology, like other scientific disciplines, cannot be divorced from (1) the research objectives, (2) the theoretical perspectives brought to bear in accomplishing those objectives, and (3) the study designs that are employed in carrying out the research. Applying the dynamic, ecologic and population perspectives of epidemiology to the problems of pain measurement provides a useful framework for considering pain assessment in epidemiologic research. For example, the dynamic (or change across time) perspective of epidemiology motivates the question of whether chronic pain assessment can be improved more readily by identifying better pain measures or by measuring pain status with measures already in use but on more than a single occasion. The population perspective suggests that understanding the spectrum of chronic pain, both across persons and within the same individual across time, may provide useful insights into pain mechanisms and pain control.

Basic epidemiologic measures of disease expression that determine prevalence rates (incidence rates, episode duration, and recurrence rates) call attention to the different ways in which two groups can come to differ in the prevalence of a pain condition. The simple distinction between incidence, duration, and recurrence points to the need for research that differentiates factors affecting onset rates from factors that influence episode duration or relapse rates. The methods of epidemiology, and epidemiologic approaches to measurement, provide bases for identifying how risk factors produce such differences in morbidity rates.

This review paid special attention to brief measures of dysfunctional chronic pain. Brief methods of measuring pain dysfunction are available that could substantially improve epidemiologic data on the distribution of chronic pain dysfunction in general population samples. These measures of pain dysfunction, when applied in longitudinal research, would provide essential new information regarding the natural history of chronic pain, and yield improved bases for identifying factors associated with the development and the maintenance of chronic pain dysfunction. In the absence of adequate empirical data on the distribution and natural history of chronic pain dysfunction in representative samples (population and primary care), both clinical and epidemiologic research concerning the causes and control of chronic pain dysfunction are handi-

capped. There is a pressing need for both epidemiologists and clinical pain researchers to begin to apply the perspectives and methods of epidemiology to the study of chronic pain and associated dysfunction.

Acknowledgment. This work was supported by grants from the Agency for Health Care Policy and Research R01 HS06168 and the National Institute of Dental Research P01 DE08773.

REFERENCES

Abramson, J.H. (1985). Cross-sectional studies. In W.W. Holland, R. Detels, & G. Knox (Eds.), *The Oxford textbook of public health; Vol. 3. Investigative methods in public health* (pp. 89–100). Oxford: Oxford University Press.

Altman, D.G. (1986). A framework for evaluating community-based heart disease prevention programs. *Social Science and Medicine, 22,* 479–487.

Bishop, Y.M.M., Fienberg, S.E., & Holland, P.W. (1978). Discrete multivariate analysis: Theory and practice. Cambridge, MA: MIT Press.

Bradburn, N.M., Rips, L.J., & Shevell, S.K. (1987). Answering autobiographical questions: The impact of memory and influence on surveys. *Science, 236,* 157–161.

Brewlow, N.E., & Day, N.E. (1980). *Statistical methods in cancer research: Vol. 1. The analysis of case-control studies.* Lyon: International Agency for Research on Cancer.

Cannel, C.F. (1977). A summary of research studies of interviewing methodology, 1959–1970. In *Vital and health statistics: Series 2. Data evaluation and methods research.* No. 69. DHEW publication (HRA) 77-1343, Washington DC: U.S. Government Printing Office.

Cobb, S., Miller, M., & Wald, N. (1959). On the estimation of the incubation period in malignant disease. *Journal of Chronic Disease, 9,* 385–393.

Cochran, W.G. (1977). *Sampling techniques* (3rd ed.) New York: Wiley.

Converse, P.E., & Traugott, M.W. (1986). Assessing the accuracy of polls and surveys. *Science, 234,* 1094–1098.

Cook, N.R., & Ware, J.H. (1983). Design and analysis methods for longitudinal research. *Annual Reviews of Public Health, 4,* 1–23.

Cox, D.R., & Oakes, D. (1984). *Analysis of survival data.* London: Chapman & Hill.

Crook, J., Rideout, E., & Browne, G. (1984). The prevalence of pain complaints in a general population. *Pain, 18,* 299–314.

Daut, R.L., Cleeland, C.S., & Flannery, R.C. (1983). Development of the Wisconsin Brief Pain Questionnaire to assess pain in cancer and other diseases. *Pain, 17,* 197–210.

Drury, T.F. (1989). Problems of meaning and measurement in cross-sectional interview surveys of chronic pain in the adult population. In C.R. Chapman & J.D. Loeser (Eds.), *Advances in pain research and therapy: Vol. 12. Issues in pain management* (pp. 498–518). New York: Raven Press.

Dworkin, S.F., Von Korff, M., & Le Resche, L. (1990). Multiple pains and psychiatric disturbance: An epidemiologic investigation. *Archives of General Psychiatry, 47,* 239–244.

Dworkin, S.F., Von Korff, M., & Le Resche, L. (1992). Epidemiologic studies of chronic pain: A dynamic-ecologic perspective. *Annals of Behavioral Medicine, 14,* 13–11.

Dworkin, S.F., Von Korff, M., Le Resche, L., & Truelove, E. (1988). Epidemiology of temporomandibular disorders. I. Initial clinical and self-report findings. In R. Dubner, G.F. Gebhart, & M.R. Bond (Eds.), *Proceedings of the Vth World Congress on Pain* (pp. 499–505). Amsterdam: Elsevier.

Eaton, W.W., & Kessler, L.G. (1985). *Epidemiologic field methods in psychiatry: The NIHM epidemiologic catchment area program.* Orlando: Academic Press.

Farquhar, J.W. (1978). The community-based model or life style intervention trials. *American Journal of Epidemiology, 108,* 103–111.

Feinlab, & Detels (1985). Cohort studies. In W.W. Holland, R. Detels, & G. Knox (Eds.), *The Oxford textbook of public health: Vol. 3. Investigative methods in public health* (pp. 101–112). Oxford: Oxford University Press.

Feinstein, A.R. (1979). Methodologic problems and standards in case-control research. *Journal of Chronic Diseases, 32,* 35–41.

Graham, J.W., Collins, L.M., Wugalter, S.E., Chung, N.K., & Hansen, W.B. (1991). Modeling transitions in latent stage-sequential processes: A substance use prevention example. *Journal of Consulting and Clinical Psychology, 59,* 48–57.

Greenberg, R.S., & Ibrahim, M.A. (1985). The case-control study. In W.W. Holland, R. Detels, & G. Knox (Eds.), *The Oxford textbook of public health: Vol. 3. Investigative methods in public health* (pp. 123–143). Oxford: Oxford University Press.

Gross, A.J., & Clark, V.A. (1975). *Survival distributions: Reliability applications in the biomedical sciences.* New York: Wiley.

Hill, A.B. (1971). *Principles of medical statistics.* New York: Oxford University Press.

Hopkins, P.N., & Williams, R.R. (1986). Identification and relative weight of cardiovascular risk factors. *Cardiology Clinics, 4,* 3–31.

Kabfleisch, J.D., & Prentice, R.L. (1980). *The statistical analysis of failure time data.* New York: Wiley.

Kerns, R.D., Turk, D.C., & Rudy, T.E. (1985). The West Haven–Yale Multidimensional Pain Inventory (WHYMPI). *Pain, 23,* 345–356.

Kish, L. (1965). *Survey sampling.* New York: Wiley.

Kleinbaum, D.G., Kupper, L.L., & Morgenstern, H. (1982).22 Epidemiologic research: Principles and quantitative methods. California: Lifetime Learning Publications.

Lilienfeld, A.M., & Lilienfeld, D.E. (1980). *Foundations of epidemiology* (2nd ed.). New York: Oxford University Press.

Llabre, M.M., Ironson, G.H., Spitzer, S.B., Gellman, M.D., Weidler, D.J., & Schneiderman, N. (1988). How many blood pressure measurements are enough? An application of generalizability theory to the study of blood pressure measurement. *Psychophysiology, 25,* 97–106.

MacMahon, B., & Pugh, T.F. (1970). *Epidemiology: Principles and methods.* Boston: Little, Brow.

Madow, W.G. (1973). Net differences in interview data on chronic conditions and information derived from medical records. In *Vital and health statistics: Series 2. Data evaluation and methods research.* No. 57. DHEW publication (HSM) 73-1331, Washington, DC: U.S. Government Printing Office.

Manton, K.G., & Stallard, E. (1988). *Chronic disease modeling: Measurement and evaluation of the risks of chronic disease processes.* New York: Oxford University Press.

Means, B., Nigam, A., Zarrow, M., Loftus, E.F., & Donaldson, M.S. (1989). Autobiographical memory for health-related events. *Vital and health statistics, Series 6. Cognitive and survey measurement,* Washington, DC: National Center for Health Statistics, PHS 89-1077.

Meinert, C.L. (1986). *Clinical trials: Design, conduct and analysis.* New York: Oxford University Press.

Morgensten, H. (1982). Uses of ecologic analysis in epidemiologic research. American Journal of Public Health, 72, 1336–1344.

Morris, J.N. (1975). *Uses of epidemiology* (3rd ed.). Edinburgh: Churchill Livingstone.

National Institutes of Health, Consensus Development Conference (1986). The integrated approach to the management of pain. NIH Consensus Development Conference Statement, Vol. 6(3). Washington, DC: U.S. Government Printing Office.

Nessleroade, J.R., & Baltes, P.B. (1979). *Longitudinal research in the study of behavior and development.* New York: Academic Press.

Osterweis, M., Kleinman, A., & Mechanic, D. (1987). *Pain and disability: Clinical, behavioral and public policy perspectives.* Washington, DC: National Academy Press.

Rose, G.A., Blackburn, H., Gillum, R.F., & Prineas, R.J. (1982). *Cardiovascular survey methods.* Geneva: World Health Organization.

Sackett, D.L. (1979). Bias in analytic research. *Journal of Chronic Diseases, 32,* 51–63.

Schlesselman, J.J. (1982). *Case-control studies: Design, conduct, and analysis.* New York: Oxford University Press.

Shavelson, R.J., & Webb, N.M. (1991). *Generalizability theory: A primer.* Newbury Park, CA: Sage.

Sherpard, D.S., & Neutra, R. (1977). A pitfall in sampling medical visits. *American Journal of Public Health, 67,* 743–750.

Sherbourne, C.D. (1992). Pain measures. In A. L. Steward & J.E. Ware (Eds.), *Measuring functioning and well-being: The medical outcomes study approach* (pp. 220–234). Durham, NC: Duke University Press.

Simon, G., & Von Korff, M. (in press). Re-evaluation of secular trends in depression rates. *American Journal of Epidemiology.*

Singer, J.D., & Willett, J.B. (in press). Modeling the days of our lives: Applying survival analysis in psychological research. *Psychological Bulletin.*

Sternbach, R.A. (1986). Survey of pain in the United States: The Nuprin Pain Report. *Clinical Journal of Pain, 2,* 49–53._

Turk, D.C., & Rudy, T.E. (1987). Toward a comprehensive assessment of chronic pain patients. *Behavior Research and Therapy, 4,* 37–249.

Turk, D.C., & Rudy, T.E. (1988). Toward an empirically derived taxonomy of chronic pain patients: Integration of psychological assessment data. *Journal of Consulting and Clinical Psychology, 56,* 233–238.

Von Korff, M. (1991). *Memory for pain in epidemiologic research: Effects of depression on back pain recall*. Proceedings of the 12th annual meeting of the Society of Behavioral Medicine. Abstract C78, p. 142.

Von Korff, M., & Dworkin, S. (1989). Problems in measuring pain by survey: the classification of chronic pain in field research. in Chapman CR & Loeser JD (Eds.) *Advances in pain research and therapy, Volume 12: Issues in pain management* (pp. 519–533). New York: Raven Press.

Von Korff, M., Dworkin, S., & Le Resche, L. (1990). Graded chronic pain status: An epidemiologic evaluation. *Pain, 40,* 279–291.

Von Korff, M., Dworkin, S., Le Resche, L., & Kruger, A. (1988). An epidemiologic comparison of pain complaints. *Pain, 32,* 173–183.

Von Korff, M., Ormel, J., Keefe, F., & Dowrkin, S.F. (in press). Grading the severity of chronic pain. *Pain*.

Von Korff, M., & Parker, R.D. (1980). The dynamics of the prevalence of chronic episodic disease. *Journal of Chronic Disease, 33,* 79–85.

Von Korff, M., Wagner, E.H., Dworkin, S.F., & Saunders, K.W. (1991). Chronic pain and use of ambulatory health care. *Psychosomatic Medicine, 53,* 61–79.

Ware, J.H. (1985). Linear models for the analysis of longitudinal data. *American Statistician, 39,* 95–101.

Whitney, C.W., & Von Korff, M. (in press). Magnitude of regression to the mean in before-after treatment comparisons of chronic pain. *Pain*.

Chapter 23

Classification Logic and Strategies in Chronic Pain

DENNIS C. TURK, PhD
THOMAS E. RUDY, PhD

A major factor that has inhibited the advancement of knowledge and treatment of chronic pain has been the absence of an accepted classification of chronic pain syndromes that is used on a systematic basis. This has resulted in the inability of investigators as well as practitioners to compare observations and results of research. Bonica (1979) referred to this state of affairs as a "tower of Babel."

In order to identify target groups, to conduct research, to prescribe treatment, to evaluate treatment efficacy, and for policy and decision-making, it is essential that some consensually validated criteria are used to describe groups of individuals who share a common set of relevant attributes. The primary purpose of classification is to describe the relationships of constituent individuals based upon their equivalence along a set of basic dimensions that represent a model about how a particular domain is structured. An infinite number of classification systems can be developed depending upon the rationale about common factors and the variables believed to discriminate among individuals.

There are two primary strategies for classification, theoretical and empirical, each with different underlying premises. The theoretical approach involves tests of a priori theoretical formulations; in contrast the empirical approach is inductive and seeks to identify naturally co-occurring sets of variables that characterize subgroups. Which of the two approaches is adopted will lead to quite different classification systems.

THEORETICAL CLASSIFICATION

A deductively derived taxonomy begins with a theoretically based statement about how individuals should differ and subsequently be categorized. Classification of diseases are usually based on a preconceived combination of characteristics (e.g., symptoms, signs, test results), with no single characteristics being both necessary and sufficient for every member of the category, yet the group as a whole possesses a certain unity (Baron & Fraser, 1968). Most classification systems used in medicine (e.g., ICD-9) are based on the consensus of a group of professionals and in that sense reflect the elimination of certain diagnostic features on which agreement could not be obtained. In theoretical classifications, preconceived categories are developed and individuals are "forced" into the most appropriate one even if not all characteristics defining the category are present. Thus, in contrast to empirical classification, theoretically based classification systems do not include the explicit formulation of the mathematical rules that should exist among the variables used in order to assign a case to a specific category.

EMPIRICAL CLASSIFICATION

An alternative approach to classification is predicated on empirical procedures. The inductive approach begins with ordering and arranging objects or events into groups or sets based on some criteria. Individual elements (e.g., symptoms, demographics) are proposed as the basis for grouping. Those who advocate the use of empirically derived taxonomies maintain that the relationships of contiguity and similarity should be sought by quantitative analysis of similarities among individuals. A number of empirical methods are available to identify categories statistically (e.g., cluster analysis) that share relationships derived directly from data versus hypothesized relationships, as is the case with deductive systems. Explicit mathematically based classification rules can then be developed from the results of identification analyses so that additional cases can be assigned to specific categories on an objective basis.

Although quantification, replication, and objectivity are the hallmarks of the inductive approach, it is important to acknowledge that because all relevant factors cannot be measured by a single classification system, the use of an inductive approach is dependent upon what the investigator chooses to measure. Thus, in practice, the inductive approach to classification is not a totally objective process that is completely atheoretical.

UNIDIMENSIONAL VERSUS MULTIDIMENSIONAL STRATEGIES

Regardless of whether a theoretical/deductive or empirical/inductive approach to classification is adopted, the nature of the information

that will be used in assigning an individual to a diagnosis or subgroup must be determined. Traditionally, the medical approach, as characterized by the ICD-9, uses signs and symptoms of physical pathology to decide upon a patient's diagnosis.

Perhaps the most commonly used classification dimensions in chronic pain has been to simply distinguish between somatogenic and psychogenic etiology. Simply put, a range of physical examination, diagnostic imaging, and laboratory tests are performed in an attempt to identify the physical basis for the report of pain. If none is found that can adequately explain the etiology and extent of the reported pain, then the symptoms, by exclusion, are viewed as being psychological in origin. In this case, a dichotomous *unidimensional* system is used, that is, physical pathology present or absent, to classify patients.

Variations on the dichotomous somatogenic versus psychogenic classification have been suggested. For example, Portenoy (1989) proposed that three primary categories of pain be used, namely, nociceptive, neuropathic, and psychogenic. Fricton (1982) proposed the use of five categories, namely, myofascial, rheumatic, causalgic, neurologic, or vascular. In the latter case patients are assigned to one of five rather than two or three categories; however, the decision regarding classification still is based on a single dimension—etiology of the pain.

Other investigators of chronic pain have suggested that patients be classified on the basis of a variety of different dimensions. For example, time course (acute, recurrent acute, chronic) or severity of pain (0–10 point scale with 0 = no pain and 10 = the worst pain can imagine). In these classifications, as those reviewed above, the system being used is still unidimensional. That is, regardless of the scale's level of measurement, nominal, ordinal, or interval, the constructs being operationalized are still one-dimensional.

An alternative to the unidimensional approaches is a *multidimensional* approach where a number of relevant dimensions serve as the basis for developing the classification system and for assigning patients to a particular subgroup. For example, the classification developed by the International Association for Pain (IASP) (Merskey, 1986) consists of a multidimensional system in which pain patients are rated on five separate axes, four of which are categorical (body region, system involved, etiology, temporal characteristics of pain and pattern of occurrence) and one that combines multidimensional features (intensity and duration of symptoms).

It is important to emphasize that the use of unidimensional or multidimensional strategies is independent of whether the classification approach is theoretical or empirical. That is, as described below, empirical approaches can be used to identify subgroups based on a single dimension (e.g., personality characteristics) or multiple dimensions (e.g., the statistical integrations of physical, psychosocial, and behavioral factors). Additionally, integrating multidimensional information need not be a purely deductive system, but can be designed on a theoretical basis rather an empirical one. Thus, two primary, independent concepts are relevant in classification. First, the logic of classification, deductive or inductive, and second, the nature of information used to create the classification system, which is then used as the basis for assigning patients to a category or subgroup. Table 23.1 illustrates this point schematically displaying four cells and includes examples that are discussed throughout this chapter. This chapter will be organized around these two concepts, logical approach to classification and methods used to develop the classification system and, subsequently, the information that is used to assign patients to subgroups.

TABLE 23.1. A Typology of Pain Taxometric Approaches

	Unidimensional	Multidimensional
Theoretical/ deductive	ICD-9 Portenoy (1989) Fricton (1982) International Headache Society (Olesen, 1988)	IASP (Merskey, 1986) Brena & Koch (1975) Waddell & Main (1984)
Empirical/ inductive	MMPI (Bradley et al., 1978) SCL-90 (Butterworth & Deardorff, 1987) Ingram et al. (1990) Keefe et al. (1990)	Turk & Rudy (1987, 1988) Rudy et al. (1989)

CLASSIFICATION OF PATIENTS BASED ON PSYCHOLOGICAL CHARACTERISTICS

A number of studies have focused on empirically identifying patient subgroups based on psychological characteristics and psychopathology. Investigators have assumed that the most important patient differences will be associated with psychological distress and personality features. Consequently, the attempts to identify subgroups have tended to rely exclusively on the use of traditional psychological measures (e.g., MMPI, Symptom Checklist-90 [SCL-90]). Some have tried to use these profiles to predict response to treatment interventions, ranging from surgery to pain clinics (e.g., Butterworth & Deardorff, 1987; Jamison, Rock, & Parris, 1988; Shutty, DeGood, & Schwartz, 1986).

Classification Based on the Minnesota Multiphasic Personality Inventory (MMPI)

In perhaps the first attempt to identify differential psychological characteristics of chronic pain patients, Sternbach (1974) described four different subgroups based on MMPI profiles. He presented descriptive information on four common MMPI profiles frequently found among chronic pain patients, which he labels (1) hypochondriasis, (2) reactive depression, (3) somatization reaction, and (4) manipulative reaction.

Sternbach (1974) made some suggestions regarding treatment for the different MMPI subgroups he reported. For example, he suggested that males and females with the elevations on Hs, D, and Hy scales might be poor candidates for operant conditioning pain clinic treatment because they may find it difficult to shift their attention away from pain toward learning to live with their pain. Similarly, the male subgroup characterized by elevations on many clinical scales indicating high levels of psychopathology might benefit from psychiatric treatment rather than traditional pain clinic treatments. Although Sternbach's attempt to identify pain patient subgroups constituted a conceptual advance, the procedures used to derive MMPI profile types were not presented, nor were statistical tests reported that were designed to evaluate the classification accuracy of assiging individuals to one of the four patient subgroups.

In the first attempt to empirically identify homogeneous subgroups of chronic pain patients based on MMPI scores, Bradley, Prokop, Margolis, and Gentry (1978) used hierarchical clustering methods with two samples of chronic low back pain patients. Within their male sample, three MMPI profile subgroups were identified. One of these subgroups had a mean profile that resembled the "hypochondriasis" configuration. A second subgroup appeared to be considerably more pathological. A third subgroup had a mean profile that looked relatively normal. Cluster analyses on a second sample of patients yielded similar profiles, although, as described later in this chapter, these analyses cannot be considered a direct replication of the results obtain on the first sample of patients.

Bradley et al.'s (1978) results suggest that the "conversion V" profile, believed by many to characterize the majority of chronic pain patients, may actually be descriptive of only a relatively small group of patients. The robustness of the patient profiles identified by Bradley et al. has generally been supported in that other investigators using exploratory cluster analytic methods have found similar patient subgroups (Armentrout, Moore, Parker, Hewett, & Felz, 1982; Bernstein & Grabin, 1983; Bradley & Van der Heide, 1984; Hart, 1984; McCreary, 1985; McGill, Lawlis, Selby, Mooney, & McCoy, 1983; Moore, Armentrout, Parker, & Kivlahan, 1986).

Classification Based on the SCL-90

Recently, attempts have been made to identify subgroups of pain patients using another psychiatric instrument, the SCL-90 (Derogatis, 1977). The SCL-90 is a 90-item self-report checklist of physical or psychiatric symptoms. The SCL-90 includes the following subscales: Somatization, Obessionality, Interpersonal Sensitivity, Depression, Anxiety, Hostility, Phobic Anxiety, Paranoia, and Psychoticism. A Global Symptom Index, which is an average of all scores, also is computed. Each item is rated on a Likert scale ranging from O, "not at all," to 5, "extremely."

Schwartz and DeGood (1983) proposed three subgroups of chronic pain patients based on responses to the SCL-90. The proposed subgroups reflected three configurations or profiles: (1) patients showing extreme somatization scores with all other scales were very low ("Psychological Denial"), (2) patients with extreme elevations on all of the scales ("Psychologically Overwhelmed"), and (3) patients with moderate elevations on all of the scales ("Psychologically Adjusted"). Subgroups one and two were characterized as presenting illness behaviors with a less likely chance of benefiting from treatment, whereas subgroup three patients were characterized as having a good prognosis. Unfortunately, no empirical evidence was presented to substantiate these patient profiles.

Jamison et al. (1988) also identified three groups based on the analysis of SCL-90 scale scores. The subgroups identified, however, differed to some extent from those reported by Schwartz and DeGood (1983). The first group (20%) demonstrated high elevations on all on the subscales displaying the greatest amount of psychological distress. The second group (44%) showed elevations of one standard deviation above the mean on the Somatization, Obsessive-Compulsive, Depression, Anxiety (similar to the neurotic triad of MMPI) and Global Symptom Index, and the third group (35%) had elevations of one standard deviation above the mean only on the Somatization scale. No significant differences were shown among the groups for demographics or physical pathology measures. The authors acknowledge that these three groups may all differ by degrees on a single factor, "general emotional distress."

Butterworth and Deardorff (1987) identified three analogous subgroups when they cluster analyzed the SCL-90 scores of craniomandibular pain patients, and suggested that the SCL-90 might be useful for the early identification of patients in need of psychological treatment "adjunctive" to a physical medicine intervention. They speculate that the no-distress subgroup and a proportion of the moderately distressed subgroup might be expected to respond favorably to a purely biomedical intervention because the patients exhibited little life disruption in other areas of functioning. On the other hand, the severely distressed group appeared to have significant emotional contributions to pain and suffering that would not respond to unilateral intervention. The moderate and severe distress groups may be appropriate candidates for a multimodal treatment approach in which all of the dimensions of pain are targets for intervention.

Unfortunately, Butterworth and Deardorff (1987) do not provide any details as to what the psychological treatment should be for Groups two and three or how psychological treatments might differ for these two groups. The lack of specificity may be due to the fact that no research has been presented that provides any indications of the specific behaviors of these subgroups of patients. As was the case with the MMPI, these suggestions are speculations that would greatly benefit from demonstration of behavioral correlates of identified and proposed subgroups.

Classification Based on Cognitive Factors

Depression is quite prevalent among chronic pain patients. Several studies have demonstrated that cognitive appraisal seems to be particularly important in mediating the pain–depression association. For example, Smith, Aberger, Follick, and Ahern (1986) reported data suggesting that the level of cognitive distortion is reliably associated with the degree of disability reported by patients with chronic low back pain. And Rudy, Kerns, and Turk (1988) have demonstrated that cognitive factors appear to mediate the association between pain and depression. These results induced Ingram, Atkinson, Slater, Saccuzzo, and Garfin (1990) to examine whether subgroups of pain patients varied on the basis of cognitive patterns associated with depression. Specifically, they used the Automatic Thoughts Questionnaire (ATQ) (Hollon & Kendall, 1980) in an attempt to differentiate pain patients on the basis of the prevalence of positive and negative thoughts and distorted thinking.

The ATQ (Hollon & Kendall, 1980) consists of 30 self-referent negative statements (e.g., "I can't finish anything," "There's something wrong with me"). Subjects are asked to rate, on a 5-point scale, how frequently each thought, or a very similar thought, has occurred during the past week. To assess positive automatic thinking, the Positive Automatic Thoughts Questionnaire (Ingram & Wisnicki, 1988) was used. This later instrument was developed as a counterpart to the ATQ in order to measure the frequency of positive self-referent thoughts ("My future looks bright," "There's nothing to worry about"), and it is identical in format to the original ATQ.

Ingram et al. (1990) found no differences among pain groups in demographics, pain intensity, duration, orthopedic diagnosis, or disease severity; however, patients experiencing depression reported more maladaptive automatic thoughts than did nondepressed subjects. These authors suggest customizing treatment to patterns of maladaptive thinking. They propose that chronic pain patients who are depressed would be appropriate for cognitive-behavioral methods that focus on correcting cognitive distortions and on modifying negative automatic thinking with more adaptive positive thoughts. Alternatively, for patients who are not depressed, these results suggest that cognitive-behavioral approaches aimed primarily at identifying and correcting negative automatic thinking and cognitive distortions are less appropriate. As with subgroups based on the MMPI and SCL-90 reviewed above, to date there are no published findings that have examined how maladaptive cognitive processes may lead to differential treatment response.

CLASSIFICATION BASED ON PAIN BEHAVIORS

The empirical classification methods reviewed up to this point have been those that have attempted to classify chronic pain patients based on self-report data derived from traditional psychological measures that were not conceptually developed or standardized on chronic pain suffers. Recently, Keefe, Bradley, and Crisson (1990) have attempted to determine whether pain patients could be classified on the basis of specific behavioral response patterns—"pain behaviors," verbal and nonverbal communications of pain, distress, and suffering (see Keefe & Williams, Chapter 16). Keefe et al. (1990) identified four subgroups. They found that 19% of back pain patients show minimal pain behavior and reported no increase in pain during standardized physical tasks. They suggest the possibility that for this group of patients, the expression of pain behaviors may be controlled primarily by social or environmental contingencies such as social reinforcement or medication, and thus an intervention focusing on pain behaviors would be expected to have greatest effect for this group.

The three other subgroups identified by Keefe et al. (1990) demonstrated moderate to high levels on differing types of pain behaviors.

In contrast to operant pain behaviors present in the first subgroup, these patients appear to be displaying respondent pain behaviors that are likely to be elicited by nociceptive influences such as physical pathology. The authors suggest that these patients are likely to respond to physical activities and decreased nociceptive input and training in the use of pain-coping strategies. Keefe et al. (1990) propose that the nature of physical activities might be individualized to the types of pain behaviors emitted by the subgroups. For example, the subgroup of patients who demonstrate high levels of "guarded" movements might benefit from training in relaxation and body mechanics.

THE NEED FOR BROADER CONCEPTUALIZATIONS OF CHRONIC PAIN PATIENTS

Each of the unidimensional conceptualizations described above contains an element of chronic pain but none is sufficient to represent this complex phenomenon. Several recent national reports and commissions have emphasized the importance of viewing chronic pain as a comprehensive, multidimensional problem. Several quotations illustrate this important point.

> How an individual experiences and manifests pain depends on a complex interaction among numerous physiological, psychological, social, and cultural variables, as well as on past pain experiences and how the pain has been handled by the practitioners the patient consults. . . . The experience of pain is more than a simple sensory process. It is a complex perception involving higher levels of central nervous system, emotional states, and higher order mental processes. . . . people who experience pain, especially pain of long duration, tend to develop behavioral and psychological responses to their symptoms. It is not always possible to identify the causes of pain, how it is expressed, and its behavioral and psychological reactions and consequences. (Osterweis, Kleinman, & Mechanic, 1987, pp. 12–13)

> Pain is a complex experience, embracing physical, mental, social, and behavioral processes which compromises the quality of life of many individual. (USDHHS, 1987, p. xii)

> Chronic pain . . . is a more complex entity with additional social and psychological factors requiring a multidimensional approach to assess the person's report of pain. (USDHHS, 1987, p. xviii)

> The experts testified that pain can really best be defined as a description of an individual's experience encompassing physical, mental, social and behavioral processes, and all dimensions involved in the pain experience need to be evaluated to make a useful determination of whether or not an individual is incapacitated by pain. Pain behavior, including verbal reports of pain, thus becomes the means to make as objective an assessment as possible of an essentially subjective area. (USDHHS, 1987, p. 82)

If we accept that chronic pain is a complex, subjective phenomenon that is experienced uniquely by each individual, then knowledge of the patients' idiosyncratic appraisals of their plight, their unique experience of pain, and their coping resources (e.g., personal, financial, social support) become critical for optimal assessment, disability determination, and treatment planning (see DeGood & Shutty, Chapter 13, and Kerns & Jacob, Chapter 14). Patients' perceptions of their life circumstances will influence their communication with significant others including health care professionals. These sources of communication will influence how others respond to them and potentially the therapeutic modalities to which people with persistent pain are and have been exposed.

In many, if not all, chronic pain syndromes it has become apparent that simply identifying physical factors and arriving at a diagnosis and subsequently prescribing somatic treatments will not provide amelioration of symptoms for a significant number of patients (e.g., Osterweis et al., 1987). Those with same medical diagnosis and ostensibly the same level of physical pathology respond quite differently to the same treatment. As a result, there has been a growing awareness of and empirical support for the importance of psychological factors in reports of pain, suffering, and disability (e.g., Gallagher et al., 1989; Murphy, Sperr, & Sperr, 1986; Waddell, Main, Morris, Paola, & Gray, 1984; Vasudevan, Chapter 7, and Waddell & Turk, Chapter 2).

For example, Cairns, Mooney, and Crane (1982) provide evidence supporting the role of variables other than medical diagnoses and identified physical pathology in treatment outcome. They commented that in their study of heterogeneous samples of chronic pain patients, initial medical diagnosis did not have prognostic value. That is, tissue pathology was not predictive of improvement of either functional activity or return to work. Similarly,

Rudy, Turk, Zaki, and Curtin (1989) noted that, at least in temporomandibular disorders (TMD), commonly used oral dysfunctional and structural abnormality assessments did not discriminate among groups of patients with different psychosocial and behavioral characteristics. Moreover, Flor and Turk (1988) found that physical factors in low back pain and rheumatoid arthritis (RA) patients did not predict pain severity, life interference, or physician visits; whereas cognitive appraisals of helplessness and hopelessness were predictive of both self-report of pain impact and behavior in response to pain.

MULTIDIMENSIONAL PERSPECTIVE

With increasing recognition that the experience of chronic pain is multidimensional, there has been an emphasis on comprehensive evaluation that includes examination of physical pathology along with a range of behavioral-functional, psychological, and psychosocial measures. The earliest attempts to measure psychological factors relied on traditional measures of psychopathology such as the MMPI (discussed above). More recently, the appropriateness and adequacy of these measures have been called into question (Turk & Rudy, 1990). A number of measures have been developed and used to assess pain patients (see other chapters in this volume and Turk & Rudy, 1987, for a review). Although this is a step in the right direction and leads to a more comprehensive evaluation of the pain patient, the difficult task is to integrate such large quantities of data in meaningful ways.

To date, there have been few attempts to develop comprehensive assessment and data integration strategies that cover the relevant dimensions of chronic pain. In the next section we review several integration and classification strategies that have been proposed.

MULTIAXIAL ASSESSMENT

A multiaxial diagnostic approach has been proposed for classification of pain syndromes (Merskey, 1986) and pain patients (Turk & Rudy, 1987). This approach involves the systematic consideration of several parameters of illness simultaneously and requires establishment of an appropriate scale or measurement approach for each parameter or axis. The multiaxial diagnostic approach attempts to present a comprehensive view of the patient's condition by articulating several parameters of disease. Multiaxial assessment may be theoretically or empirically derived. The determination of the most appropriate number of axes in a multiaxial system depends on the scope of clinical information required to reach a comprehensive diagnosis of and treatment plan for the patient.

Up to this point, the attempts to identify subgroups of chronic pain patients reviewed have focused on single factors such as demographics, psychopathology, idiosyncratic thinking patterns, and behavioral expression. Rehabilitative outcome, however, is likely to be determined by the interactive effects of multiple factors, as single factors may not account for a statistically significant or clinically meaningful proportion of the variance in outcome. Thus, measures such as the MMPI are not likely to be predictive of outcome on a consistent basis. Several studies that included measures of both physical and psychological functioning have reported interactive effects of biopsychosocial factors on the outcome of low back pain patients (Beals & Hickman, 1972; Frymoyer, Rosen, Clements, & Pope, 1985; Pope, Rosen, Wilder, & Frymoyer, 1980; Reesor & Craig, 1988).

IASP Classification

The IASP Subcommittee on Taxonomy has published a theoretically based multiaxial classification of chronic pain (Merskey, 1986) that is designed to serve as a preliminary attempt to standardize descriptions of relevant pain syndromes and as a point of reference. The proposed classification system is based on evaluation of each pain syndrome on five separate axes believed by the Subcommittee to be relevant to the diagnosis of the entire range of chronic pain states. As noted earlier, the five axes include: (1) Axis I, the body region or site affect by pain; (2) Axis II, the body system whose abnormal functioning produces the pain; (3) Axis III, the temporal characteristics of pain; (4) Axis IV, the patient's statement of pain intensity and time of onset; and (5) Axis V, the presumed etiology of the pain problem.

The IASP classification is not an assessment procedure per se but rather a heuristic, multiaxial guide emphasizing the consideration of both signs and symptoms. It does not, however, include assessment of psychosocial or behavioral data.

The Emory Pain Estimate Model

Perhaps the first attempt at an empirical integration of multiaxial assessment information was initiated by Steven Brena and his colleagues at Emory University (Brena & Koch, 1975; Brena, Koch, & Moss, 1976). Brena developed a two-dimensional strategy that is referred to as the Emory Pain Estimate Model (EPEM). The dimension are somewhat arbitrarily labeled "pathology" and "behavior." The pathology dimension includes the quantification of physical examination procedures (e.g., ratings of joint mobility, muscle strength) as well as assigning numerical indices to reflect the extent of abnormalities determined from diagnostic procedures such as radiographic studies. The behavioral dimension is comprised of a composite of activity levels, pain verbalizations, drug use, and measures of psychopathology based on the elevations of MMPI scales.

Using median divisions on the pathology and behavior dimensions, the EPEM defines four "classes" of chronic pain patients (see Figure 23.1). Class I patients are characterized by higher scores on the behavior dimension and lower scores on the pathology dimension. These patients are described as displaying low activity levels, high verbalizations of pain, prominent social and psychological malfunctions, and frequent misuse of medications. Class II patients are those who display lower scores on both the pathology and behavioral dimensions. These patients are described as displaying highly dramatized pain complaints with ill-defined anatomical patterns who, however, do not display significant behavioral dysfunction. Class III is comprised of patients with higher scores on both dimensions, and these patients are characterized as showing clear evidence of physical pathology and high-intensity illness behavior. Finally, Class IV patients are those who have higher scores on the pathology dimension and lower scores on the behavior dimension and thus are described as demonstrating "competent" coping in the presence of a physical pathological condition.

Although Brena and his colleagues have appropriately emphasized the importance of integrating physical and psychological data in order to develop a classification system for chronic pain patients, some of the basic theoretical and quantitative characteristics of the EPEM are problematic, and the model might best be viewed as a conceptual model rather than an adequately operationalized empirical one. For example, from a theoretical standpoint, the inclusion of activity levels, pain verbalizations, and measures of psychopathology under a single dimension labeled "behavioral" is troubling in that research suggests that there is little association between pain behaviors and psychopathology. Thus, the "behavioral" dimension is most likely not unidimensional and, therefore, cannot be considered to measure behavior directly.

Examination of the empirical aspects of the scoring and classification system used in the EPEM highlights additional problems. For example, the weights assigned to specific medical–physical findings were based on an a priori weighting system and were not empirically derived. Moreover, applying median divisions to the two dimensions, although intuitively appealing, artificially creates four classes of patients; that is, there is no statistical demonstration that four nonoverlapping groups of pain patients "naturally exist" in these data or that, in fact, the pathology and behavioral dimensions are independent.

Review of the 2 × 2 grid displayed in Figure 23.1 reveals that within the EPEM extreme scores are treated the same as scores near the medians. For example, the scores of patients 1 and 2, depicted as points in Figure 23.1, would both be assigned to Class III, whereas those of patients 3 and 4 would be classified in Class II. In reality, however, the scores of patients 2 and 3 are more similar than they are with the scores of patient 1 or patient 4. Thus, this method of establishing classification rules may lead to er-

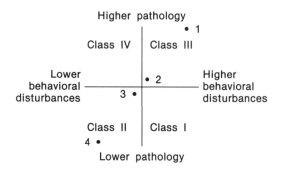

FIGURE 23.1. The Emory pain estimate model.

roneous or nonindependent patient assignments because it is derived from artificial and external mathematical criteria rather than from divisions or clusterings that occur naturally within patients' scores.

The Waddell Approach

Although not intended to be a patient classification system as in the EPEM approach, research by Waddell and his colleague (Waddell & Main, 1984; Waddell et al., 1984; see also Waddel & Turk, Chapter 2) have addressed the interdependencies among physical and psychological assessment findings in chronic low back pain patients as well as how are these related to illness behavior. A central theme of this research has been evaluation of the association between "objective" physical impairment and "subjective" disability. Waddell and Main (1984) empirically identified nine basic physical activities in daily living that are frequently restricted by back pain (e.g., lifting, sitting, walking, sleeping). Patients' reports of their loss of ability or limitations on these activities are recorded in an interview format and are used to form a Chronic Disability Index. This index is then related to clinical findings of physical impairment, which is comprised of physician ratings related to the appropriateness or inappropriateness of patients' descriptions of their pain pattern, evaluation of patients' degree of lumbar flexion, straight leg raising, root compression signs, and previous lumbar surgeries. It is interesting to note that other physical signs of deformity, muscle tenderness, other spinal movements, and radiological findings of degeneration did not improve upon their physical impairment index.

MULTIDIMENSIONAL, EMPIRICALLY DERIVED CLASSIFICATION OF PAIN PATIENTS—MULTIAXIAL ASSESSMENT OF PAIN PATIENTS

Three central assessment questions would appear to capture the complex nature of chronic pain, and any chronic condition for that matter, namely,

1. What is the extent of the patient's physical pathology (physical impairment)?

2. What is the magnitude of the patient's disability (suffering and inability to enjoy usual activities)?

3. Is the patient's behavior consistent with the pathology identified, or is there evidence of amplification of symptoms for any of a variety of psychological, social, or economic purposes?

Based on these questions, and as an alternative to the rational approaches to classification adopted by Brena and his colleagues (Brena & Koch, 1975; Brena et al., 1976), IASP (Merskey, 1986), and the Intentional Headache Society (Olesen, 1988) and the unidimensional empirical models described above (i.e., Bradley et al., 1978; Butterworth & Deardorff, 1987; Ingram et al., 1990; Keefe et al., 1990), Turk and Rudy (1987) have suggested that an approach and inductive strategy where empirical strategies are used to classify patients might alleviate some of the problems inherent in such deductive and unidimensional approaches.

Specifically, Turk and Rudy (1987) have proposed a classification system for chronic pain patients based on the empirical integration of biomedical, psychosocial, and behavioral data that they labeled the Multiaxial Assessment of Pain (MAP) patients. They also suggested that a taxonomy of pain patients based on psychosocial and behavioral data alone could be developed (Rudy et al., 1989; Turk & Rudy, 1988) and might complement more traditional diagnosis that is based largely on physical findings. The primary hypotheses were that certain modal psychosocial and behavioral response patterns recur in chronic pain patients and that these patterns represent homogeneous subgroups of chronic pain patients, at least to some extent, independent of medical diagnoses. The MAP (Turk & Rudy, 1987) approach is described below to illustrate how multidimensional assessment of pain patients can be operationalize, conducted, and integrated to provide comprehensive assessment.

A number of instruments and assessment procedures, many described throughout this volume, have been developed to address each or some of these questions. Some of these have been described earlier (e.g., MMPI, pain behavior) but have not been integrated in a systematic assessment package. The Multidimensional Pain Inventory (MPI) (Kerns, Turk, & Rudy, 1985) is a 64-item self-report questionnaire comprised of three parts. The first two parts are related to patients' appraisals of pain and the impact of pain on different domains of their lives and perceptions of the responses of significant others to their distress and suffering. The last part relates to the frequency that patients indicate that they perform specific common activities. The first part was specifically designed to assess: (1) reports of pain severity; (2) perceptions of pain interference with family and marital functioning, work and social-recreational activities; (3) dissatisfaction with present levels of functioning in each of the ares listed in (2); (4) appraisal of support provided by significant others; (5) perceived life control, ability to solve problems, and feelings of personal competence; and (6) affective distress. Part II consists of ratings by patients of the frequency with which significant others respond to their expressions of pain by (1) punishment (e.g., irritability), (2) solicitousness (e.g., freeing patients from their usual chores), and (3) distraction (e.g., encouraging patients to engage in activities). Part III of the MPI assess the performance of such common activities as household chores and socializing with family and friends (see Kerns & Jacob, Chapter 14).

The MPI has the advantage of having been standardized on a population of patients with persistent pain complaints, with normative data available for pain syndromes based on IASP Axis 1 (body location) classification. The MPI also has been demonstrated to be easy to administer and score, including a microcomputer program that provides scoring and database management facilities for up to three assessment times for each patient, and to be a reliable and valid instrument for assessment of chronic pain patients. Moreover, it has been demonstrated to be sensitive to change following rehabilitation (Kerns, Turk, Holzman, & Rudy, 1986).

Turk and Rudy (1988) reported the results of two studies suggesting that psychological assessment data incorporating cognitive, affective, and behavioral information can be integrated using numerical taxometric methods and can serve as the basis for the identification of an empirically derived classification system of chronic pain patients. Utilizing cluster-analytic and multivariate classification methods, three homogeneous subgroups of chronic pain patients have been identified and replicated across a wide range of medical diagnoses (e.g., back pain temporomandibular disorders, headache).

The three groups' distinct patient profiles were labeled (1) "Dysfunctional," characterized by patients who perceive the severity of their pain to be high, reported that pain interfered with much of their lives, reported higher degree of affective distress, and low levels of activity (see also Von Korff, this volume); (2) "Interpersonally Distressed," characterized by a common perception that significant others were not very understanding or supportive of their problems; and (3) "Adaptive Copers," characterized by high levels of social support, relatively low levels of pain, perceived interference, affective distress, and higher levels of activity and perceived control. The percentages of patients in each group were 43%, 28%, 29%, for Dysfunctional, Interpersonally Distressed, and Adaptive Copers, respectively.

To establish the external validity of the MPI patient profiles, multivariate and univariate analyses of variance for reliable, conceptual related measures not used in the clustering solutions (e.g., McGill Pain Questionnaire, Melzack, 1975; Pain Behavior Checklist, Turk, Wack, & Kerns, 1985; Beck Depression Inventory, Beck, Ward, Mendelson, Mock, & Erbaugh, 1961) were used to test for significant differences across the three patient clusters. Patient demographic characteristics and medical findings also were included in these analyses. The patient subgroups were found to be independent of age, gender, and duration of pain, and there remained significant group differences even when the effects of physical pathology was statistical controlled.

As hypothesized, significant subgroup differences were found on (1) Pain Behavior Checklist (Turk, Wack, & Kerns, 1985), (2) the frequency of using prescription analgesic medication, (3) the amount of time spent in bed, and (4) employment status. The Dysfunctional patients displayed more pain behaviors, used pain medications more frequently, spent more time in bed due to pain, and were more likely to be unemployed than Cluster II and III patients who did not differ from each on these measures. The Interpersonally Distressed group (Cluster II) differed significantly from the other two groups on marital satisfaction, being less satisfied with their marital relationship. In sum, the use of measures that were external to the clustering procedures used to developed the three patient profiles provided evidence that these three groups were unique and distinct, that is, were neither random nor an artifact of the measures used in profile development.

A recent study (Rudy et al., 1989) provided additional confirmation of the MAP taxonomy and the three patient profiles described above. In this study a sample of patients diagnosed as having temporomandibular disorders revealed the three same profiles as the original study of pain clinic patients (Turk & Rudy, 1988) and in roughly the same proportion. Similarly, in this study the three profiles appeared to be independent of patients' age, duration of pain, oral dysfunction, and structural abnormalities based on CT scans. As displayed in Table 23.2, analyses based on measures external to the measures used in taxometric development demonstrated the uniqueness and validity of the three TMD patient subgroups identified.

We also have evaluated the robustness of the MAP taxonomy across several different pain syndromes, specifically, chronic low back pain (CLBP), head pain (H), and temporomandibular disorders (TMD) (Turk & Rudy, 1990). Classification accuracy, multivariate generalized distance functions and Bayesian approaches to empirical classification were applied to patients' MPI scale scores to assign them into one of the three patient profiles. Ninety-five percent of CLBP, 94% of TMD, and 92% of the H patients could be classified accurately into one of the three profiles.

As would be expected, the mean scores on each of the MPI scales were significantly different for each of these three patient samples.

However, when mean differences were statistically removed, the MPI scale intercorrelations among the three patient groups were equivalent. This finding provided evidence of the structural invariance of the MPI scale scores across diverse patient samples and, therefore, the feasibility and statistical appropriateness of testing a common set of multivariate classification rules across diverse chronic pain samples. The results of these analyses are displayed in Table 23.3 and indicated (1) a higher percentage of CLBP patients were classified as Dysfunctional when compared with the patients from the TMD and H samples; (2) a higher percentage of TMD and H patients compared with CLBP patients were classified as Adaptive Copers; and (3) no significant between group differences were found for the Interpersonally Distressed classification across the three patient samples.

It is important to note that the three syndrome groups were represented in each of the MAP clusters. Thus, it is possible that TMD, H, and CLBP patients who are classified within the same subgroup may be psychologically more similar to each other than patients with the same diagnosis but who are classified within different subgroups. In other words, patients' psychosocial and behavioral response patterns to their pain problems were found to be similar despite different medical and dental diagnoses.

To summarize, the classification system developed by Turk and Rudy (1988) focused on similarities among chronic pain patients regard

TABLE 23.2. Results of External Validation of MPI Clusters

Variable	Mean scores by cluster			F-test	P
	I	II	III		
Mean pain rating from dental exam	1.82	1.40	1.13	$F(2,123) = 11.07$	$<0.001^a$
Pain Behavior Checklist	4.98	3.31	2.78	$F(2,104) = 7.18$	$<0.001^b$
CES Depression Scale	21.74	14.52	9.54	$F(2,144) = 25.36$	$<0.001^a$
POMS Depression Scale	15.09	10.88	4.60	$F(2,144) = 17.11$	$<0.001^a$
POMS Total Score	48.39	29.09	5.04	$F(2,144) = 23.03$	$<0.001^a$
Daily Hassles Scale	73.56	51.71	44.73	$F(2,117) = 8.49$	$<0.001^a$
Wahler Physical Symptoms	1.60	1.29	1.13	$F(2,84) = 4.24$	$<0.05^b$
Locke-Wallace Marital Scale	103.04	83.71	106.92	$F(2,51) = 3.98$	$<0.005^c$
Age	32.15	33.46	30.65	$F(1,144) = 0.99$	n.s.
Duration of pain (in years)	4.74	5.89	5.95	$F(2,144) = 0.72$	n.s.
Number of TMJ symptoms from exam	1.18	1.16	1.38	$F(2,137) = 1.72$	n.s.
Max. interincisal opening (mm)	30.23	30.31	32.09	$F(2,131) = 0.55$	n.s.
Proportional abnormal CT findings	0.44	0.52	0.47	$\chi^2(2) = 0.45$	n.s.

[a]Cluster 1> cluster II> cluster III.
[b]Cluster 1> cluster II> and cluster III.
[c]Cluster II> cluster I and cluster III.

TABLE 23.3. Profile Proportions by Patient Sample

Profile classification	CLBP subjects	TMD subject	H subjects
Dysfunctional	0.62	0.46	0.44
Interpersonally distressed	0.18	0.22	0.25
Adaptive coper	0.20	0.32	0.31

less of their medical diagnosis. Moreover, the taxonomy was empirically derived and makes no assumptions about the classification of chronic pain patients other than acknowledging the relevance of cognitive, affective, and behavioral data for establishing group membership and that multivariate classification rules can be used to accurately assign patients to specific profiles. Additionally, the MAP classification system appears to have good reliability and external validity, and was cross-validated on several heterogeneous as well as homogeneous samples of chronic pain patients. The proposed taxonomy has the added strength of using psychometrically sound measures developed on and normed for chronic pain patients. Thus, it may have greater utility than approaches that are based on instruments that were never developed for this population. However, as with all of the classification systems discussed throughout this paper, no studies have as yet evaluated the efficacy of matching treatment to the MAP subgroups identified.

Integrating Biomedical Findings

The empirical classification methods described above did not consider the potential influence of biomedical findings on the integration of psychological and behavioral patient assessment findings. As a first step toward integrating biomedical findings with the MPI subgroups described above, we (Turk & Rudy, 1987) combined the MPI scale scores of 46 patients with physical pathology scores derived from the Medical Examination Diagnostic Information Coding System (MEDICS) (Rudy, Turk, & Brena, 1988; Rudy, Turk, Brena, Stieg, & Brody, 1990, and Rudy, Turk, & Brody, Chapter 25). An analysis of variance indicated that the Dysfunctional subgroup of patients, compared with patients classified as Interpersonally Distressed and Adaptive Co-

pers, were found to have significantly more abnormal medical-physical findings. A reclustering of the MPI scores along with the inclusion of MEDICS scores resulted in the Dysfunctional subgroup further dividing into two groups of approximately equal size. Similar to the Dysfunctional profile, the new patient subgroup that emerged appeared to reflect a group of patients who were characterized by higher levels of pain, negative life impact, and psychological distress, and lower levels perceived control and activity; however, these findings also were coupled with higher levels of physical pathology. Thus, the sole difference between this new subgroup and the previously identified Dysfunctional subgroup was the extent of the physical pathology identified. We have tentatively labeled this fourth patient subgroup as "Impaired."

Some might question, as we have, the appropriateness of combining physical pathology with psychological and behavioral data. Turk (1990) has described a possible alternative that he labeled "polydiagnostic." A polydiagnostic approach would include multiple classifications simultaneously. It might be suggested that physical assessment should be directed toward the syndrome classification (e.g., IASP taxonomy) and that psychosocial-behavioral taxometric findings could be most useful in treatment planning, with these separate assessment strategies providing unique information.

For example, a person with persistent pain might have diagnoses on two different but complementary taxonomies (e.g., IASP and MAP). Thus, a patient might be classified as suffering from Reflex Sympathetic Dystrophy (IASP code 203.91: Axis I Region = Upper Shoulder and Upper Limbs, Axis II System = Nervous System, Axis III Temporal Characteristics of Pain: Pattern of Occurrence = Continuous, Axis IV Intensity and Time of Onset = Severe, more than 6 months, Axis V Aetiology = Trauma) and simultaneously be classified as Dysfunctional by the MAP taxometric approach. A second patient might have the same IASP classification but be classified as an Adaptive Coper on the MAP taxonomy. The extent of disability as well as the most appropriate treatments for these two patients might vary considerably.

Adopting a polydiagnostic approach would serve the valuable function of encouraging clinicians as well as researchers to think concurrently in terms of two different but complementary diagnostic systems, biomedical and psychosocial-behavioral. Empirical studies would be needed to evaluate the efficacy of individualized treatments based on the poly-diagnostic approach.

CUSTOMIZING TREATMENT BASED ON EMPIRICAL CLASSIFICATION

The results of the studies reviewed above provide support for the hypothesis that there are different subgroups of pain patients and that treating them all the same may dilute the ability to demonstrate treatment efficacy. That is, specific interventions may have their greatest utility with particular subgroups of patients. Combining heterogeneous samples in treatment outcome studies without statistically controlling for subgroup differences (e.g., by blocking) may result in nonsignificant or only modest therapeutic gains.

The results reported above suggest that greater attention should be given to using the identification of patient characteristics and how these profiles are predictive of patients who improve as a result of a particular treatment intervention and those who do not. Furthermore, the ability to identify characteristics of patients who do not benefit from specific treatment should facilitate the development of innovative treatment approaches tailored to the needs of those patients who do not benefit from existing programs.

Many forms of medical and psychological treatment, and more commonly multidisciplinary rehabilitation programs, have been partially successful in reducing suffering and disability accompanying persistent pain problems. The results of these diverse treatments, however, are highly variable. Despite the reported successes, many studies report that there remains a significant proportion of patients who do not demonstrate substantial treatment gain (40%–60%)—interestingly, these results are similar to the outcomes reported for back surgery, (Wiesel, Feffer, & Rothman, 1979); whereas other patients who report immediate gains do not retain the improvements following discharge. These studies are examined in recent reviews (Holroyd & Penzien, 1986; Turk, Flor, & Fydrich, 1990; Turk & Rudy, 1990).

Although subgroups have been identified, few attempts have been made to evaluate the differential efficacy of treatments that are customized to specific patient characteristics. Bradley and Van der Heide (1984) have called for studies concerning the responses of different subgroups to pharmacological, medical, and behavioral treatments. The studies that have been conducted have used retrospective methods rather than looking prospectively at differential response to the same treatment (e.g., Guck, Meilman, Skultety, & Poloni; 1988; McGill et al., 1983; Moore et al., 1986).

The absence of empirical data that consistently link chronic pain patient characteristics with successful treatment and rehabilitation has impeded the design of individual treatment plans. Consequently, despite an increasing awareness among researchers and clinicians of the importance of collecting multiaxial assessment information, chronic pain patients still tend to be considered as a homogeneous group when it comes to treatment planning. Treating all patients with persistent pain in the same manner has been abetted by the attempt to view chronic pain as a specific syndrome (Black, 1975; Florence, 1981). This has been referred to as a "patient uniformity myth" (Fordyce, 1976). Such patient homogeneity has been opposed by the Institute of Medicine (IOM) as "There has been no demonstration of a common etiology, a predictable natural history, a clearly defined constellation of symptoms, or a specific treatment for the various pain conditions that would suggest a basis for positing a single chronic pain syndrome" (p. 8). The IOM committee further criticized this view "Because of the considerable differences in types of pain and patients, it is inappropriate to speak of 'the' chronic pain patients as if there were only one type . . . implies a homogeneity among conditions that are actually quite different" (Osterweis et al., 1987, pp. 12–13).

In sum, the delineation of homogeneous subgroups among pain patients may provide an important framework for the development of specific, optimal treatment regimens for these subgroups of patients. Of course, the notion of matching diagnosis to treatment is not new, but has been of central importance in clinical medicine as well as psychological therapy for a number of years. However, given the complexity of chronic pain and the multidimensional impact on patients' lives, establishing a better link between multiaxial diagnosis and treatment planning remains a substantial challenge.

RECOMMENDATIONS AND FUTURE DIRECTIONS

Developing a meaningful and scientifically sound empirical classification for chronic pain is a daunting task. The minimum requirements include:

1. Identifying the necessary and sufficient constructs that are theoretically related to the purposes of the taxonomy.
2. Developing the necessary methodology to operationalize the constructs selected.
3. Establishing the psychometric adequacy of the measurement strategies selected for each construct.
4. Conducting exploratory data analyses to determine whether distinct, conceptually meaningful patterns or clusters exist in the data.
5. Constructing objective, mathematically based classification rules, based on the exploratory analyses, so that these rules can be used in replicating the obtained structure on a new sample.
6. Establishing the validity and utility of the derived classification system.
7. Testing the generalizability and limitations of the classification system across different chronic pain syndromes (Turk & Rudy, 1988).

Psychometric Considerations

The general utility of any proposed empirical taxonomy is closely linked to the psychometric properties of the measures, scales, or instruments used to derive the classification system. Because these are the building blocks used to generate profiles or clusterings, the reliability and validity of the classification system is dependent, in part, on the psychometric quality of the measures used. Because reliability and validity coefficients are generic terms, consideration needs to be given to the specific psychometric techniques used to evaluate a measure's "psychometric properties" (see Dworkin & Whitney, Chapter 24, and Rudy, Turk, & Brody, Chapter 25). Because there are multiple ways of demonstrating the reliability and validity of measures, the more psychometric support there is for a measure, the more likely it will perform well when used in taxometric identification and classification procedures.

Nonetheless, it is important to realize that using highly reliable and valid measures in profile development does not ensure that the resulting profiles derived from these measures are themselves reliable and valid. Extreme cases or "outliers," cluster analyzing an inappropriate distance measures, selecting the wrong clustering algorithm for the data under question, small sample sizes, deciding to retain too few or too many profiles, inclusion of irrelevant variables, and so forth, all can lead to unreliable and invalid profiles. Conger (1982) provides several methods that can be used to compute the multivariate reliability of profiles, which are based on the intercorrelations among the measures used and their individual reliabilities. Additionally, replication of classification accuracy on new samples and demonstrating substantial, statistically significant differences across patient profiles for conceptually related measures *external* to the measures used to develop the profiles are some of the best ways to demonstrate the reliability and validity of empirically derived profiles.

Common Statistical Pitfalls

Many clinical investigators interested in empirical classification methods do not appear to be aware of the immense amount of activity and advances in the field of classification. The reason, in part, is that the literature on clustering methodology is segmented, with authors in one academic discipline often isolated from research in other fields. Fortunately, several recent comprehensive reviews of clustering methods and developments have helped to bridge this gap (e.g., Aldenderfer & Blashfield, 1984; Milligan & Cooper, 1987). In the sections that follow, we will briefly review several common problems that are encountered with using clustering methods to develop empirical classification systems and some of the solutions that have been proposed.

The Number-of-Clusters Problem

Similar to the number-of-factors problem in exploratory factor analysis, determining the correct number of clusters to retain from a dataset retains a thorny and unresolved issue in clustering methodology. Currently, there are no satisfactory methods for determining the number of clusters or profiles that are present in a dataset for any type of cluster analysis, in that there are no definitive statistical tests that exist to inform the experimenter whether the "true" number of clusters have been achieve by the clustering algorithm. However, most clustering procedures require the user to specify or to determine the number of clusters to retain in the final solution.

Ordinary significance tests, such as the *F*-test that results from the analysis of variance, are not valid for testing differences between clusters because clustering methods attempt to maximize differences among clusters. Thus, the assumptions of the usual significance tests for both parametric and nonparametric procedures are seriously violated. In fact, the clustering of completely random data frequently results in highly significant *F*-tests between clusters (Aldenderfer & Blashfield, 1984). Thus, traditional significance testing between the computed clusters on the *same* measures used to create the clusters or patient profiles are *useless*.

The difficulty in determining the correct number of clusters in a dataset has led to the development of over 30 criteria that can be used. Milligan and Cooper (1985, 1986) compared the performance of these criteria across a wide variety of currently used clustering algorithms, including a diverse set of hierarchical and partitioning approaches. Their findings, as well as the results of computer simulation studies by others, are summarized in Milligan and Cooper (1987). Basically, most of the criteria that have been proposed for determining the number of clusters in a dataset performed poorly. Several criteria, however, were found to be generally robust in identifying the correct number of clusters in a dataset, even in the presence of "noisy" data. These criteria included the techniques developed by Baker and Hubert (1975), Calinski and Harabasz (1974), Duda and Hart (1973), Beale (1969), and the cubic clustering criterion used in the statistical software package SAS (Sarle, 1983).

Our recommendations are as follows:

1. Since the term "cluster analysis" is a generic term and over 100 different clustering algorithms have been developed, pain researchers reporting the results of a cluster analysis should explicitly report which specific algorithm or clustering procedure was used (e.g., the phase "hierarchical clustering" is too broad because there are numerous approaches that have been developed to achieve hierarchical solutions).

2. Similarly, the author should report explicitly what criterion was used to determine the number of clusters to retain.

3. A minimum of one of the criteria listed above should be used whenever possible, at least until better procedures are developed.

4. When addressing problems similar to those in published literature, keeping an a priori number of clusters in one's dataset because another author kept a specific number is inappropriate and unjustified. We recommend using more objective statistical decision rules, rather than another investigator's decision rules, which may have been subjective and in error. This is because, as described below, the vast majority of cluster analytic applications are exploratory rather than confirmatory in nature.

Identification, Classification, and Replication

Considerable confusion exists in the applied classification literature between the concepts of identification and classification, and, consequently, replication (Breckenridge, 1989). To clarify this confusion it is important to recognize that cluster analysis, despite the specific algorithm used, yields only partitioned data. As such, it only can be considered an exploratory method to identify potential clusters or profiles that exist *in a specific dataset*. In other words, cluster-analytic methods do not provide information that is independent of the data analyzed. Thus, although cluster analysis can be used appropriately in identification of subgroups, this methodology is not suitable for the additional purposes of classification and replication.

The process of classification from an empirical standpoint assumes that group profiles or clusters of common attributes or symptoms have already been identified and the desire is to assign cases, perhaps from a new sample, to one of the already identified profiles. For example, in order to classify the scores obtained from a pain patient into an empirically based taxonomy, explicit mathematical rules need to be applied to the patient's scores to determine the similarity between the patient's scores and the scores that characterize each of the derived profiles. Thus, in contrast to cluster analysis, the mathematical results of many multivariate procedures used in classification (e.g., discriminant functions, regression equations) can be expressed independently of the data analyzed. Once explicit mathematical rules for creating a cluster partition have been specified, the classification is "objective in the sense of being repeatable by anyone less invested in the findings" (Gordon, 1981, p. 9).

Commonly used parametric multivariate classification methods, sometimes referred to as classificatory discriminant analysis, are discussed in most texts on multivariate statistics (e.g., Overall & Klett, 1972; Tatsuoka, 1971). More recent advances in nonparametric multivariate classification methods are discussed in Silverman (1986), and Breckenridge (1989) compares the relative performance of several parametric approaches with a nonparametric approach when applied to cluster replication studies.

The process of identifying or discovering profiles as a result of cluster analysis and then developing multivariate classification rules from the clustering results has important implications for replication methods, which are essential for establishing the reliability, validity objectivity, and generalizability of an empirical taxonomy. For example, the common practice of simply repeating the cluster analysis in a second sample and inferring replication from visual inspection of cluster mean profiles (e.g., Bradley et al., 1978) cannot be treated as scientific evidence of cross-validation (Breckenridge, 1989). More precise evidence of the fit between the cluster structures identified in one sample and the similarity of those in a second sample is needed.

Perhaps one of the best cluster replication methods, based on the logic of cross-validation as used in regression analysis, is the strategy proposed by McIntyre and Blashfield (1980). Their methodology can be summarized as follows:

1. Obtain two samples for clustering purposes. If one dataset is sufficiently large, randomly divide it into two samples.
2. The first sample is cluster analyzed. From this analysis, the centroids (mean values) for the clusters are computed and a multivariate classification model is developed.
3. This classification model is then applied to the cases in the second sample to assign each case to one of the clusters developed in the first sample.

4. The second sample is then directly cluster analyzed without regard to the results obtained from the first sample. Thus, for the second sample there are two clusterings for comparison purposes.
5. Some measure of agreement (e.g., kappa) is used to measure the similarity between the two partitions of the same data. The consistency between the original cluster solution and the cross-validated cluster classifications indicates the stability of the obtained profiles.

To summarize, cluster-analytic procedures should not be confused with empirical classification techniques. Clustering procedures help to identify profile structures in a dataset, while classification methods establish the mathematical rules among the variables that can be used to recreate the same or very similar profile structures in independent datasets or for additional individual cases. Cluster analysis should be considered an exploratory statistical technique, whereas multivariate classification procedures are more confirmatory and permit a direct replication of the cluster-analytic results. In other words, although prevalent in the pain literature, "one cluster analysis does not a taxonomy make."

Classification Caveat

It is unreasonable to believe that a small number of typical patterns or clusters, as have been described throughout this chapter, can represent *all* patient profiles that might result from the complex interactions involved in the pain experience. Similarly, it is unreasonable to believe that a single empirically derived classification system can reliably and accurately classify patients regardless of the specific pain syndrome. For example, the pain behavior taxonomy developed by Keefe et al. (1990) may work well for classifying back pain patients but may be of limited utility for headache patients. Similarly, the MAP taxonomy that we have developed (Rudy et al., 1989; Turk & Rudy, 1988) and described above appears to provide accurate and useful classifications for back, headache, and TMD pain patients but may not, at least in its present form, reliably classify groups of patients who are quite different from the sample used in the original subgroup identification study, for example, with pain associated with cancer.

The basic point is best described in the title

of an article by Bergman (1988), "You Can't Classify All of the People All of the Time," who concludes that any empirical classification system should allow for "leftovers." A common pitfall is that investigators attempt to cluster and/or classify all patients in the dataset. Not only does this practice reduce the accuracy of many clustering algorithms (e.g., Scheibler & Schneider, 1985) and, consequently, the mathematical rules derived from them, but makes the unwarranted assumption that the data of all patients can be accounted for or explained by these statistical procedures. This simply is not possible. Cases that are "outliers" can have a serious, negative impact on clustering methods. Further, these atypical cases can be the result of numerous influences, ranging from a rare but valid profile, to an invalid profile, perhaps the result of random or aberrant responding or "faking bad." Without very large datasets, additional patient profiles that occur infrequently simply cannot be detected.

Thus, although multidimensional, empirically derived classification systems have many advantages over theoretically-based systems, whether unidimensional or multidimensional, we recommend that any empirical classification system for chronic pain patients provides a explicit mechanism, usually in the form of decision rules based on probability theory, for not classifying cases that simply "do not fit" any of the patient profiles. For example, in the MAP classification system we label these cases "anomalous," which accounts for about 5–7% of the pain patients that we have tested. Additionally, it is recommended that developers of empirical taxometric systems in chronic pain provide more information about the limitations of their systems, particularly in terms of the appropriateness and accuracy of applying it to different pain syndromes. More specifically, it is important to recognize that the null hypothesis is that the classification system *does not fit* any other patient sample than the one used in it development. In other words, the validity of applying the classification system to a new sample cannot be assumed; it has to be empirically demonstrated.

CONCLUSION

Conceptualizations about pain and dysfunction will influence the methods and types of assessment procedures performed and the interpretation of the results of these procedures. We have suggested throughout this chapter that chronic pain is not simply a result of objective tissue damage nor can simple intensity measures of pain capture the range of factors that describe the perception of pain. Moreover, separate psychological, behavioral, and motivational factors are inadequate to explain the experience of chronic pain. Rather, persistent pain, from whatever cause, by definition extends over time and affects all aspects of an individual functioning—social, familial, psychological, vocational, as well as physical. Because pain persists over time it needs to be viewed as a dynamic process with reciprocal interactions among physical, psychological, social, and behavioral components that both influence and are influenced by one another.

The multiaxial approach to the assessment of pain and dysfunction described earlier would appear to be a reasonable strategy to adopt. Once the comprehensive set of physical and functional capacity data are collected, the strategy of matching patients to existing classification systems could serve as a basis for disability determination. The use of the polydiagnostic approach seems to hold promise because it incorporates biomedical, psychosocial, and behavioral data in the assignment of patients to empirically derived categories. Additional research, however, is needed to relate patient classification with performance on standardized physical capacity assessment protocols, rehabilitation, and ability to engage in gainful employment and regular homemaking activities.

The utility of any classification system is best determined by actually using it to classify individuals. Does assignment of an individual to a class facilitate treatment decisions or predictions of future behavior? Few of the taxometric systems described in this paper qualify as empirical classification systems, and none has demonstrated its utility in predicting treatment outcome (Turk, 1990).

The construction of empirical classification systems and their eventual use are inherently psychological processes, no matter how mathematically elegant they may seem. From the decision of what measures to use in the development of a taxonomy to the interpretation of the final statistical results, the investigator's biases and theoretical preferences clearly influence the final product. What has been described in this paper are classification approaches based on deductive and inductive perspectives based on unidimensional or multidimensional strategies that have been used to group (diagnose, subdivide) chronic pain patients, common statistical pitfalls that are encountered during the development of these systems, and the use of polydiagnostic and multiaxial approaches. Some of the advantages and disadvantages of these strategies were noted. The important point, however, is the fundamental need to develop and evaluate taxometric systems that can facilitate communication, understanding, and treatment. If there are, indeed, different subgroups or clusters of patients, then matching of treatment to patient characteristics would seem a reasonable alternative to treating all patients with the same diagnosis as a homogeneous group (Turk, 1990).

Acknowledgments. Preparation of this paper was supported in part by Grant 2R01AR38698 from the National Institute of Arthritis and Musculoskeletal and Skin Diseases and Grant 2R01DE07514 from the National Institute of Dental Research.

REFERENCES

Aldenderfer, M.S., & Blashfield, R.K. (1984). *Cluster analysis* (Sage University Paper series on Quantitative Applications in the Social Sciences, 07-044). Beverly Hills, CA: Sage.

Armentrout, D.P., Moore, J.E., Parker, J.C., Hewett, J.E., & Felz, C. (1982). Pain patient MMPI subgroups: The psychological dimensions of pain. *Journal of Behavioral Medicine, 1,* 201–211.

Baker, F. B., & Hubert, L. J. (1975). Measuring the power of hierarchical cluster analysis. *Journal of the American Statistical Association, 70,* 31–38.

Baron, D.N., & Fraser, P.M. (1968). Medical applications of taxonomic methods. *British Medical Journal, 24,* 236–240.

Beale, E. M. L. (1969). *Cluster analysis.* London: Scientific Control Systems.

Beals, R.K., & Hickman, N.W. (1972). Industrial injuries of the back and extremities. *Journal of Bone Joint Surgery, 54A,* 1593–1611.

Beck, A.T., Ward, C.H., Mendelson, M., Mock, J., & Erbaugh, J. (1961). An inventory for measuring depression. *Archives of General Psychiatry, 4,* 561–571.

Bergman, L. R. (1988). You can't classify all of the people all of the time. *Multivariate Behavioral Research, 23,* 425–441.

Bernstein, I.H., & Grabin, C.P. (1983). Hierarchical clustering of pain patients' MMPI profiles: A replication note. *Journal of Personality Assessment, 47,* 171–172.

Black, R.G. (1975). The chronic pain syndrome. *Surgery Clinics of North America, 55,* 999–1011.

Bonica, J.J. (1979). The need of a taxonomy, *Pain, 6,* 247–252.

Bradley, L.A., Prokop, C.K., Margolis, R., & Gentry, W.D. (1978). Multivariate analyses of the MMPI profiles of low back pain patients. *Journal of Behavioral Medicine, 1,* 253–272.

Bradley, L.A., & Van der Heide, L.H. (1984). Pain-related correlates of MMPI profile subgroups among back pain patients. *Health Psychology, 3,* 157–174.

Breckenridge, J. N. (1989). Replicating cluster analysis: Method, consistency, and validity. *Multivariate Behavioral Research, 24,* 147–161.

Brena, S.F., & Koch, D.L. (1975). A "pain estimate" model for quantification and classification of chronic pain states. *Anesthesia Review, 2,* 8–13.

Brena, S.F., Koch, D.L., & Moss, R.M. (1976). Reliability of the "pain Estimate" model. *Anesthesia Review, 3,* 28–29.

Butterworth, J.C., & Deardorff, W.W. (1987). Psychometric profiles of craniomandibular pain patients: Identifying specific subgroups. *Journal of Craniomandibular Practice, 5,* 225–232.

Cairns, D., Mooney, V., & Crane, P. (1982). Spinal pain rehabilitation: Inpatient and outpatient treatment results and development of predictors for outcome. *Spine, 9,* 91–95.

Calinski, R. B., & Harabasz, J. (1974). A dendrite method for cluster analysis. *Communications in Statistics, 3,* 1–27.

Conger, A. J. (1982). Multivariate reliability: Implications for evaluating profiles. In N. Hirschberg & L. G. Humphreys (Eds.), *Multivariate applications in the social sciences* (pp. 5–60). Hillsdale, NJ: Erlbaum.

Derogatis, L.R. (1977). *SCL-90 administration, scoring and procedures manual.* Baltimore, MD: Johns Hopkins University Press.

Duda, R. O., & Hart, P. E. (1973). *Pattern classification and scene analysis.* New York: Wiley.

Flor, H., & Turk, D.C. (1988). Chronic back pain and rheumatoid arthritis: Predicting pain and disability from cognitive variables. *Journal of Behavioral Medicine, 11,* 251–265.

Florence, D.W. (1981). The chronic pain syndrome: A physical and psychologic challenge. *Postgraduate Medicine, 70,* 218–228.

Fordyce, W.E. (1976). *Behavioral methods for chronic pain and illness.* St. Louis, MO: Mosby.

Fricton, J.R. (1982). Medical evaluation of patients with chronic pain. In J. Barber & C. Adrian (Eds.), *Psychological approaches to the management of pain* (pp. 37–61). New York: Brunner/Mazel.

Frymoyer, J.W., Rosen, J.C., Clements, J., & Pope, M.H. (1985). Psychologic factors in low back pain disability. *Clinical Orthopedics and Related Research, 195,* 178–84.

Gallagher, R.M., Rauh, V., Haugh, L.D., Milhous, R., Callas, P.W., Langelier, R., McClallen, J.M., & Frymoyer, J. (1989). Determinants of return-to-work among low back pain patients. *Pain, 39,* 55–67.

Gordon, A.D. (1981). *Classification: Methods for the exploratory analysis of multivariate data.* London: Chapman & Hall.

Guck, T.P., Meilman, P.W., Skultety, F.M., & Poloni, L.D. (1988). Pain-patient Minnesota Multiphasic Personality Inventory (MMPI) subgroups: Evaluation of long-term treatment outcome. *Journal of Behavioral Medicine, 111,* 159–169.

Hart, R. (1984). Chronic pain: Replicated multivariate clustering of personality profiles. *Journal of Clinical Psychology, 40,* 129–132.

Hollon, S.D., & Kendall, P.C. (1980). Cognitive self-statements in depression: Development of an Automatic Thoughts Questionnaire. *Cognitive Therapy and Research, 4,* 383–395.

Holroyd, K.A., & Penzien, D.B. (1986). Client variables and the behavioral treatment of recurrent tension headache: a meta-analytic review. *Journal of Behavioral Medicine, 9,* 515–36.

Ingram, R.E., Atkinson, J.H., Slater, M.A., Saccuzzo, D.P., & Garfin, S.R. (1990). Negative and positive cognition in depressed and nondepressed chronic pain patients. *Health Psychology, 9,* 300–314.

Ingram, R.E., & Wisnicki, K.S. (1988). Assessment of positive automatic cognitions. *Journal of Consulting and Clinical Psychology, 56,* 898–902.

Jamison, R.N., Rock, D.L., & Parris, W.C.V. (1988). Empirically derived Symptom Checklist 90 subgroups of chronic pain patients: a cluster analysis. *Journal of Behavioral Medicine, 11,* 147–158.

Keefe, F.J., Bradley, L.A., & Crisson, J.E. (1990). Behavioral assessment of low back pain: identification of pain behavior subgroups. *Pain, 40,* 153–160.

Kerns, R.D., Turk, D.C., Holzman, A.D., & Rudy, T.E. (1986). Comparison of cognitive-behavioral and behavioral approaches to the outpatient treatment of chronic pain. *Clinical Journal of Pain, 4,* 195–206.

Kerns, R.D., Turk, D.C., & Rudy, T.E. (1985). The West Haven–Yale Multidimensional Pain Inventory (WHYMPI). *Pain, 23,* 345–356.

McCreary, C. (1985). Empirically derived MMPI profile clusters and characteristics of low back pain patients. *Journal of Consulting and Clinical Psychology, 54,* 558–560.

McGill, J.C., Lawlis, G.F., Selby, D., Mooney, V., & McCoy C.E. (1983). The relationship of Minnesota Multiphasic Personality Inventory (MMPI) profile cluster to pain behaviors. *Journal of Behavioral Medicine, 6,* 77–92.

McIntyre, R. M., & Blashfield, R. K. (1980). A nearest-centroid technique for evaluating the minimum-variance clustering procedure. *Multivariate Behavioral Research, 2,* 225–238.

Melzack, R. (1975). The McGill Pain Questionnaire: Major properties and scoring methods. *Pain, 1,* 277–299.

Merskey, H. (1986). Classification of chronic pain. Descriptions of chronic pain syndromes and definitions. *Pain* (Suppl. 3), S1–S225.

Milligan, G. W., & Cooper, M. C. (1985). An examination of procedures for determining the number of clusters in a data set. *Psychometrika, 50,* 159–179.

Milligan, G.W., & Cooper, M.C. (1986). A study of the comparability of external criteria for hierarchical cluster analysis. *Multivariate Behavioral Research, 21,* 441–458.

Milligan, G. W., & Cooper, M. C. (1987). Methodology review: Clustering methods. *Applied Psychological Measurement, 11,* 329–354.

Moore, J.E., Armentrout, D.P., Parker, J.C., & Kivlahan D.R. (1986). Empirically derived pain-patients MMPI subgroups: Prediction of treatment outcome. *Journal of Behavioral Medicine, 9,* 51–63.

Murphy, J.K., Sperr, E.V., & Sperr, S.J. (1986). Chronic pain: An investigation of assessment instruments. *Journal of Psychosomatic Research, 30,* 289–296.

Olesen J. (1988). Classification and diagnostic criteria for headache disorders, cranial neuralgias and facial pain. *Cephalalgia, 8*(Suppl. 7), 9–96

Osterweis, M., Kleinman, A., & Mechanic, D. (1987). *Pain and disability: Clinical, behavioral, and public policy perspectives.* Washington, DC: National Academy Press.

Overall, J. E., & Klett, C. J. (1972). *Applied multivariate analysis.* New York: McGraw-Hill.

Pope, M.H., Rosen, J.C., Wilder, P.G., & Frymoyer, J.W. (1980). The relationship between biomechanical and psychological factors in patients with low back pain. *Spine, 9,* 137–138.

Portenoy, R.K. (1989). Mechanisms of clinical pain. Observations and speculations. *Neurologic Clinics of North America, 7,* 205–230.

Reesor, K.A., & Craig K.D. (1988). Medically incongruent chronic back pain: Physical limitations, suffering and ineffective coping. *Pain, 32,* 35–45.

Rudy, T.E., Kerns, R.D., & Turk, D.C. (1988). Chronic pain and depression: Toward a cognitive-behavioral mediational model. *Pain, 35,* 129–140.

Rudy, T.E., Turk, D.C., & Brena, S.F. (1988). Differential utility of medical procedures in the assessment of chronic pain patients. *Pain, 34,* 53–60.

Rudy T.E., Turk, D.C., Brena, S.F., Stieg, R.L., Brody, M.C. (1990). Quantification of biomedical findings of chronic pain patients: Development of an index of pathology. *Pain, 42,* 167–182.

Rudy, T.E., Turk, D.C., Zaki, H.S., & Curtin, H.D. (1989). An empirical taxometric alternative to traditional classification of temporomandibular disorders. *Pain, 36,* 311–320.

Sarle, W. S. (1983). *Cubic clustering criterion (Tech. Rep. A-108).* Cary, NC: SAS Institute.

Scheibler, D., & Schneider, W. (1985). Monte carlo tests of the accuracy of cluster analysis algorithms—A comparison of hierarchical and nonhierarchical methods. *Multivariate Behavioral Research, 20,* 283–304.

Schwartz, D.P., & DeGood, D.E. (1983). An approach to the psychosocial assessment of the chronic pain patient. *Current Concepts in Pain, 1,* 3–11.

Shutty, M.S., DeGood, D.E., & Schwartz, D.P. (1986). Psychological dimensions of distress in chronic pain patients: A factor analytic study of Symptom Checklist-90 responses. *Journal of Consulting and Clinical Psychology, 54,* 836–842.

Silverman, W.B. (1986). *Density estimation for statistics and data analysis.* New York: Chapman & Hall.

Smith, T.W., Aberger, E.W., Follick, M.J., & Ahern, D.K. (1986). Cognitive distortion and psychological distress in chronic low back pain. *Journal of Consulting and Clinical Psychology, 54,* 573–575.

Sternbach, R. (1974). *Pain patients: Traits and treatments.* New York: Academic Press.

Tatsuoka, M.M. (1971). *Multivariate analysis.* New York: Wiley.

Turk, D.C. (1990). Strategies for classifying chronic orofacial pain patients. *Anesthesia Progress, 37,* 155–160.

Turk, D.C., Flor, H., & Fydrich T. (1990). *Are interdisciplinary pain treatments efficacious? A meta-analytic evaluation.* Paper presented at the First International Congress of Behavioral Medicine, Uppsala, Sweden.

Turk, D.C., & Rudy, T.E. (1987). Toward the comprehensive assessment of chronic pain patients. *Behavior Therapy and Research, 25,* 237–249.

Turk, D.C., & Rudy, T.E. (1988). Toward an empirically derived taxonomy of chronic pain patients: Integration of psychological assessment data. *Journal of Consulting and Clinical Psychology, 56,* 233–538.

Turk, D.C., & Rudy, T.E. (1990). The robustness of an empirically derived taxonomy of chronic pain patients. *Pain, 43,* 27–36.

Turk, D.C., Wack, J.T., & Kerns, R.D. (1985). An empirical examination of the "pain behavior" construct. *Journal of Behavioral Medicine, 8,* 119–130.

U.S. Department of Health and Human Services (1987). *Report of the Commission on the Evaluation of Pain* (SSA Pub. No 64–031). Washington, DC: U.S. Government Printing Office.

Waddell, G., & Main, C.J. (1984). Assessment of severity in low-back disorders. *Spine, 9,* 204–208.

Waddell, G., Main, C.J., Morris, E.W., Paola, M.D., & Gray, I.C.M. (1984). Chronic low-back pain, psychological distress, and illness behavior. *Spine, 9,* 209–213.

Wiesel, S.W., Feffer, H.L., & Rothman, R.H. (1979). Industrial low-back pain: A prospective evaluation of a standardized diagnostic and treatment protocol. *Spine, 9,* 199–203.

Chapter 24

Relying on Objective and Subjective Measures of Chronic Pain: Guidelines for Use and Interpretation

SAMUEL F. DWORKIN, DDS, PhD
CORALYN W. WHITNEY, PhD

As the organization and content of this book attest, it is now well established that human pain is a multidimensional experience (Melzack & Wall, 1982). One immediate clinical and research implication of this multidimensional perspective, first recognized by Bonica (1977), is that pain assessment in health care settings must be multidisciplinary in nature. Capturing the multidimensional aspects of pain can mean measurement of basic biologic processes spanning anatomy, neurophysiology, and biochemistry. In clinical settings, chronic pain assessment translates to assessments involving multiple biomedical specialities (e.g., orthopedics, neurology, anesthesiology, dentistry, therapeutics) and extends to biobehavioral and psychosocial domains, invoking measurement of such diverse dimensions as sensory psychophysiology, cognition, affect, pain behavior, and adoption of the sick role.

The purpose of this chapter is to present a pragmatic framework for evaluating the usefulness of pain measures generated to assess the multiple dimensions of pain. We first present a recently developed model (Dworkin, Von Korff, & LeResche, 1992) for depicting the various levels at which pain-relevant variables may be measured over time. Using this overall organization, we then discuss, from a practical perspective, critical issues concerning the reliability, validity, and interpretation of pain-related measures. The principal targets of this discussion are selected issues that influence the measures we use to assess signs and symptoms of chronic pain in research and clinical treatment settings.

DECIDING WHAT TO MEASURE: THE LEVELS OF PAIN MEASUREMENT

The first issue to be confronted relates to the multiple levels at which it is possible to measure pain—that is, deciding which of the diverse manifestations of chronic pain a measure has been designed to assess. The model depicted in Figures 24.1 and 24.2 was developed to help us

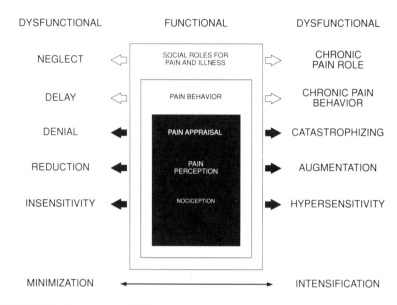

FIGURE 24.1. Ecological model for chronic pain and dysfunction: multidimensional aspects.

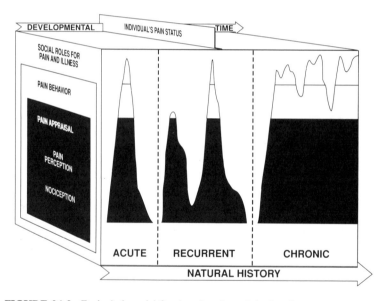

FIGURE 24.2. Ecological model for chronic pain and dysfunction: temporal aspects.

(Dworkin et al., 1992) depict the relationships among physiologic, psychologic, behavioral, and social factors that interact in chronic pain, as elaborated by influential workers in the field (Fields, 1987; Fordyce, 1976; Kleinman, 1988; Mechanic, 1986; Melzack & Wall, 1965; Parsons, 1975; Petrie, 1967; Pilowski & Spence, 1983; Turk & Rudy, 1988).

The model depicts pain phenomenolgy as emerging from the subjective perception of noxious physiologic events that are appraised for their personal meaning to the individual and that then get acted upon through behaviors shaped by social and cultural contexts to yield the role of a pain patient (Loeser, 1980). These processes can go on within normal limits or can be maladaptively intensified. By and large, each pain measure attempts to assess only one of these levels (e.g., pain perception), although some measures assess adaptation at multiple levels (e.g., appraisal and behavior).

Moreover, this essentially ecologic view of

pain as an integration of objective, subjective, and environmental influences is also dynamic— that is, it recognizes that pain states change over time, as depicted in Figure 24.2. Pain experience may be influenced by time-dependent stages of development, from infancy through childhood, adolescence, maturity, and senescence. Only recently, for example, has attention been drawn to the special challenges encountered when attempting systematic measurement of pain in children (McGrath, 1990; see also McGrath & Brigham, Chapter 17, and Craig, Prkachin, & Grunau, Chapter 15). Independently, pain experience over time may be acute, recurrent, or chronic, and pain measures must be responsive to the course of pain fluctuation in its natural history or in its clinical course when treatments are provided. Our current state of knowledge leaves unresolved many aspects of the longitudinal measurement of pain.

Nociception and Physiologic versus Clinical Measurements of Chronic Pain

Our model assumes, at the biologic level, that pain report is associated with information, or signals, being transmitted in the nervous system that has the potential for being perceived and appraised as noxious, aversive, or painful. In most settings in which human pain data are gathered, however, it is not possible to obtain information at the level of basic nociceptive processes (such as neurotransmitter concentrations, specifity of neural pathways being discharged). In clinical settings, the equivalent of the nociceptive level of measurement is the physical level of recording objective pain-related clinical signs through physical examination and to a lesser extent, through laboratory tests (see Vasudevan, Chapter 7, Polatin & Mayer, Chapter 3, and Waddell & Turk, Chapter 2). The resultant findings, commonly labeled ''signs,'' are generally thought of as objective measures of the physical components of pain because they do not appear to require subjectively derived self-report. Common clinical measures include, for example, assessment of range of motion for musculoskeletal pains, use of radiographs and other imaging methods to detect abnormal structural changes, and laboratory tests for indications of painful systemic diseases, such as rheumatoid arthritis or ischemic cardiac pain. While many of these measures are truly free of the patient's

subjective report they are not necessarily free of examiner bias when interpreting these clinical findings, which we discuss below.

In any event, it remains one of the major enigmas of pain assessment that measurements at the physical level, typically clinical signs in the case of pain patients, are often inconsistent with or inadequate to explain subjective reports of persistent pain and suffering accompanied by frequently dysfunctional chronic pain behaviors (Sternbach, 1990; see also Waddell & Turk, Chapter 2).

Measuring Pain Perception

Because pain is a uniquely personal experience, the first opportunity to measure the subjective experience is at the perceptual level. We simply elicit from the person a communication indicating whether pain is present. Measurable nociceptive physiological responses presumed to reflect the presence of pain cannot be used to define whether or not a person is in pain, although they yield valuable information concerning the body's status when pain is reported. The International Association for the Study of Pain (IASP) defines pain as a subjective experience described in terms of bodily damage—that is, pain involves both the perception and subjective report of a noxious bodily state, but the formal definition of pain does not require that a pathologic process be confirmed (Merskey, 1986).

The most common form of assessing pain experience is at the perceptual level, using self-report measures. Measurement at this level attempts to assess the quality and quantity of pain by inquiring into perceived sensory attributes: intensity, location, duration, and sensory qualities (e.g., burning, throbbing, dull, or sharp). The most common measures of pain perception include Visual Analogue Scales (VASs) of pain intensity and the sensory scales of common pain measures, notably, the McGill Pain Questionnaire (MPQ) (Melzack, 1975) and verbal descriptor scales based on psychophysical methods, such as the Verbal Descriptor Scale (Gracely & Dubner, 1987) and the Pain Perception Profile (Tursky, 1976; see Jensen & Karoly, Chapter 9, Price & Harkins, Chapter 8, and Melzack & Katz, Chapter 10).

When pain perception is intensified beyond adaptive levels, it is often assessed as inappropriate augmentation of physical sensations (Petrie, 1967), symptom amplification (Barsky,

1979), or somatization (Simon & Von Korff, in press). In the case of somatization, intensified pain perception may reflect a more generalized tendency to report multiple physical symptoms (e.g., numbness, tingling, shortness of breath, pounding heart), perhaps modifying the diagnostic saliency of the observed pain report (Dworkin, Von Korff, & LeResche, 1990b).

Measuring Pain Appraisal

The measurement of pain perception is known to be influenced by underlying physiologic processes that create large individual differences in pain thresholds and tolerance levels. In addition, pain perception is known to be heavily influenced by "higher order" processes that characterize the cognitive and emotional appraisal of pain—what people feel and think about their pain and its fate. These pain appraisal factors include consideration of the interpersonal context in which pain is encountered (e.g., when with friends or when alone), the emotional significance to patients of their pain (the presence of attendant anxiety or depression), the cognitive attributions they make concerning its origins, the best way to treat the pain and their capacity to control or otherwise cope with the pain problem (see Bradley, Haile, & Janorski, Chapter 12, Kerns & Jacob, Chapter 14, and DeGood & Shutty, Chapter 13).

The cognitive and emotional influences on pain perception are well known and briefly summarized here as a reminder of the need to keep in mind the particular aspects of pain for which measurement is sought. The recent advances in conceptualizing pain as multidimensional have yielded numerous measures of the cognitive (Turk & Flor, 1984) and emotional (Romano & Turner, 1985) components of pain, many of which are reflected in chapters in this volume. When measures of cognitive appraisal reveal excessive intensification, as indicated in Figure 24.1, the pain patient is characterized as catastrophizing or may be assessed as hypochondriacal. When measures of emotional status are intensified, the pain patient may be assessed as clinically depressed or anxious.

Pain Behaviors

The nociceptive, perceptual, and appraisal processes underlying pain experience depicted in

Figure 24.1 and discussed so far reflect intrapersonal, or covert events happening within the individual and hence not yet observable. Overt pain behaviors—behaviors that can be measured by an observer—typically fall into two categories: (1) self-reported or verbal behaviors, as when one responds to a questionnaire or interview, and (2) nonverbal behaviors, as observed facial expressions, bodily posture, gross motor movements, and physical activities (see Keefe & Williams, Chapter 16, and Craig, Prkachin, & Grunau, Chapter 15). Largely due to the efforts of Fordyce (1976) and later, Keefe (Keefe, Gil, & Rose, 1986), measures of pain behavior have emerged as potent indicators of current pain status and as measures of change in response to treatment. Measuring pain in terms of observable behavior at the level of physical activity (e.g., range of motion studies, facial expression, activity level, and treatment-seeking behaviors) offers the possibility of assessing the status of the pain patient without recourse to subjective self-report. However, as we shall see, many behavioral measurements, although not directly involving verbal self-report, nevertheless are contingent on subjective pain experience, as for example, when the patient is instructed to "Bend over and touch your toes." The range of motion, commonly thought of as a clinical sign assessed in objective units of measurement, is nevertheless often implicitly limited by the patient's subjective experience of pain symptomatology.

Intensification of avoidant pain behaviors, as measured by decreased activity levels, increased pain-related interference with tasks of daily living, and excessive treatment-seeking behavior are major factors in assessing chronic pain patients as dysfunctional (Von Korff & Dworkin, 1989). Much of pain therapy, especially in specialized pain clinics, is directed largely at modifying dysfunctional chronic pain behaviors (see Figure 24.1 and 24.2). The aim of such behaviorally focused therapies is to elicit measurable changes in pain behavior, principally as measurably increased activity levels, with less concern for demonstrating comparable changes in self-report measures of perceived pain intensity or affect.

Others have argued the inadequacy of primarily focusing on measuring behavioral change to the exclusion of assessing changes in affective status and pain attributions. The multiaxial pain assessment approach offered by Turk and

Rudy (1987; and Chapter 23) is an example of a widely used approach integrating measurement of the cognitive, affective, behavioral, and interpersonal sequelae associated with chronic pain. The approach of Von Korff et al. (in press) to grading chronic pain integrates measures of pain severity, pain interference, and activity limitations, representing an attempt to assess multiple dimensions of chronic pain in a theoretically integrated manner.

Social Roles in Chronic Pain: Measuring the Impact

Chronic pain behaviors are embedded in social roles for pain patients (see Figure 24.1) that sanction temporary withdrawal from personal and work responsibilities while acknowledging the need for an appropriate increase in treatment seeking. The notion of a sick role, first elaborated by Parsons (1975), implies measuring the reciprocating impact of pain on both the person and the environment. The Sickness Impact Profile (Bergner, Bobbitt, Carter, & Gilson, 1981) measures the social impact of chronic illness and has been applied to the study of impairment, disability, and dysfunction associated with chronic pain. The intensification of the sick role for chronic pain patients is also measured as the increased amount of time and expense associated with loss of productive work together with the heightened costs of medical, surgical, and pharmalogical treatment which the dysfunctional chronic pain patient encumbers. The societal costs due to chronic pain are acknowledged to be very high. Both the Institute of Medicine (Osterweis, Kleinman, & Mechanic, 1987) and the Social Security Administration (1984) have labeled chronic pain as a problem of major societal significance. Attempts to measure the cost of chronic pain and chronic pain dysfunction to the U.S. economy place those societal costs at billions of dollars annually.

RELYING ON PAIN MEASURES: THE CENTRAL ISSUES OF RELIABILITY AND VALIDITY

A schematic model for organizing the levels at which pain can be assessed has been presented because we believe that evaluating pain measures for their usefulness begins with assessing which level(s) of pain—for example, percep-

tion, appraisal, behavior—the measure purports to tap. The next step is to evaluate how well the measure actually performs. We now turn to a more detailed discussion of underlying issues that influence the performance and interpretation of pain measures, focusing specifically on the most basic properties of any measurement instrument, namely, reliability and validity. The emphasis is not on the statistical or psychometric principles and methods that underlie the measurement of pain (or any other aspect of health and illness), although statistical and psychometric issues are engaged. Rather, the focus is on sharing an approach we find useful when evaluating and interpreting chronic pain measurement methods described in the literature or when designing studies requiring the selection of measures at one or more levels of chronic pain assessment.

Reliability and Validity: An Overview

Reliability and validity are the basic underpinnings of all pain measures because they reflect the quality, or "goodness," of a measure. A commonly cited analogy used to clarify the distinction between reliability and validity involves the possibilities when shooting at a target with a bulls-eye at its center. The marksman who is both reliable and valid as a sharpshooter hits the bulls-eye every time; the marksman who is reliable but not valid consistently hits the same point on the target, but it is not the bulls-eye; the unreliable and invalid marksman sprays shots all over the place.

Reliability and validity indices express the extent to which we can depend on a pain measure to (1) assess current status, (2) contribute to a useful diagnosis, (3) yield rational treatment decisions, and (4) evaluate the course of a pain condition over time. *Reliability* (Anastasi, 1988) of a measure refers to consistency of measurement—the ability of a measure to yield comparable results on repeated administrations. Replicability, reproducibility, and consistency can be thought of as useful synonyms for reliability of measurement. A score on any measure is understood to be a combination of the "true" score and some random, or measurement, error. When the measure is repeated, if measurement error is small and random, and if between administrations nothing has changed in the subjects being tested, then the initial scores will be closely related to (i.e., highly correlated with) scores on the repeated measurement and the measure will be assessed as having high reliability. Otherwise, the reliability may be questionable.

Validity (Anastasi, 1988) of a measure is often defined as the extent to which a test measures what it is supposed to measure. If reliability reflects the correlation of a measure with itself, then validity reflects the correlation of a measure with external criteria. A clinical measure such as joint palpation pain may lead to a diagnosis of joint pathology. To determine if the measure is reliable, it may be repeated. To determine if the joint palpation measure is valid for diagnosing joint pathology, results are compared to findings from an external criterion measure; for example, radiographic studies of the joint, which serves as an acceptable standard of comparison. If the palpation pain measure and the radiographic interpretation agree, because the radiograph is the so-called "gold standard," the palpation measure is assessed as highly valid for detecting joint pathology (see also Rudy, Turk, & Brody, Chapter 25).

It is obvious that reliability and validity are intimately associated. A measure that is not consistent with itself (i.e., is unreliable) cannot be consistent with some other measure (hence, invalid). Statistically, reliability and validity are most often expressed as correlation coefficients. The maximum validity that could be achieved using a particular measure is the square of its reliability coefficient. Most helpful would be to provide the reliability of both the measure and the external criterion. The maximum validity that is possible can be determined as the product of the square roots of the reliability of each measure. In our previous example, if the reliability of assessing joint sounds was reported as 0.64 and the reliability of interpreting joint radiographs was given as 0.81, then the maximum validity of the diagnosis using joint palpation pain as the measure and radiographic interpretation as the criterion is $0.8 \times 0.9 = 0.72$. A simple approach to assessing the accuracy of prediction of this measure is to square the resulting "validity" coefficient; that is, the correlation of the measure with its criterion. In this case, about a 50% reduction (0.72^2) in error, compared to guessing, would result when predicting joint pathology from the joint palpation measure (McDowell & Newell, 1987). As we shall see, many clinical measures

of pain are not associated with such high levels of reliability or, perforce, validity.

Finally, it should be emphasized that reliability and validity concerns are heightened when the data being accumulated relate to subjective experience, such as when pain intensity and dysfunctional chronic pain levels are measured and where no objective standard for comparison is available. By contrast, when measurements are derived at the physiologic level, reliability of measurement is generally not a problem because measuring instruments (e.g., thermometers, scintillation counters) which gather objective data can be calibrated to known and very high levels of reproducibility of measurement. For such objective physiologic measures, reliability and validity are replaced by degree of precision and accuracy as the measurement concerns.

Reliability

Two general forms of reliability are of concern. One form assesses repeatability and consistency of a measure and has received considerable attention from those constructing pain measures (McDowell & Newell, 1987). The second form of reliability, interexaminer reliability, infrequently addressed in the pain literature, assesses whether different clinical raters or examiners, assessing the same person would obtain the same results when using the same examination procedures. Intraexaminer reliability, an additional form of examiner reliability, assesses the consistency of observers with themselves on repeated trials; intraexaminer reliability is not discussed here because it is generally considered to be high relative to interexaminer reliability and is not viewed as a significant source of measurement error for most types of clinical research. Recognizing the inherent problems in clinical assessment, the World Health Organization (1971) recommends that reliability indices be routinely incorporated in all health survey reports.

Consistency and Repeatability

This traditional aspect of reliability has received adequate attention in the development of pain measures (McDowell & Newell, 1987). The most common index of consistency or repeatability is the simple correlation coefficient. Two approaches to assessing the reliability of pain measures have been employed. One uses a test–retest method, repeating the measure and expressing the results as a test–retest reliability (correlation) coefficient. Reliability coefficients in the range of 0.8 or higher are considered acceptable, however test–retest coefficients of around 0.9 are preferred (Anastasi, 1988; McDowell & Newell, 1987). As a rule, the measures most commonly in use to assess the sensory, affective, coping, and other behavioral levels of pain show good reliability. For example, Scott and Huskisson (1976) report test–retest reliability of 0.99 for VASs measuring pain intensity. Test–retest reliability of the Illness Behavior Questionnaire (IBQ) (Pilowski & Spence, 1983), which has been used to assess maladaptive responses to chronic pain, reveals reliability coefficients around 0.84 and the Back Pain Classification Scale (Leavitt, 1983) showed test–retest reliability of 0.86.

As many reviewers have noted, test–retest methods for assessing reliability of pain measures appear simple but are deceptively complex in interpretation. For example, in order to ensure minimal fluctuations in pain levels, repeated administrations should be close together in time. Such a procedure introduces the possibility that the repeated assessments are not independent; that is, the subject may be remembering and then repeating the same values given in the relatively recent prior administration. When repeated administrations of the same measure are spaced further apart in time, and different values are obtained, it is difficult to separate instability of pain levels from unreliability of the measure. We shall return to this issue of distinguishing change or instability from unreliability of measurement when we discuss the reliability of clinical examination measures.

Internal Consistency

Partly in response to the complex issues associated with repeated administrations alluded to above, a second approach to assessing reliability examines pain measures for their internal consistency. Internal consistency indices assess the extent to which the individual items or elements of the measure are correlated with each other, and hence presumably measuring the same thing. One form of assessing internal consistency of the items in a measure is to compare results from one-half of the measure

with results from the other half. Several methods for assessing "split-half" reliability have emerged (e.g., comparing odd- and even-numbered items), but the most common methods estimate the correlations among all possible pairs of items. The most frequently used reliability coefficients to assess internal consistency of a measure are derived from methods of Kuder-Richardson and Cronbach (Anastasi, 1988). These approaches, which assess interitem correlations, are in effect assessing the correlation between different versions of the same test. High correlations among items indicate homogeneity of the measure, which is likely to yield consistent results. Generally, acceptable levels for these internal consistency measures of reliability hover around .85, although it may be difficult to achieve these higher values when assessing pain at the level of dysfunctional behaviors. It must be emphasized that if a pain measure is also used to assess change over time, then high levels of consistency (e.g., reliability) are important to be able to distinguish a real change from random fluctuations in pain. At a minimum, the measure should be able to predict itself (McDowell & Newell, 1987).

The preceding sections have discussed various aspects of consistency and repeatability of results as fundamental issues underlying measures of pain and dysfunction. For the most part, measures considered so far are identified as self-report measures or paper-and-pencil measures because they are delivered by interview or in self-administered form. Typically these are in the form of well-standardized scales or tests, for example, the MPQ or the Minnesota Multiphasic Personality Inventory (MMPI) scales used in pain assessment, and the field of pain measurement has been reviewed favorably for the attention it pays to assessing the reliability and validity of self-report pain measures.

Examiners need to interact with patients very little in the case of self-administered pain measures. Similarly, well-standardized formats have been developed for conducting data-gathering interviews. As a result, the examiner typically has limited opportunity to bias the outcome of self-report pain measures. By marked contrast, clinical examination has multiple opportunities for successive examiners to differ in detecting, rating and reporting clinical signs—that is, measurement of clinical findings is associated with reliability issues of a different type (Chilton, 1982; Fleiss, Slakter, Fischman, Park, & Chilton, 1979; Koran 1975).

Consistency Among Examiners: Interexaminer Reliability

A concern of paramount importance for both pain clinicians and researchers is that clinical examiners must also be reliable in their methods or the clinical findings they generate will not be reproducible by others and hence invalid for forming diagnoses and treatment plans or for evaluating treatment outcomes. As we shall see, the problem of interrater reliability in assessment of physical signs and symptoms is a generic one, not limited by any means to pain measurements. Nevertheless, it is fair to say that interexaminer reliability can be expected to be poor in many clinical areas of direct relevance to pain measurement, unless deliberate procedures are taken to ensure that when two or more clinicians examine the same patient for the same purpose, they come away with comparable sets of findings. Nor is poor interexaminer reliability limited to measuring physical signs directly from examination of patients. Studies have demonstrated that radiographic interpretation for clinical problems as diverse as detecting pulmonary lesions (Yerushalumy, 1969), dental caries, and periapical dental conditions (Reit & Hollender, 1986) is associated with surprising low levels of interexaminer agreement.

Statistical Methods for Analyzing Reliability

Because the issues associated with interexaminer reliability in the area of pain measurement have not received so much attention, we will describe more fully some of the statistical methods used to assess interexaminer agreement. We will next present data on this issue, using for these purposes our own studies of the reliability of examinations for painful temporomandibular disorders (TMDs) as well as data from examinations for other painful conditions and conclude the discussion of this topic with some recommendations to maximize interexaminer agreement among pain clinicians and researchers.

The most common statistics used to assess interexaminer agreement are the intraclass correlation coefficient (ICC) (Shrout & Fleiss, 1979) and the kappa statistic (Fleiss, 1981). In

fact, in certain study designs, the two have been shown to be virtually equivalent. Empirically, the particular statistic used depends upon the scale of the pain measurement. The ICC is used for continuous measurements, and the kappa statistic is used for categorical. A continuous measure has, theoretically, an infinite number of possible values. The VAS for pain intensity and the amount, in millimeters, the jaw can open until pain is experienced are both examples of continuous measures. If there are only a few possible values associated with a measure, then the measure is categorical. An example of a categorical measure would be the simple measure of pain coded as either present or absent, or the presence of pain could be further classified into four descriptive categories such as none (scored 0), mild (scored 1), moderate (scored 2), or severe (scored 3), yielding a 0–3 measure of pain.

For either of these statistics, a key assumption behind reliability measures is the independence of the examiner assessments. If the measures are not independent, then it is not possible to determine how much of the agreement is due to the actual measure and how much is due to the biases of the examiners.

Intraclass Correlation

The intraclass correlation coefficient can be used to assess the agreement between two or more examiners on a continuous measure. The exact calculation of the ICC depends on the design (Shrout & Fleiss, 1979) of the reliability study as well as how these reliability results are to be interpreted and used. There are two general study designs: (1) Each subject is evaluated by a different set of examiners, and (2) each subject is evaluated by the same set of examiners. The first case does not allow us to sort out the differences in results due to examiners because there is no overlap between examiners and subjects. Thus, the effects associated with examiners cannot be sorted out from random error.

The second design, much preferred, allows us to sort out the variability due to the subjects, examiners, and the random error. For this second design, the formula for calculating the ICC for a group of examiners depends on the ultimate use of the examiners—that is, whether data will be analyzed for each examiner separately or whether measurements obtained from all examiners will be pooled. For example, a longitudinal study of TMD pain that we conducted over a 5-year period encompassed several hundred subjects and required up to five calibrated (see below) dental hygienist/field examiners to collect measures of pain and related characteristics by performing clinical exams and interviews in the field. Each hygienist/examiner collected data from a different subset of research subjects. For the analysis phase, we needed to assume the hygienist/examiners were interchangeable so that the data could be pooled and analyzed as a whole, not separately by examiner/hygienist. We assessed reliability of our examiners by conducting several studies, already mentioned (Dworkin, Le Resche, & DeRouen; 1988; Dworkin, Le Resche, De-Rouen, & Von Korff, 1990). High ICC indicates that all examiners would have come up with the same measurements if they had all measured one another's subjects. For the remainder of this section the focus is on this latter example of assessing reliability of a group of examiners calibrated to be interchangeable. If examiners are not equally reliable, then the results of the study are questionable.

Examiners will be in good agreement if for each patient (subject) evaluated, the measured responses differ very little from examiner to examiner. If, however, measures obtained by the examiners are quite discrepant, then obviously agreement is poor. The extent of agreement needs to be evaluated in light of the amount of variability that is observed among all the examiner measurements taken on all the subjects. If the examiners are in high agreement, then most of the variability observed among all the measurements is attributed to subjects having different pain experiences (plus some measurement error), rather than to differences in how examiners go about measuring pain. Examiner reliability is quantified as the proportion of variability that can be attributed to sources (subjects, errors) other than the examiners. In statistical terms, this constitutes the ratio of variances and covariances associated with subjects relative to the total observed variability and is called the intraclass correlation coefficient. The following example demonstrates the principles involved in determining and interpreting ICC.

We wanted to measure, in millimeters, the extent to which subjects (normal and TMD) could open their mouths before pain occurred. This measure was determined on $n = 25$ subjects by $k = 5$ separate examiners. To

calculate the ICC we performed a two-way ANOVA to estimate the variability due to subjects (BMS), due to examiners (JMS), and measurement error (EMS). From this we observed the following:

Source of variation	Mean square error
Subjects (BMS)	434.43
Examiners (JMS)	26.30
Error (EMS)	17.89

$$\text{ICC} = \frac{\text{BMS} - \text{EMS}}{\text{BMS} + (k - 1)\text{EMS} + \dfrac{k(\text{JMS} - \text{EMS})}{n}}$$

This example of intraclass correlation indicates high agreement among the five examiners. Moreover, because ICC can be thought of as a ratio of variances, it can be interpreted to represent the amount of variability explained by subjects versus examiners. Thus, in the above example, an ICC of 0.82 means that 82% of the variability in measurements was due to the subjects differing in extent of jaw opening and only 18% of variability in measurement (100–82%) was due to differences among hygienist/examiners plus measurement error. These findings are interpreted to mean that vertical range of jaw opening can be assessed with high reliability by these calibrated hygienist/examiners.

Kappa Statistic

The kappa statistic also measures the extent of agreement, but for categorical data, and does so by comparing the observed agreement between two examiners to the agreement that would be expected if the examiners merely guessed at what the measure should be. Examiners could agree just by chance alone, especially if there are only a few choices available. If there are only two choices, for example, pain present or pain absent, in a pain clinic, just by guessing "pain" all the time, examiners would show high agreement but, because pain is so prevalent in this setting, the apparent agreement would not reflect high reliability of examiners.

The kappa statistic is calculated as follows:

$$\text{kappa} = (p_o - p_e)/(1 - p_e)$$

where p_o is the actual proportion of agreement observed between two examiners and p_e is the proportion of agreement that would be expected merely by chance alone.

A low kappa can reveal poor study design where almost all subjects evaluated fall into one category, such as being largely pain-free. Such situations have a greater proportion of agreement by chance alone as compared to a study where a greater variety of pain levels among subjects is being evaluated. Kappa also affords the opportunity to observe whether a particular examiner tends to disagree with other examiners in a particular direction. (Davies & Fleiss, 1982). The following examples demonstrate some of the issues involved in the calculation and interpretation of kappa.

A group of 25 subjects were evaluated for presence or absence of posterior temporalis muscle pain upon palpation and the following table of results was observed:

		Examiner 2	
		Yes	No
	Yes	2	1
Examiner 1			
	No	1	21

Here, the observed proportion of agreement, obtained by adding the values in the diagonal when both examiners find muscle pains is 92% [(2 + 21)/25)]. However, the expected agreement (calculated as for chi-square test of independence) by chance alone is 79%, which is high also. Adjusting for this chance agreement yields a kappa = 0.62, indicating substantial agreement between examiners 1 and 2. Now, however, suppose we observed the following instead:

		Examiner 2	
		Yes	No
	Yes	1	1
Examiner 1			
	No	1	22

One observation was moved from Yes/Yes to No/No combination. The overall proportion of agreement is still 92% but the expected proportion of agreement is 85%. This increase in the agreement expected by chance alone is reflected in a moderate estimate of reliability with kappa = 0.47.

These examples have the same proportion of agreement (92%), hence the same proportion of disagreement, but the kappa estimates are quite different. Thus, the resulting kappa needs

to be interpreted in light of the distribution of the subjects being evaluated with regard to the pain characteristic being measured.

This is to be compared with a set of 25 subjects who were varied in their actual presence/absence of pain characteristics. For example, we might have observed:

		Examiner 2	
		Yes	No
	Yes	9	0
Examiner 1			
	No	2	14

The percent observed agreement is still 92% but the expected percent agreement due to chance alone is only 52% resulting in a kappa = 0.83. Such a kappa indicates "almost perfect" agreement (Landis & Koch, 1977).

Despite problems associated with interpreting kappa (all statistics are associated with problems of interpretation), kappa remains the preferred statistic for assessing interexaminer reliability, especially preferred over those statistics such as percent agreement, which do not correct for agreement occurring by chance.

The intraclass correlation of the type considered here can range from 0 to 1. The kappa statistic can range from -1 to $+1$; however, the values of interest are in the range of 0 to 1. A kappa less than 0 indicates the examiners agree less often than would be expected by chance alone. If the ICC or kappa statistic is 1, then there is perfect agreement among the examiners. On the other hand, if the estimate of reliability is 0, then there is no agreement among the examiners. The general guidelines (Landis & Koch, 1977) for characterizing these reliability coefficients are as follows: 0.00–0.20 indicates none to slight agreement, 0.21–0.40 indicates fair agreement, 0.41–0.60 is moderate, 0.61–0.80 is substantial, and anything greater than 0.80 is almost perfect agreement. Our own criteria for reliability of pain measurements obtained in our own studies are somewhat more stringent. We view ICC levels below 0.80 and kappa values below 0.6 as not acceptable levels of reliability.

The problem of attaining acceptable interexaminer agreement when conducting objective assessments of physical findings, pervades virtually every domain of clinical research, For example, disagreement at about the 30% level was reported by radiologists interpreting serial radiographs for pulmonary shadows (Yerushalumy, 1969). Dentists in a reliability study of their ability to detect, radiographically, defective restorations or associated secondary caries showed levels of disagreement around 34% and found comparably large variations in observer agreement regarding the assessment of periapical conditions and the adequacy of endodontic therapy as assessed by status of root canal fillings (Reit & Hollender, 1986).

Closer to present concerns, Nelson, Allen, Clamp, and de Dombal (1990) found high levels of observer error (e.g., about 33% disagreement), in a study of the reliability and reproducibility of clinical findings in low back pain. They concluded that more precise definition and a sharper focus on what is being measured are necessary to decrease the unreliability in their examination and history data gathered to diagnose and treat back and leg pain. Stam and van Crevel (1990), in a study of the reliability of examination of non-pain-related tendon reflexes conducted with neurologists, found agreement on reflex scores as measured by ICC to be high among three examiners (ICC = 0.70–0.88), with agreement highest for knee jerks; whereas agreement of reflex symmetry was poor, especially for the triceps (ICC = 0.32).

Similarly, interexaminer reliability among three chiropractors was poor for misalignment palpation (kappas hovering around .00) and was highest (kappas in the range 0.57–0.65) for palpation pain in soft tissues, especially in the lumbar region. The authors concluded that subjective pain reports may be gathered with more reliability than clinical spinal observations (Keating, Bergmann, Jacobs, Finer, & Larson, 1990).

In a series of reliability studies (Dworkin et al., 1988; Dworkin, LeResche, et al., 1990), we reported excellent interexaminer reliability for certain clinical signs of TMDs and poor to marginal reliability for other clinical signs associated with this chronic orofacial pain condition. For example, maximum vertical range of jaw motion was a highly reliable measurement among four calibrated examiners (ICC = 0.90–0.98), whereas examination to detect temporomandibular joint (TMJ) sounds was associated with a marginally acceptable kappa (= 0.62). This pattern of certain TMD signs being associated with high interexaminer reliability whereas others are not is in substantial agreement with findings from reliability studies conducted by Liu, Alan, Clark, and Flask (1989) and Fricton and Schiffman, (1986).

The relevance of these studies, taken together, is that they point to the possibility of using interexaminer reliability studies to make decisions concerning the usefulness of some clinical measurements over others. Additionally, these studies have been selected to emphasize the point that reliability of clinical measurement is acknowledged to be associated with difficulties that cut across clinical disciplines and such diverse clinical examination methods as radiographic interpretation, assessment of physical findings, and even interpretation of electrocardiograms and laboratory tests (Koran, 1975). Several methods for maximizing such examiner agreement are discussed in the following sections.

Obtaining Dependable Clinical Pain Measurements

Interexaminer reliability can be significantly improved by attending to several basic procedures. These procedures for obtaining reliable clinical measurements are especially relevant to clinical researchers who must communicate their methods as well as their data, to allow replication by others. Basic guidelines are available for assessing the confidence one can have in the reliability of clinical measurements (Anastasia, 1988; Chilton, 1987; Dworkin et al., 1988):

Criterion Definition

A clear definition, in measurable terms, of the clinical sign being assessed is absolutely essential. As an example, the detection of unequivocal asymmetry of knee jerks in a neurologic examination was assessed in a reliability study by Stam and van Crevel (1990), who defined reflex asymmetry as a right–left difference of at least 2 mm. Waddell and colleagues (see Waddell & Turk, Chapter 2) have been especially attentive of the need to develop clear clinical criteria and then submit them to reliability assessment. They have paid special attention to establishing criteria that distinguish among physical signs, psychological disturbance, and illness behaviors as each may be manifest in chronic pain populations.

The need to define, in as reproducible a fashion as possible, the clinical signs being assessed should be self-evident, because it is the fundamental basis for determining reliability of measurement. For assessing reliability of measurement it is not sufficient, for example, to simply report that "range of motion" was measured; unfortunately, the criteria for defining a clinical sign are too often stated in such vague or imprecise terms that one cannot be confident about what has been measured.

Examination Specifications

Having defined what is to be measured, the next step is to specify the procedures for obtaining the measurements. The assessment of reliability of clinical findings requires a set of examination procedures stated in clear behavioral terms so methods for obtaining measurements can be reproduced by others. For example, methods for conducting an examination of muscle palpation tenderness should specify locations on the muscle to be palpated, the amount and rate of pressure application, and if palpation pressure is delivered digitally or through mechanical devices of specified size and type. In our own work, for example, we found it absolutely essential to have developed carefully detailed examination methods and specifications, which provide operational criteria for training examiners to conduct reliable assessments of clinical findings associated with TMD. (Dworkin, Huggins, et al., 1990; Dworkin et al., 1988; Dworkin, Le Resche et al., 1990).

Calibration of Examiners

Clinical examiners, even experienced clinician-specialists, must be calibrated to the criteria being used to define clinical variables under study and to the examination methods used to measure those clinical variables. Calibration of examiners refers to specific training procedures undertaken by examiners in preparation for determining if clinical data will be gathered in consistent fashion among the examiners. These training procedures include exposure to specific clinical criteria and examination methods all examiners will use, observing the consistency among examiners on a small sample of subjects and using the feedback from these trial assessments to further ensure agreement on what is

being measured and how the measurements are gathered.

Calibrating examiners to a common set of criteria and methods turns out to be one of the most effective ways to ensure maximum reliability of clinical measurement. It also turns out to be an approach that encounters strong initial resistance, especially among experienced clinicians, who find it difficult to believe they need training in examination methods in order to produce reliable clinical findings. To emphasize that this phenomenon is not restricted to pain clinicians, Yerushalumy (1969) reports a fascinating series of studies involving the ability of radiologists to assess pulmonary shadows and lesions on radiographic examination. Experienced radiologists, feeling "they knew whether a lesion was . . . fuzzy or sharply defined . . . what its shape was" (p. 390) were incredulous to learn of the difficulty in finding a reliable classification for the roentgenographic appearance of the quality of a tuberculosis pulmonary lesion. In our own studies of the reliability of clinical measurements associated with pain of TMDs, we found that calibrated dental hygienists, trained to a common set of clinical criteria and examination methods by expert clinicians, were more reliable in their clinical measurements than were the clinicians themselves when each clinician "went his or her own way" rather than following a common set of measurement methods. Subsequent calibration of the specialist examiners significantly improved their reliability of assessment. For example, reliability of detecting TMJ joint sounds initially yielded kappa = 0.39, which on retraining improved to at least marginally significant levels of kappa = 0.62. Kappa coefficients for uncalibrated examiners ranged from 0.13–0.54 across a broad range of clinical variables. Calibrated examiners showed a range of kappa = 0.52–0.78 for the same distribution of clinical assessments.

It should be emphasized that calibration of examiners is widely recognized as essential to maximize interrater reliability, and the capacity to do so is completely under the control of the examiners. It is also the case that interexaminer reliability is influenced by all of the factors being reviewed here.

Selecting Appropriate Clinical Samples

When reliability estimates are provided, it is necessary to know if an adequate representation of clinical signs was present in the sample being reported on. In a study of muscle tenderness to palpation, Duinkerke, Lureijn, Bouman, and deJons (1986) reported high reliability among examiners using a sample of normal, healthy volunteers and reported excellent (ranging from 83 to 100%) agreement among examiners. Using Scott's (1955) pi, a measure related to kappa, it was demonstrated that the high degree of percentage agreement among examiners was unduly inflated for many measurements (pi ranged from 0.13–1.00) because, in this instance, most of the subjects did not have the clinical sign being investigated; namely, most subjects were pain free. It is clear that reliability studies must include a distribution of subjects with appropriate signs and must also include subjects without those signs, so the reliability of appropriately detecting signs (sensitivity) when they are present and not detecting them when they are absent (specificity) can be most meaningfully assessed; this was illustrated in the earlier section on the kappa statistic.

Assessing Unreliability versus Instability

Wherever possible, studies assessing the reliability of examiners should assure that examiners assess subjects in random order, to control for the effects of repeated examinations and the passage of time. Many clinical signs important to pain clinicians may vary as a function of repeated examination.

Palpation tenderness, joint sounds, and range of motion are all examples of physical signs related to several pain conditions that may yield different measurements when the first and last in a series of repetitions are compared. Thus, the first examiner may discover restricted range of motion associated with a particular joint, while subsequent examiners may report more nearly adequate range of motion, as a function of repeated use of the joint associated with the repeated reliability measurements. To demonstrate this problem, we asked pairs of examiners to simultaneously assess the same TMJ for the presence of a clinically relevant joint sound, either a discrete click or more prolonged grating and crepitus sounds in the joint. Examiners used "dual-headed" stethoscope to ensure that each member of the examiner-pair was assessing the same joint movement. We found that when successive pairs of examiners reported perfect intrapair

agreement, on about 50% of the trials, the results from each pair differed with respect to the immediately preceding pair—that is, joint sounds heard by both members of one pair were different from joint sounds heard by the next pair. We interpret these results to mean that TMJ sounds can change, even over very brief periods of time, perhaps as a result of repeated observations. These findings are more consistent with instability of joint sounds than with unreliability of clinical examiners. To best control for the possibility that unreliability of examiners is confounded with instability, or change, in the clinical sign itself, it is essential that examiners assess subjects in random order and that each examiner assess every subject. Such practices will not eliminate instability of clinical findings, but will better disengage the confounding of interexaminer unreliability from instability of the clinical sign.

Validity

It may appear obvious that a pain measure should reflect, or be derived from, a conceptual or theoretical basis. After all, what is the measure measuring? Validity is associated with just such a questions: If we are measuring pain, what do we mean by "pain." The intended meaning of pain should be revealed by the measures used. Therefore, the validity of a pain measure is an indication of the "goodness of fit" or relevance of the pain measure to the underlying dimension of pain being assessed.

However, as we have seen, pain is a concept invoking multiple dimensions, and as the model we presented earlier depicts (see Figures 24.1 and 24.2), these dimensions of pain are dynamically integrated. Not surprisingly, then, validating a pain measure is much more complex than establishing its reliability (McDowell & Newell, 1975) (which, as we have seen, is not necessarily so straightforward, either).

In order to evaluate if a pain measure is measuring what it is supposed to measure, scores on the measure are compared to external criteria or standards. The most common way to express validity, statistically, is in terms of validity coefficients, which represent the correlation between performance on a pain measure and performance on a criterion measure. Validity coefficients are thus comparable to reliability coefficients, except, as we have seen, reliability coefficients evaluate the consistency of a measure with itself, whereas validity coefficients evaluate the "consistency" of a pain measure with some outside standard.

Evaluating the "goodness of fit" between a pain measure and its conceptual basis is defined as establishing construct validity and is the most intangible aspect of validity to assess. The additional aspects of validity usually assessed include (1) content validity, (2) concurrent validity, (3) predictive validity, and (4) discriminant validity (Anastasi, 1988; Cronbach & Meehl, 1955).

Content Validity

Content validity essentially refers to how well the specific elements, items, or questions contained in a pain measure or in a clinical procedure relate to the aims of the measure. Content validity is usually assessed informally, not statistically. The most common approach is to ask experts to furnish items or to use experts to confirm (i.e.,validate) the clarity, organization, and suitability of a series of items. When specific external criteria are available, item analysis statistics can be used to assess how well each item in the pain measure is related to the external measure, thus giving an index of the validity of specific items.

Concurrent Validity

Sometimes called correlational or criterion validity, concurrent validity involves comparing the pain measure with results from a related measure that serves as a criterion for assessing a comparable aspect of the concept of pain. For example a correlation of .75 is reported between VAS for pain and a 4-point descriptive pain scale criterion measure. Similarly, using the MPQ as a criterion measure, correlations ranging from .60–.63 were obtained between a pain VAS and the MPQ (Huskisson, 1982).

Predictive Validity

Predictive validity is examined through longitudinal or prospective studies, in which changes in pain are expected, either as the result of natural history or as the result of an intervention. The idea is that if a pain measure is valid, it should predict the future course of the pain condition; for example, a measure of postoperative pain is expected to show decreases in pain intensity with the passage of time. If the comparison of baseline and subse-

quent pain measures does not reveal the predicted decrease, then the measure may be invalid for the assessment of postoperative pain. Another possibility, of course, is that the pain status did not change. Hence, once again, it is clear that an external, or criterion measure is needed that serves as the standard for determining whether or not the pain "really" changed. Suffice it to say that assessing the predictive validity of a pain (or any other) measure is difficult, involving complex longitudinal study designs and so, in fact, is rarely done.

Discriminant Validity

In lieu of assessing how well tests predict future outcomes, pain measures can be assessed for their discriminant validity by sophisticated statistical methods such as factor analysis and discriminant analysis. Factor analysis, technically not usually considered under discriminant validity, is placed here for convenience. It is a statistical method that analyzes all the possible intercorrelations of items in a test to determine if these items fall into groups, or factors, that are consistent with the underlying dimensions that form the conceptual basis for the test. In this sense, factor analysis may be thought of as a procedure for determining if independent groupings of items can be discriminated from one another. Factor analysis is typically applied to multidimensional tests that were designed to measure different aspects or dimensions of the pain experience. The MPQ is an excellent example of a multidimensional measure of pain, which has as its conceptual basis, the Gate-Control Theory of Pain. The MPQ purports to measure the sensory, affective and evaluative dimensions of pain experience. Factor-analytic studies of the MPQ have essentially validated its multidimensional structure, finding that the measure does dependably yield useful separate factors, or dimensions (see Melzack & Katz, Chapter 10). The clearest findings relate to the validity of distinguishing between the sensory and affective dimensions; less agreement is reported with regard to the validity of the evaluative dimension (McDowell & Newell, 1987).

Discriminant analysis, a separate statistical method, can be used to validate a pain measure by statistically evaluating the measure's ability to group persons (as opposed to test items, in the case of factor analysis) according to some underlying characteristic they share. It seeks to classify individuals into mutually exclusive groups based on their responses to a series of supposedly related items or measures and compares this new classification to a gold standard. For example, discriminant analysis of the Back Pain Classification Scale (Leavitt & Garron, 1980) was conducted to determine the ability of the test to positively identify persons whose pain was due to psychological distress. The scale correctly classified 132/159 cases (83%). In a sample of low back pain patients without organic disease comprised of persons who showed clinical signs of psychological disturbance and some who did not, the scale correctly classified 78% of patients into those psychologically disturbed versus those not showing such psychological symptoms. The MMPI Low Back Scale was not as effective in discriminating among these two groups, achieving only a 37% correct classification.

Although these more sophisticated statistical methods for assessing the validity of pain measures have an intuitive appeal, it is nevertheless fair to say that assessing the validity of a measure remains at least as much art as science. The challenge seems even greater in the complex area of pain measurement, where the need is to uncover the relative contributions to pain experience of the physical stimulus, the characteristics of the person, and the social environment. Suggested guidelines for the construction of good validation studies emphasize the need for (1) clear statements of hypotheses and the methods used to test them; (2) inclusion of methods that demonstrate what the test does not measure, showing its ability to reject reasonable competing hypotheses, instead of being restricted to confirmations of what the test does measure; and (3) most importantly, use of a variety of approaches rather than relying on a single type of validation procedure.

SUMMARY AND CONCLUSION

A few key issues have been identified as most salient when determining the extent to which a clinician or researcher can rely on measures of pain reported in the literature. Guidelines for evaluating how well pain measures address these issues have been discussed to assist the researcher or clinician in these efforts. First and foremost, it is necessary to be clear concerning the level of pain experience being measured.

Because pain is a multidimensional and complex human experience, it is now understood that relevant pain information can be assessed at the physical (biologic), subjective (psychological), behavioral, and social (environmental) levels. In addition, renewed attention has been called to the temporal dimension of pain, in terms of pain as it arises in successive developmental stages and in terms of its acute, recurrent, or chronic natural history.

Broadly speaking, three classes of pain measures can be identified: one assesses physical signs of pain, reported singly or aggregated into clinical indices. A second type of pain measure assesses subjective experience, typically using self-report questionnaire or interview formats that can inquire into aspects of pain as diverse as subjective perception of pain intensity, extent of affective disturbance or somatization, cognitive appraisal of pain etiology and pain course, and social or cultural influences that shape pain interpretation and coping responses. The third class of pain measurement, and the most recent to emerge as central to our complete understanding of pain is behavioral observation. Behavioral measures have been elaborated, notably by Keefe (Keefe, Gil & Rose, 1986; see also Keefe & Williams, Chapter 16) for assessing the extent to which pain is reflected as disturbances in gross motor movements, including physical appearance, gait, and range of motion. A more finely tuned approach has been developed by LeResche (LeResche & Dworkin, 1988) as well as by Craig and Prkachin (1983; see also Craig, Prkachin, & Grunau, Chapter 15), which examines movement of facial muscles to identify facial expressions of pain associated with different developmental stages, varying interpersonal contexts, and self-reported pain intensity, duration and location.

A prime requirement of any pain measurement instrument is that it clearly denote the level or levels of pain it has been designed to assess. This is nothing less than saying that pain measures should have a conceptual basis and be derived from a relevant body of theory. When empirical approaches are used to derive new pain measures (e.g., Turk and Rudy's, 1988 MAP, see also Turk & Rudy, Chapter 23; or Von Korff's graded classification of chronic pain, see also Von Korff, Chapter 22), it is reasonable to expect those measures to be subjected (as the examples cited have) to independent tests of their reliability and validity using methods such as those discussed earlier.

The fundamental determinants of a pain measure's usefulness resides in its reliability and validity. Reliability assessment evaluates the extent to which a measure is consistent with itself and synonyms for reliability are consistency and reproducibility. A limiting factor for the validity of a pain measure is its reliability—an unreliable measure of pain cannot be a valid one. The most common methods for assessing reliability are to examine a measure's internal consistency (Kuder-Richardson and Cronbach's alpha) and to measure its repeatability over time (test–retest reliability).

A special set of concerns arise over the reliability of clinical findings presumed relevant to pain. The most important concern regards interexaminer reliability. Interexaminer reliability refers to the extent to which successive clinical examiners of the same patient can be viewed as interchangeable in terms of the consistency of the data they each report. Interexaminer reliability among pain clinicians, indeed, throughout medical practice, is known to be unsatisfactory unless steps are taken to ensure that examiners use a common set of examination methods and specifications, have been previously calibrated in the use of these methods, and their reliability assessed through independent reliability studies. The issues surrounding the assessment of reliability in general and clinician reliability in particular are complex because differences in successive measurements can be due to unreliability of examiners or instability of clinical signs due to normal biologic variation, treatment effects, or disease remission/exacerbation.

Validity refers to the ability of a measure to assess an underlying concept or theoretical construct. Informally, the definition of validity is expressed as "Does the test measure what it is supposed to?" The validity of the MPQ, for example, rests on its ability to measure several related but unique dimensions of pain deduced from a theoretical conceptualization (the Gate Control Theory) of pain as multidimensional. The validity of any measure cannot be assessed by a single method or in a single study. The essence of establishing the validity of any instrument to measure pain is that the measurement of its validity must be approached from several perspectives: the measure must be relevant to a conceptual dimension of pain (construct validity); experts must agree that the components of the measure follow directly from the underlying dimensions being measured (content validity); the measure must

relate to independent measures of the same concept, while remaining unconfounded from other variables (concurrent validity); and the measure should be predictive (predictive validity), and should adequately discriminate those who carry the phenomenon of interest from those who do not (discriminative validity). No currently available pain measure adequately meets all of these validity criteria, but this state of affairs applies at present to all aspects of measuring health.

Finally, a great deal of attention is currently being paid to developing more sophisticated methods for improving reliability of measurement (Guyatt, Walter, & Novman, 1987; Ormel, Koster, & van den Brinker, 1989; van Belle, Uhlmann, Hughes, & Larson, 1990; see also Rudy, Turk, & Brody, Chapter 25) and, even more specifically, to increasing the ability of clinicians and researchers to more precisely identify components of change in health measurements that arise from improvement, deterioration, decline, and loss or gain in physical or psychosocial functioning, thus separating observed change in clinical status from issues of reliability of measurement (van Belle et al., 1990). Examples of these approaches, including approaches to reliability addressed by Cronbach's generalizability theory, are contained in this text (e.g., see Rudy, Turk, & Brody, Chapter 25, and Von Korff, Chapter 22). Taken together, these newer methods hold much promise for improving our understanding of the complexly determined and multidimensional nature of human pain experience.

REFERENCES

Anastasi, A. (1988). *Psychological testing*. New York: Macmillan.

Barsky, A.J. (1979). Patients who amplify bodily sensations. *Annals of Internal Medicine, 91,* 63–70.

Bergner, M., Bobbitt, R.A., Carter, W.B., & Gilson, B.S. (1981). The Sickness Impact Profile: Development and final revision of a health status model. *Medical Care, 19,* 787–805.

Bonica, J.J. (1977). Basic principles in the management of chronic pain. *Archives of Surgery, 112,* 783–778.

Chilton, N.W. (1982). Reliability studies. In *Design and analysis in dental and oral research* (2nd ed., p. 421). New York: Praeger.

Craig, K.D., & Prkachin, K.M. (1983). Nonverbal measures of pain. In R. Melzack (Ed.), *Pain measurement and assessment* (pp. 173–179). New York: Raven Press.

Cronbach, L.J., & Meehl, P.E. (1955). Construct validity in psychological tests. *Psychological Bulletin, 52,* 281–302.

Davies, M., & Fleiss, J.L. (1982). Measuring agreement for multinomial data. *Biometrics, 38,* 1047–1051.

Duinkerke, A.S.H., Luteijn, F., & de Jons, H.P. (1986). Reproducibility of a palpation test for the stomatognathic system. *Community Dentistry and Oral Epidemiology, 14,* 80–85.

Dworkin, S.F., Huggins, K.H., LeResche, L., Von Korff, M., Howard, J., Truelove, E., & Sommers, E. (1990). Epidemiology of signs and symptoms in temporomandibular disorders: clinical signs in cases and controls. *Journal of the American Dental Association, 120,* 273–281.

Dworkin, S.F., LeResche, L., & DeRouen, T. (1988). Reliability of clinical measurement in temporomandibular disorders. *Clinical Journal of Pain, 4,* 89–99.

Dworkin, S.F., LeResche, L., DeRouen, T., & Von Korff, M. (1990). Assessing clinical signs of temporomandibular disorders: reliability of clinical examiners. *Journal of Prosthetic Dentistry, 63,* 574–579.

Dworkin, S.F., Von Korff, M., & LeResche, L. (1990). Multiple pains and psychiatric disturbance. *Archives of General Psychiatry, 47,* 239–244.

Dworkin, S.F., Von Korff, M., & LeResche, L.L. (1992). Epidemiologic studies of chronic pain: A dynamic-ecologic perspective. *Annals of Behavioral Medicine, 14*:3–11.

Fields, H. (1987). *Pain.* New York: McGraw Hill.

Fleiss, J.L. (1981). *Statistical methods for rates and proportions.* New York: Wiley.

Fleiss, J.L., Slakter, M.J., Fischman, S.L., Park, M.H., & Chilton, N.W. (1979). Inter-examiner reliability in caries trials. *Journal of Dental Research, 58,* 604–609.

Fordyce, W.E. (1976). *Behavorial methods in chronic pain and illness.* St. Louis, MO: Mosby.

Friction, J.R., & Schiffman, E.L. (1986). Reliability of a craniomandibular index. *Journal of Dental Research, 65,* 1359–1364.

Gracely, R.H., & Dubner, R. (1987). Reliability and validity of verbal descriptor scales of painfulness. *Pain, 29,* 175–185.

Guyatt, G., Walter, S., & Norman, G. (1987). Measuring change over time: Assessing the usefulness of evaluative instruments. *Journal of Chronic Diseases, 40,* 171–178.

Huskisson, E.C. (1982). Measurement of pain. *Journal of Rheumatology, 9,* 768–769.

Keating, J.C., Bergmann, T.F., Jacobs, G.E., Finer, B.A., & Larson, K. (1990). Interexaminer reliability of eight evaluative dimensions of lumbar segment abnormality. *Journal of Manipulative and Physiologic Therapeutics, 13,* 463–469.

Keefe, F.J., Gil, K.M., & Rose, S. (1986). Behavioral approaches in the multidisciplinary management of chronic pain: Programs and issues. *Clinical Psychology Review, 6,* 87.

Kleinman, A. (1988). *The illness narrative: Suffering, healing and the human condition.* New York: Basic Books.

Koran, L.M. (1975). The reliability of clinical methods, data and judgments. *New England Journal of Medicine, 293,* 642–646.

Landis, R.J., & Kock, G.G. (1977). The measurement of observer agreement for categorical data. *Biometrics, 33,* 159–174.

Leavitt, F. (1983). Detecting psychological disturbance using verbal pain measurement: the Back Pain Classification Scale. In R. Melzack (Ed.), *Pain measurement and assessment* (pp. 79–84). New York: Raven Press.

Leavitt, F., & Garron, D.C. (1980). Validity of a back pain classification scale for detecting psychological disturbance as measured by the MMPI. *Journal of Clinical Psychology, 36,* 186–189.

LeResche, L., & Dworkin, S.F. (1988). Facial expressions of pain and emotions in chronic TMD patients. *Pain, 35,* 71–78.

Liu, C., Alan, S., Clark, G., & Flack, K.V. (1989). Reliability of a method of detecting TMJ sounds. *Journal of Dental Research, 68* (abstract), 232.

Loeser, J.D. (1980). Perspectives on pain. In *Proceedings of the First World Congress on Clinical Pharmacology and Therapeutics* (pp. 313–316). London: Macmillan.

McDowell, I., & Newell, C. (1987). *Measuring health.* New York: Oxford University Press.

McGrath, P.A. (1990). *Pain in children: Nature, assessment, treatment.* New York: Guilford Press.

Mechanic, D. (1986). Illness behavior: An overview. In S. McHugh & T. M. Vallis (Eds.), *Illness behavior: A multidisciplinary model* (pp. 101–110). New York: Plenum Press.

Melzack, R. (1975). The McGill Pain Questionnaire: Major properties and scoring methods. *Pain, 1,* 277–299.

Melzack, R., & Wall, P.D. (1965). Pain mechanics: A new theory. *Science, 150,* 971–979.

Melzack, R., & Wall, P.D. (1988). *The challenge of pain.* New York: Basic Books.

Merskey, H. (1986). Classification of chronic pain—descriptions of chronic pain syndromes and definitions of pain terms. *Pain* (Suppl), S1–S225.

Nelson, M.A., Allen, P., Clamp, S.E., & de Dombal, F.T. (1990). Reliability and reproducibility of clinical findings in low-back pain. *Spine, 4,* 97–100.

Ormel, J., Koeter, M.W.J., & van den Brink, W. (1989). Measuring change with the General Health Questionnaire (GHQ). The problem of retest effects. *Social Psychiatry and Psychiatry Epidemiology, 24,* 227–2323.

Osterweis, M., Kleinman, A., & Mechanic, D. (1987). *Pain and disability: Clinical, behavioral and public policy perspectives.* Washington, DC: National Academy Press.

Parsons, T. (1975). The sick role and role of the physician reconsidered. *Milbank Memorial Fund Quarterly, 53,* 257–278.

Petrie, A. (1967). *Individuality in pain and suffering.* Chicago: University of Chicago Press.

Pilowsky, I., & Spence, N.D. (1983). *Manual for the Illness Behaviour Questionnaire (IBQ)* (2nd ed.). Adelaide. University of Adelaide.

Reit, C., & Hollender, L. (1986). On decision making in endodontics. *Swedish Dental Journal* (Suppl. 41):3–30.

Romano, J.M., & Turner, J.A. (1985). Chronic pain and depression: Does the evidence support a relationship? *Psychological Bulletin, 97,* 18–26.

Scott, J., & Huskisson, E.C. (1976). Graphic representation of pain. *Pain, 2,* 175–184.

Scott, W.A. (1955). Reliability of context analysis: The case of nominal scale coding. *Public Opinion Quarterly, 19,* 321–325.

Shrout, P.E., & Fleiss, J.L. (1979). Intraclass correlations: Uses in assessing rater reliability. *Psychological Bulletin, 86,* 420–428.

Simon, G. E., & Von Korff, M. (in press). Somatization in psychiatric disorder in the ECA study. *American Journal of Psychiatry.*

Social Security Administration. (1984). *National study of chronic pain syndrome.* Office of Disability, Washington, DC.

Stam, J., & van Crevel, H. (1990). Reliability of the clinical and electromyographic examination of tendon reflexes. *Journal of Neurology, 237,* 427–431.

Sternbach, R.A. (1990). *The psychology of pain.* New York: Raven Press.

Turk, D.C., & Flor, H. (1984). Etiological theories and treatments for chronic back pain: II. Psychological models and interventions. *Pain, 19,* 209–233.

Turk, D.C., & Rudy, T.E. (1987). Toward comprehensive assessment of chronic pain patients: a multiaxial approach. *Behavior Research and Therapy, 25,* 237–249.

Turk, D.C. & Rudy, T.E. (1988). Toward an empirically derived taxonomy of chronic pain patients: Integration of psychological assessment data. *Journal of Consulting and Clinical Psychology, 56,* 233–238.

Tursky, B. (1976). The development of pain perception profile: A pyschophysical approach. In M. Weisenberg & B. Tursky (Eds.), *Pain: New perspectives in therapy and research* (pp. 171–194). New York: Plenum Press.

Van Belle, G., Uhlmann, R.F., Hughes, J.P., & Larson, E.B. (1990). Reliability estimates of changes in mental status performance in senile dementia of the Alzheimer type. *Journal of Clinical Epidemiology, 43,* 589–595.

Von Korff, M., & Dworkin, S.F. (1989). Problems in measuring pain by survey: The classification of chronic pain. In C. R. Chapman & J. Loeser (Eds.), *Issues in pain measurement* (pp. 519–533). New York: Raven Press.

Von Korff, M., Ormel, J., & Keefe, F.S. (in press). Graded chronic pain status: Concepts, uses and validity. *Pain.*

World Health Organization (1971). *Oral health surveys—basic methods.* Geneva: World Health Organization.

Yerushalumy, J. (1969). The statistical assessment of the variability in observer perception and description of roentgenographic pulmonary shadows. In W. J. Tuddenham (Ed.), *Radiologic clinics of North America.* (pp. 376–392) Philadelphia: Saunders.

Chapter 25

Quantification of Biomedical Findings in Chronic Pain: Problems and Solutions

THOMAS E. RUDY, PhD
DENNIS C. TURK, PhD
MICHAEL C. BRODY, MD

The diagnosis and treatment of chronic pain is still one of the most perplexing and unrewarding problems to deal with in clinical medicine (McCombe, Fairbank, Cockersole, & Pynsent, 1989). Medical management of the individual patient traditionally has been based on the clinical history and physical findings, and how these findings correlate with laboratory results. This classical approach to medicine assumes that the data obtained from interview, examination, and laboratory procedures provide reliable measures that permit valid diagnostic interpretations. However, difficulties in assessing and quantifying the medical signs and symptoms that may be related to patients' reports of pain are well recognized, and there are no universally accepted criteria for scoring the presence, absence, extent, or importance of the results of a particular medical finding or diagnostic procedure (Brand & Lehmann, 1983; Rudy, Turk, & Brena, 1988).

As in other areas of medicine, the importance of clinical data in chronic pain assessment lies in their utility for understanding, diagnosis,

and treatment planning. In the field of chronic pain, however, the successful completion of these goals has been seriously hindered by the unreliability and questionable validity of many of the clinical procedures used to evaluate patients. In fact, some medical investigators have suggested that much of the clinical information obtained from the medical evaluation of pain patients is so unreliable as to be scientifically useless (e.g., Waddell et al., 1982; Dworkin & Whitney, Chapter 24).

The wide variability among practitioners in interpreting clinical data is not unique to chronic pain. Low interrater reliabilities have been found in areas as diverse as respiratory medicine (Spitteri, Clark, & Cook, 1988), psychiatry (Fisch, Hammond, Joyce, & O'Reilly, 1981), radiology (Herman & Hessel, 1975), and interpretation of laboratory specimens (Koran, 1975). Several important methodological and statistical problems exist in studies designed to determine the reliability of physical and laboratory procedures that have resulted in the questionable acceptance of some procedures as "reliable" and others as not. Thus, the first primary objective of this chapter is to highlight some of the sources of error that can result when clinical data are collected, scored, interpreted, and analyzed, and how these factors can substantially impact on the conclusions drawn about a measure's reliability.

Historically, physicians had to make their patient management decisions based on very limited data. More recently, significant advances in medical technology have resulted in the availability of an enormous mass of information to physicians, often with no guidance for systematically organizing the mass of data. As a result, they must rely on intuition and ad hoc decision rules that can result in less-than-optimal decision making. The sheer quantity of information also has resulted in a new set of problems. Foremost among these is the problem of interpreting and integrating information from many different tests. Physicians faced with a vast array of data may actually experience information overload. In fact, some studies have found that providing clinicians with too much data can lead to lower diagnostic accuracy than providing them with what might appear to be too little data (e.g., Sisson, Schoomaker, & Ross, 1976). As Simon (1978) says, "we cannot afford to attend to information simply because it is there" (p. 13).

Given the diversity of biomedical findings collected to evaluate the pain patient, the second major focus of this chapter is to address some of the data integration methods that have been proposed for chronic pain and some of the substantive questions that result from integration methods. Should clinical and laboratory findings be summed in some way to create an overall pathology index? Should the range of findings be weighted differentially? If the answer to the previous question is yes, should this weighting be based on (1) a statistically derived model, (2) clinical consensus as to the importance of each finding, or (3) the purpose of the examination (e.g., diagnosis vs. disability determination)?

Before proceeding it is important to emphasize that our intent in this chapter is not to review the relative merits of specific diagnostic procedures that are used to assess different pain syndromes, because this is covered in depth by other authors in this volume (see Polatin & Mayer, Chapter 3, Gerwin, Chapter 5, Laskin & Greene, Chapter 4, and Waddell & Turk, Chapter 2). Rather, our plan is to review

quantification methods that have been used to record the results of these assessments and highlight some of the potential difficulties that arise from measuring biomedical findings in chronic pain patients and provide the reader with recommendations for resolving these difficulties.

BIOMEDICAL QUANTIFICATION PROCEDURES IN CHRONIC PAIN

A quotation from a popular textbook on medical diagnosis makes this task seem straightforward, "diagnosis requires marshalling all the facts . . . an unprejudiced analysis . . . and a logical conclusion" (Harvey, Bordley, & Barondess, 1979, p. 3). Quantifying biomedical findings that may be related to patients' complaints of pain is, however, an extremely difficult task.

Gathering data ("marshalling the facts") is more complicated than simply conducting a history and physical examination and ordering a set of laboratory tests. The diagnostician must know what to look for in the first place, which remains a difficult and controversial topic in pain patients (see Polatin & Mayer, Chapter 3, and Waddell & Turk, Chapter 2). The information collected also must be systematically recorded, accurately and consistently assessed, and then interpreted appropriately so that valid inferences can be drawn. In sum, the diagnostic process requires a system consisting of at least three separable parts: data-collection devices (e.g., physical, laboratory tests), an observer to record the data collected, and a decision maker to decide what the data mean (Swets & Pickett, 1982). Whatever the method of collection, the resulting data are imperfect, as all data contain some degree of uncertainty and inaccuracy, including the so-called "objective" tests (see Turk & Melzack, Chapter 1, and Waddell & Turk, Chapter 2.

Common Difficulties in Quantifying Biomedical Findings

In our review of over 50 studies designed to undertake the complex task of quantifying biomedical findings in chronic pain and to evaluate the reliability and utility of these findings, several important features that were common across the majority of studies emerged. These features can be summarized as follows:

1. Studies designed to test the association among examination and laboratory findings often neglect to consider or report the reliability of the findings being compared.
2. Some studies that do report "reliability coefficients" have made use of an inappropriate index of interrater reliability (e.g., Pearson correlations).
3. Studies often present reliability statistics (e.g., kappa) without considering sensitivity, specificity, and base rate (prevalence) indices, which may lead to inaccurate conclusions about the accuracy of a specific examination or laboratory procedure.
4. Many scales developed to quantify biomedical findings are rather arbitrary and unique to a specific study.
5. Most investigators do not consider how the number of rating categories selected can impact reliability indices and the sample sizes necessary to have adequate statistical power to test these indices.
6. The large majority of reliability studies of biomedical procedures adhere to classical measurement theory, which does not permit evaluation of the many potential sources of measurement error.
7. Few pain investigators have used statistical procedures (e.g., signal detection theory) that have been proven to be useful in establishing the reliability and accuracy of diagnostic tests in other areas of biomedical research (e.g., radiology).
8. Few studies that evaluate the reliability of biomedical procedures used in the examination of pain patients have considered methodological problems that can limit the generalizability of their findings (e.g., lack of control or "normal" groups to establish base rates, the potential temporal instability of examination findings).

Although it is impossible to address each of these issues in depth within the limits of this chapter, nonetheless in the sections that follow we will attempt to highlight some of the problems and propose some solutions.

Failure to Establish the Reliability of Procedures

All medical data are collected with some degree of uncertainty and inaccuracy in that no test is completely free of measurement error. Thus, the reliability (i.e., replicability, reproducibility, and consistency) of medical tests is a matter of degree. One of the primary reasons for establishing the reliability of measures is the important influence that reliability can have on the conclusions of experimental findings. Measures that demonstrate good reliability are at least as important a component of a well-designed study as are randomization, double blinding, controlling, when necessary, for prognostic factors, and so forth. The use of unreliable measures can have numerous untoward consequences, including the need to use larger sample sizes to obtain adequate statistical power, statistical analyses that result in biased estimates (e.g., correlations that are greatly reduced in size), and even the selection of biased clinical samples (see Fleiss, 1986). In *all* instances, it must be assumed that a biomedical measure is unreliable until proven otherwise.

Unfortunately, some investigators hold to the arbitrary distinction between "objective" and "subjective" measures, with the implicit assumption that the reliability of "objective" measures is assured, or at least cannot contain the same degree of measurement error as patients' self-reports. The impact of subjective bias (i.e., the tendency to respond in a particular way) on measurement error, however, is not restricted to patients alone. All biomedical findings are "subjective" because they involve human interpretation. Thus, the potential for bias and interpretational variability among diagnosticians is always present.

For example, physicians have been found to disagree when interpreting electrocardiograms (Segall, 1966), electroencephalograms (Woody, 1968), and even determining the peripheral pulse of patients (Meade, Gardner, & Cannon, 1968). Additionally, not only have physicians been found to disagree with one another, they sometimes will disagree with their own previous judgments. For example, Coppleson, Factor, Strum, Graff, and Rapaport (1970) asked pathologists to examine the same tissue sample on two different occasions and found that their dichotomous conclusions (malignant or benign) differed 28% of the time.

Inappropriate Interrater Reliability Statistics

A considerable body of literature and consensus among statisticians now exists in terms of what *are not* appropriate statistical procedures to use to quantify interrater reliability. What *are* appropriate statistical procedures remains more controversial, because statisticians continue to develop "new and improved" methodologies as well as evaluate the potential limitations of traditional wisdom.

Briefly, measures of association commonly used in correlational experimental designs *are not* appropriate measures of interrater reliability. These include the use of chi-square for dichotomous and ordinal types of measures, and the Pearson product moment or Spearman rank order correlation for continuous measures. Also, coefficient alpha, a well-known measure of internal consistency among items within a particular test or subtest, is not a suitable index of interrater reliability.

In our review of pain-related biomedical quantification studies, the most frequent problem encountered was the use of the Pearson correlation coefficient to measure the interrater reliability for continuous measures. The Pearson coefficient as an index of interrater reliability has been criticized because it merely measures similarity in judges' ratings of subjects rather than *levels* of interrater agreement per se (e.g., Bartko & Carpenter, 1976). The Pearson correlation coefficient does not identify systematic error, so the coefficient can be high even when there is considerable systematic error. For example, two clinicians can have remarkably different scores, but if the differences follow a consistent pattern (i.e., systematic error) the correlation coefficient will, nonetheless, be very high. In fact, Whitehurst (1984) has demonstrated that two clinicians can be in complete disagreement, but a Pearson correlation coefficient of 1.0 (i.e., complete agreement) can nevertheless result.

The following questions should be asked when selecting an interrater reliability statistic:

1. Does the statistic measure levels of interrater reliability rather than similarity in the ordering of responses?
2. Does the statistic correct for the amount of agreement between raters expected on the basis of chance alone?
3. Is the statistic applicable to the situation in which different groups of subjects are rated by different groups of raters (i.e., not all raters rate all patients)?
4. In addition to providing reliability coefficients, does the statistical procedure permit the investigator to evaluate the magnitude and direction of any interrater bias?
5. Can the statistic be applied to the types of measurement scales frequently used in biomedical research (i.e., dichotomous, ordinal, and continuous)?
6. Are statistical tests of significance available to evaluate the reliability values derived?

Only the intraclass correlation coefficient, when used within the framework of generalizability theory (described below), meets the six conditions listed above. The kappa statistic, when applied to dichotomous and ordinal data (with some cautions noted below), meets most of them.

The Adverse Impact of Prevalence on Reliability Statistics

The kappa (x) statistic (Cohen, 1960; Dworkin & Whitney, Chapter 24), and the related weighted kappa statistic (Bartko & Carpenter, 1976) have become popular measures to calculate interrater concordance when evaluating the reliability of biomedical diagnostic procedures used in chronic pain assessment. The popularity of x stems from at least three useful properties. First, as opposed to correlations or other measures of association, it can be interpreted as a measure of the amount of agreement between two raters or between a rater and a known "true" state. Second, x values, which can range from -1.0 to 1.0, do not simply reflect the amount of raw agreement but the amount of agreement corrected for chance. Thus, a x value close to 1.0 indicates near perfect agreement, whereas negative values denote less than chance agreement. And third, the variance of each x value can be computed and used to test whether a particular value is significantly different from zero.

Despite these apparent strengths, there is increasing evidence that kappa suffers from some rather serious problems (e.g., Grove, Andreasen, McDonald-Scott, Keller, & Shapiro, 1981; Spitznagel & Helzer, 1985). At the heart of the problem is that the value of the x statistic varies simultaneously with sensitivity, specificity, and the illness or abnormality base rate (prevalence). That is, the same diagnostic process may yield different values of kappa depending on the proportions of positive and negative cases in the sample. Thus, differing values of x may be due entirely to differences in prevalence, rather than reliability differences between diagnostic procedures.

To help clarify the x base rate problem and to refresh the reader's memory regarding how sensitivity and specificity are defined for a diagnostic test, Table 25.1 presents the classic 2 × 2 decision matrix. As displayed in Table 25.1, a test's *sensitivity* is defined as the proportion of "true" abnormal cases that the test correctly identifies as abnormal (i.e., the rate of true-positive diagnoses), and its *specificity* is defined as the proportion of "true" normal cases that the test correctly identifies as normal (i.e., the rate of true-negative diagnoses). Ideally, a diagnostic test should have both high levels of sensitivity and specificity. Usually, however, there is a trade-off between these two indices. That is, if the criteria for making a positive diagnosis is lowered so that no abnormal cases are missed, the sensitivity of a test is increased but its specificity is decreased because an increased number of normal cases will be diagnosed as abnormal (i.e., false positives).

Although sensitivity and specificity are frequently used to summarize the predictive merits of a specific diagnostic procedure, they do not take into account the prevalence or base rate for abnormalities in the population under question. That is, another critical factor in evaluating a test's utility is the probability of the occurrence of abnormalities in the population being evaluated. The procedure for computing base rates is displayed in Table 25.1.

The basic problems that have been identified for the x statistic center on the complex interaction between sensitivity, specificity, and base rate (prevalence) values. Although theoretically the maximum possible value of a reliability coefficient like x is always 1.0, indicating perfect agreement, if the sensitivity and specificity of a diagnostic procedure are not perfect (some false-positive and some false-negative errors oc-

cur), the value of x and estimates of base rates will both be affected (Kraemer, 1979). To illustrate the practical importance of the interdependencies among sensitivity, specificity, base rates, and the maximum possible values of x, we can consider the case where a diagnostic procedure used to evaluate pain patients has a sensitivity of 0.50, a specificity of 0.99, and a "true" base rate of 25% of patients displaying abnormal findings. Under these conditions, the maximum x value that can possibility be achieved is only 0.39. Other examples are given in Table 25.2, and formulas for computing additional values are provided by Grove et al. (1981).

As Grove et al. (1981) demonstrated, the x statistic is not a single reliability index but a whole series of reliabilities, one for each set of base rates. In general, as base rates decline so too does the maximum possible value of x. Thus, it is quite possible that an investigator will conclude that a diagnostic procedure is unreliable on the basis of the x value when it is in fact a rather good diagnostic procedure. Additionally, x values obtained from samples with different base rates may *not* be comparable. Similarly, when sample base rates are not representative of population base rates, generalizations of a sample x value to populations may be similarly subject to error (Uebersax, 1987).

A rather striking example of the inappropriateness of comparing x values with different base rates in a chronic back pain sample is provided by Coste, Paolaggi, and Spira (1991), who evaluated the reliability of interpreting plain lumbar spine radiographs. Of the 36 diagnostic categories (e.g., disc space narrowing at L3-L4) evaluated for interrater reliability, 15 categories were found to have x values < 0.40.

TABLE 25.1. General Decision Matrix to Evaluate the Results of a Diagnostic Test

		Test results	
		Abnormal	Normal
"True" state	Abnormal	A	B
	Normal	C	D

Sensitivity = $A/(A + B)$
Specificity = $D/(D + C)$
Base rate (prevalence) = $(A + B)/(C + D)$

TABLE 25.2. The Influence of Selected Sensitivity, Specificity, and Base Rates Values on the Kappa Reliability Coefficient

Sensitivity	Specificity	Base rate	Maximum x
.95	.95	.50	.81
.95	.95	.25	.76
.95	.95	.01	.14
.50	.99	.50	.32
.50	.99	.25	.39
.50	.99	.01	.16
.99	.50	.50	.32
.99	.50	.25	.19
.99	.50	.01	.01

However, 11 of the 15 categories (73%) had abnormal readings reported for less than 15% of the 115 patients evaluated. Thus, concluding that some radiographic procedures have low reliability without considering the ceiling imposed on x values due to low prevalences may have led to incorrectly rejecting certain radiographic interpretations as unreliable.

Two basic solutions to the problems with computing x values for diagnoses with low base rates have been proposed, using kappa-related procedures that correct for the base rate problem when the prelavence rate is low and abandoning the kappa approach entirely. Spitznagel and Helzer (1985), who endorse the correction approach, suggest that what is needed is a quantification of interrater agreement that takes chance agreement into account but that does not confound base rate with sensitivity and specificity. They recommend the use of the Y coefficient of colligation (Yule, 1912) because this statistic is stable over differing base rates and is directly comparable with the x statistic. Using the cell lettering for the 2 × 2 decision matrix illustrated in Table 25.1, the Y statistic is defined as follows:

$$Y = \frac{\sqrt{AD} - \sqrt{BC}}{\sqrt{AD} + \sqrt{BC}}$$

An example may help to highlight the different values for x and Y that can be obtained when the base rate for abnormal findings are low. Suppose that a physician conducts clinical examinations of 108 back pain patients and uses the examination findings to rate the presence or absence of lateral spinal stenosis. Suppose also that MR imaging procedures also were available for these patients and a radiologist independently judges the presence or absence of lateral spinal stenosis. Based on the sensitivity and specificity of radiographic studies used in diagnosing spinal disorders reported by Andersson (1991) and the prevalence rate of lateral spinal stenosis in chronic low back pain patients reported by Haldeman, Shouka, and Robboy (1988), the "realistic" hypothetical results that might be obtained from this study are displayed in Table 25.3. If MR findings are considered the "gold standard," the sensitivity of the physical exam to detect lateral stenosis is 0.875, its specificity is 0.90, the prevalence in this sample is 8%, and, overall, diagnoses based on neurological findings were in agreement 90% of the time with MR findings. However,

TABLE 25.3. An Example of the Effects of Low Base Rate on x and Y Reliability Coefficients

		Neurological findings	
		Present	Absent
MRI findings	Present	7 (A)	1 (B)
	Absent	10 (C)	90 (D)

Sensitivity = $A/(A + B)$ = $7/(7 + 1)$ = .875
Specificity = $D/(D + C)$ = $90/(10 + 90)$ = .90
Base rate (Prevalence) = $(A + B)/(C + D)$ = (7 + 1)/(10 + 100) = 0.080
Kappa = .051, Yule Y = 0.78

the computed x value is only 0.51, which some published guidelines for interpreting x values would suggest is too low to indicate adequate reliability (e.g., Dworkin & Whitney, Chapter 26). On the other hand, the Y statistic is not influenced by the low base rate and provides a more accurate and acceptable reliability index of .78. Thus, interpreting the results of this hypothetical study would lead to opposite conclusions depending on whether x or the Y statistic was used.

There appears to be an increasing number of statisticians advocating abandoning x as a measure of interrater reliability. A wide range of alternative approaches to interrater agreement and its measurement have been proposed, including (1) the use of log-linear models or contingency table analysis (e.g., Tanner & Young, 1985); (2) relational agreement models that do not assume that different raters necessarily use the measurement scales in the same way (e.g., Stine, 1989); and (3) a Rasch item response theory (IRT) measurement approach, described below, to interrater reliability (Linacre, 1989).

Issues Related to Selecting the Number of Categories in a Rating Scale

Often in quantifying biomedical findings in chronic pain, clinical interpretation of examination and/or laboratory findings (the dependent variables of interest) may take on only a limited number of values. Unfortunately, the clinical investigator has no satisfactory solution to the fundamental a priori problem of deciding how many rating categories should be used in forming a rating scale to quantify measurements (Cicchetti, Showalter, & Tyrer, 1985).

The number of categories selected to quantify biomedical findings in pain runs the gamut from the simplest "absent" or "present" of clinical signs and symptoms (e.g., McCombe et al., 1989) to the ordinal category format of "absent," "mild," "moderate," "severe" (e.g., Hendler et al., 1985) and, finally, to the "continuous" scale formats (e.g., degree of pathology from 0.0 to 2.5, Brena, Koch, & Moss, 1976; amount of palpation pressure required to produce pain, Wolfe et al., 1990).

It is important to note that these scales, regardless of the number of categories, all have an underlying metric, that is, a continuous or dimensional scale format. In other words, all are based on at least ordinal levels of measures in that higher numbers reflect a greater magnitude. The discussion that follows regarding issues in selecting the number of rating categories only applies to these types of scales; it does not apply to categorical scales that have no underlying metric (i.e., scales that consist of discrete, mutually exclusive groups that do not bear any magnitude relationships to one another—nominal measurement).

In a computer simulation study, Cicchetti et al., (1985) evaluated how dichotomous, ordinal, and continuous scales of measurement (i.e., the number of categories or scale points ranged from 2 to 100) impacted the magnitude of the intraclass R interrater reliability coefficient. Their study found that reliability increased steadily from a 2-point scale to a 7-point scale and then leveled off after the 7-point scale. The most dramatic increase occurred between the 2-point and the 3-point scale. These findings are consistent with the caveats expressed by Cohen (1983), who quantified the substantial losses in accuracy that can occur when a continuous scale of measurement is dichotomized.

Cicchetti et al.'s (1985) findings, however, should not be taken as indicating that more categories are always better. Rather, they suggest that if the investigator has insufficient information available for deciding what number of scale points is optimal for studying a given clinical phenomenon, choosing more categories (e.g., between 4 and 7) is a better place to start than selecting a 2-point scale. Following data collection, an analysis of scale responses may indicate that two are indeed adequate for the intended measurement purposes, as illustrated in the fibromyalgia study by Wolfe et al. (1990). These investigators,

after considering the over 40 history and physical measures used, concluded that the presence of 11 of 18 tender points (defined dichotomously) provided the most sensitive, specific, and accurate criteria for the diagnosis of fibromyalgia.

How is a researcher to know the appropriate number of rating categories to select? Typically, the number of rating categories is selected a priori, the data are collected from multiple raters, reliability coefficients are computed (e.g., x), and if these values are below a particular cutoff point, the biomedical finding in question is deemed as "unreliable." This practice, however, may lead to "throwing out the baby with the bath water."

As suggested above, it is quite possible that interrater reliability may be good for some categories (e.g., normal) but not for others (e.g., "moderate"). As a practical illustration, consider the interrater frequency data presented in Table 24.4. These data were collected from two radiologists who independently evaluated the results of CT scans of 60 patients with complaints of temporomandibular joint pain (TMJ). The radiologists, in addition to quantifying several more detailed aspects of the scan, made an overall judgment of abnormality on a 4-point scale, 0 = normal, 1 = mild abnormalities, 2 = moderate abnormalities, and 3 = severe abnormalities.

As displayed in Table 25.4, there appeared to be good agreement in terms of the normal and severe categories, but substantial disagreements in terms of the use of the mild and moderate categories. A more detailed analysis of the reliability of each category can be undertaken using a computer program developed by Heavens and Cicchetti (1978). The program not only computes x values for each rating category in the original scale, but also permits the user to ask questions regarding the x values that would result if specific categories are combined.

TABLE 25.4. An Example of Interrater Disagreement for Specific Rating Categories

		Rater 1			
	Category	Normal	Mild	Moderate	Severe
Rater 2	Normal	11	0	0	0
	Mild	2	12	9	0
	Moderate	0	7	6	2
	Severe	0	0	2	9

The results of these analyses are displayed in Table 25.5. As can be seen in the top section of Table 25.5, as hypothesized good interrater agreement was present for the normal ($x = 0.90$) and severe ($x = 0.78$) categories, but not for the mild or moderate categories ($x = 0.34$ and 0.15, respectively). The row labeled "Totals" indicated that the overall x value was 0.50. This value indicates only a moderate level of interrater reliability, and would be classified as unacceptable by some recommendations for interpreting x values (e.g., Dworkin & Whitney, Chapter 24).

The reanalysis of the radiologists' rating data when the mild and moderate categories are combined is displayed in the lower portion of Table 25.5. As can be seen in Table 25.5, the x values for the normal and severe categories are unchanged, however, combining the mild and moderate abnormality categories into one category resulted in a x value of 0.79. Additionally, the overall x value was found to be 0.82.

This example illustrates that overall reliability indices may not tell the whole story about the level of agreement among raters. Investigators should not be too hasty in their rejection of some biomedical quantification procedures as "unreliable," because the number of categories to use in quantifying a particular finding is frequently a "best guess." Like any guess or hypothesis, it should be tested. Additionally, conducting analyses of individual rating categories can provide the investigator with further information about other sources of measurement error, ambiguities in the criteria used to define response categories, and/or the need for more training or calibration of raters (see Dworkin & Whitney, Chapter 24).

The last issue we will attempt to answer in terms of the number of rating scale categories to use relates to the minimal sample size required for assessing the reliability of a rating scale. Cicchetti and Fleiss (1977) evaluated rating scale formats from between 3 and 7 ordinal points and demonstrated that even when raters are extremely different in their use of a particular rating scale, weighted kappa still produced valid results provided that certain sample sizes, based on the number of categories, are used. Specifically, they determined that the minimal sample size (N) necessary is approximately $N > 2k^2$, where k is the number of categories. Based on these findings, this produces sample sizes ranging between about 20 cases for 3-point rating scales to about 100 cases for 7-point scales. The 4-, 5-, and 6-point scales, then, require minimal sample sizes of about 30, 50, and 75. respectively.

The Many Sources of Measurement Error

The two most common experimental methods for determining the reliability of biomedical procedures used in pain assessment involve (1) obtaining two or more separate scorings of the same instrument (interrater reliability), and (2) obtaining two scores from two or more separate administrations of the same instrument (test–retest reliability). Reliability statistics for these scores, based on the classical psychometric approach to reliability, then are computed (e.g., kappa, intraclass correlation).

It is important, however, for the investigator to realize that the central theoretical concept that underlies this psychometric view of reliability is that every obtained test score is composed of two parts, a *true score* variance, which

TABLE 25.5. An Example of Kappa Analyses for Individual Rating Categories

Category	No. Times selected	Average usage frequency	Index of rater agreement		
			Obtained	Expected	Kappa
Normal	24	.200	.917	.199	.896
Mild	42	.350	.571	.347	.344
Moderate	32	.267	.375	.266	.149
Severe	22	.183	.818	.183	.777
Totals	120	1.00	.633	.266	.501
Normal	24	.200	.917	.199	.896
Mild to Moderate	74	.617	.919	.616	.789
Severe	22	.183	.818	.183	.777
Totals	120	1.00	.900	.453	.817

reflects the presence or extent of some patient characteristic, plus an *error score* variance, which is random and independent of the true score (Nunnally, 1978). Reliability from this perspective, then, is expressed as

$$\text{reliability} = \frac{\text{true score variance}}{\text{true score variance + error variance}}$$

The primary difficulty with the classical approach to reliability is that error variance is not a monolithic construct. Measurement error arises from multiple sources, some of which is random, and some of which is systematic based on the experimental design (e.g., differences among raters, changes over time). Classical reliability theory confounds these sources of error by lumping all error into a single term. For example, (1) reliability coefficients based on two scorings of the same instrument (interrater reliability) confound random subject error with differences between raters, and (2) coefficients for the same instrument administered on two occasions (test–retest reliability) confound measurement errors with real changes in subjects that occur between the two administrations.

Generalizability Theory

In contrast to the restrictive and difficult to satisfy measurement error assumptions in classical theory (CT), generalizability theory (GT) (Cronbach, Gleser, Nanda, & Rajaratnam, 1972; Shavelson & Webb, 1981, 1991) provides a flexible, practical framework for examining the dependability of measurements. GT extends CT by (1) estimating the magnitude of multiple sources of measurement error, (2) modeling the use of a measurement for both norm-referenced and domain-referenced decisions, (3) providing reliability (generalizability) coefficients tailored to the proposed uses of the measurement, and (4) isolating major sources of error so that a cost-efficient measurement design can be built (Shavelson et al., 1989). In sum, GT recognizes that there are multiple sources of measurement error, estimates each source separately, and provides a mechanism for optimizing the reliability. The concept of reliability in CT is replaced in GT by the broader notion of generalizability. Instead of asking how accurately observed scores reflect their corresponding true scores, GT asks how accurately observed scores permit us to generalize about patient findings to a defined universe of testing situations.

Computation of reliability and error estimates in GT are based on factorial applications of the familiar analysis of variance (ANOVA) model. By applying factorial instead of simple one-way ANOVA, GT acknowledges that multiple factors contribute to variance in data by partitioning data into segments corresponding to each factor, to the interactions among them, and to random error. The result of these calculations leads to a reliability or generalizability coefficient as well as a measurement model that describes potential sources of systematic or nonrandom measurement error (e.g., significant differences between items in a scale, interrater variation, time effects in test–retest reliability).

The use of the ANOVA model provides GT with greater flexibility than CT approaches in that crossed, repeated measures, and nested designs can all be used to determine reliability coefficients. For example, reliability studies can be designed so that different raters can be used across different subjects, a methodology quite difficult or impossible in other approaches to reliability. Additionally, GT constitutes a framework within which "the theory of 'reliability' and the theory of 'validity' coalesce; the analysis of generalizability indicates how validly one can interpret a measure as representative of a certain set of possible measures" (Cronbach, Rajarathnam, & Gleser, 1963, p. 231). GT suggests modifications of a design to reduce error and improve reliability, which also can be considered as a means to improve validity.

To date, only a handful of studies have applied GT to the study of biomedical data (e.g., Lankhorst, van de Stadt, Vogelaar, van der Korst, & Prevo, 1982; Looney, Smith, & Srinivasin, 1990). Thus, an illustration should help to highlight the strengths of applying GT to the reliability assessment of biomedical measures. Suppose that an investigator is interested not only in the interrater reliability of determining tender points in patients with fibromyalgia, but also whether examination findings have stability between separate examination occasions. The seven potential sources of variability that can be estimated for this experimental design from within the GT framework are displayed in Table 25.6.

Similar to CT, one source of variability, attributable to the object of measurement, is individual differences among patients in terms

TABLE 25.6. An Example of Generalizability Theory in Interrater Reliability Research

Source of variability	Type of variation	Estimated variance components	Percentage of total variance
Patients (p)	Universe-score variance (object of measurement)	1.84	43.5
Raters (r)	Constant effect for all patients due to differences between raters	0.11	2.6
Occasions (o)	Constant effect for all patients due to inconsistencies from one occasion to another	0.59	13.9
$p \times r$	Inconsistencies of raters' evaluation of particular patients	0.03	.70
$p \times o$	Inconsistencies from one occasion to another in particular patients	0.27	6.4
$r \times o$	Constant effect for all patients due to differences between raters from one occasion to another	0.21	5.0
$p \times r \times o, e$	Residual consisting of the unique combination of p, r, o; unmeasured facets that affect the measurement; and/or random variance	1.18	27.9

of the presence of tender points. As displayed in Table 25.6, GT also estimates six additional sources of variability. In the parlance of ANOVA, "main effects" variance for raters and occasions can be estimated, as can their interaction with each other and with the patients factor. Finally, the last source of variability is the residual that includes the unique combination of patients, raters, and occasions, unmeasured sources of variation in this particular data-collection design, and random events.

Table 25.6 also presents hypothetical estimated variance components that may result from the analysis of this example. Because the estimated variance components depend on the scale of measurement used in a specific study, it is common to interpret variance components by their *relative* magnitudes (Shavelson & Webb, 1991). As a heuristic in interpreting the relative magnitude of estimated variance components, the sum of the variance components can be computed and then used to create percentages by dividing each component by this value. This creates an index that indicates how much total variance is accounted for by each component that is independent of the types of measurement scales used.

These percentages are displayed in Table 25.6. As can be seen in Table 25.6, the largest variance component was for the patients factor and accounted for 43.5% of the total variance in scores. This variance can be interpreted as reflecting that patients systematically differed in the number of tender points present. Additionally, the variance for the patients factor can also be used to compute an intraclass correla-

tion reliability coefficient (R_I). In this example, R_I was computed to be 0.71, which was statistical significant at the 0.0001 level (a sample size of 100 was used in this simulation).

Similar to the use of ANOVA to test for significant effects for the independent variables in other types of experimental designs, F-tests can be computed to test whether the amount of variance for each component in a GT study is statistically significant. As displayed in Table 25.6, the percentage of total variance for the raters factor and the three two-way interactions ($p \times r$, $p \times o$, and $r \times o$) were relatively small. Assume for the purposes of the example all of the F-tests for these components were nonsignificant. A particularly important aspect of these findings would be that no significant, systematic bias in terms of assigning scores to patients were found between the raters. This finding would provide strong evidence that the raters were well trained and calibrated in that they reached highly similarly conclusions from their examinations of patients.

Table 25.6, however, indicates that the rating occasions factor accounted for 13.9% of the variance. Provided that we had an adequate sample size (e.g., ≥ 50 patients), a magnitude of this size would most likely be statistically significant. This finding would indicate that the presence of tender points systematically varied for patients from the first examination to the second, suggesting some instability in the presentation of tender point symptoms. However, this finding does not appear severe enough to cause the overall assessment of tender points to be unreliable, as indicated by the relatively high R_I value of 0.71. Additionally, these analyses also suggest that changes in tender points occur systematically for all patients, rather than only for a subset of patients. If the latter had occurred, the $p \times o$ interaction would have been found to be statistically significant.

Finally, Table 25.6 indicates the variance component for the residual showed that a substantial proportion of the variance (27.9%) was due to the three-way interaction between persons, raters, and occasions and/or other unsystematic or systematic sources of variation that were not measured in this study. In other words, this experimental design, like any design, could not account for all of the sources of measurement error.

Methodological Considerations

The ability of GT-type of analyses to identify multiple sources of measurement error is not a substitute for careful attention to methodological aspects that may reduce sources of error *before* a study is conducted. For example, some of the variability in the information obtained in medical histories and interviews is the result of how people perceive their current state of health. Some patients simply do not consider their symptoms very important while others bring even the most trivial problems to the attention of their doctors. Patients' perceptions influence more than just their responses to verbal questions; they can also affect their responses to procedures that are part of most physical examinations. For example, when an examiner presses part of the patient's body and asks if it feels painful, it is the patient's definition of pain, which varies widely among individuals, that will determine whether the answer is yes or no. How a patient interprets a physician's questions, the patient's background and education, and the patient's attitude toward symptoms and disease can all affect the quality and accuracy of the data the physician receives. Thus, the wording of questions should be standardized and careful attention needs to be given to the language used. A striking example of patients' misunderstanding of language was provided by Lilienfeld and Graham (1958), who reported that 35% of their sample of 192 men gave an inaccurate answer to the question, "Are you circumcised?"

Other methodological considerations also can help to reduce the amount of measurement error that is present is a reliability study. These include (1) development of careful, written specifications for examination procedures; (2) developing careful, detailed definitions for the criteria that should be used to measure each clinical variable (e.g., what defines categories such as normal, mild, moderate, and severe); (3) training of examiners in the use of examination procedures and criteria for measurement; and (4) appropriate selection of a study sample to ensure that clinical signs and symptoms are indeed present with sufficient prevalence to determine if examiners can detect them dependably (Dworkin, LeResche, & DeRouen, 1988).

It is important to reiterate that history and clinical examination data are not the only types of biomedical data that may contain unforeseen measurement error. Numerous methodological problems also can affect the quality of laboratory data. Aside from the obvious errors that can occur between raters when interpreting these data, myriad more errors also can occur. For example, different positioning of patients can lead to different interpretations of x-rays; blood samples may be stored, labeled, or taken incorrectly; diagnostic machines may not be accurately or regularly calibrated; worker-related errors can occur in conducting assays, measuring or recording values, and so forth. In fact, Spilker (1986) reviews over 50 common laboratory errors that can lead clinicians to reach invalid conclusions about test results. Needless to say, the reliability of interpreting laboratory data is dependent, in part, on the quality control used to collect these data.

INTEGRATION OF BIOMEDICAL DATA

The inherent subjectiveness of integrating a diversity of biomedical data as well as human information-processing limitations have lead some pain investigators to recommend quantitatively derived approaches to information integration (e.g., Brand & Lehmann, 1983; Rudy, Turk, Brena, Stieg, & Brody, 1990; Waddell & Main, 1984). These recommendations remain controversial (e.g., Million, Wall, Nilsen, Baker, & Jayson, 1982); however, the source of dispute is not whether biomedical data should be integrated, but how and under what conditions. More specifically, physicians evaluating pain patients for the purpose of diagnosis or disability determination rarely, if ever, base their conclusions on a single finding. Rather, the diagnostician collects multiple findings and implicitly integrates this information before reaching a decision. Each finding is not considered separate and independent of the others. Thus, for example, an abnormal lumbar spine x-ray finding without significant physical findings (e.g., range of motion limitations, neurological impairment) is interpreted in a different light than if physical findings are present to substantiate or clarify the meaning of the abnormal x-ray finding.

Despite the recognition that the diagnostician needs to integrate medical findings in some way, at least two common objections are raised to formal, quantitative approaches to data integration. The first objection is that because every patient presents in unique ways, it is not possible to compute scores that are comparable across patients. More specifically, a common clinical position is that the results of laboratory tests can only, or at least most accurately, be interpreted in the context of unique information from the patient's history, physical examination, and underlying pathophysiology (e.g., Spilker, 1986). Thus, it is concluded that the complex interaction among medical data remains distinctive for each patient.

A second objection, which is more specific to chronic pain, is that physical signs and symptoms frequently are uncorrelated. This lack of correlation is viewed as indicating that there is not a statistical basis for integrating findings and, therefore, substantiates many clinicians' distrust of simply adding together biomedical findings in order to compute a total severity score (e.g., Million et al., 1982).

Despite these objections, there has been increased interest and research efforts in recent years to develop quantification methods to integrate biomedical findings. Several common rationales exist among investigators developing systematic data integration methods. These include: (1) integrated, quantitative measures of dysfunction, based on consensus among specialists rather than arbitrary, idiosyncratic systems used by individual evaluators, should lead to improved clinical management, more consistent and reliable impairment ratings, and more equitable disability determinations (e.g., Brand & Lehmann, 1983; Clark et al., 1988; Rudy et al., 1988); (2) an inherent requirement of the conceptualization of chronic pain syndromes is that these are highly complex disorders that require the adoption of statistical methods that are sufficiently sophisticated to cope with this complexity (e.g., Burton & Tillotson, 1991; Rudy, 1989); and (3) improved measurement approaches for evaluating the severity of pain disorders would facilitate more accurate patient selection and, therefore, the scientific basis for treatment trials (e.g., Waddell & Main, 1984; Turk & Rudy, Chapter 23).

Although a diversity of summation or aggregation procedures have been used to combine diffuse sets of biomedical findings in order to compute an overall "index" that estimates the extent of patients' pathology, impairment, or disability, an issue that is common to all approaches is how different findings should be weighted. To date, three weighting strategies have been developed: (1) a simple summation approach that assigns all biomedical findings equal weights, (2) differential weighting schemes in which the weights for biomedical findings are determined arbitrarily by the investigators or from the survey results of experts, and (3) weights derived from statistical models (e.g., regression or discriminant analyses).

Equal Weighting Approaches

Perhaps the most common integration approach to pain-related biomedical findings is to create a total score by simply summing the results of the individual biomedical procedures conducted. This aggregation approach implicitly assigns all procedures an equal weighting of one. For example, the physician-based pathology score developed by Hendler et al. (1985) is derived by summing the results of electromyography, nerve conduction velocity studies, thermography, myelograms, x-rays, and CT scans to create a total "physical findings" score for each patient. This summation approach implies, at least in determining an overall pathology score, that all findings are of equal importance.

The creation of summed pathology scores in the Hendler et al. (1985) study, as in others (e.g., Rudy et al., 1990), was complicated by the fact that not all of these physical findings were available for all patients. This highlights a common problem when creating integrated biomedical scores. Although from a statistical standpoint it would be best to have all biomedical findings that comprise a summed scale available for all patients, from a clinical perspective certain tests may not be relevant or indicated for certain patients. In other words, for heterogeneous samples, ordering all tests for all patients would not be in the best interest of patients (e.g., unnecessary contrast radiographs) and also would be quite costly.

When all findings are not available for all patients, the summation of the number of abnormal findings is inappropriate because simply summing the number of abnormal findings without adjusting for the number of procedures conducted on an individual patient does not permit comparison of total scores across patients. For example, a patient who has 2 abnormal findings out of 4 procedures conducted cannot be considered to be equivalent to a patient who has 2 abnormal findings out of 8 procedures conducted because the probabilities of receiving abnormal results are different for these two patients.

One common solution to the dilemma of an unequal number of procedures being conducted across patients is to form a proportion by dividing the number of abnormal findings by the total number of procedures that were performed. Using this approach would lead to the conclusion that the first patient, in the example above, had a higher pathology score than the second patient. That is, $2/4 = 0.50$, which is greater than $2/8 = 0.25$. However, proportions (1) produce skewed or nonlinear distributions (Wright & Masters, 1982), (2) may grossly underestimate the "true" correlation between proportions and other measures (Mosteller & Tukey, 1977), and (3) produce widely fluctuating or unstable variances because the variance of a proportion is dependent on the denominator of the fraction and thus may produce misleading statistical results (Agresti, 1984).

The most frequent solution to the statistical dilemmas created by proportions is to transform them into logit scores (Armitage & Berry, 1987). The logit transformation of proportions corrects the variance, range restriction, and nonlinear distributional problems. This type of data transformation also is common in other areas of medicine. For example, many laboratory tests of analytes have to be transformed because they do not have a normal (Gaussian) distribution (Spilker, 1986). Additionally, research by Rudy et al. (1990) has demonstrated that logit scoring approaches to biomedical findings that include the differential weighting of procedures, based on a consensus survey (see

below), can lead to a reliable integrated pathology index when all findings are not available for all patients.

The formula to compute logit scores are available in most medical statistics books (e.g., Armitage & Berry, 1987; Fleiss, 1986). It should be noted, however, a difficulty with applying logit scoring approaches to aggregating biomedical findings is that when all findings are normal or abnormal, the computed logit scores take on the value of negative and positive infinity, respectively. Because at least one of these conditions is likely to occur when quantifying pain-related biomedical findings, a modified logit formula provided by Mosteller and Tukey (1977) can be used so that a score can be derived for all patients. This formula is:

$$x = \log_e \frac{k + c}{(n - k) + c}$$

where x is the transformed summated score in logits, $\log_e$ is the natural logarithm, k is the number of abnormal findings, n is the number of procedures conducted, and c is a constant. Although any constant greater than zero can be used, for simple counts (e.g., the number of abnormal findings) the value of .1667 (1/6) is recommended (Mosteller & Tukey, 1977). Application of this logit scoring approach by Rudy et al. (1990) for 263 chronic pain patients and 18 biomedical procedures resulted in summated scores that were analogous to standardized z scores in that the logit scores ranged from -2.849 to 2.849 with a mean of 0.01 and a S.D. of 1.1.

Consensus Weighting Approaches

The simple aggregation of biomedical data to create an overall pathology index has been criticized because it is based on the unwarranted or at least untested assumption that each test result or sign is of equal importance (Rudy et al., 1988). The utility of using a weighted summation procedure that reflects consensual agreement among expert clinicians as to the relative importance of each medical finding in the evaluation of chronic pain patients has been suggested as an alternative to either using equally weighted linear combinations or relying on weights determined by the preferences of individual investigators (e.g., Brand & Lehmann, 1983; Clark et al., 1988).

A commonly used research design to determine "consensus weights" has been to conduct surveys of medical practitioners who have specialized in the area of interest (e.g., impairment ratings, treatment of chronic pain). For example, Rudy et al. (1988) surveyed 80 physicians who specialized in the assessment and treatment of chronic pain (i.e., members of the American Academy of Pain Medicine) and asked them to rank order 18 commonly used physical examination and diagnostic procedures in terms of their usefulness in evaluating chronic pain patients. Coefficients of concordance indicated that these physicians displayed substantial agreement as to the differential utility of the 18 procedures. Based on the relative utility assigned to each procedures by these specialists, weights for each of the 18 procedures were derived by multidimensional scaling statistical techniques. These weights, displayed in Table 25.7, accounted for over 80% of the variance in the experts' judgments.

As displayed in Table 25.7, an abnormality detected during a neurological examination was perceived as being of substantially greater importance in assessing the chronic pain patient than, for example, positive plain x-ray findings. The results of this study suggest that the identification of neurological abnormalities in a patient reporting prolonged pain is perceived to have greater utility and thus should be given more emphasis or weight in chronic pain patients than an abnormality detected by x-ray. It is important to note, however, the data presented in Table 25.7 should not be interpreted as indicating that some biomedical findings are unimportant in the physician's general medical management of a patient, but rather that some procedures are *relatively* less useful than others for establishing the extent of pathology that may be associated with pain complaints.

The results of the survey study by Rudy et al. (1988) were then used in a second study (Rudy et al., 1990) that developed the Medical Examination and Diagnostic Information Coding System (MEDICS), based on the procedures listed in Table 25.7, and tested the interrater reliability of this biomedical quantification system. Additionally, we evaluated the reliability of a total pathology score derived from the MEDICS, tested the influence of unequal numbers of procedures performed across 263 chronic pain patients on the reliability of total pathology scores, and evaluated whether a differentially weighted integration scoring approach, based on the survey results, was superior to a simple summation approach.

TABLE 25.7. Linear Weights for 18 Medical Procedures Used in Chronic Pain Assessment

Standardized weight[a]	Percentage of total[b]	Medical procedure
0.394	15.5	Neurological examination
0.364	13.2	Observation of gait and posture
0.354	12.5	Assessment of spinal mobility
0.339	11.5	Examination of muscular function (tone, mass, strength)
0.317	10.0	Examination of soft tissue
0.301	9.1	Assessment of mobility of weight-bearing joints
0.260	6.8	Assessment of joint mobility other than weight bearing
0.239	5.7	Pain radiography
0.219	4.8	CT scan
0.196	3.8	Electromyography
0.166	2.8	Contrast radiography
0.134	1.8	Examination of internal organs (inspection, palpation, auscultation, percussion)
0.107	1.1	Nuclear medicine
0.082	0.67	Laboratory tests (other than blood)
0.071	0.50	Blood count
0.039	0.15	Thermography
0.009	0.008	Electroencephalography
0.007	0.005	Electrocardiography

Note: Based on a survey of 80 physician specializing in patient treatment from Rudy et al. (1988). Copyright 1988 Elsevier Science Publishers. Reprinted by permission.

[a]These weights have been standardized so that when squared they sum to 1.00.

[b]These numbers represent the standardized weights as percentages and reflect the degree to which each finding contributes to a weighted total index of pathology.

The results of the studies reported by Rudy et al. (1990) demonstrated that physicians can reliably rate the presence of abnormalities (positive findings) of the 18 common biomedical procedures that comprise the MEDICS. Additionally, we found that not all biomedical procedures on the MEDICS need to be performed on all patients, nor do the same set of procedures have to be available for all patients to formulate a reliable total pathology score. Further, our results indicated that a subset of procedures can be used to create a reliable pathology score that is relatively unbiased by the types or absolute number of the procedures performed. This finding offers a solution to a major problem in the quantification of biomedical findings across patients with disparate numbers of assessment procedures.

Similar survey studies of physicians that were designed to evaluate consensus and derive weighting systems have been conducted for impairment and disability ratings. For example, Brand and Lehmann (1983) asked orthopedic surgeons in the state of Iowa to give their average impairment ratings, usual duration of impairment after acute back pain and spinal surgery, and the factors (e.g., history, physical exam, x-rays, psychosocial) that influenced their impairment decisions. Large differences were found for average impairment ratings, although the mean consensus for nonoperative cases was 13 ± 8%. Only 3 of the 67 respondents reported using fewer than 5 factors in determining impairment ratings. Findings obtained from physical examinations, roentgenograms, history, and response to treatment received the highest consensus among the respondents as the factors that they considered most frequently in making their ratings of impairment.

To test the consistency of disability evaluations among independent medical examiners (IMEs) in the state of California, Clark et al. (1988) conducted a set of three survey studies. In the first survey, Clark et al. found that IMEs provided with the same hypothetical case information displayed widely discrepant disability ratings that ranged from 0% to 70%. In the second survey, each IME was requested to evaluate 10 actual, complete case histories that included physical examination, x-ray, and other laboratory test results. Again, they found considerable variability in terms of the disability ratings provided by IMEs when presented with the same reports. In the third survey, specific functional capacity findings related to a patient's ability to work, as required by the California disability schedule, were also contained with the reports provided to IMEs. As was the case in the first two surveys, the disability conclusions reached by the IMEs indicated great variability.

Clark et al. (1988) concluded that their survey findings revealed unacceptable interexaminer inconsistency using the current California disability rating system, a system with which the IMEs surveyed were supposedly experts. After determining that the current rating system did not work, a list of 82 different factors that may be present in the history, examination, and laboratory testing (e.g., history of surgery, positive myelogram, positive bone scan) was mailed to 73 IMEs, who rated on a 5-point scale how important they thought each factor was in determining disability ratings. Although Clark et al. reported that there was general agreement among IMEs on the ratings given most of the factors, no statistical tests were computed to confirm this impression, nor were descriptive statistics other than mean scores for each factor reported. Additionally, the final weighted disability scoring system developed by Clark et al. was *not* based on consensus weights computed from their survey of IMEs, but rather were derived by the authors. Thus, although the survey results were used to help determine what biomedical findings should be included in disability evaluations, the final scoring system that resulted for determining disability scores was based on the subjective preferences of the authors.

Statistically Derived Weighting Approaches

In contrast to deriving differential weights for biomedical data based on the consensus survey approach, some investigators have used statistical models to determine how medical findings should be weighted. For example, Waddell and Main (1984) used multiple linear regression to determine the relative importance or influence of physical examination findings on patients' reports of disability. The beta weights that resulted from the regression analysis were then used to develop a "simplified" weighted scoring system for physical examination findings. Similarly, Burton and Tillotson (1991) used discriminant analysis to determine the differential contribution of 13 examination findings to the treatment outcome of 109 chronic low back pain patients at 1 month, 3 months, and 1 year posttreatment.

Studies that use regression approaches to evaluate the differential utility of biomedical findings are not without significant statistical and conceptual problems. In addition to the problems that can result when ordinal and categorical types of measures are used in statistical procedures that are designed to determine the linear associations among interval level measures (e.g., Agresti, 1989), the primary difficulty with using regression approaches to determine differential weights for biomedical procedures is that the beta weights derived are highly dependent on (1) the patient sample used in the regression analyses and (2) the other factors or variables involved in the regression equations.

For example, in the Waddell and Main (1984) study highly discrepant weights for physical examination findings may have occurred if these findings were used to predict, for example, the test results of standardized functional capacity tests, rather than patients' self-reports of disability. Thus, regression analyses, including discriminant approaches, evaluate how biomedical findings correlate with other findings and the "best" set of weights that should be applied to biomedical findings so that the correlation of these findings as a set with the variables on the opposite side of the regression equation is maximized. In other words, these statistical models do not evaluate directly the relative utility of each biomedical findings independent of other variables and, therefore, do not determine the optimal weights per se that should be used to score biomedical findings.

Item Response Theory

Although the findings reviewed above hold promise for the integration of biomedical findings, to date the "mathematical appropriateness" of adding together a diversity of results from examination and/or diagnostic tests has *not* been tested directly. The following fundamental measurement questions have not been addressed. What is the relationship of each individual item (biomedical finding), independent of the other items, to the derived total scale score? Do some items provide a better "fit" or operationalization of the total scale score than others? How should item fit be tested? Should some items be eliminated from computing the total score because they contain too much measurement error or simply do not measure the intended total score construct (e.g., disability)? Do different response scoring formats across items (dichotomous, ordinal, continuous) bias the computation of a total score and, if so, can this bias be corrected? Is a

total score appropriate to compute for the test results of some patients but not others?

These and other questions that might be raised about summing biomedical findings to create a total scale score are critical questions to answer before an investigator can be confident that a total score really is measuring anything useful. In other words, although it is easy to create summed scores, weighted or otherwise, the result of this simple mathematical operation may produce meaningless results. For example, the sum of a person's age, weight, and height, although mathematically possible, produces as unintelligible, worthless number. However, it is important to recognize that our current discussion is not related to determining the validity of a total score, although of course this also is an important consideration. Rather, we are raising a more fundamental concern with data integration procedures; that is, are the mathematical operations performed on the numbers that result from these procedures to form a total scale score justifiable?

Addressing the questions raised above is impossible from the perspective of classical psychometric theories of measurement because of their primary focus on the association (e.g., correlation) among items in a scale. Thus, for example, measures of internal consistency (e.g., alpha) and factor-analytic procedures do not test directly the mathematical appropriateness of creating summed scale scores (e.g., Hambleton, Swaminathan, & Rogers, 1991; Lord, 1980). In reaction to the serious limitations of classical psychometric theories of test development, item response theory (IRT) emerged in the 1960s. At the present time IRT is having a major impact on the field of test development and psychometrics. For example, large-scale testing programs such as Educational Testing Services's Scholastic Aptitude Tests use IRT models to equate test forms. Major test publishers such as CTB/McGraw-Hill and the Psychological Corporation are using IRT models to develop tests and to equate test scores. They are also using IRT models to help produce standardized achievement tests. IRT-based tests are currently employed by the U.S. Armed Services. Over 800 organizations (e.g., medical, allied health, insurance) have initiated certification, recertification, and/or licensing exams for assessing professional competencies and awarding certificates, licenses, and the like, based on IRT approaches (Hambleton, 1986).

Basically, the major psychometric advances that are achieved by IRT include:

1. Unlike classical test theory, IRT is focused not on scores that result from the combination of individual test items, but on the responses of individuals to individual test items, *before* these items are combined to form a scale score. Each item that comprises a scale can be evaluated for its bias, its level of difficulty, its discriminate ability, and its relationship to other conceptually similar individual items collected by a different method. The results of these analyses can be incorporated into the creation of a common scale score.

2. IRT directly addresses measurement bias and provides a system to create scores that are free from biases that are inherent in different methods of data collection. IRT scoring methods provide "scale-free measures" that allow scores from differing scales to be brought together in a statistical sense in order to improve interpretation of test results. The scoring models used in IRT are predicated on a family of mathematical algorithms which, by design, are scale-free and bias-free. *Scale-free* means that the scale measures that result from IRT approaches to test scoring are not bound by the original units of measurements, which may not be equivalent across test items. *Bias-free* refers to the ability to separate the important underlying characteristics of the respondent from the immediate confines of the test taken.

3. IRT approaches create psychometric or item parameters that are *sample independent*. The presence of a "person parameter" in item response models is used to remove the effect of specific persons on specific tests. This has opened up the possibility of creating testing banks of "calibrated" items from which can be selected items that are optimal for measuring specific constructs in specific measurement situations. Additionally, item response methodology, because of the independence of item parameters, allows the simultaneous testing of multiple or parallel forms or methods of a test, and when some common items are added to each form for the purpose of "linking," all of the test items designed to measure a particular construct across all forms can be compared on a *common measurement scale*.

4. IRT models, unlike classical psychometric models, are *falsifiable* models. A specific IRT model may or may not be appropriate for a

particular set of test data. In other words, specific mathematical models are tested to evaluate whether the observed data are appropriate for a specific model. If so, the model and not the data determines what mathematical operations can be performed legitimately on the obtained data (e.g., simple summation). Additionally, IRT provides explicit tests for the quality of fit between an individual test item and the total scale score that are independent of other items in the scale, as well as tests for the appropriateness of creating scale scores for individual subjects that are independent of other subjects and the items used.

5. Finally, IRT approaches provide explicit methods to score subjects who have missing data on some items as well as statistical tests to determine whether the derive scale score is, nonetheless, "legitimate."

Several investigators have applied IRT methods to pain measurement. Kalinowski (1985) used the ratings of 53 chronic low back patients on 25 of the 78 adjectives found in Part 2 of the original McGill Pain Questionnaire (MPQ) (Melzack & Torgerson, 1971) and evaluated the fit of the one-parameter IRT model (Rasch model) to these data. Kalinowki demonstrated the measurement superiority of using the Rasch model to create a pain intensity scale score and found that the model fit the data of all but two patients. McArthur, Cohen, and Schandler (1989) also used IRT approaches to evaluate the MPQ, and McArthur, Cohen, and Schandler (1991) demonstrated the advantages of scoring pain behaviors with IRT methods, particularly in measuring changes over time (e.g., posttreatment and follow-up).

Although the flexibility of IRT approaches appear particularly well-suited to testing and developing scale scores for biomedical findings in chronic pain, to our knowledge IRT methods have not been used to evaluate the quantification of biomedical data. Thus, as a preliminary attempt to test the potential of IRT techniques of scoring biomedical findings, we evaluated the results of 12 biomedical findings collected by examining physicians for 1,012 back pain patients.

The 12 findings collected for these patients are displayed in Table 25.8. Findings were scored dichotomously (0 = normal or absent versus 1 = abnormal or present). The BIG-STEPS computer program (Wright & Linacre,

TABLE 25.8. An Example of Applying Item Response Theory to Biomedical Findings (N = 1,012)

Biomedical item	Abnormal probability	Infit t statistic	Outfit t statistic	δ Parameter estimate	Standard Error
Spinal mobility	0.713	−0.30	0.40	−1.238	0.075
Mobility of weight-bearing joints	0.372	−0.80	−0.70	0.600	0.073
Joint mobility other than spine or weight bearing	0.310	1.06	0.50	0.909	0.077
Gait and posture	0.870	−0.40	−0.50	−2.455	0.099
Muscle tone	0.288	−0.20	−0.30	1.044	0.075
Muscle mass	0.177	−0.60	−0.50	1.819	0.088
Muscle strength	0.416	−1.10	−1.00	0.342	0.070
Trigger points	0.668	2.10	2.20	−0.974	0.068
Neurological findings	0.533	0.00	0.30	−0.258	0.068
Electrodiagnostic studies	0.363	0.60	0.60	0.665	0.138
Plain x-rays	0.522	−0.50	−0.40	−0.136	0.091
CT scans	0.566	0.10	0.50	−0.329	0.101

1991) was used to test whether these data fit the Rasch IRT model (e.g., Andrich, 1988). Specifically, this program provided separate statistical tests for evaluating (1) the overall goodness-of-fit between the observed data and the Rasch measurement model for the 12 procedures and the 1,012 patients, (2) the goodness-of-fit of each biomedical finding to the formation of an overall physical pathology scale score, and (3) the appropriateness of computing a physical pathology score for each patient. Additionally, the program also permits missing data, so that all biomedical findings were not needed for all patients.

Although space limitations do not permit a comprehensive discussion of IRT analytic approaches to these data, the primary results of these analyses are summarized below. First, the overall fit index for the 12 biomedical procedures was found to be 1.00 (SD = 0.11) and 1.00 (SD = 0.38) for the 1,012 patients. The expected value for these statistics are 1.00, with values substantially less than 1.00 indicated too much dependency (redundancy) in the data, and values substantially greater than 1.00 indicating too much "noise" in the data. An additional finding was that the overall separation reliability index (equivalent to the KR-20 internal consistency coefficient) for the 12 biomedical procedures was computed to be 0.99. Thus, these overall fit statistics indicated that the observed data provided an excellent fit to the mathematical assumptions of the Rasch measurement model.

More detailed analyses for each of the 12 biomedical procedures are presented in Table

25.8. Column 2 provides the proportion of patients in this sample that had abnormal findings for each of the 12 biomedical procedures. As displayed in Table 25.8, gait and posture was the most frequent abnormal finding, and abnormal muscle mass was least frequent.

Columns 3 and 4 in Table 25.8 present two separate t-statistic fit indices for each of the 12 biomedical procedures. The t-statistic labeled "infit," displayed in column 3, is used to test whether a particular item in a scale contains excessive "noise," that is, responses that are not in line with the conditional probabilities predicted by other items in the scale. The "outfit" t-statistic (column 4, Table 25.8) is used to test whether a specific item is unduly influenced by the presence of unexpected outlier or "extreme" cases in the data. Taken together, these two fit statistics can be used to determine whether specific items should be deleted from a scale. As displayed in Table 25.8, all 12 biomedical procedures were substantially below the significant cutoff value of ± 2.0, with the exception of trigger point findings. This evaluation procedure failed both goodness-of-fit t-tests, which indicated that trigger point findings were too noisy and unreliable to be incorporated within an overall physical pathology scale score.

Analogous to the β (beta) weights that result from regression analysis, the Rasch analysis of data produces a δ (delta) parameter for each item in a scale. In should be noted, however, the β values that result from regression analysis are usually linear, while the δ values that result from IRT analyses are nonlinear. Columns 4 and 5 in Table 25.8 present the δ parameter estimates computed by the BIGSTEPS programs, as well as the standard error of these estimates.

Basically, the δ parameter, frequently referred to as the "difficulty" index, for each item in a scale is computed by evaluating its conditional probabilities with all the other items in a scale. For our present purposes, the item δ parameters presented in Table 25.8 represent the point on the physical pathology scale, measured in logits, where the probability of an abnormal response for this procedure is 0.50. Thus, this parameter is a location parameter with respect to the measurement scale and in IRT applications is frequently represented by a data plot called an item characteristic curve (ICC). The ICC function is central to a basic postulate of IRT that states the relationship between subjects' performances on a set of test items and the set of traits or characteristics that underlie performance can be described by a monotonically increasing function; that is, the ICC function (Hambleton et al., 1991).

Figure 25.1 presents ICC plots for 4 of the 12 biomedical findings. The functions plotted in Figure 25.1 indicate that as the level of physical pathology increases, the probability of an abnormal response to a procedure similarly increases. Also, ICC functions predict that patients with higher levels of physical pathology should have higher probabilities of

abnormal findings, and as might be anticipated, abnormal findings with lower probabilities of occurrence, when present, should lead to higher levels of physical pathology. Thus, at the heart of IRT approaches to scale development is the explicit testing of whether the obtained data fit the expected probabilities predicted by ICC functions.

As can be seen in Figure 25.1, the location of ICC functions differ according to each item's δ parameter. The dotted lines in Figure 25.1 correspond to the parameter estimates displayed in Table 25.8. Figure 25.1 illustrates that biomedical procedures with higher positive δ values require higher levels of physical pathology for the probability of an abnormal finding on *that* procedure to reach 0.50. At the extreme in Table 25.8 is abnormal muscle mass, which has a δ value of 1.82. The ICC plot for this procedure (Figure 25.1) indicates that the probability of abnormal muscle mass in this patient sample is quite low unless the total physical pathology score is high. In other words, the high δ value for muscle mass indicates that in these data there is a very low probability of finding abnormal muscle mass without the presence of abnormalities on at least some of the other procedures.

On the other hand, biomedical procedures with lower negative δ values indicate that less physical pathology needs to be present for the probability of an abnormal finding on these procedures to reach 0.50. Two of the 12 procedures, gait and posture and spinal mobility, had δ values of < −1.2, which would be anticipated given their high abnormality rates (see Table 25.8). Figure 25.1 displays the ICC function for spinal mobility.

In sum, the wide range of δ values, from −2.45 (gait and posture) to 1.82 (muscle mass), found for these 12 biomedical procedures indicates that they provide a good, diverse operationalization of physical pathology. In other words, selecting procedures that all had high or low abnormality rates would not lead to a physical pathology measurement scale with a very wide range and, therefore, would not be capable of measuring diverse levels of physical pathology across a patient sample.

Goodness-of-fit statistics for evaluating the appropriateness of scoring individual patients indicated that 28 of 1,012 patients (2.8%) had biomedical finding profiles that were too "atypical" or "noisy" to compute valid physical pathology scores. The BIGSTEPS com-

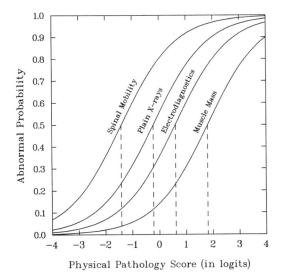

FIGURE 25.1. Item characteristic curves for four biomedical findings.

puter program was used to compute physical pathology scores for the remanding 984 patients (excluding trigger point findings) and these scores are plotted in Figure 25.2. As displayed in Figure 25.2, the consequence of calculating physical pathology scores for these patients resulted in a normally distributed range of pathology scores, another indication of the quality of measurement that resulted by scoring these biomedical data with the Rasch model.

To conclude this example, the data and statistical analyses described above provide strong evidence that IRT approaches to scoring biomedical findings in chronic pain patients appear to hold considerable promise in that IRT measurement models provide detailed information about the quantitative appropriateness of using specific procedures to derive a total pathology score. Further, despite the more rigorous testing of the statistical fitness of biomedical findings to the quantification of overall pathology indices that is inherent within IRT methods, this example demonstrates that what appears to be primitive scoring methods (e.g., dichotomous) to quantify biomedical findings in chronic pain patients are, nonetheless, adequate to meet the eloquence and mathematical challenges of newer psychometric methods.

CONCLUSIONS

Evaluating the nature, extent, and importance of physical pathology has been particularly problematic in the assessment of chronic pain.

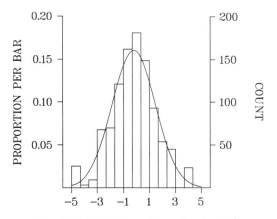

Physical Pathology Score (in logits)

FIGURE 25.2. Distribution of physical pathology scores resulting from the Rasch scoring approach to 11 biomedical procedures for 984 back pain patients.

For many chronic pain syndromes, as opposed to symptoms of acute pain, the etiology, nature, and extent of pathophysiology is often unclear or clouded by other factors. The choice of what biomedical procedures to perform may be more associated with physician preference, conservatism, and experience rather than consensus (Brand & Lehmann, 1983). In sum, there is often little agreement as to the appropriateness and necessity of specific biomedical procedures to evaluate pathology that may be associated with chronic pain. Furthermore, relatively little attention has been given to the methods used to quantify these procedures and their corresponding reliability and validity.

Throughout this chapter we have focused on quantification approaches to biomedical findings per se, rather than on the relative merits of specific procedures. Our intent was to highlight two primary points. Conceptually, quantifying biomedical findings that may be related to patients' complaints of pain is not an uncomplicated process that involves simply assigning some numbers to test results. Rather, we have emphasized that the quantification enterprise is in reality part of a complex, multidimensional decision-making process. At a minimum, quantifying biomedical data requires that investigators (1) determine what biomedical data are appropriate to collect, (2) what are the best data collection methods to use, (3) how these data should be scored, (4) who and what methods and guidelines should be used to interpret these data, and (5) what statistical analyses should be performed on these data once they are collected in order to evaluate if the quantification procedures used produced reliable and valid measures.

Given the complexity of the quantification process, there are numerous potential pitfalls along the way. In this chapter we attempted to present some solutions to these pitfalls, with particular emphasis on how quantification procedures can have an adverse impact on the reliability of biomedical findings and, therefore, the conclusions drawn about the utility of specific procedures.

A second and perhaps more sensitive issue raised throughout this chapter was that many of the statistical procedures that have been used by pain investigators are inappropriate or inadequate to analyze biomedical findings. Specifically, many "traditional" psychometric and statistical models, particularly those taught in introductory courses, are not well-suited to analyzing the types of biomedical measurements collected by most pain investigators and, therefore, can provide deceptive answers to investigators' hypotheses. Fortunately, major advances in statistics and psychometrics have been developed that have direct relevance to improving pain measurement. We have highlighted how some of these advances have direct relevance to improving the quantification of biomedical findings.

It is important to recognize, however, that the newer approaches discussed in this chapter will not cure all of the ills that have afflicted the quantification of biomedical findings in chronic pain. In fact, these newer approaches have their own set of limitations (e.g., Rudy, 1989). Of practical significance to the pain investigator is that much of the literature describing these statistical approaches is highly technical, and assumes a rather advanced level of statistical knowledge on the part of the reader. Additionally, some of the psychometric methods that we have discussed (e.g., IRT) are not contained within standard, widely available statistical software packages. Finally, IRT approaches to measurement require large sample sizes (e.g., over 1,000 cases for some of the more complex IRT models).

Despite these formidable concerns, if we hope to advance the field of pain, it will be necessary for us to develop a passing knowledge of these newer approaches. Moreover, there will be an even greater need for collaborative research teams that include sophisticated methodologists and statisticians, along with the clinical investigators. Familiarity with the newer psychometric and statistical concepts and advances and greater attention to these methods within the pain literature will facilitate understanding and make these approaches more palatable as well as more consumable.

Acknowledgment. Preparation of this chapter was supported in part by Grant 2RO1AR38698 from the National Institute of Arthritis and Musculoskeletal and Skin Diseases and Grant 2RO1DE07514 from the National Institute of Dental Research. We are grateful to Richard A. E. Assaf, M.B., B.Ch., Ph.D., Department of Anaesthesia, St. Vincents Hospital, Dublin, Ireland, for his helpful comments and suggestions to an earlier draft of this chapter.

REFERENCES

Agresti, A. (1984). *Analysis of ordinal categorical data.* New York: Wiley.

Agresti, A. (1989). Tutorial on modeling ordered categorical response data. *Psychological Bulletin, 105,* 290–301.

Andersson, G. B. J. (1991). Sensitivity, specificity, and predictive value: A general issue in the screening for disease and in the interpretation of diagnostic studies in spinal disorder. In J. W. Frymoyer (Ed.), *The adult spine: Principles and practice* (pp. 277–287). New York: Raven Press.

Andrich, D. (1988). *Rasch models for measurement.* Beverly Hills, CA: Sage.

Armitage, P., & Berry, G. (1987). *Statistical methods in medical research* (2nd ed.). Oxford: Blackwell Scientific Publications.

Bartko, J. J., & Carpenter, W. T. (1976). On the methods and theory of reliability. *Journal of Nervous and Mental Disease, 163,* 307–317.

Brand, R. A., & Lehmann, T. R. (1983). Low-back impairment rating practices of orthopaedic surgeons. *Spine, 8,* 75–78.

Brena, S. F., Koch, D. L., & Moss, R. M. (1976). Reliability of the "Pain Estimate" model. *Anesthesiology Review, 3,* 28–29.

Burton, A. K., & Tillotson, K. M. (1991). Prediction of the clinical course of low-back trouble using multivariable models. *Spine, 16,* 7–14.

Cicchetti, D. V., & Fleiss, J. L. (1977). Comparison of the null distributions of weighted kappa and the C ordinal statistic. *Applied Psychological Measurement, 1,* 195–201.

Cicchetti, D. V., Showalter, D., & Tyrer, P. J. (1985). The effect of number of rating scale categories on levels of interrater reliability: A monte carlo investigation. *Applied Psychological Measurement, 9,* 31–36.

Clark, W. L., Haldeman, S., Morris, J. J., Schulenberger, C., Trauner, D., & White, A. (1988). Back impairment and disability determination: Another attempt at objective, reliable rating. *Spine, 13,* 332–341.

Cohen, J. (1960). A coefficient of agreement for nominal scales. *Educational and Psychological Measurement, 20,* 37–46.

Cohen, J. (1983). The cost of dichotomization. *Applied Psychological Measurement, 7,* 249–253.

Coppleson, L. W., Factor, R. M., Strum, S. B., Graff, P. W., & Rapaport, H. L. (1970). Observer disagreement in the classification and histology of Hodgkin's disease. *Journal of the National Cancer Institute, 45,* 731–740.

Coste, J., Paolaggi, J. B., & Spira, A. (1991). Reliability of interpretation of plain lumbar spine radiographs in benign, mechanical low-back pain. *Spine, 16,* 426–428.

Cronbach, L. J., Gleser, G. C., Nanda, H., & Rajaratnam, N. (1972). *The dependability of behavioral measurements: Theory of generalizability of scores and profiles.* New York: Wiley.

Cronbach, L., Rajaratnam, N., & Gleser, G. (1963). Theory of generalizability: A liberalization of reliability theory. *British Journal of Mathematical and Statistical Psychology, 16,* 137–163.

Dworkin, S. F., LeResche, L., & DeRouen, T. (1988). Reliability of clinical measurement in temporomandibular disorders. *Clinical Journal of Pain, 4,* 89–99.

Fisch, H. U., Hammond, K. R., Joyce, C. R. B., & O'Reilly. (1981). An experimental study of the clinical judgment of general physicians in evaluating and prescribing for depression. *British Journal of Psychiatry, 138,* 100–109.

Fleiss, J. L. (1986). *The design and analysis of clinical experiments*. New York: Wiley.

Grove, W. M., Andreasen, N. C., McDonald-Scott, P., Keller, M. B., & Shapiro, R. W. (1981). Reliability studies of psychiatric diagnosis. *Archives of General Psychiatry, 38,* 408–413.

Haldeman, S., Shouka, M., & Robboy, S. (1988). Computed tomography, electrodiagnostic and clinical findings in chronic workers' compensation patients with back and leg pain. *Spine, 13,* 345–350.

Hambleton, R. K. (1986). The changing conception of measurement: A commentary. *Applied Psychological Measurement, 10,* 415–421.

Hambleton, R. K., Swaminathan, H., & Rogers, H. J. (1991). *Fundamentals of item response theory.* Newbury Park, CA: Sage.

Harvey, A. M., Bordley, J. I., & Barondess, J. A. (1979). *Differential diagnosis: The interpretation of clinical evidence* (3rd ed.). Philadelphia: Saunders.

Heavens, R., & Cicchetti, D. V. (1978). A computer program for calculating rater agreement and bias statistics using contingency table input. *Journal of the American Statistical Association, 21,* 366–370.

Hendler, N., Mollett, A., Vierstein, M., Schroeder, D., Rybock, J., Campbell, J., Levin, S., & Long, D. (1985). A comparison between the MMPI and the ''Mensana Clinic Back Pain Test'' for validating the complaint of chronic back pain in women. *Pain, 23,* 243–251.

Herman, P. G., & Hessel, S. J. (1975). Accuracy and its relationship to experience in the interpretation of chest radiographs. *Investigative Radiology, 10,* 62–67.

Kalinowski, A. G. (1985). Measuring clinical pain. *Journal of Psychopathology and Behavioral Assessment, 7,* 329–349.

Koran, L. M. (1975). The reliability of clinical methods, data and judgments. *New England Journal of Medicine, 293,* 642–646, 695–701.

Kraemer, H. C. (1979). Ramifications of a population model for x as a coefficient of reliability. *Psychometrika, 44,* 461–472.

Lankhorst, G. J., van de Stadt, R. J., Vodeelaar, T. W., van der Korst, J. K., & Prevo, A. J. H. (1982). Objectivity and repeatability of measurements in low back pain. *Scandavanian Journal of Rehabilation Medicine, 14,* 21–26.

Lilienfeld, A., & Graham, S. (1958). Validity of determining circumcision status by questionnaire as related to epidemiological studies of cancer of the cervix. *Journal of the National Cancer Institute, 21,* 713–770.

Linacre, J. M. (1989). *Many-faceted Rasch measurement.* Chicago: MESA Press.

Looney, M. A., Smith, S. L., & Srinivasan, S. (1990). Establishing reliability of biomechanical data using univariate and multivariate approaches. *Research Quarterly for Exercise and Sport, 61,* 154–160.

Lord, F. M. (1980). *Applications of item response theory to practical testing problems.* Hillsdale, NJ: Erlbaum.

McArthur, D. L., Cohen, M. J., & Schandler, S. L. (1989). A philosophy for measurement of pain. In C. R. Chapman, & J. D. Loeser (Eds.), *Advances in pain research and therapy* (pp. 37–50). New York: Raven Press.

McArthur, D. L., Cohen, M. J., & Schandler, S. L. (1991). Rasch analysis of functional assessment scales: An example using pain behaviors. *Archives of Physical Medicine and Rehabilitation, 72,* 296–304.

McCombe, P. F., Fairbank, J. C. T., Cockersole, B. C., & Pynsent, P. B. (1989). Reproducibility of physical signs in low-back pain. *Spine, 14,* 908–918.

Meade, T. W., Gardner, M. J., & Cannon, P. (1968). Observer variability in recording the peripheral pulses. *British Heart Journal, 30,* 661–665.

Melzack, R., & Torgeson, W. (1971). On the language of pain. *Anesthesiology, 34,* 50–59.

Million, R., Wall, W., Nilsen, K., Baker, R., & Jayson, M. (1982). Assessment of the progress of the back pain patient. *Spine, 7,* 204–212.

Mosteller, F., & Tukey, J. W. (1977). *Data analysis and regression.* Reading, MA: Addison-Wesley.

Nunnally, J. C. (1978). *Psychometric theory.* New York: McGraw-Hill.

Rudy, T. E. (1989). Innovations in pain psychometrics. In C. R. Chapman & J. D. Loeser (Eds.), *Advances in pain research and therapy* (pp. 51–61). New York: Raven Press.

Rudy, T. E., Turk, D. C., & Brena, S. F. (1988). Differential utility of medical procedures in the assessment of chronic pain patients. *Pain, 34,* 53–60.

Rudy, T. E., Turk, D. C., Brena, S. F., Stieg, R. L., & Brody, M. C. (1990). Quantification of biomedical findings of chronic pain patients: Development of an index of pathology. *Pain, 42,* 167–182.

Segall, H. N. (1966). The electrocardiogram and its interpretation: A study of reports by 20 physicians on a set of 100 electrocardiograms. *Canadian Medical Association Journal, 82,* 2–6.

Shavelson, R. J., & Webb, N. M. (1981). Generalizability theory: 1973–1980. *British Journal of Mathematical and Statistical Psychology, 34,* 133–166.

Shavelson, R. J., & Webb, N. M. (1991). *Generalizability theory: A primer.* Newbury Park, CA: Sage.

Shavelson, R. J., Webb, N. M., & Rowley, G. L. (1989). Generalizability theory. *American Psychologist, 44*(6), 922–932.

Simon, H. A. (1978). Rationality as a process and product of thought. *The American Economic Review, 68,* 1–16.

Sisson, J. C., Schoomaker, E. B., & Ross, J. C. (1976). Clinical decision analysis: The hazard of using additional data. *Journal of the American Medical Association, 236,* 1259–1263.

Spilker, B. (1986). *Guide to clinical interpretation of data.* New York: Raven Press.

Spitteri, M. A., Clark, S. W., & Cook, D. G. (1988). Reliability of eliciting physical signs in examination of the chest. *Lancet, 1,* 873–875.

Spitznagel, E. L., & Helzer, J. E. (1985). A proposed solution to the base rate problem in the kappa statistic. *Archives of General Psychiatry, 42,* 725–728.

Stine, W. W. (1989). Interobserver relational agreement. *Psychological Bulletin, 106,* 341–347.

Swets, J. A., & Pickett, R. M. (1982). Evaluation of diagnostic systems. New York: Academic Press.

Tanner, M. A., & Young, M. A. (1985). Modeling agreement among raters. *Journal of the American Statistical Association, 80,* 175–180.

Uebersax, J. S. (1987). Diversity of decision-making models and the measurement of interrater agreement. *Psychological Bulletin, 101,* 140–146.

Waddell, G., & Main, C. J. (1984). Assessment of severity in low-back disorders. *Spine, 9,* 204–208.

Waddell, G., Main, C. J., Morris, E. W., & Venner, R. M., Rae, P. S., Sharmy, S. H., & Galloway, H. (1982). Normality and reliability in the clinical assessment of backache. *British Medical Journal, 284,* 1519–1523.

Whitehurst, G. J. (1984). Interrater agreement for journal manuscript reviews. *American Psychologist, 39,* 22–28.

Woody, R. H. (1968). Interjudge reliability in clinical electroencephalography. *Journal of Clinical Psychology, 24,* 251–256.

Wolfe, F., Smythe, H. A., Yunus, M. B. et al. (1990). The American College of Rheumatology 1990 criteria for the classification of fibromyalgia. *Arthritis and Rheumatism, 33,* 160–172.

Wright, B. D., & Linacre, J. M. (1991). *BIGSTEPS: Rasch model computer program.* Chicago: Mesa Press.

Wright, B. D., & Masters, G. N. (1982). *Rating scale analysis: Rasch measurement.* Chicago: Mesa Press.

Yule, G. U. (1912). On the methods of measuring association between two attributes. *Journal of the Royal Statistical Association, 75,* 581–642.

SUMMARY

Chapter 26

Trends and Future Directions in Human Pain Assessment

DENNIS C. TURK, PhD
RONALD MELZACK, PhD

> When the right thing can only be measured poorly, it tends to cause the wrong thing to be measured only because it can be measured well. And it is often much worse to have good measurement of the wrong thing—especially when, as is so often the case, the wrong thing will IN FACT be used as an indicator of the right thing—than to have poor measurement of the right thing.
>
> Tukey (1979, p. 786)

The chapters in this volume attest to the wealth of attention that has been given to the issues of pain measurement, and more broadly, assessment of the person with pain. A variety of new instruments have become available for use with people with pain, and new ones are constantly being offered. It is altogether fitting at this point to heed Tukey's admonition cited above and to consider the current trends and issues in human pain assessment as well as to consider some future directions.

PAIN > SENSORY INTENSITY

It is evident from the chapters in this volume that major advances have been made in developing sophisticated procedures designed to quantify the subjective experience of pain. A great deal of attention has been given to the fact that pain is a multidimensional perception and not a simple sensation. Thus, appropriate measurement of pain needs to include motivational-affective and cognitive-evaluative contributions.

The question most frequently asked by physicians when a patient complains of pain is some variation of "How much does it hurt?" A wealth of research demonstrates that the response to the simple numerical response to this question involves a cognitive-evaluational (meaning) component associated with the processing of pain-relevant information, as well as sensory and emotional qualities.

QUANTIFICATION OF PAIN VERSUS ASSESSMENT OF THE PERSON WHO EXPERIENCES PAIN

It is apparent that the experience and report of pain are influenced by multiple factors such as cultural conditioning, expectancies, current so-

473

cial contingencies, and the like. Physical pathology and the resulting nociception is thus only one, albeit very important, contributor to the experience of and subsequent response to pain. Rather than focusing exclusively on the assessment of pain many contributors have urged that adequate assessment, especially of chronic pain patients, needs to be comprehensive, attending to patients' beliefs, attitudes, coping resources, mood state, behaviors as they related to the impact of pain on daily life, as well as physical pathology. To understand the individual's pain obviously requires much greater knowledge of the various domains that have an impact on the patient and influence not only his or her report of pain intensity but also responses to pain.

SUBJECTIVITY VERSUS OBJECTIVITY

Pain is a subjective experience that has concerned investigators and clinicians for many years. There have been continued searches for objective measures of pain that would not be biased by the patient. Thus, many efforts have attempted to develop performance testing to assess strength, lifting capacity, and trunk muscle function. However, there is little evidence that physical examination and various biomechanical measurements are highly associated with pain. Motivational and cognitive factors affect performance in these tests. Similarly, the association between psychophysiological parameters and pain has not been demonstrated. As Sternbach (1968) noted, "Because of the variability of responses elicited by different pain stimuli, and because of the additional variance contributed by individual differences in response-stereotype, it is difficult to specify a pattern of physiological responses characteristic of pain" (p. 57). Similarly, studies of the association between observable pain behaviors and self-reports of pain have reported equivocal results. These efforts have not provided the objective measures of pain that many desire.

It is essential to acknowledge the importance of the self-reports by the patients; we will never be able to evaluate pain without reliance on these patients' subjective reports. These reports are also important because they influence how patients are responded to by their families as well as health-care providers. Moreover, pa-

tients' self-reports have been shown to be related to functional behavior (e.g., Deyo & Diehl, 1983; Riley, Ahern, & Follick, 1988), return to work (e.g., Bigos et al., 1991), use of the health-care system (Flor & Turk, 1988), and response to treatment (e.g., Shutty & DeGood, 1990). Thus, we anticipate future refinements in self-report measures but do not expect them to be replaced. It is also important to realize that many of the physical measurements that are viewed as objective are probably influenced by the patient's motivation, effort, and psychological state (Pope, Rosen, Wilder, & Frymoyer, 1980).

The research to date suggests that patients' performances on physical and biomechanical measures are not associated with the risk of acute pain evolving into chronic pain (Bigos et al., 1991) or with return to work (e.g., Gallagher et al., 1989). Thus, the suggestion that objective measurement based on performance, using sophisticated apparatus designed to assess functional capacity, will predict disability or will identify malingers is probably inappropriate. Furthermore, the relationship between this performance return to work has yet to be demonstrated. Investigators and clinicians must be cautious in not overselling these expensive pieces of equipment.

GOING BEYOND THE PSYCHOMETRIC PROPERTIES OF INSTRUMENTS AND ASSESSMENT PROCEDURES

The importance of psychometric characteristics has long been acknowledged, and careful attention to reliability and validity is required for the development of any new assessment instrument. Several chapters in this volume (e.g., Dworkin & Whitney, Chapter 24, and Rudy, Turk, & Brody, Chapter 25) focus a great deal of discussion on the reliability of instruments and procedure. Considerably less attention has been given to the issue of validity. Is the instrument or procedure appropriate, meaningful, and useful for making specific inferences? The question is whether the test is valid for the purposes and samples for which it is to be used. Proxy measures should be demonstrated to be related to meaningful criteria. Do pain behaviors relate to clinically meaningful criteria such as return to work or increased function? Does the presence of a specific coping response predict treatment outcome? Do the patient's beliefs predict dropping out of treatment? Do x-ray findings relate to pain and disability? Do elevated patterns on various psychophysiological measures relate to physical functioning? The research described throughout this volume is beginning to address these types of questions. More recently, there has been growing emphasis on the importance of demonstrating that the diverse range of physical assessment and laboratory procedures commonly used in evaluating patients are reliable, valid, and useful.

It has been emphasized in a number of chapters in this volume that greater attention must be given to the combination of sets of physical information and to the processes whereby decisions are made about the extent of pathology present, the amount of impairment, the degree of disability, and the appropriateness of different treatment alternatives. Further research is needed to demonstrate the interrelationships among pathology, impairment, disability, and pain. It is essential that research address how individual characteristics of patients and their social environment affect responses to impairment, development of disability, and differential responses to alternative treatment interventions.

There is a need to demonstrate the association of various physical measures (e.g., EMG activity) and any meaningful criteria such as functional status and actual behavior (Deyo, 1988). Similarly, it is essential that the association between psychological measures and meaningful behaviors be established. What is the relationship between the frequency of rubbing a pain body part and uptime, use of the health care system, or functional capacity? Does differential responding on the MMPI correlate with specific behaviors that can be addressed in treatment? Does spinal mobility relate to disability?

One trend that can be observed is the translation of assessment instruments originally developed in one language to others. Just because the questions comprising the instruments can be translated, however, does not mean that the concepts being measured are equivalent in different cultures. Consequently, because an instrument has be shown to be valid for one sample of patients is not a guarantee that it is valid for another sample with different characteristics. This was demonstrated by Deyo (1984) when he showed the pitfalls of simply translating an assessment instrument into another language and assuming that the validity of the two languages (English and Spanish) was comparable. It is not sufficient to demonstrate that a specific assessment instrument is reliable and valid on a single patient sample.

NORMATIVE INFORMATION

The appropriateness of norms of tests has rarely been considered in the pain literature. In the absence of normative information, the raw score on any test is meaningless. To observe that a patient with migraine headaches scores a "10" on a Visual Analog Scale (VAS) of pain intensity conveys little or no information. However, if it is known that the average pain severity for 100 migraine headache patients is 5.4 with a standard deviation of 1.0, this information would permit the conclusion that this patient is expressing a very high level of pain relative to other migraine headache sufferers. However, if the only available normative evidence was based on cancer patients and their mean was 5.4 with a standard deviation of 1.0, then it is not known how the patient rated his or her pain relative to a group of migraine patients. Is the patient's pain report atypical for migraine sufferers? Without appropriate normative information it will not be possible to answer this question.

In all areas of pain assessment, it is important to be cognizant of the population for whom normative information is available and the appropriateness of generalizing from the original sample used to establish the reliability. In many cases, instruments that were developed for use with physically healthy or psychiatrically impaired individuals have been used with chronic pain patients. This can lead to erroneous conclusions. For example, the MMPI (see Bradley, Haile, & Jaworsky, Chapter 12) was originally developed to diagnose personality types associated with psychopathology.

Several studies have directly addressed concerns about the item content of the MMPI scales and interpretations of elevations of the first three scales for medical patients. Pincus, Callahan, Bradley, Vaughn, and Wolfe (1986) asked 18 rheumatologists to predict which of the 117 statements that comprise the first three MMPI scales would be answered differently by patients with rheumatoid arthritis (RA) and normal subjects, without regard to psychological status. The predictions of the rheumatologists were analyzed by actually comparing the responses of RA patients and the healthy subjects. The findings suggest that in RA, elevated scores on the MMPI hypochondriasis (Hy), Depression (D), and Hysteria (Hs) scales result from chronic disease rather than from psychological abnormality.

Naliboff, Cohen, and Yellin (1982, 1983) have demonstrated that chronic pain patients produce MMPI profiles that are quite similar to those produced by patients with chronic illnesses such as hypertension and diabetes. These investigators have also shown that 20–30% of the variance in patients' Hy, D, and Hs scale scores are determined by functional disability. Brennan, Barrett, and Garretsen (1986–1987) report that correlations between MMPI and outcome appear to be a direct association between the MMPI and pain-related characteristics, perhaps as a result of "artifactual" elevations due to pain-related items on these scales. When the predictive value of initial pain and disability are statistically accounted for, psychological test scores tend not to produce a further significant increment in predictability of pain clinic treatment outcome. In short, there is a strong possibility that pain patients' elevations on certain MMPI scales may be primarily a function of their disease or injury per se, its sequelae, and medication used, rather than the experiences reflected by those same scales when used with psychiatric patients.

Before using the norms of an instrument, it is important to demonstrate the invariance of the factor structure of the new instrument for the new population. For example, Turk and Rudy (1988) demonstrated that subgroups of pain patients can be identified based on their responses on the West Haven–Yale Multidimensional Pain Inventory (WHYMPI) (Kerns, Turk, & Rudy, 1985; see also Kerns & Jacob, Chapter 14, and Turk & Rudy, Chapter 23). The original sample consisted of a heterogeneous group of pain patients evaluated at a pain clinic. Do the same subgroups generalize to other medical diagnoses, or are the results idiosyncratic to the original sample of patients? Turk and Rudy (1990) demonstrate that although the mean scores on the different scales of the MPI and the percentage of patients comprising the subgroup differ among low back pain, headache, and temporomandibular

disorder pain patients, the correlation matrices among the scales are invariant. Thus, although different normative values should be used based on diagnosis, the subgroups identified seem to transcend medical/dental diagnosis, thus validating the generalizability of the patterns of the scales that characterize the subgroups.

As many chapters in this volume illustrate, measures that were never developed for pain samples but that were used because they were readily available are being replaced by ones that are specifically developed and normed with specific samples of pain patients. Future research needs to demonstrate that these pain-specific measures are both psychometrically acceptable and clinically useful.

The incremental validity of any new instrument should also be considered. That is, do the new instruments add anything to existing measures, or do they place less demand upon the patient? When two measurement instruments are shown to be measuring the same thing, all others things being equal, the one that requires less time and effort to complete may be preferred.

PROLIFERATION OF MEASURES

It is appropriate to be cautious when noting the proliferation of measurement instruments that have appeared in the literature. The development of new assessment instruments and procedures is a laborious task requiring large samples of patients. It is all too easy to avoid this task by making use of published instruments that appear to measure constructs related to our interest. It is also possible that the availability of instruments may shape the research questions that we ask.

The wealth of available pain assessment measures and procedures described throughout this volume can be both a blessing and a curse. Not only must the clinician or investigator choose the set of procedures to use but he or she most also decide how to integrate the large amount of information obtained (see Rudy et al., this volume). Many questions should be considered in determining an assessment battery. Which measures should be included in the assessment of the pain patient? Have the measures been shown to be psychometrically sound? Can the information be aggregated into a single score?

Are these measurements reproducible and sensitive enough to detect clinical response to therapy? Does each measure, regardless of its name, assess a unique variable, or is it merely a measure that duplicates an existing measure that has a different label but assesses the same domain? Are norms available and are they appropriate?

Those who select from the array of assessment instruments must ask themselves, "Assessment for what purpose—classification, diagnosis, treatment planning, decision making, prediction, outcome criteria?" Although some criteria for evaluating the appropriateness of a specific instrument cross these different purposes, this is not always the case. For example, if an investigator wishes to evaluate the efficacy of a treatment based on changes from pretreatment to posttreatment, he or she needs to be concerned about whether the instruments selected to evaluate success are subject to change. Related to this is the sensitivity of an instrument to detect small changes. The purpose of the assessment should guide the selection of the measurement instrument or guide the decision regarding the need to develop a new instrument.

Related to question of purpose is that of what to assess. In clinical areas there should be some relation between the instruments selected and treatment. It is unfair to ask patients to complete a lengthy assessment battery or to submit to a large number of laboratory tests if the information collected is simply entered in the patient's file but has no impact on treatment. Insufficient attention has been devoted to customizing treatments to important characteristics of patients (Turk, 1990). Even less effort has been devoted to evaluating whether such customizing of treatment leads to any differential outcome. The new measures that are described in this volume may help to answer the questions of customizing of treatment.

DEVELOPMENT OF STANDARDIZED PROCEDURES

It has long been debated whether standardized instruments and methods of aggregating data are better than clinicians' judgments. Many clinicians resist the use of standaradized assessment instruments in assessing pain, emphasizing the nuances of clinical judgment. For example, Foley (1984, p. 22) advocates that clinical assessment of oncology patients adhere to nine principles:

1. Believing in the patient's pain complaint
2. Taking a careful history of the pain complaint
3. Assessing the psychosocial status of the patient
4. Performing a careful medical and neurological examination
5. Ordering and personally reviewing the appropriate diagnostic procedures
6. Evaluating the extent of the patient's disease
7. Treating the pain to facilitate the diagnostic study
8. Considering alternative methods to pain control during the initial evaluation
9. Reassessing the pain compliant during the prescribed therapy

This approach relies heavily on clinical judgment. The availability of standardized assessment methods and strategies for aggregating data, such as those described throughout this volume, can be complementary to the clinician's judgment and need not be viewed as mutually exclusive.

FEASIBILITY

There is a growing concern about feasibility of various assessment procedures for different populations. There may be an ideal measure but one that is not appropriate. For example, it may not be possible to administer a lengthy pain questionnaire on a frequent basis to pain patients in the terminal stage. Young children may be unable to respond to questions in the same way that adults can. Older people display different "pain behaviors" from younger adults and may not be able to engage in some biomechanical tests. Particular consideration must be give to the special characteristics of different populations in determining what assessment procedures can reasonably be used. The comparability of measures that are ostensibly designed to measure the same things but in demographically very different samples need to be demonstrated.

CONCLUSION

It is less than a decade since Melzack's (1983) volume on pain assessment first appeared. In the time since the publication of that book, there has been a veritable explosion of research devoted to the development of techniques to measure pain and assess people who experience it. The chapters contained in this volume present the state of the art as of this point in time.

It is precarious to predict how pain assessment will evolve. Rather than make a set of prognostications, we will enumerate a "wish list" of what we would like to see occur in human pain assessment over the next decade.

- We hope that the trends we have described in this chapter will continue. New instruments and procedures will be developed in an effort to measure domains that are believed to be important in understanding pain and the individual who experiences it.
- We hope to witness the consolidation of instruments that may be measuring similar concepts, as well as the replacement of some described in this volume by new approaches that have been demonstrated to be more appropriate (reliable, valid, less demanding on patients).
- We hope that greater emphasis will be placed on relating assessment instruments and procedures to important behaviors rather than focusing primarily on psychometric properties.
- We hope that more attention will be given to innovative strategies for integrating diverse sets of information.
- We hope that greater emphasis will be given to prescribing treatments based on patient characteristics derived from assessment data rather than treating all pain patients as basically the same or matching treatment exclusively to medical diagnosis.
- We hope that there will be greater effort to demonstrate the generalizability of different instruments to new populations rather than assume that the instrument can be used with samples that differ from the original sample.
- We hope that recent advances in test theory (e.g., item response theory) will be used in evaluating pain assessment instruments and procedures.

One primary goal of this volume has been to provide practical and useful information for clinical investigators and health-care providers. It is our hope that the discussions initiated throughout this volume will serve to inspire additional research. The continuing evolution of human pain assessment is essential for success in the search for treatments for those who continue to suffer.

REFERENCES

Bigos, S.J., Battie, M.C., Spengler, D.M., Fisher, L.D., Fordyce, W.E., Hansson, T.H., Nachemson, A.L., & Wortley, M.D. (1991). A prospective study of work perceptions and psychosocial factors affecting the report of back injury. *Spine, 16,* 1–6.

Brennan, A.F., Barrett, C.L., & Garretson, H.D. (1986–87). The prediction of chronic pain outcome by psychological variables. *International Journal of Psychiatry in Medicine, 16,* 373–387.

Deyo, R.A. (1984). Pitfalls in measuring the health status of Mexican Americans: Comparative validity of the English and Spanish Sickness Impact Profile. *American Journal of Public Health, 6,* 560–573.

Deyo, R.A. (1988). Measuring the functional status of patients with low back pain. *Archives of Physical Medicine and Rehabilitation, 69,* 1044–1053.

Deyo, R.A., & Diehl, A.K. (1983). Measuring physical and psychosocial function in patients with low-back pain. *Spine, 8,* 635–647.

Flor, H., & Turk, D.C. (1988). Chronic pain and rheumatoid arthritis: Predicting pain and disability from cognitive variables. *Journal of Behavioral Medicine, 11,* 251–265.

Foley, K.M. (1984). Assessment of pain. In R.G. Twycross (Ed.), *Pain relief in cancer* (pp. 17–31). London: Saunders.

Gallagher, R.M., Rauh, V., Haugh, L.D., Milhous, R., Callas, P.W., Langelier, R., McClallen, J.M., & Frymoyer, J. (1989). Determinants of return-to-work among low back pain patients. *Pain, 39,* 55–67.

Kerns, R.D., Jr., Turk, D.C., & Rudy, T.E. (1985). The West Haven–Yale Multidimensional Pain Inventory (WHYMPI). *Pain, 23,* 345–356.

Melzack, R. (Ed.). (1983). *Pain measurement and assessment.* New York: Raven Press.

Naliboff, B.D., Cohen, M.J., & Yellin, A.M. (1982). Does the MMPI differentiate chronic illness from chronic pain? *Pain, 13,* 333–341.

Naliboff, B.D., Cohen, M.J., & Yellin, A.M. (1983). Frequency of MMPI profile types in three chronic illness populations. *Journal of Clinical Psychology, 39,* 843–847.

Pincus, T., Callahan, L.F., Bradley, L.A., Vaughn, W.K., & Wolfe, F. (1986). Elevated MMPI scores for hypochondriasis, depression, and hysteria in patients with rheumatoid arthritis reflect disease rather than psychological status. *Arthritis and Rheumatism, 29,* 1456–1466.

Pope, M.H., Rosen, J.C., Wilder, D.G., & Frymoyer, J.W. (1980). Relation between biomechanical and psychological factors in patients with low-back pain. *Spine, 5,* 173–178.

Riley, J.F., Ahern, D.K., & Follick, M.J. (1988). Chronic pain and functional impairment: Assessing beliefs about their relationship. *Archives of Physical Medicine and Rehabilitation, 69,* 579–582.

Shutty, M.S., & DeGood, D.E. (1990). Patient knowledge and beliefs about their pain and its treatment. *Rehabilitation Psychology, 35,* 43–54.

Sternbach, R. (1968). *Pain: A psychophyiological analysis.* New York: Academic Press.

Tukey, J.W. (1979). Methodology and the statistician's responsibility for both accuracy and relevance. *Journal of the American Statistical Association, 74,* 786–793.

Turk, D.C. (1990). Customizing treatment for chronic pain patients: Who what, and why. *Clinical Journal of Pain, 6,* 225–270.

Turk, D.C., & Rudy, T.E. (1988) Toward an empirically derived taxonomy of chronic pain patients: Integration of psychological assessment data. *Journal of Consulting and Clinical Psychology, 56,* 760–768.

Turk, D.C., & Rudy, T.E. (1990). The robustness of an empirically derived taxonomy of chronic pain patients. *Pain, 43,* 27–35.

Index